Principles and Practice of Image-Guided Radiation Therapy of Lung Cancer

IMAGING IN MEDICAL DIAGNOSIS AND THERAPY

Series Editors: Andrew Karellas and Bruce R. Thomadsen

Published titles

Quality and Safety in Radiotherapy
Todd Pawlicki, Peter B. Dunscombe, Arno J. Mundt, and Pierre Scalliet, Editors
ISBN: 978-1-4398-0436-0

Adaptive Radiation Therapy
X. Allen Li, Editor
ISBN: 978-1-4398-1634-9

Quantitative MRI in Cancer
Thomas E. Yankeelov, David R. Pickens, and Ronald R. Price, Editors
ISBN: 978-1-4398-2057-5

Informatics in Medical Imaging
George C. Kagadis and Steve G. Langer, Editors
ISBN: 978-1-4398-3124-3

Adaptive Motion Compensation in Radiotherapy
Martin J. Murphy, Editor
ISBN: 978-1-4398-2193-0

Image-Guided Radiation Therapy
Daniel J. Bourland, Editor
ISBN: 978-1-4398-0273-1

Targeted Molecular Imaging
Michael J. Welch and William C. Eckelman, Editors
ISBN: 978-1-4398-4195-0

Proton and Carbon Ion Therapy
C.-M. Charlie Ma and Tony Lomax, Editors
ISBN: 978-1-4398-1607-3

Physics of Mammographic Imaging
Mia K. Markey, Editor
ISBN: 978-1-4398-7544-5

Physics of Thermal Therapy: Fundamentals and Clinical Applications
Eduardo Moros, Editor
ISBN: 978-1-4398-4890-6

Emerging Imaging Technologies in Medicine
Mark A. Anastasio and Patrick La Riviere, Editors
ISBN: 978-1-4398-8041-8

Cancer Nanotechnology: Principles and Applications in Radiation Oncology
Sang Hyun Cho and Sunil Krishnan, Editors
ISBN: 978-1-4398-7875-0

Image Processing in Radiation Therapy
Kristy Kay Brock, Editor
ISBN: 978-1-4398-3017-8

Informatics in Radiation Oncology
George Starkschall and R. Alfredo C. Siochi, Editors
ISBN: 978-1-4398-2582-2

Cone Beam Computed Tomography
Chris C. Shaw, Editor
ISBN: 978-1-4398-4626-1

Computer-Aided Detection and Diagnosis in Medical Imaging
Qiang Li and Robert M. Nishikawa, Editors
ISBN: 978-1-4398-7176-8

Cardiovascular and Neurovascular Imaging: Physics and Technology
Carlo Cavedon and Stephen Rudin, Editors
ISBN: 978-1-4398-9056-1

Scintillation Dosimetry
Sam Beddar and Luc Beaulieu, Editors
ISBN: 978-1-4822-0899-3

Handbook of Small Animal Imaging: Preclinical Imaging, Therapy, and Applications
George Kagadis, Nancy L. Ford, Dimitrios N. Karnabatidis, and George K. Loudos Editors
ISBN: 978-1-4665-5568-6

IMAGING IN MEDICAL DIAGNOSIS AND THERAPY

Series Editors: Andrew Karellas and Bruce R. Thomadsen

Published titles

Comprehensive Brachytherapy: Physical and Clinical Aspects
Jack Venselaar, Dimos Baltas, Peter J. Hoskin, and Ali Soleimani-Meigooni, Editors
ISBN: 978-1-4398-4498-4

Handbook of Radioembolization: Physics, Biology, Nuclear Medicine, and Imaging
Alexander S. Pasciak, PhD., Yong Bradley, MD., J. Mark McKinney, MD., Editors
ISBN: 978-1-4987-4201-6

Monte Carlo Techniques in Radiation Therapy
Joao Seco and Frank Verhaegen, Editors
ISBN: 978-1-4665-0792-0

Stereotactic Radiosurgery and Stereotactic Body Radiation Therapy
Stanley H. Benedict, David J. Schlesinger, Steven J. Goetsch, and Brian D. Kavanagh, Editors
ISBN: 978-1-4398-4197-6

Physics of PET and SPECT Imaging
Magnus Dahlbom, Editor
ISBN: 978-1-4665-6013-0

Tomosynthesis Imaging
Ingrid Reiser and Stephen Glick, Editors
ISBN: 978-1-138-19965-1

Ultrasound Imaging and Therapy
Aaron Fenster and James C. Lacefield, Editors
ISBN: 978-1-4398-6628-3

Beam's Eye View Imaging in Radiation Oncology
Ross I. Berbeco, Ph.D., Editor
ISBN: 978-1-4987-3634-3

Principles and Practice of Image-Guided Radiation Therapy of Lung Cancer
Jing Cai, Joe Y. Chang, and Fang-Fang Yin, Editors
ISBN: 978-1-4987-3673-2

Principles and Practice of Image-Guided Radiation Therapy of Lung Cancer

Edited by
Jing Cai, PhD
Joe Y. Chang, MD, PhD
Fang-Fang Yin, PhD

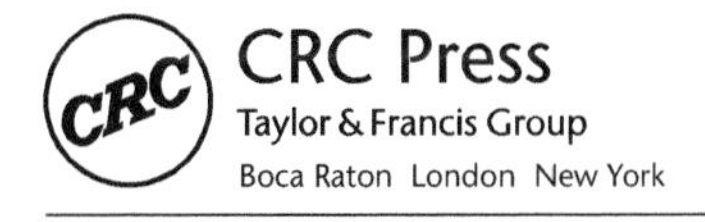

CRC Press is an imprint of the
Taylor & Francis Group, an **informa** business

CRC Press
Taylor & Francis Group
6000 Broken Sound Parkway NW, Suite 300
Boca Raton, FL 33487-2742

First issued in paperback 2021

ISBN 13: 978-0-367-78186-6 (pbk)
ISBN 13: 978-1-4987-3673-2 (hbk)

Library of Congress Cataloging-in-Publication Data

Names: Cai, Jing (Radiation oncologist), editor. | Chang, Joe Y., editor. | Yin, Fang-Fang, editor.
Title: Principles and practice of image-guided radiation therapy of lung cancer / [edited by] Jing Cai, Joe Y. Chang, Fang-Fang Yin.
Other titles: Imaging in medical diagnosis and therapy.
Description: Boca Raton : Taylor & Francis, 2017. | Series: Imaging in medical diagnosis and therapy | Includes bibliographical references.
Identifiers: LCCN 2017014457 | ISBN 9781498736732 (hardback : alk. paper)
Subjects: | MESH: Lung Neoplasms—radiotherapy | Radiotherapy, Image-Guided
Classification: LCC RC280.L8 | NLM WF 658 | DDC 616.99/424—dc23
LC record available at https://lccn.loc.gov/2017014457

Visit the Taylor & Francis Web site at
http://www.taylorandfrancis.com

and the CRC Press Web site at
http://www.crcpress.com

Contents

Series Preface

Advances in the science and technology of medical imaging and radiation therapy are more profound and rapid than ever before, since their inception over a century ago. Further, the disciplines are increasingly cross-linked as imaging methods become more widely used to plan, guide, monitor and assess treatments in radiation therapy. Today the technologies of medical imaging and radiation therapy are so complex and so computer-driven that it is difficult for the persons (physicians and technologists) responsible for their clinical use to know exactly what is happening at the point of care, when a patient is being examined or treated. The persons best equipped to understand the technologies and their applications are medical physicists, and these individuals are assuming greater responsibilities in the clinical arena to ensure that what is intended for the patient is delivered in a safe and effective manner.

The growing responsibilities of medical physicists in the clinical arenas of medical imaging and radiation therapy are not without their challenges, however. Most medical physicists are knowledgeable in either radiation therapy or medical imaging, and expert in one or a small number of areas within their discipline. They sustain their expertise in these areas by reading scientific articles and attending scientific talks at meetings. In contrast, their responsibilities increasingly extend beyond their specific areas of expertise. To meet these responsibilities, medical physicists periodically must refresh their knowledge of advances in medical imaging or radiation therapy, and they must be prepared to function at the intersection of these two fields. How to accomplish these objectives is a challenge.

At the 2007 annual meeting of the American Association of Physicists in Medicine in Minneapolis, this challenge was the topic of conversation during a lunch hosted by Taylor & Francis Group and involving a group of senior medical physicists (Arthur L. Boyer, Joseph O. Deasy, C.-M. Charlie Ma, Todd A. Pawlicki, Ervin B. Podgorsak, Elke Reitzel, Anthony B. Wolbarst, and Ellen D. Yorke). The conclusion of this discussion was that a book series should be launched under the Taylor & Francis banner, with each volume in the series addressing a rapidly advancing area of medical imaging or radiation therapy of importance to medical physicists. The aim would be for each volume to provide medical physicists with the information needed to understand technologies driving a rapid advance and their applications to safe and effective delivery of patient care.

Each volume in the series is edited by one or more individuals with recognized expertise in the technological area encompassed by the book. The editors are responsible for selecting the authors of individual chapters and ensuring that the chapters are comprehensive and intelligible to someone without such expertise. The enthusiasm of volume editors and chapter authors has been gratifying and reinforces the conclusion of the Minneapolis luncheon that this series of books addresses a major need of medical physicists.

Imaging in Medical Diagnosis and Therapy would not have been possible without the encouragement and support of the series manager, Lu Han of CRC Press/Taylor & Francis Group. The editors and authors, and most of all I, are indebted to his steady guidance of the entire project.

William Hendee, Founding Series Editor
Rochester, MN

Preface

Lung cancer remains a leading cause of cancer death in the United States and worldwide. Multidisciplinary approaches including radiation therapy have had a crucial role in the management strategy for patients affected with lung cancer, but local control and survival rates are still poor. The effectiveness of radiation therapy can be hindered by challenges in accurately localizing and delineating targets as well as delivering the radiation. Recent developments in image-guided radiation therapy (IGRT), which uses imaging technologies such as x-ray and optical imaging to direct the delivery of radiation, offer additional accuracy and the potential for increasingly aggressive treatments, with consequent improvements in local control and perhaps survival. In this book, we address the field of IGRT for lung cancer, including a brief history, step-by-step guidelines for clinical implementations, a summary of major recent technical advances, and an introduction of next-generation technologies. Readers will benefit from the in-depth explanations of the benefits and limitations of current IGRT techniques, informed interpretation of the quality and safety issues related to IGRT in clinical practice, and stimulating discussions about cutting-edge IGRT technologies that are promising to improve clinical outcomes for patients with lung cancer.

The techniques used for IGRT have improved greatly over the past 10 years in terms of both practical optimization and technical advances. Understanding of the benefits and limitations of IGRT techniques has also increased tremendously during this period as IGRT techniques have become more widely used in the clinic. Having a single book dedicated to addressing these important changes is extremely valuable as it serves as a reference for all of the issues associated with IGRT for lung cancer. Our intent in this book is to provide a complete practical guide coupled with data-driven methods for developing this important paradigm in radiation therapy.

The technologies used for IGRT have also experienced substantial change in parallel with changes in techniques over recent years, especially the advances associated with 4D imaging and multimodality image guidance. A great deal of clinical experience and knowledge on IGRT has been gained during this period because of the widespread use of and extensive research on IGRT. Several recently developed IGRT technologies are highly promising, particularly magnetic resonance imaging–guided IGRT, adaptive radiation therapy, and functional imaging for response assessment. All of these topics are comprehensively described in this book.

The materials in the book have been thoughtfully prepared and carefully organized by the logical progression of simple to complex, basic to comprehensive, practical to investigational, and current to future. Our hope is that this organization will help to maximize the reading and learning experience for readers with various backgrounds in IGRT.

This book consists of four parts, each detailing an important aspect of IGRT for lung cancer. The first part consists of an overview of IGRT and the history of IGRT for lung cancer. The second part describes the principles of IGRT for lung cancer in a step-by-step process, from imaging simulation to treatment planning, verification, and delivery, and on to quality assurance. The third part describes the unique features and processes of IGRT for lung cancer using specialized machines and technologies. The fourth part introduces new directions for IGRT and the promise of those directions for lung cancer treatment.

We anticipate that this volume will be a good reference for a broad range of professionals, including radiation oncologists, medical physicists, radiation therapists, medical dosimetrists, and oncology nurses as well as researchers, educators, and physicians working in the field of lung cancer, medical imaging, and oncology management. Its authors include both physicians and physicists to ensure that the content and format meet the needs of clinicians and others in related fields.

We, the editors, sincerely thank the contributing authors of this book, all of whom are nationally and internationally recognized medical physicists and radiation oncologists with expertise in IGRT and lung cancer radiation therapy. Readers will greatly benefit from their sharing their experience in developing and clinically implementing state-of-the-art IGRT techniques.

Editors

Jing Cai, PhD, is an associate professor of radiation oncology at Duke University Medical Center, Durham, North Carolina. His research is focused on developing and clinically implementing novel image-guided radiation therapy techniques. He has published more than 60 peer-reviewed journal articles and over 190 conference abstracts. He regularly provides scientific reviews for journals and conferences, and serves as expert reviewer for grant applications. His research has received federal, charitable, and industrial funding.

Joe Y. Chang, MD, PhD, is a professor in the department of radiation oncology at The University of Texas MD Anderson Cancer Center in Houston, Texas. He is also clinical section chief for thoracic radiation oncology and director of the stereotactic radiotherapy program. He earned his PhD in cancer biology at the University of Texas MD Anderson Cancer Center, and his MD from Shanghai Medical College in China. He performed clinical residency at Rush-Presbyterian St. Luke Medical Center in Chicago, Illinois. He is board certified in radiation oncology and is the recipient of numerous honors and is an active member of several professional organizations.

Fang-Fang Yin, PhD, is chief of the division of radiation physics and professor of radiation oncology at Duke University, Durham, North Carolina, since 2004. He is also the director of the Medical Physics graduate program at Duke Kunshan University. The author of more than 250 refereed publications and book chapters, Yin's research interests include image-guided radiation therapy, informatics in cancer treatment, advanced planning and delivery techniques, and quality assurance. Yin is a Fellow of the American Association of Physicists in Medicine (AAPM) and Fellow of American Society for Radiation Oncology (ASTRO). He earned his PhD. in medical physics from the University of Chicago, Illinois.

Contributors

Peter Balter
Department of Radiation Physics
UT MD Anderson Cancer Center
Houston, Texas

Stanley Benedict
Department on Radiation Oncology
UC Davis Medical Center
Sacramento, California

Kristy K. Brock
Department of Imaging Physics
UT MD Anderson Cancer Center
Houston, Texas

Andrew Cardin
Radiation Physics Solutions, LLC
Garnet Valley, Pennsylvania

Zheng Chang
Department of Radiation Oncology
Duke University
Durham, North Carolina

Quan Chen
Department of Radiation Oncology
University of Virginia
Charlottesville, Virginia

Indrin Chetty
Department of Radiation Oncology
Henry Ford Health System
Detroit, Michigan

Kamila Nowak Choi
Department of Radiation Oncology
Thomas Jefferson University
Philadelphia, Pennsylvania

Martina Descovich
Department of Radiation Oncology
University of California
San Francisco, California

Josh Evans
Department of Radiation Oncology
Virginia Commonwealth University
Richmond, Virginia

Jing Feng
Philadelphia CyberKnife Center
Havertown, Pennsylvania

Hong Ge
Department of Radiation Oncology
Henan Cancer Hospital
Zhengzhou, China

Carri K. Glide-Hurst
Department of Radiation Oncology
Henry Ford Health System
Detroit, Michigan

Steven J. Goetsch
San Diego Gamma Knife Center
La Jolla, California

Clemens Grassberger
Department of Radiation Oncology
Massachusetts General Hospital
Boston, Massachusetts

Lauren Henke
Department of Radiation Oncology
Washington University
St. Louis, Missouri

David Hoffman
Department of Radiation Medicine and Applied Sciences
University of California
La Jolla, California

Mischa Hoogeman
Radiotherapy
Erasmus University Rotterdam
Rotterdam, The Netherlands

Long Huang
Department of Radiation Oncology
University of Utah
Salt Lake City, Utah

Rojano Kashani
Department of Radiation Oncology
Washington University
St. Louis, Missouri

Chris R. Kelsey
Department of Radiation Oncology
Duke University
Durham, North Carolina

Taeho Kim
Department of Radiation Oncology
Virginia Commonwealth University
Richmond, Virginia

Feng-Ming (Spring) Kong
Department of Radiation Oncology
Indian University
Indianapolis, Indiana

Tim Lautenschlaeger
Department of Radiation Oncology
Indian University
Indianapolis, Indiana

Guang Li
Department of Medical Physics
Memorial Sloan Kettering Cancer Center
New York, New York

Mei Li
Department of Radiation Oncology
Shantou University Medical College
Shantou, China

Ruijiang Li
Department of Radiation Oncology
Stanford University
Stanford, California

Xing Liang
Radiation Physics Solutions, LLC
Garnet Valley, Pennsylvania

Yilin Liu
Department of Radiation Physics
UT MD Anderson Cancer Center
Houston, Texas

Virginia Lockamy
Department of Radiation Oncology
University of Pennsylvania
Philadelphia, Pennsylvania

Daniel Low
Department of Radiation Oncology
University of California at Los Angeles
Los Angeles, California

Wei Lu
Department of Medical Physics
Memorial Sloan Kettering Cancer Center
New York, New York

Martha M. Matuszak
Department of Radiation Oncology
University of Michigan
Ann Arbor, Michigan

Harald Paganetti
Department of Radiation Oncology
Massachusetts General Hospital
Boston, Massachusetts

Tinsu Pan
Department of Imaging Physics
UT MD Anderson Cancer Center
Houston, Texas

Julian Perks
Department on Radiation Oncology
UC Davis Medical Center
Sacramento, California

Julianne M. Pollard-Larkin
Department of Radiation Physics
UT MD Anderson Cancer Center
Houston, Texas

Lei Ren
Department of Radiation Oncology
Duke University
Durham, North Carolina

Gregory C. Sharp
Department of Radiation Oncology
Massachusetts General Hospital
Boston, Massachusetts

Ke Sheng
Department of Radiation Oncology
University of California at Los Angeles
Los Angeles, California

Karen Chin Snyder
Department of Radiation Oncology
Henry Ford Health System
Detroit, Michigan

Robert Timmerman
Department of Radiation Oncology
UT Southwestern
Dallas, Texas

Irina Vergalasova
Department of Radiation Oncology
Rutgers Robert Wood Johnson Medical School
New Brunswick, New Jersey

EnMing Wang
Department of Neurosurgery
Huashan Hospital
Shanghai Medical College
Fudan University
Shanghai, China

Jing Wang
Department of Radiation Oncology
UT Southwestern Medical Center
Dallas, Texas

Ning Wen
Department of Radiation Oncology
Henry Ford Health System
Detroit, Michigan

Krishni Wijesooriya
Department of Radiation Oncology
University of Virginia
Charlottesville, Virginia

Lei Xing
Department of Radiation Oncology
Stanford University
Stanford, California

Jun Yang
Philadelphia CyberKnife Center
Havertown, Pennsylvania
and
Department of Radiation Oncology
Drexel University College of Medicine
Philadelphia, Pennsylvania

Yan Yu
Department of Radiation Oncology
Thomas Jefferson University
Philadelphia, Pennsylvania

PART 1

INTRODUCTION

1

Overview of IGRT

FANG-FANG YIN, YU YAN, AND ROBERT TIMMERMAN

1.1 INTRODUCTION

Recently, there has been a global movement toward using targeted therapy to treat a variety of human afflictions including lung cancer. While most of this effort has been in the realm of drug discovery, a similar philosophy is being implemented using local modalities such as surgery and radiotherapy. In the realm of radiotherapy, an explosion of useful, computer-aided technologies have taken center stage, potentially allowing more geometrically targeted therapy. Still, accurate delineation of treatment targets critical organ volumes, personalized prescription of treatment dose associated with the delineated volumes, optimal design of treatment planning, and precise delivery of prescribed dose to the target. These remain major technical challenges for the precision radiation therapy of cancers.

1.2 GOAL OF IGRT

The primary goal of image-guided radiation therapy (IGRT) is to improve local control and reduce impending side effects [1]. Uncertainties can arise from inter- and intrafractional motions [2]. During treatment or even sometimes prior to, the imaging provides direct confirmation that the beams are targeting the exact location of the tumor. Any shifts or corrections detected by the imaging can be made to ensure the proper treatment. Highly conformal, highly modulated, and escalated dosing schemes are being used more routinely. If slight errors are not detected prior to the execution of treatment, there is a possibility of under- or overdosing not only the intended area, but critical structures as well. IGRT provides the ability to ensure that the tumor is being properly targeted while limiting toxicities to normal structures.

1.3 BENEFITS OF IGRT

The overall goal of any radiation treatment is to deliver the prescribed dose to the tumor volume while limiting harm to any other tissues. The negligible variation in the dose being delivered versus the dose that is prescribed when IGRT is used for treatments is its main benefit. Protocols can benefit from the inclusion of IGRT by ensuring a uniform radiation dose is truly being delivered based on IGRT usage and reducing the heterogeneity of responses seen among the control and treatment groups [2]. The reduction in dose variability may also lead to better clinical outcomes and help researchers draw conclusions that are based on outcomes, and not other outcomes that could be caused in treatment variation.

Another benefit of IGRT is the ability to know what was delivered to both tumor and normal tissues. Certain systems allow the isodose lines from the plan to be displayed on the imaging obtained during the IGRT procedure. Based on this knowledge, clinicians can adjust accordingly in setup prior to treatment based on position of the target and critical structures. This could lead to a better understanding of normal tissue toxicity relationships and tumor control probabilities by understanding where the dose is being delivered daily. Other benefits include tighter margins for tumors and being able to account for target motion, whether the motion is inter- or intrafractional.

The current role of IGRT in radiation therapy is depicted in Figure 1.1 [3]. The circle on the left represents the patient's cycle in the radiation oncology process. The clinical objective is determined by the physician based on the intent of the plan and the intended dose to be delivered. This is followed by the therapy design, which includes a treatment planning CT, contouring of the tumor(s) as well as normal and critical structures, plan development, and any necessary quality assurance (QA). Upon initiation of treatment, IGRT can be used to assess the accuracy of the patient's alignment as well as continually monitor the tumor. An intervention based on IGRT may be required due to setup errors or shifts in the tumor, which could lead to reassessment. If an offline review of the images is performed by the physician, the error might not be detected until after that day's treatment. Online or real-time image reviews are faster at detecting potential errors and making the needed corrections.

1.3.1 Tighter margins

Margins for tumors have become increasingly tighter with the addition of IGRT to the treatment regimen. This has also led to more focused doses to the tumor volume(s) and a decrease in doses to normal tissue. The dose delivery is now more accurate and reliable when including IGRT. The benefit of including IGRT with

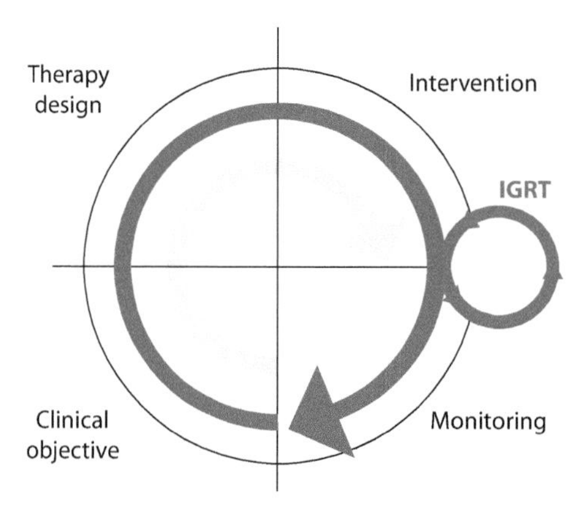

Figure 1.1 Advancement of radiation therapy from a three-step approach (as indicated by light blue) to one of a full-feedback approach (dark blue). The intervention step can include correcting for setup error and/or tumor shifts, replanning, or even discontinuation of current treatment plan. The image review can be performed offline, online, or even real time. IGRT uses the full-feedback approach to ensure precise delivery of the treatment. (Reprinted with permission from Dawson, L.A. and D.A. Jaffray, *J Clin Oncol*, 25, 938–46. © 2007 by American Society of Clinical Oncology. All rights reserved.)

treatment is to reduce any residual geometric uncertainties (e.g., differences between targeting and treatment delivery), so that there is essentially no clinical significance between the planned dose and what is actually delivered (Kim et al., 2011).

1.3.2 Target motion

With the inclusion of IGRT as part of the treatment, the uncertainties arising from target motions can be reduced, whether from inter- or intrafractional motion. Possible IGRT techniques that can be used include, but are not limited to, kV imaging (whether on the linear accelerator or ceiling/floor-mounted units), MV imaging, MV or kV cone beam computed tomography (CBCT), four-dimensional (4D) CBCT, CT-on-rails, on-board magnetic resonance imaging (MRI), and ultrasound guidance.

As with any new technology, the question is how efficient and accurate will the systems perform. This certainly applies to all advances that have been made in IGRT. Multiple groups have suggested that the key capabilities for an ideal IGRT system should include the following:

1. Three-dimensional (3D) imaging of soft tissues and tumors
2. 3D images that can be acquired and compared in an efficient and timely manner
3. An effective process to apply corrections based on imaging [4,5]

Patient's imaging data can be monitored and assessed at multiple points. Online assessments can be made prior to turning on the beam, real-time occurs as the treatment is being delivered, and off-line occurs after the treatment has been delivered [1]. Figure 1.2 demonstrates the image registration performed at the linear accelerator console following a CBCT (green) to the original treatment planning CT (purple). Physicians may also review these images and the registration in the record and verify system (R&V), as seen in Figure 1.3. Each of these assessments provides the clinicians insight as to the daily dose delivery and allows them to make any adjustments as they see fit. These changes may range from as small as having the patient moved to as large as deciding that the patient needs to be rescanned and reassessed based on the image review.

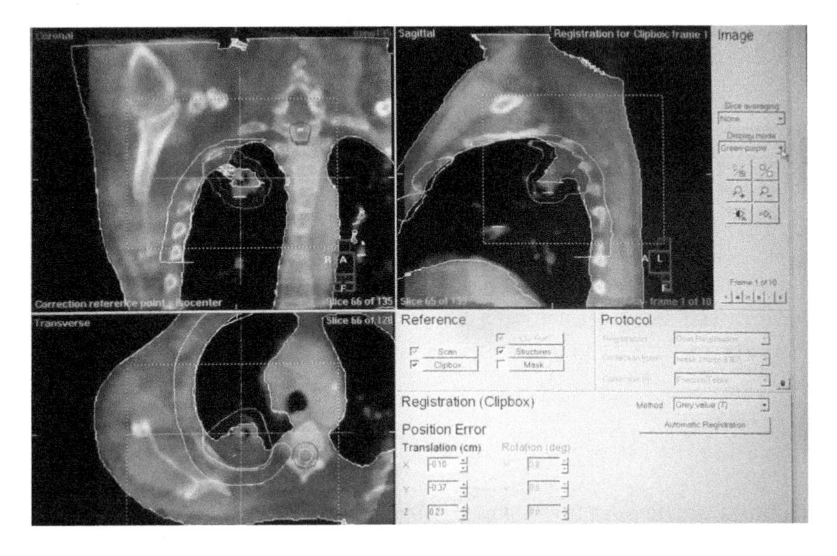

Figure 1.2 Image registration performed following a CBCT at the treatment console. The treatment planning CT is depicted in purple while the acquired CBCT is in green. Images are used to determine the necessary shifts prior to treatment. In this case, the positional error is shown in the lower-right portion. These translational shifts are performed prior to treatment. The tumor volume, planning target volume (PTV), spinal cord, and planning risk volume (PRV) for the spinal cord, lungs, and chest wall contours are displayed on the planning CT. (Image courtesy of Yan Yu, Thomas Jefferson University, Pennsylvania.)

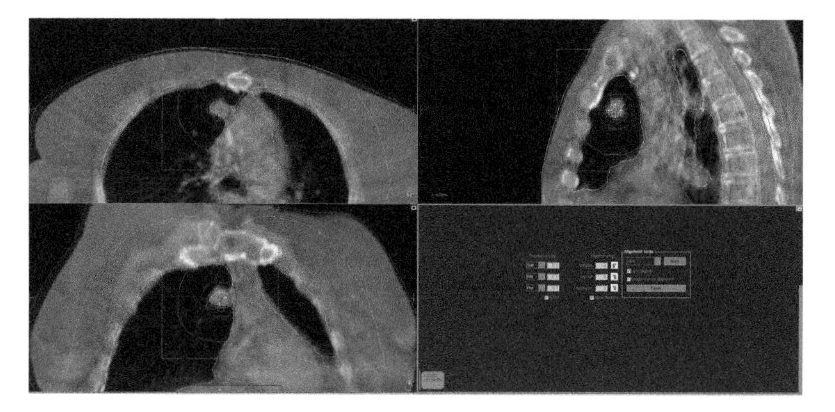

Figure 1.3 Image review of registration following a CBCT in the record and verify system. The treatment planning CT is depicted in purple while the acquired CBCT is in green. Images are used to determine the necessary shifts prior to treatment. In this case, the positional error is shown in the lower-right portion. These translational shifts are performed prior to treatment. (Image courtesy of Yan Yu, Thomas Jefferson University, Pennsylvania.)

1.3.3 Intrafractional adjustments

With the implementation of IGRT into the treatment procedure, intrafactional motion errors can be reduced by imaging the patient prior to or even during treatment, to determine the extent of the tumor motion (due to breathing, peristalsis, and other normal functions) as well as the position of critical structures. Imaging techniques useful for this include orthogonal images (kV or MV) or CBCTs (kV or MV). This will allow patient positional changes to be made to ensure proper dosing of the tumor while limiting the dose to the normal surrounding tissues.

1.3.4 Interfractional adjustments

Over the course of treatment, patients may experience weight loss or tumor shrinkage, which may be detected with the use of IGRT. It has also been noted that soft tissue tumors tend to shift positions more frequently relative to adjacent bone anatomy [6,7]. Since margins have become tighter and the use of highly modulated plans and dose escalation has increased over the years, IGRT has become a useful tool for detecting any necessary interfractional adjustments. 3D, intensity-modulated radiotherapy (IMRT) and volumetric modulated arc therapy (VMAT) plans are much more sensitive to organ geometry or anatomic changes in the patient [1]. Undetected changes in the patient can lead to underdosing of the tumor as well as unintended higher doses to critical structures. Without IGRT, the benefits of using such plans would be nonexistent because these differences would not have been detected prior to treatment initiation.

In the event that interfractional adjustments are needed, the patient can be repositioned and imaged again prior to treatment. If repositioning is not enough to ensure proper treatment, the patient can be rescanned and reassessed to alleviate these issues.

1.4 PROCESS OF IGRT

Effective management of these challenges penetrates the entire treatment process, including consultation, simulation, planning, quality assurance, pretreatment target localization, delivery, and assessment [8], as shown in Figure 1.4. At present, various image-guidance techniques play an important role in each of these processes. It is critical to understand what these technologies are and how they can optimally be used in these processes for lung radiation therapy as well as their impact on the success of each step in the treatment process.

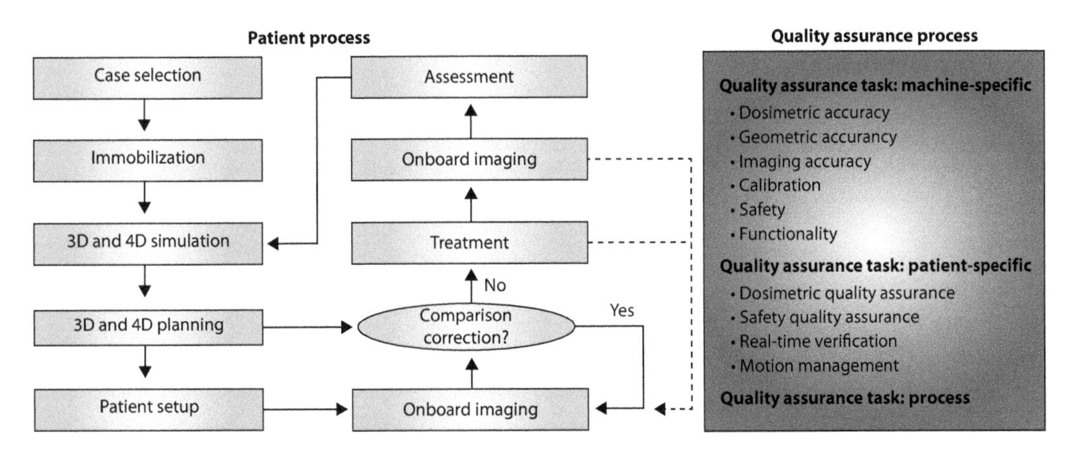

Figure 1.4 Integrated process for the IGRT for lung cancer. (From Salama, J.K., J.P. Kirkpatrick, and F.F. Yin, *Nat Rev Clin Oncol*, 9(11): 654–65, 2012.)

At consultation, a multidisciplinary team determines the feasibility of applying radiation therapy to the specific type of lung cancer and the potential for integration with other therapies. If radiotherapy is indicated, the treatment team, led by a radiation oncologist, will formulate a patient-specific immobilization method and suggest simulation images needed for treatment planning and a possible approach for managing organ motion based on the patient condition as well as a review of previous diagnostic imaging and patient information.

The process of simulation involves patient positioning, immobilization, and imaging to define how the patient will be treated. The stability and reproducibility of the simulation will have substantial impact on the precision of the radiation therapy. The prior experience/knowledge of the treatment team as well as the patient's performance and compliance also play important roles. Various techniques can be used to achieve the goals of stabilizing patient and organ movements. Motion management involves two distinct processes: motion assessment and, if necessary, motion control [9,10].

Motion assessment mainly involves acquiring information about target motion to allow formulating a methodology of modulating radiation for optimizing target coverage while minimizing normal tissue irradiation. The motion information may be multifactorial but is typically acquired using four-dimensional computed tomography (4D-CT) [11–13] or/and 4D magnetic resonance imaging (4D-MRI) [14–16] as well as x-ray fluoroscopic imaging. While fluoroscopic imaging provides real-time motion information, it only provides two-dimensional (2D) information and often may not be able to see the real target due to overlaid anatomic structures. 4D-CT and 4D-MRI generated with the same type of retrospective sorting techniques are then used for organ motion representation. However, it should be noted that the current reconstruction techniques only give one breathing cycle for each patient and the motion information can only be an approximation when an irregular breathing pattern is associated with the patient.

In turn, motion control is required if inherent motion exceeds thresholds to allow optimized planning. One approach for minimizing the normal tissue irradiation is the use of gating technologies which involves application of sophisticated imaging methods for planning and verification. Gating is well tolerated, and as long as the extension of time associated with its duty cycle does not lead to positional errors, patient discomfort is unlikely. Other methods, including abdominal compression, active breath-hold, and target tracking, also have been implemented in large published series.

The process of planning is aimed at determining the volumes for moving target and critical organs, the prescriptions for doses and associated volumes, and the radiation beam design and delivery strategy, as well as the verification methods used in the treatment room. Target volume is determined based on simulation images and available diagnostic images. Precision target delineation, dose calculation, and optimal delivery technique are all decided in this process. The prescription is related to these volumes [17–20].

The process of target localization in the treatment room involves verification of treatment targets and patient positioning as planned. Several technologies are available for this task. Some are based on 2D plane images while others are based on 3D tomographic images and 4D images with a selected motion management technique. Images could be taken using classic x-ray sources, optical systems, ultrasound units, and MRI and electromagnetic imaging systems, etc. Different imaging modalities have different pros and cons for different treatment sites and should wisely be selected for each specific type of diseases. Verification of moving targets is always challenging. Real-time fluoroscopic imaging, 4D-CBCT [21–23], and electromagnetic tracking as well as 4D-MRI are some of the powerful tools used for this purpose. Imaging prior to and post-delivery of radiation is a way of examining patient immobilization and organ motion management [24].

The process of precise delivery of prescribed radiation involves management, monitoring or tracking, and verification of target motion, as well as possible intervention strategies as needed. This is critical, because the whole process of radiation therapy will not be optimal if there is no confirmation that the dose is appropriately delivered. Several imaging and guidance technologies are available for selection. X-ray-based imaging, such as CBCT, provides not only 3D information about the patient, but also the motion information such as internal target volume (ITV). This process should be carefully thought out while engaging in the treatment planning. It is important that motion information be carefully validated with a minimal imaging dose. Although image guidance is critical for precision targeting, it also introduces imaging doses as well as interventional time. Optimization of these factors also should be considered in lung cancer radiation therapy [25,26].

Adaptive treatment planning based on the image-on-the-day involves dose calculation accuracy and image quality for target delineation. Both real-time and non-real-time adaptation could be completed for improved therapeutic efficacy [2]. The process of adaptation involves imaging (using x-ray, MRI, positron emission tomography (PET), etc.) of treatment responses of target as well as normal tissue toxicities. This process is critical because it checks how effective radiation therapy is for the specific lung disease. These treatments are traditionally done through personal interpolation of the data by physicians. However, the emerging approach is the use of analytics of all possible data obtained during and after the treatment, which is the application of big data analytics in radiation therapy [27].

Finally, a process of quality assurance (QA) should be emphasized. Optimal QA should be literally engrained into the treatment team's culture, particularly as treatments become more potent and sophisticated. In addition to performance of conventional machine-specific and patient-specific QA, process-specific and evidence-based QA should be emphasized. The training and performance of the staff performing the latter two should be checked periodically [28–30].

1.5 SUMMARY

The process of managing lung cancers with radiation therapy is rapidly evolving as technologies and techniques are continuously advancing. Introduction of new image-guidance technologies and techniques such as real-time 4D-CT and MR imaging, enhanced imaging of both biological and physical markers, and tracking of physical and biological targets, continues to modify the treatment paradigm for precision radiation therapy for lung cancer, eventually leading to evidence-based and personalized treatment with improved clinical outcomes.

Methodologies, techniques, and technologies described in the subsequent chapters should be very useful and instructive in performing precision lung radiation therapy. We hope the entire processes of lung cancer radiation therapy can be analytically optimized based on prior knowledge of specific disease treatments and current knowledge of the specific patient conditions.

REFERENCES

1. Kim, J., J.L. Meyer, and L.A. Dawson, Image guidance and the new practice of radiotherapy: What to know and use from a decade of investigation, in *IMRT, IGRT, SBRT—Advances in the Treatment Planning and Delivery of Radiotherapy*, J.L. Meyer, Editor. 2011, Basel: Karger, pp. 196–216.

2. Wu, Q.J. et al., Adaptive radiation therapy: Technical components and clinical applications. *Cancer J*, 2011. **17**(3): 182–9.
3. Dawson, L.A. and D.A. Jaffray, Advances in image-guided radiation therapy. *J Clin Oncol*, 2007. **25**(8): 938–46.
4. Ling, C.C., E. Yorke, and Z. Euks, From IMRT to IGRT: Frontierland or neverland? *Radiother Oncol*, 2006. **78**(2): 119–22.
5. Greco, C. and C.C. Ling, Broadening the scope of image-guided radiotherapy (IGRT). *Acta Oncol*, 2008. **47**(7): 1193–200.
6. Hugo, G. et al., Changes in the respiratory pattern during radiotherapy for cancer in the lung. *Radiother Oncol*, 2006. **78**(3): 326–31.
7. Case, R.B. et al., Inter-and intrafraction variability in liver position in non-breath-hold stereotactic body radiotherapy. *Int J Radiat Oncol Biol Phys*, 2009. **75**(1): 302–8.
8. Salama, J.K., J.P. Kirkpatrick, and F.F. Yin, Stereotactic body radiotherapy treatment of extracranial metastases. *Nat Rev Clin Oncol*, 2012. **9**(11): 654–65.
9. Yin, F. et al., Extracranial radiosurgery: Immobilizing liver motion in dogs using high-frequency jet ventilation and total intravenous anesthesia. *Int J Radiat Oncol Biol Phys*, 2001. **49**(1): 211–6.
10. Keall, P.J. et al., The management of respiratory motion in radiation oncology report of AAPM Task Group 76. *Med Phys*, 2006. **33**(10): 3874–900.
11. Low, D.A. et al., A method for the reconstruction of four-dimensional synchronized CT scans acquired during free breathing. *Med Phys*, 2003. **30**(6): 1254–63.
12. Pan, T., Comparison of helical and cine acquisitions for 4D-CT imaging with multislice CT. *Med Phys*, 2005. **32**(2): 627–34.
13. Pan, T. et al., 4D-CT imaging of a volume influenced by respiratory motion on multi-slice CT. *Med Phys*, 2004. **31**(2): 333–40.
14. Cai, J. et al., Four-dimensional magnetic resonance imaging (4D-MRI) using image-based respiratory surrogate: A feasibility study. *Med Phys*, 2011. **38**(12): 6384–94.
15. Liu, Y. et al., Four dimensional magnetic resonance imaging with retrospective k-space reordering: A feasibility study. *Med Phys*, 2015. **42**(2): 534–41.
16. Liu, Y. et al., T2-weighted four dimensional magnetic resonance imaging with result-driven phase sorting. *Med Phys*, 2015. **42**(8): 4460–71.
17. McGuire, S.M. et al., A methodology for using SPECT to reduce intensity-modulated radiation therapy (IMRT) dose to functioning lung. *Int J Radiat Oncol Biol Phys*, 2006. **66**(5): 1543–52.
18. Chen, S. et al., Investigation of the support vector machine algorithm to predict lung radiation-induced pneumonitis. *Med Phys*, 2007. **34**(10): 3808–14.
19. Tian, Y. et al., Dosimetric comparison of treatment plans based on free breathing, maximum, and average intensity projection CTs for lung cancer SBRT. *Med Phys*, 2012. **39**(5): 2754–60.
20. Ge, H. et al., Quantification and minimization of uncertainties of internal target volume for stereotactic body radiation therapy of lung cancer. *Int J Radiat Oncol Biol Phys*, 2013. **85**(2): 438–43.
21. Bergner, F. et al., Autoadaptive phase-correlated (AAPC) reconstruction for 4D CBCT. *Med Phys*, 2009. **36**(12): 5695–706.
22. Qi, Z. and G.H. Chen, Extraction of tumor motion trajectories using PICCS-4DCBCT: A validation study. *Med Phys*, 2011. **38**(10): 5530–8.
23. Zhang, Y. et al., A technique for estimating 4D-CBCT using prior knowledge and limited-angle projections. *Med Phys*, 2013. **40**(12): 121701.
24. Wang, Z. et al., Refinement of treatment setup and target localization accuracy using three-dimensional cone-beam computed tomography for stereotactic body radiotherapy. *Int J Radiat Oncol Biol Phys*, 2009. **73**(2): 571–7.
25. Yin, F. et al., *AAPM REPORT NO. 104: The Role of In-Room kV X-Ray Imaging for Patient Setup and Target Localization*. 2009, College Park, MD: American Association of Physicists in Medicine.
26. Ren, L., Y. Zhang, and F.F. Yin, A limited-angle intrafraction verification (LIVE) system for radiation therapy. *Med Phys*, 2014. **41**(2): 020701.

27. Liu, J. et al., From active shape model to active optical flow model: A shape-based approach to predicting voxel-level dose distributions in spine SBRT. *Phys Med Biol*, 2015. **60**(5): N83–92.
28. Klein, E.E. et al., Task Group 142 report: Quality assurance of medical accelerators. *Med Phys*, 2009. 36(9): 4197–212.
29. Benedict, S.H. et al., Stereotactic body radiation therapy: The report of AAPM Task Group 101. *Med Phys*, 2010. 37(8): 4078–101.
30. Solberg, T.D. et al., Quality and safety considerations in stereotactic radiosurgery and stereotactic body radiation therapy: Executive summary. *Pract Radiat Oncol*, 2012. 2(1): 2–9.

2

History and future of IGRT in lung cancer

JOE Y. CHANG

2.1 INTRODUCTION

After its discovery by Wilhelm Roentgen in 1895, radiation started to be used as a diagnostic and therapeutic modality for cancer (Table 2.1). A patient with superficial breast cancer was treated with kilovoltage (kV)- range radiotherapy (RT) in 1896, but it was not until 1951 when the first cancer patient was treated with Cobalt-60 radiation. In 1956 when megavoltage (MV) energy-based linac was developed at Stanford University, it became possible to treat deep tumors. As a result of the development of computed tomography (CT) technology in the early 1970s, imaging techniques for cancer advanced significantly from 1970 to 1980. Finally, three-dimensional (3D) CT imaging and RT planning were widely implemented in the 1990s, revolutionizing RT.

Modern RT plays a crucial role in the management of lung cancer in definitive, neoadjuvant, and adjuvant settings. In the past two decades, emerging cutting-edge technologies have enabled radiation oncologists to deliver a radiation dose using either photons or charged particles, conformal to the target while sparing the surrounding critical normal structures [1,2]. The primary goal of radiotherapy is to achieve tumor local/regional control with acceptable side effects. Several major factors contribute to local and regional recurrence, distant failure, and normal tissue toxicity after RT:

1. Target misses because of imprecise imaging staging and RT planning
2. Geographic misses due to lung tumor motion and anatomic changes during RT
3. Inadequate radiation doses that lead to residual viable cancer cells and therefore local recurrence and metastasis
4. Biological heterogeneity that results in radiation-resistant residual disease, circulating tumor cells, or a compromised immune response. To improve the therapeutic ratio of RT, we must focus high doses to targets and curve them away from critical normal structures—a practice known as conformality [2].

Image-guided RT (IGRT) is crucial to conformality. It has led to improved RT accuracy and clinical outcomes (1), particularly with the use of positron emission tomography (PET)/CT, four-dimensional (4D)-CT (for evaluating the tumor's location, motion, and anatomy before and during RT), and on-board image-guided adaptive RT. These techniques have enabled us to aim radiation precisely at the target and minimize the dose to surrounding critical structures (1, 2). IGRT makes it is possible to widely implement cutting-edge technologies such as stereotactic ablative RT/stereotactic body RT (SABR/SBRT), intensity-modulated RT (IMRT), volumetric modulated arc therapy (VMAT), and particle therapy in lung cancer, which typically presents as a moving target. Although we are entering a new era of molecular biology and immunology-based personalized medicine, it remains investigated about how to define the optimal RT dose and volume individually based on genomic profiling and how to combine RT with immunotherapy and molecularly targeted therapy in individual patients [3,4]. In this chapter, we review the history of IGRT (Table 2.1), as well as its status and future directions.

2.2 CT SIMULATION AND 3D-CRT HAVE REVOLUTIONIZED RT IN LUNG CANCER

Modern RT began with the implementation of a CT-based RT planning system in the 1990s that helps us view tumors three-dimensionally and view their relationship with normal critical structures. Previously,

Table 2.1 History of radiotherapy and image-guided radiation therapy in lung cancer

Event	Year	Source
Discovery of radiation	1895	German physicist Wilhelm Roentgen, first Nobel Prize in Physics 1901
First use of diagnostic radiation	1896	Dartmouth College
First use of radiation to treat breast cancer	1896	Chicago medical student Emil Grubbe
Gamma rays from radium	1903	Physicists Marie and Pierre Curie, Nobel Prize in Physics
Nuclear particle cyclotron	1929	Ernest Lawrence, Nobel Prize in Physics 1939
Stereotactic radiosurgery	1951	Swedish neurosurgeon Lars Leksell
First patient treated on an MV linac	1956	Henry Kaplan at Stanford University
Concept of CT	1972	British engineer Sir Godfrey Hounsfield and Allan Cormack, Nobel Prize for Physiology or Medicine 1979
First PET image	1973	Edward Hoffman, Michael Pogossian, and Michael E. Phelps at Washington University
First MRI	1977	Raymond Damadian and Paul Lauterbur at SUNY Stony Brook
First 3D treatment planning	1990	Physicist Wendel Renner in Indianapolis
First CT simulator	1993	Picker International
First IMRT	1993	Physicists Thomas Bortfeld and Art Boyer at MD Anderson
First use of stereotactic radiotherapy in lung cancer	1995	Blomgren et al. [19], Karolinska Hospital, Sweden
Concept of IMPT	1999	Lomax et al. [15], Paul Scherrer Institut, Switzerland
First passive scattering proton therapy in lung cancer	1999	Bush et al. [21], Loma Linda
First 4D-CT	2003	Low et al. [22], Washington University; Pan et al. [23], GE Medical; Keall et al. [24], MD Anderson
First MRI-linac	2008	Lagendijk et al. [35], University Medical Center, Utrecht, The Netherlands
First clinical report of IMRT in lung cancer	2011	Yom et al. [30], MD Anderson
First clinical report of IMPT in lung cancer	2014	Chang et al. [18], MD Anderson

two-dimensional (2D) RT planning was used to obtain tumor measurements and the information was copied to orthogonal "simulation films" (typically anterior to posterior and lateral films). Radiation oncologists were known to carry different-colored markers in their pockets to draw target volumes in simulation films. Using 2D techniques, it was established that a total dose of 60–66 Gy could be delivered to a lung cancer target with acceptable toxicity. However, this dose was associated with local control of only 30% to 50% (Radiation Therapy Oncology Group (RTOG) 7410) [5] and 35% grade 3 and higher esophagitis and pneumonitis when concurrent chemotherapy was given (RTOG 9410) [6].

By the late 1990s, CT-based RT planning was widely used, enabling the development of 3D conformal RT (3D-CRT) for lung cancer (Table 2.1). 3D-CRT evaluates different beam angles and weightings three-dimensionally and calculates doses for both the target and each critical normal tissue structure [7]. 3D-CRT remains the current "standard" of RT in lung cancer in many countries, although it is being gradually replaced by IMRT/VMAT [2,7].

2.3 4D-CT MILESTONE OF HIGHLY CONFORMAL RT IN MOVING TARGETS

One of the greatest challenges in RT of lung cancer is respiration-induced target motion (also called intra-fractional tumor motion); it adds considerable geometric uncertainty to treatment [8,9], particularly when using highly conformal RT techniques such as IMRT/VMAT, SABR/SBRT, and particle therapy. In IMRT/VMAT, each treatment field or arc may cover only a portion of the target, and motion could lead to a geographical target miss [10,11]. The implementation of IMRT/VMAT in lung cancer was delayed until 4D-CT became available [7]. In SABR/SBRT, the target volume is typically small and has significant motion; it is easy to miss the target, which can result in significant target underdosing and local treatment failure [12]. In addition, due to the high doses being used, it is critical that the dose to the surrounding normal tissues is minimized [13]. Particle therapy, such as proton therapy, is more sensitive to motion and tissue density changes than photon therapy [14]. Robust motion management is crucial, particularly for intensity-modulated proton therapy (IMPT) [15–18].

Several approaches have been developed to address respiration-induced motion and minimize the risk of missing or overdosing critical structures. Based on simplified motion control techniques such as case selection, a large motion margin, surrogate-guided respiratory gating, and abdominal compression, SABR/SBRT [19,20] and passive scattering proton therapy [21] were developed before the application of modern 4D-CT-based motion management in 2003 (Table 2.1) [22–24]. With its multi-slice detectors and fast-imaging reconstruction, 4D-CT performs image acquisition while the patient is breathing, thus allowing for the assessment of individual organ and target motion. Using 4D-CT, we can determine optimal motion management strategy, including the use of iGTV, breath-hold, respiratory gating, and tumor tracking [1]. In addition, 4D-CT simulation significantly improves RT accuracy in moving targets and trig wide acceptance and implementation of IMRT/VMAT, SABR/SBRT, and proton therapy, particularly IMPT [1,18].

2.4 ADAPTIVE RT

Developed in the early 2000s, daily on-board kV images using bony structures have improved location accuracy and reduced daily set-up uncertainty in RT. The wide use of kV imaging led to decreased planning of target volume margins that spared more critical structures and reduced toxicities. However, lung cancer typically cannot be visualized by kV imaging. The motion and anatomy of tumors can change significantly during RT, which can lead to targets being missed and normal tissues being overtreated [25]. Thus, an initial simulation-based treatment plan may not match the daily treatment delivered. Volumetric in-room or on-board imaging such as cone beam CT or CT on-rails, implemented in the early 2000s, can reveal these changes and guide daily setup [26,27]. Re-planning of RT using repeat 4D-CT images to adapt to changes in patient anatomy and organ motion between treatment fractions might be warranted for selected highly mobile tumors to reduce the potential for missing the target in highly conformal RT [28].

4D-CT-based motion management and volumetric image-based adaptive RT provide the basis for modern RT in lung cancer (i.e., IMRT/VMAT, SABR/SBRT, and particle therapy) [1]. Thanks to these developments, lung cancer outcomes have significantly improved, including survival and toxicities. Image-guided SABR/SBRT was found to improve local control and overall survival in medically inoperable stage I non-small-cell lung cancer (NSCLC) [12] and has become the standard of care. It is also emerging as a non-invasive treatment option for medically operable stage I NSCLC [29]. IMRT has been gradually adapted in the clinic for lung cancer and shows improved toxicity and quality of life [30–32]. Better image staging and the implementation of 3D-CRT, IMRT have been shown to improve overall survival. In a national research protocol, the median overall survival duration increased from 17 months in RTOG 9410 to 28 months in RTOG 0617 [33].

4D-CT only samples a snapshot of tumor motions on the simulation day; the motion and shape/volume can vary significantly at different times and on different days, particularly with the conventional 30 fractions of RT. The ideal solution to this problem is to track the tumor in real time during treatment and correct the beam position to match the location of the target [34]. This approach has been used with the Calypso® system and CyberKnife®, with implemented fiducials as a surrogate. It is now possible to perform volumetric imaging during treatment delivery with true "real-time" tumor tracking using MRI-based linac [35].

2.5 MRI-GUIDED RT

There are two disadvantages in using CT for RT:

1. Some soft tissue targets, such as esophageal cancer, liver cancer, prostate cancer, and rectal cancer, cannot be visualized clearly using CT because surrounding normal tissues have similar soft tissue densities on built-in "on-board" volumetric images.
2. There is no real-time imaging during radiation delivery at present.

Although MRI was invented in the 1970s, its use in radiation oncology was delayed due to cost and technique complexity. It has been extensively used to evaluate metastatic disease in the brain in patients with lung cancer. It has substantially improved the diagnostic accuracy for certain cancers, including liver, prostate, head/neck, and lung cancers that invade soft tissues. MRI-linac or MRI-Cobalt machines have recently been implemented and have great potential to improve the therapeutic ratio in selected cancer cases. Functional MRIs can provide unique biological information about the target and surrounding critical structures. Additional research is ongoing as more MRI-based simulation, MRI-Linac/Cobalt machine procedures are implemented clinically [35,36].

2.6 CANCER BIOLOGICAL CONFORMALITY: INDIVIDUALIZED DOSE PAIRING BASED ON QUANTITATIVE FUNCTIONAL AND MOLECULAR IMAGING

The improved capabilities of MRI, spectroscopy, and PET have provided physiological and functional images of tumors and their surrounding normal tissues that can be used to guide RT, optimizing dose boosts and sparing critical structures. PET/CT imaging improves lung cancer staging and improves RT target accuracy by 25% to 50% (37). PET/CT imaging upstaged and downstaged lung cancer in 25% of patients [37]. Studies examining the utility of FDG-PET and hypoxic imaging as radiographic biomarkers for treatment failure have shown that regions with a high standardized uptake value (such as >13.8) or hypoxia are more likely to have local recurrence after a standard dose of RT [38].

Biologically, tumors are heterogeneous: clones and tumor subregions may contain different dominant driving gene mutations, tumor-associated antigens, and different enrichments of cancer stem cells. In addition, the microenvironment, such as blood endothelial cells, of each subregion can differ. Therefore, not only should we treat each patient individually based on his or her tumor's histological type, size, location, and motion but also based on the targeted subregion microenvironment, metabolism, gene profile, and immune reaction.

IMRT/VMAT, including IMPT, allows for non-homogenous dose distribution, thereby providing the means to selectively paint the dose to subregions within the target using quantitative functional images and to further customize the delivered dose distribution [39]. Dose escalation to regions at high risk of tumor recurrence may further improve local control—and potentially survival—while protecting large areas of normal tissue from high doses of radiation. Currently, the RTOG is evaluating this approach in stage III NSCLC using PET imaging to boost the volume to up to 86 Gy during 30 fractions of RT. CT imaging voxel-based prescriptions of deliberately non-uniform dose distributions that are based on quantitative molecular imaging (i.e., dose-painting RT) can map the image data intensities to prescribed doses [40,41]. IMRT has significantly improved physical conformality in RT, but quantitative functional imaging has launched a new era of biological conformality and additional studies are ongoing.

There is emerging information about the molecular and immune profiles of cancer that will lead to changes in treatment. Molecular imaging based on this information will reveal biological and immunological traits of tumors at the genotype and phenotype levels. These developments will converge to provide significant opportunities for enhancing the success of RT. Computer-based technologies, such as CT, PET/CT, 4D-CT and 4-D PET/CT, have revolutionized RT in the past decades. The combination of biology and technology will certainly provide more opportunities to revolutionize RT. For example, the combination of immunotherapy and SABR/SBRT holds promise for improving the therapeutic ratio compared with either treatment alone. It might lead to more cures of stage I to IV cancers, including lung cancer [3]. Molecular markers, quantitative functional imaging [42] including radiomics [43], IGRT, and the combination of emerging immunotherapies and molecularly targeted therapies [3,4] will be the next research focuses in radiation oncology. IGRT will play more of a role in lung cancer management in the coming decades. There is no better time in radiation oncology to have an impact on the management of lung and other cancers.

REFERENCES

1. Chang, J.Y. et al., Image-guided radiation therapy for non-small cell lung cancer. *J Thorac Oncol*, 2008. **3**(2): 177–86.
2. Chang, J.Y. and J.D. Cox, Improving radiation conformality in the treatment of non-small cell lung cancer. *Semin Radiat Oncol*, 2010. **20**(3): 171–7.
3. Zeng, J. et al., Combination of stereotactic ablative body radiation with targeted therapies. *Lancet Oncol*, 2014. **15**(10): e426–34.
4. Bernstein, M.B. et al., Immunotherapy and stereotactic ablative radiotherapy (ISABR): A curative approach? *Nat Rev Clin Oncol*, 2016. **13**(8): 516–24.
5. Perez, C.A. et al., A prospective randomized study of various irradiation doses and fractionation schedules in the treatment of inoperable non-oat-cell carcinoma of the lung. Preliminary report by the Radiation Therapy Oncology Group. *Cancer*, 1980. **45**(11): 2744–53.
6. Curran, W.J., Jr. et al., Sequential vs. concurrent chemoradiation for stage III non-small cell lung cancer: Randomized phase III trial RTOG 9410. *J Natl Cancer Inst*, 2011. **103**(19): 1452–60.
7. Chang, J.Y., Intensity-modulated radiotherapy, not 3 dimensional conformal, is the preferred technique for treating locally advanced lung cancer. *Semin Radiat Oncol*, 2015. **25**(2): 110–6.
8. Liu, H.H. et al., Assessing respiration-induced tumor motion and internal target volume using four-dimensional computed tomography for radiotherapy of lung cancer. *Int J Radiat Oncol Biol Phys*, 2007. **68**(2): 531–40.
9. Schwarz, M. et al., Impact of geometrical uncertainties on 3D CRT and IMRT dose distributions for lung cancer treatment. *Int J Radiat Oncol Biol Phys*, 2006. **65**(4): 1260–9.
10. Bortfeld, T. et al., Effects of intra-fraction motion on IMRT dose delivery: Statistical analysis and simulation. *Phys Med Biol*, 2002. **47**(13): 2203–20.

11. Timmerman, R. et al., Stereotactic body radiation therapy for inoperable early stage lung cancer. *JAMA*, 2010. **303**(11): 1070–6.
12. Timmerman, R. et al., Excessive toxicity when treating central tumors in a phase II study of stereotactic body radiation therapy for medically inoperable early-stage lung cancer. *J Clin Oncol*, 2006. **24**(30): 4833–9.
13. Engelsman, M., E. Rietzel, and H.M. Kooy, Four-dimensional proton treatment planning for lung tumors. *Int J Radiat Oncol Biol Phys*, 2006. **64**(5): 1589–95.
14. Kang, Y. et al., 4D Proton treatment planning strategy for mobile lung tumors. *Int J Radiat Oncol Biol Phys*, 2007. **67**(3): 906–14.
15. Lomax, A., Intensity modulation methods for proton radiotherapy. *Phys Med Biol*, 1999. **44**(1): 185–205.
16. Seco, J. et al., Breathing interplay effects during proton beam scanning: Simulation and statistical analysis. *Phys Med Biol*, 2009. **54**(14): N283–94.
17. Li, Y. et al., Selective robust optimization: A new intensity-modulated proton therapy optimization strategy. *Med Phys*, 2015. **42**(8): 4840–7.
18. Chang, J.Y. et al., Clinical implementation of intensity modulated proton therapy for thoracic malignancies. *Int J Radiat Oncol Biol Phys*, 2014. **90**(4): 809–18.
19. Blomgren, H. et al., Stereotactic high dose fraction radiation therapy of extracranial tumors using an accelerator. Clinical experience of the first thirty-one patients. *Acta Oncol*, 1995. **34**(6): 861–70.
20. Uematsu, M. et al., Focal, high dose, and fractionated modified stereotactic radiation therapy for lung carcinoma patients: A preliminary experience. *Cancer*, 1998. **82**(6): 1062–70.
21. Bush, D.A. et al., Proton-beam radiotherapy for early-stage lung cancer. *Chest*, 1999. **116**(5): 1313–9.
22. Low, D.A. et al., A method for the reconstruction of four-dimensional synchronized CT scans acquired during free breathing. *Med Phys*, 2003. **30**(6): 1254–63.
23. Pan, T. et al., 4D-CT imaging of a volume influenced by respiratory motion on multi-slice CT. *Med Phys*, 2004. **31**(2): 333–40.
24. Keall, P.J. et al., Acquiring 4D thoracic CT scans using a multislice helical method. *Phys Med Biol*, 2004. **49**(10): 2053–67.
25. Britton, K.R. et al., Assessment of gross tumor volume regression and motion changes during radiotherapy for non-small-cell lung cancer as measured by four-dimensional computed tomography. *Int J Radiat Oncol Biol Phys*, 2007. **68**(4): 1036–46.
26. Bissonnette, J.P. et al., Cone-beam computed tomographic image guidance for lung cancer radiation therapy. *Int J Radiat Oncol Biol Phys*, 2009. **73**(3): 927–34.
27. Knap, M.M. et al., Daily cone-beam computed tomography used to determine tumour shrinkage and localisation in lung cancer patients. *Acta Oncol*, 2010. **49**(7): 1077–84.
28. Koay, E.J. et al., Adaptive/nonadaptive proton radiation planning and outcomes in a phase II trial for locally advanced non-small cell lung cancer. *Int J Radiat Oncol Biol Phys*, 2012. **84**(5): 1093–100.
29. Chang, J.Y. et al., Stereotactic ablative radiotherapy versus lobectomy for operable stage I non-small-cell lung cancer: A pooled analysis of two randomised trials. *Lancet Oncol*, 2015. **16**(6): 630–7.
30. Yom, S.S. et al., Initial evaluation of treatment-related pneumonitis in advanced-stage non-small-cell lung cancer patients treated with concurrent chemotherapy and intensity-modulated radiotherapy. *Int J Radiat Oncol Biol Phys*, 2007. **68**(1): 94–102.
31. Liao, Z.X. et al., Influence of technologic advances on outcomes in patients with unresectable, locally advanced non-small-cell lung cancer receiving concomitant chemoradiotherapy. *Int J Radiat Oncol Biol Phys*, 2010. **76**(3): 775–81.
32. Movsas, B. et al., Quality of life analysis of a radiation dose-escalation study of patients with non-small-cell lung cancer: A secondary analysis of the Radiation Therapy Oncology Group 0617 randomized clinical trial. *JAMA Oncol*, 2016. **2**(3): 359–67.
33. Bradley, J.D. et al., Standard-dose versus high-dose conformal radiotherapy with concurrent and consolidation carboplatin plus paclitaxel with or without cetuximab for patients with stage IIIA or IIIB non-small-cell lung cancer (RTOG 0617): A randomised, two-by-two factorial phase 3 study. *Lancet Oncol*, 2015. **16**(2): 187–99.

34. Suh, Y. et al., Four-dimensional IMRT treatment planning using a DMLC motion-tracking algorithm. *Phys Med Biol*, 2009. **54**(12): 3821–35.
35. Lagendijk, J.J. et al., MRI/linac integration. *Radiother Oncol*, 2008. **86**(1): 25–9.
36. Yang, Y. et al., Longitudinal diffusion MRI for treatment response assessment: Preliminary experience using an MRI-guided tri-cobalt 60 radiotherapy system. *Med Phys*, 2016. **43**(3): 1369–73.
37. Bradley, J. et al., A phase II comparative study of gross tumor volume definition with or without PET/CT fusion in dosimetric planning for non-small-cell lung cancer (NSCLC): Primary analysis of Radiation Therapy Oncology Group (RTOG) 0515. *Int J Radiat Oncol Biol Phys*, 2012. **82**(1): 435–41. e1.
38. Ling, C.C. et al., Towards multidimensional radiotherapy (MD-CRT): Biological imaging and biological conformality. *Int J Radiat Oncol Biol Phys*, 2000. **47**(3): 551–60.
39. Galvin, J.M. and W. De Neve, Intensity modulating and other radiation therapy devices for dose painting. *J Clin Oncol*, 2007. **25**(8): 924–30.
40. Bowen, S.R. et al., On the sensitivity of IMRT dose optimization to the mathematical form of a biological imaging-based prescription function. *Phys Med Biol*, 2009. **54**(6): 1483–501.
41. Bentzen, S.M., Radiation therapy: Intensity modulated, image guided, biologically optimized and evidence based. *Radiother Oncol*, 2005. **77**(3): 227–30.
42. Ohri, N. et al., Pretreatment 18F-FDG PET textural features in locally advanced non-small cell lung cancer: Secondary analysis of ACRIN 6668/RTOG 0235. *J Nucl Med*, 2016. **57**(6): 842–8.
43. Aerts, H.J. et al., Decoding tumour phenotype by noninvasive imaging using a quantitative radiomics approach. *Nat Commun*, 2014. **5**: 4006.

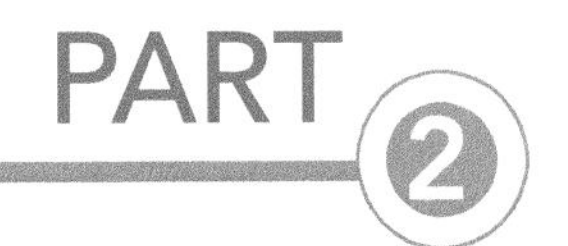

PRINCIPLES OF IGRT FOR LUNG CANCER

3

Imaging simulation for lung cancer IGRT

DANIEL LOW, TINSU PAN, NING WEN, AND CARRI K. GLIDE-HURST

3.1 INTRODUCTION

Advances in image-guided radiation therapy (IGRT) and intensity-modulated radiation therapy (IMRT) have enabled the generation and delivery of highly conformal radiation dose distributions. These conformal techniques facilitate target dose escalation with the aim of improving survival and normal tissue sparing. The accuracy of the conformal techniques is, however, limited by the uncertainties in patient positioning and internal tumor and normal tissue motion. This issue is particularly critical in IGRT of lung cancer where the respiratory motion is an inherent source of uncertainty. Four-dimensional computed tomography (4D-CT) imaging technologies have shown that significant motion can occur during radiation treatments. If left uncompensated, such motion can lead to significant dose delivery errors.

Breathing-induced motion is relatively fast. In computed tomography (CT), respiratory motion causes artifacts because tissues move in and out of the CT slice window during image acquisition. Modern CT scanners have rotation periods of between 0.3 s and 0.5 s. For a slice thickness of 1 mm, this implies that tissue velocities greater than 2 mm/s will cause at least minor blurring. Different types and magnitude of artifacts have been reported by Yamamoto et al. [1]. Sub-optimal image quality can cause target volumes to be inaccurately delineated, leading to inconsistencies between the actual tumor shape and the high radiation dose regions.

During the treatment, respiratory motion of the tumor also leads to the degradation of the prescribed dose distribution [2]. This is typically reflected by blurring of the dose distribution. The amount of blurring depends on the amplitude and characteristics of the breathing motion and is most often independent of the specific delivery technique. When the delivery techniques involve moving beams or moving apertures, such as IMRT delivered with a multileaf collimator, interplay effects between the moving beams and organs can further distort the radiation dose distributions. The resulting dose distribution can also be deformed by the motion of internal heterogeneities [3], but it has been found that dose deformations and interplay effects are relatively small, and the dominant effect is the blurring of the dose distributions. Given the adverse impact that respiratory motion can have on both imaging and treatment delivery, it is important to understand the motion characteristics and the different motion reduction/compensation strategies during imaging simulation to develop optimal treatment plan. This chapter discusses the methodologies for characterizing respiratory motion, measuring respiratory motion, and motion management strategies for IGRT of lung cancer.

3.2 4D-CT

Since respiration can be both voluntary and involuntary, there can be significant variation in the extent of the tissue motion. Breathing patterns are patient specific and, coupled with the differing locations of diseased tissues, large variations can be observed. The range and variation of organ motion has been reported extensively, e.g., Keall et al. (Table 3.1) [4]. Nevertheless, there are some observations that generally apply to respiration-induced organ motion.

- Organs translate and deform due to respiration.
- Tissue motion hysteresis, shift in baseline position, and cardiac-induced tissue motion as well as change in respiratory patterns have been observed. Figure 3.1 [5] shows examples of regular and irregular breathing motion.
- In the lungs, the largest displacement is generally observed in the cranio-caudal direction and the least in the lateral direction.

4D-CT was one of the most important developments in radiation oncology in the last decade. Its early development in single-slice CT (SSCT) and commercialization in multi-slice CT (MSCT) have radically changed our practice in radiation treatment of lung cancer and have enabled the stereotactic radiosurgery of early stage lung cancer. In this section, we will document the history of 4D-CT development, detail the data sufficiency condition governing the 4D-CT data collection, present the designs, and compare the differences of the helical and cine 4D-CTs.

3.2.1 History of 4D-CT

Helical CT was developed in 1990 [6] to allow simultaneous data acquisition and table translation. Prior to that, CT data were obtained in the axial mode where the table was stationary during data acquisition. It was clear that helical CT saved time in data acquisition because it avoided the stop-and-shoot acquisitions of the axial CT. The x-ray beam width was ≤10 mm in the table direction and the fastest gantry rotation time was 1 s. Often, the

Table 3.1 Variation in respiration induced motion of organs in the thorax and abdomen in literature

	Direction		
Observer	**SI**	**AP**	**LR**
Barnes (Ref. 74): Lower lobe	18.5 (9–32)	–	–
Middle, upper lobe	7.5 (2–11)	–	–
Chen (Ref. 73)	(0–50)	–	–
Ekberg (Ref. 22)	3.9 (0–12)	2.4 (0–5)	2.4 (0–5)
Engelsman (Ref. 24)	–	–	–
Middle/upper lobe	(2–6)	–	–
Lower lobe	(2–9)	–	–
Erridge (Ref. 104)	12.5 (6–34)	9.4 (5–22)	7.3 (3–12)
Ross (Ref. 60): Upper lobe	–	1 (0–5)	1 (0–3)
Middle lobe	–	0	9 (0–16)
Lower lobe	–	1 (0–4)	10.5 (0–13)
Grills (Ref. 80)	(2–30)	(0–10)	(0–6)
Hanley (Ref. 61)	12 (1–20)	5 (0–13)	1 (0–1)
Murphy (Ref. 77)	7 (2–15)	–	–
Plathow (Ref. 65): Lower lobe	9.5 (4.5–16.4)	6.1 (2.5–9.8)	6.0 (2.9–9.8)
Middle lobe	7.2 (4.3–10.2)	4.3 (1.9–7.5)	4.3 (1.5–7.1)
Upper lobe	4.3 (2.6–7.1)	2.8 (1.2–5.1)	3.4 (1.3–5.3)
Seppenwoolde (Ref. 50)	5.8 (0–25)	2.5 (0–8)	1.5 (0–3)
Shimizu (Ref. 75)	–	6.4 (2–24)	–
Sixel (Ref. 79)	(0–13)	(0–5)	(0–4)
Stevens (Ref. 49)	4.5 (0–22)	–	–

Source: Keall, P.J. et al., *Med Phys.*, 33, 3874–900, 2006.
Mean displacement (minimum-maximum) in mm.

CT scanner had to pause for the tube to cool down prior to another scan. We call these types of CT scanners SSCT as opposed to the MSCT introduced in 1998 when the CT simulation was about to become clinically popular [7]. MSCT was a technological revolution over SSCT because it allowed for the reconstruction of slices less than 5mm thickness with >20mm craniocaudal detector coverage. The major improvements from SSCT to MSCT were larger detector coverage, faster gantry rotation, and a larger capacity x-ray tube. These technological advances were originally designed to support cardiac imaging. The fastest gantry rotation cycle was 0.28 s per revolution. Dual source CT further has further reduced cuts the scan time by half and can improve the temporal resolution to 75 ms [8]. The largest coverage in one CT rotation is typically 16 cm to allow imaging of the coronary arteries in one cardiac cycle or cerebrovascular perfusion imaging of the whole brain for about a minute [9].

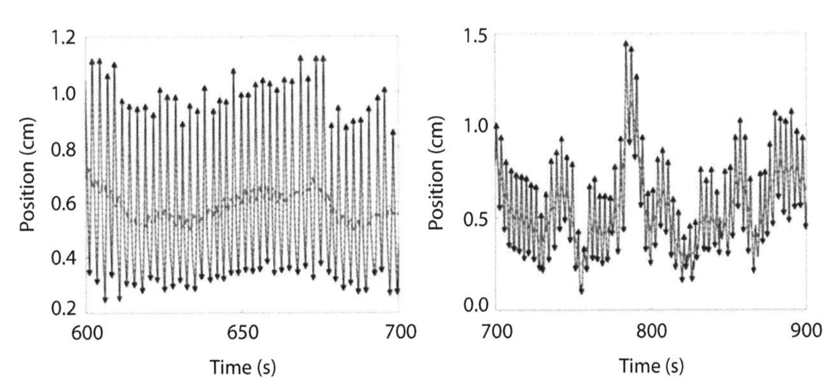

Figure 3.1 Examples showing the tumor position variability. These patient datasets were acquired using CyberKnife® Synchrony®. (From Suh, Y. et al., *Phys Med Biol.*, 53, 3623–640, 2008.)

SSCT was not practical for clinical 4D-CT imaging because of its limited detector coverage and slow gantry rotation [10]. Routine clinical 4D-CT was not practical until MSCT became available in 1998. With a detector coverage of more than 1 cm, a single rotation of a 4-slice CT scanner could produce four 2.5 mm thick slices much faster than a SSCT. Almost as significant as the development of MSCT was the introduction of the gantry rotations of 0.5 s, which was designed to support coronary artery CT imaging, with a spatial resolution of less than 0.5 mm and a temporal resolution of faster than 250 ms. 64-slice CT has become popular in both diagnostic imaging and radiation oncology. Currently, the scanner with the largest detector coverage is the Aquilion ONE 320-slice CT scanner (Toshiba America Medical Systems, Tustin, CA), with a coverage of 16 cm per gantry rotation [11,12]. It was shown in a phantom study that the 320-slice MSCT can help characterize tumor motion more accurately than a 16-slice MSCT [13]. Its clinical application in 4D-CT is promising. The scanner with the highest temporal resolution (< 100 ms) is the SOMATOM dual-source CT scanner [8] (Siemens Medical Solutions USA, Malvern, PA). The first 4D-CT application was the cardiac CT, a non-invasive procedure to image the coronary arteries.

The first application of 4D-CT imaging of the lung tumor subject to the respiratory motion was first published by Vedam et al. [10] and Ford et al. [14], using the AcQSIM SSCT scanner (Philips Medical Systems, Andover, MA). The smallest pitch, defined as the ratio of the table travel per 360 degree gantry rotation to the width of the imaging x-ray beam, on this scanner was 0.5. Given the relatively small radiation beam width, using the maximum gantry rotation speed would not allow the patient to be scanned rapidly enough to complete a single breathing cycle. Therefore, the gantry rotation rate was slowed to 1.5 s [15]. However, the table speed in this design was still too fast for 4D-CT. Also, the long acquisition time of up to 7 min per respiratory phase due to the limited coverage of the SSCT scanner was not well suited for routine clinical 4D-CT.

The first clinical use of 4D-CT was presented at the AAPM 2002 Annual Meeting in Montreal, Canada, using the GE MSCT scanners (GE Healthcare, Waukesha, WI) [15]. They utilized the cine CT scan protocol already available on the GE MSCT scanner, which could scan at the same location for multiple gantry rotations to provide cine (or movie) CT images, which were correlated with a respiratory surrogate (Real-time Position Management (RPM) respiratory gating system (Varian Medical Systems, Palo Alto, CA). Both Phillips and Siemens later modified their low-pitch helical cardiac CT scanning mode for their 4D-CT design [16]. This design was commercialized in 2006 on MSCT scanners with at least 16 slices. In comparison, all the GE MSCT scanners manufactured since 1998 and with at least 4 slices and that were configured with cine CT scan capability have been able to conduct 4D-CT.

3.2.2 4D-CT IMAGE ACQUISITION

The goal of 4D-CT in to derive a time sequence of the 3D anatomy of interest over a respiratory cycle. The data collection is typically obtained through synchronized acquisition of a patient respiratory signal and the anatomical image data. The respiratory signal can be acquired using devices that track patient surface positions or breathing tidal volume [14,17]. In addition, internal surrogates have been introduced, such as body area [18], combined image features [19], and diaphragm positions [20].

There are two basic methodologies for 4D-CT imaging: helical and cine image acquisitions [21–24]. In both cases, a breathing surrogate is measured simultaneously to CT acquisition. Helical scanning involves the couch translates as the CT gantry rotates. The patient passes through the bore once, and the CT projections are sorted per breathing trace and breathing cycle definition (amplitude or phase-angle). The requirement for 4D-CT data collection is to acquire the data at each slice location for at least one breath cycle of approximately 4–5 s. As the patient passes through the scanner, the couch moves slowly, so projections are acquired at each location for at least one breath cycle. For example, a typical CT simulator has a rotation period of 0.5 s and uses a pitch of 0.06. Therefore, each location is scanned for 8.3 s, longer than a typical breathing cycle. As the scanner rotates, CT projections are stored and then re-sorted according to the breathing phase during which they were collected. The second technique is cine. In this case, the couch is stationary and the CT scanner acquires repeated cine scans. Once sufficient scans have been acquired, the CT couch moves to an abutting position and the scanning is repeated.

Both helical and cine 4D-CT scans need to meet the requirement of data sufficiency condition to ensure there is at least one respiratory cycle of data at each location. Unlike cine 4D-CT, helical 4D-CT tends to result in thicker slices due to data interpolation and a longer workflow because image reconstruction cannot start until the respiratory signal of the helical 4D-CT scan has been completely acquired. Commercial helical 4D-CT can be performed by MSCT scanners of 16-slice or up, while cine 4D-CT can be done using MSCT scanners with 4-slice or up. A very important quality control step in 4D-CT is to ensure accuracy in identifying the end-inspiration phases of the respiratory signal because inaccurate identification of the end-inspiration phases will cause 4D-CT to generate incorrect data.

3.2.2.1 HELICAL 4D-CT

The challenge in 4D-CT imaging is to capture a complete breath cycle of the lung motion in CT imaging. Since no CT detector can cover the whole lungs, and the conventional scan speeds for diagnostic CT and cardiac CT imaging are still too fast for 4D-CT of the lungs. Special care must be taken to ensure the scanner parameters such as pitch value, gantry rotation time, table speed or table translation per rotation and detector configuration are suitable for 4D-CT imaging. Figure 3.2 is an illustration of a helical CT scan. An x-ray source sends out a cone-like radiation field illuminating a multi-row detector. This cone-like radiation field

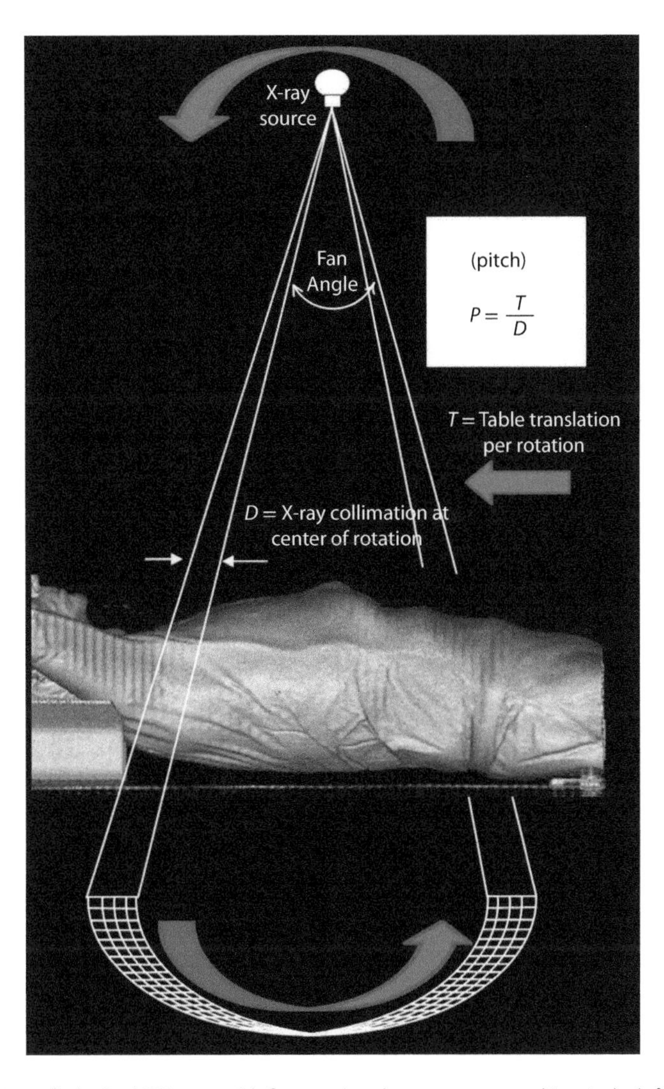

Figure 3.2 Illustration of a helical CT scan with four active detector rows and its pitch definition.

is characterized by the in-plane fan angle of about 60 degrees and the x-ray collimation (the active detector width) at the center of rotation. Since the patient table is moving while the CT gantry is rotating, the illumination field follows a helical course in a patient-centric coordinate system. Table motion and gantry rotation speed must be selected in a way that the targeted lung area is covered in the x-ray beam for at least one complete breath cycle, which is the data sufficiency condition of 4D-CT [22].

The time needed to acquire one image is equal to one gantry rotation cycle for full-scan reconstruction (FSR) or half of a gantry rotation cycle plus fan-angle for half-scan reconstruction (HSR) [25], which is 180 degrees plus about 60 degrees, roughly 2/3 gantry rotations. Additional data acquisition is needed because it takes at least 2/3 of a gantry rotation cycle in CT for an image reconstruction and to ensure that there are images at both ends of a complete breath cycle. This additional data acquisition is not necessary for projection x-ray imaging such as fluoroscopy, in which each projection is an image without image reconstruction like in CT [26]. To satisfy the data sufficiency condition, the pitch value p needs to fulfill the following conditions;

$$p \le \frac{Tg}{T_b + T_g} \tag{3.1}$$

$$p \le \frac{Tg}{T_b + \frac{2}{3}T_g} \tag{3.2}$$

where equations 3.1 and 3.2 correspond to FSR and HSR, respectively. Where T_g and T_b are the durations of the gantry rotation cycle and the breath cycle, respectively. If the breath cycle T_b is the same as the gantry rotation cycle T_g, then after one T_g (e.g., $T_b = T_g = 4$ s), the detector moves in and out of the x-ray beam in exactly one T_b. Considering the extra acquisition of T_g for one image reconstruction, $p = ½$. If the breath cycle T_b is 4 times of T_g (i.e., $T_b = 4$ s, $T_g = 1$ s), then $p = 0.2$. Typically, $T_b = 4$ s and $T_g = 0.5$ s and $p = 0.11$, almost the same as the typical pitch factor of 0.1 or less in the helical 4D-CT in Tables 3.2 and 3.3. Similar reasoning can be applied to Equation 3.2 for HSR.

One important observation of the pitch value selection is that the longer the breath cycle T_b or the shorter the gantry rotation cycle T_g is, the smaller the pitch factor p becomes. In diagnostic CT imaging, the pitch value with patient breath-hold and without gating, p is about 1, which is 10 times faster than the pitch employed in helical 4DCT.

Philips and Siemens employ helical 4D-CT. Both implementations were derived from the low-pitch helical CT scan of cardiac CT, which has the pitch values p of 0.2–0.3 for a targeted heart rate of about 60 beats per minute. By lowering p to 0.1 or less, and replacing the electrocardiographic monitor with a respiratory monitor, the helical 4D-CT for imaging the thorax under the condition of respiratory motion of 10–20 cycles per minute (corresponding to a 3- to 6-s respiratory cycle) becomes possible. The slower the respiratory motion, the smaller the pitch value p must be to meet the data sufficiency condition and to avoid undersampling in helical 4D-CT.

The pitch values p of the Philips CT scanners [27] and calculated values by Equation 6.1 for the breathing cycles of 3–6 s and gantry rotations of 0.44 and 0.5 s for FSR are listed in Table 3.2. Both values match closely. When the gantry rotation time changes from 0.5 to 0.44 s, pitch values p become smaller because the shorter gantry rotation time allows the scanner to cover a larger volume for the same duration at the same pitch, which may cause the scanner to scan too fast and violate the data sufficiency condition. Equation 3.1 can be used to calculate the gantry rotation cycles and the breath cycle durations other than those listed in Table 3.2.

The Siemens pitch values [28] and calculated values from Equation 3.1 are listed in Table 3.3. This scanner uses a single pitch value of 0.1 and two gantry rotation cycles of 0.5 and 1.0 s [29]. Since the pitch values p stay the same, the gantry rotation time must be increased with the increase of the breath cycle duration. This design is different from that of the Philips CT scanner, whose pitch value becomes smaller when the breath cycle becomes longer. In the Siemens design, a longer gantry rotation cycle of 1.0 s is required to slow down the scan speed to accommodate for a breath cycle of ≥6 s with the same p of 0.1. One disadvantage in this

Table 3.2 Pitch Values p for the Philips CT scanner and calculated values from equation 3.1 at the given gantry rotation cycles T_g and breath cycles of 3–6 s

	Philips design		Calculated values with FSR	
T_b	p @ $T_g = 0.5$	p @ $T_g = 0.44$	p @ $T_g = 0.5$	p @ $T_g = 0.44$
3	0.15	0.12	0.14	0.13
4	0.11	0.10	0.11	0.10
5	0.09	0.08	0.09	0.08
6	0.075	0.065	0.077	0.068

Table 3.3 Pitch Values p for the Siemens CT scanner and calculated values from equation 3.1 at given gantry rotation cycles T_g and breath cycles of 3–6 s

	Siemens design		Calculated values with FSR	
T_b	p @ $T_g = 0.5$	p @ $T_g = 1.0$	p @ $T_g = 0.5$	p @ $T_g = 1$
3	0.1	N/A	0.14	0.25
4	0.1	N/A	0.11	0.20
5	0.1	N/A	0.09	0.17
6	N/A	0.1	0.077	0.14

design is that each CT image will have a temporal resolution of 1 s for FSR and 0.5 s for HSR. Longer breath cycles tend to have a longer duration of expiration than shorter cycles do. A decrease of the temporal resolution will increase image blurring in the CT image, particularly for the images acquired in the transition of the end-expiration phase to the end-inspiration phase, which tends to have the largest motion during respiration.

3.2.2.2 CINE 4D-CT

Cine 4D-CT was the first 4D-CT commercially available on MSCT. Instead of using the pitch factor of less than ~0.1 to achieve the data sufficiency condition in helical 4D-CT, the scan duration (or cine duration) of each cine CT scan is set at one breath cycle plus 1 s, and the scan coverage of each cine CT scan is 1-cm (= 4 slices of 2.5 mm) on a 4-slice or 2 cm (= 8 slices of 2.5 mm) on an 8-slice or a 16-slice CT scanner. An illustration of cine 4D-CT is shown in Figure 3.3 for an 8-slice CT scanner. A cine 4D-CT scan consists of multiple cine CT scans of 1 or 2 cm to cover the whole lungs. This cine CT scan capability has been available on the GE MSCT scanners since 1998, and was first applied to 4D-CT in 2002 (AAPM 2002 Annual Meeting in Montreal, Canada) on the GE MSCT scanner (GE Healthcare, Waukesha, WI) [15]. Because the GE cine 4D-CT is based on the cine CT scan mode already available on their MSCT scanner, it does not require any hardware or software modification on the MSCT scanner, and it only needs an image sorting software, which correlates the same phase of CT images over the multiple cine scan positions for a single phase of 4D-CT images. The GE MSCT allows for the prescription of a large coverage of over 30 cm in a single scan setup, convenient for the application of 4D-CT. Radiation dose in the thorax application of 4D-CT is generally less than 50 mGy. Low et al. [30] proposed a similar cine 4D-CT technique on a Siemens 4-slice CT using a spirometer to measure the respiratory signal. In their approach, each cine CT scan of 1-cm coverage requires a new scan setup [17,22]. It takes 15 scans of 0.5 s (7.5 s total x-ray on time) per position to scan over one respiratory cycle of data. There was an inter-scan delay of 0.25 s between two consecutive 0.5-s scans. In total, 11.25 s per step was needed, considering the inter-scan delay time. A scanning pause of about 2 min after 7 scans was required for the user to re-program another sequence of 7 scans. Although this approach could achieve 4D-CT, it was not practical for a large coverage of over 30 cm due to the inconvenience of setting up the scan protocol.

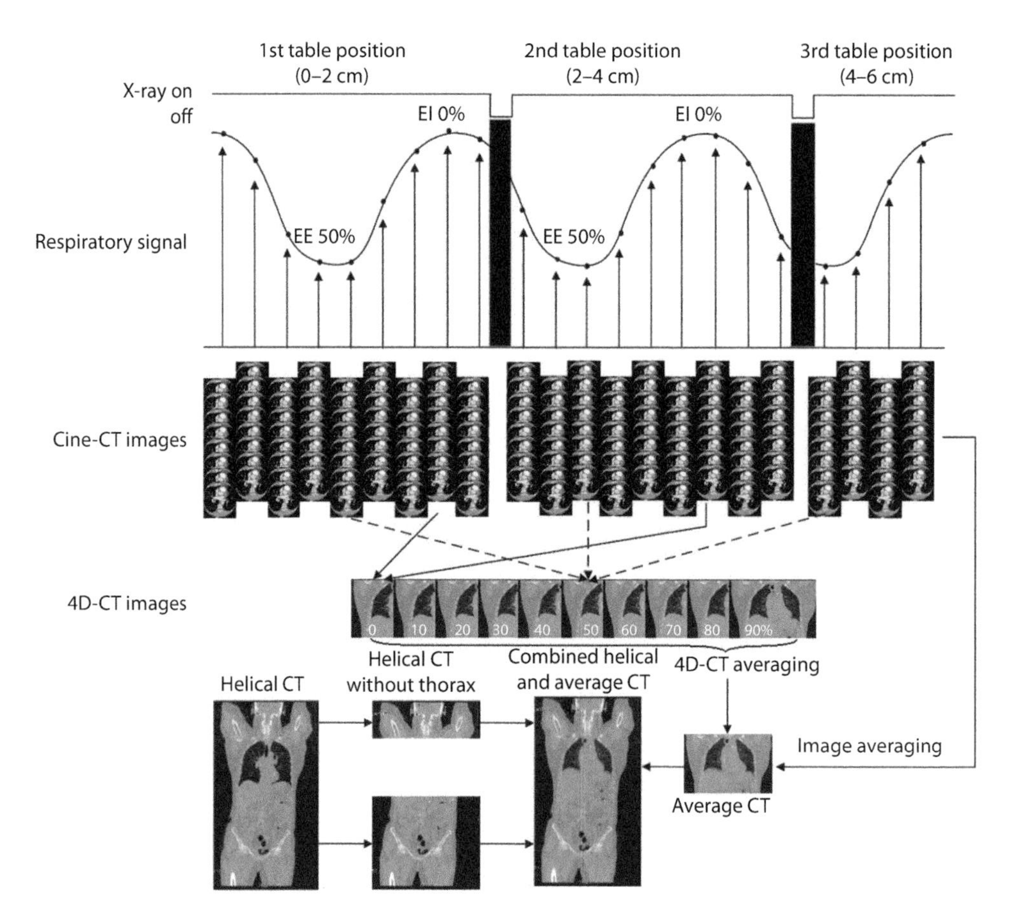

Figure 3.3 Cine 4D-CT data acquisition on an 8-slice CT scanner with 2-cm cine acquisition of one breath cycle plus 1 s per table position. The end-inspiration and end-expiration phases are EI and EE, respectively. The cine CT images are correlated with the respiratory signal to become 10 phases of 4D-CT images, which can be averaged to become average CT for attenuation correction of the PET data. Alternatively, average CT can be averaged directly from the cine CT images. One approach to making attenuation correction of PET work is to replace the thorax portion of the helical CT images with the average CT images.

3.2.2.3 COMPARISON OF HELICAL 4D-CT AND CINE 4D-CT

The helical 4D-CT scan data allow for CT image reconstruction at any location by permitting data interpolation between two neighboring detector elements (Figure 3.4), whereas the cine 4D-CT scan data allow for reconstructions only at the scan positions. When using 4D-CT to scan lung cancer patients, it is important to have a complete coverage of the lungs for tumor delineation and dose calculation. Typical image slice thicknesses in radiation treatment planning are 2–3 mm. Data interpolation in helical 4D-CT widens the slice sensitivity profile, a measure of the slice thickness of the CT image. It is important to use the thin slice collimation of 16 × 1.50 mm or below in helical 4D-CT on a 16-slice MSCT scanner because data interpolation will widen a slice thickness of 1.50 mm to almost 2.7 mm. The 8 × 2.50 mm collimation in cine 4D-CT will generate the slices of 2.5 mm because no data interpolation is in the cine CT image reconstruction. In diagnostic imaging, data interpolation causes only about 20% widening when the pitch is greater than 0.5; the amount of widening reaches 180% when the pitch is less than 0.2. To better understand this, we can take two independent slices of 2.5 mm at two neighboring locations in cine 4D-CT and interpolate for an image located right between the two slices; in such a case, interpolation would assign 50% weight to each image, and the composite image will become a 5.0-mm slice (resulting in 200% broadening of the slice thickness). Image reconstruction at pitch values of less than 0.1 in helical 4D-CT significantly thickens the CT images [22]. Once the pitch factor p becomes 0, helical CT interpolation is no longer needed and the helical

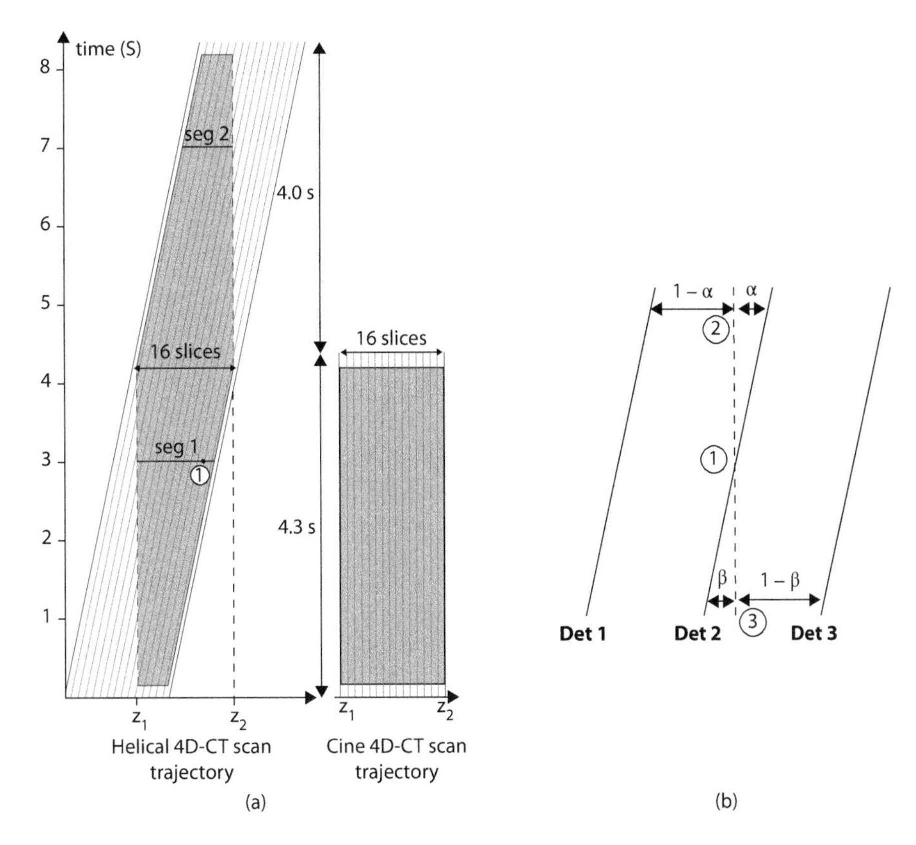

Figure 3.4 Illustration of data interpolation widening the slice thickness. The scanning trajectories of helical and cine 4D-CTs for a breath cycle of 4 s are shown in (a). The data in both seg 1 and seg 2 correspond to the same respiratory phase. Data interpolation of the helical CT data around point 1 in seg 1 is illustrated in (b). The two gray regions in (a) indicate the 4D-CT data between the two locations of z_1 and z_2. To scan only one breath cycle of 4D-CT data, helical acquisition needs to scan for 8.3 s, whereas cine acquisition only needs 4.3 s, assuming the gantry rotation cycle of $T_g = 0.5$ s. Helical CT data interpolation is illustrated in (b). There is only one data point from Det 2 ("Det" stands for detector) for data point 1 (no interpolation is needed); two data points of Det 1 and Det 2 are weighted by $(1 - \alpha)$ and α for data point 2; and two data points of Det 2 and Det 3 are weighted by β and $(1 - \beta)$ for data point 3. The location of the reconstructed image is at the dashed line.

4D-CT becomes cine 4D-CT. That is the reason that the typical detector configuration in a 16-slice MSCT is 16×1.50 mm to keep the slice thickness < 3 mm.

The fan angle of the CT detector arc is about 60 degrees. If the breath cycle is 4 s, and the gantry rotation cycle is 0.5 s, a cine 4D-CT acquisition will take 4.3 s and a helical 4D-CT acquisition 8.3 s to cover 2 cm on a 16-slice MSCT scanner (Figure 3.4). The 8.3 s was from a 4-s breath cycle, 0.3 s of 180 degrees plus 60 degrees of gantry rotation and additional 4-s to allow for a complete breath cycle at the location of interest between z_1 and z_2. The longer acquisition time needed for helical 4D-CT is due to the additional time needed for the table to translate to acquire the data over one respiratory cycle. Since the 4D-CT acquisition for the lung cancer typically covers the whole lung, this overhead in the helical 4D-CT acquisition is not significant. It contributes to a small amount of extra time required in acquisition and a small amount of extra radiation exposure to the patient. Overall, helical 4D-CT is faster than cine 4D-CT for imaging the thorax because in cine 4D-CT the table will be paused to allow the table to move to the next position; the accumulated pause time lengthens the overall acquisition time required for cine 4D-CT, making helical 4D-CT a faster 4D-CT. The speed up (in favor of helical 4D-CT) and extra radiation (in favor of cine 4D-CT) are both very small.

In helical 4D-CT, once the pitch factor is determined from either Table 3.2 or Table 3.3, collections of the helical 4D-CT data and the respiratory signal proceed simultaneously. Reconstruction of the helical 4D-CT images will not start until completion of the review of the respiratory signal for accurate identification of the end-inspiration phases, which may also require editing by the operator. This process slows down the helical 4D-CT workflow but allows for the reconstruction of the 4D-CT images at the specified phases. A suggestion to start image reconstruction before completion of data acquisition is possible. However, any change of image selection through editing of the end-inspiration locations will result in additional image reconstruction. Due to this, the multiple phases of helical 4D-CT may not be available for several minutes after the patient leaves the 4D-CT acquisition session.

Data processing is generally faster for cine 4D-CT than helical 4D-CT to generate the 4D-CT images. Once the average duration of the respiratory signal is determined, the cine scan duration per location is set to the average duration plus 1 s. This additional 1 s is recommended in case the patient's breathing slows down during data acquisition. Image reconstruction starts immediately when there are data for image reconstruction. The time interval between two CT image reconstructions should be less than T_g so that the image correlation with the respiratory signal will have a better chance of getting the images at the targeted phases.

In general, phase selection accuracy is better with helical 4D-CT than with cine 4D-CT because the reconstruction of a specific phase is determined before image reconstruction in helical 4D-CT, but not in cine 4D-CT. However, the difference is very small because 4D-CT is primarily used to depict the extent of tumor motion and the temporary resolution or time span of each CT image itself can cover more than 10% of a respiratory cycle. For example, a CT image from one 0.5-s gantry rotation of data is 12.5 % of a 4-s breath cycle and 10% of a 5-s cycle. A difference of several percentages in image selection will not impact the utility of cine 4D-CT.

One important quality control measure that must be undertaken in 4D-CT is to ensure that identification of the end-inspiration phases by the respiratory monitoring device is accurate. If phase calculation or identification is not accurate, both helical and cine 4D-CTs will generate erroneous data, not representative of the breathing motion. One example of this is illustrated in Figure 3.5. Some end-inspiration phases in (A) were incorrectly identified or missing. The correct identification of the phases is shown in (B). This step of ensuring accurate identification of end-inspiration phases is critical and should be checked in every 4D-CT data processing.

The basic assumption of 4D-CT is that the respiratory motion is reproducible throughout the data acquisition and the duration of data acquisition at any location is at least one breath cycle plus the duration for one image reconstruction, which is one or 2/3 of a CT gantry rotation. Anything deviating from this assumption can cause artifacts manifested as (1) irregular respiratory motion or (2) missing data if the scan duration is less than one breath cycle due to an underestimate of the patient's breath cycle duration. A higher helical pitch p in the Philips helical 4D, a faster CT gantry rotation in the Siemens helical 4D, or a shorter cine scan duration in GE cine 4D could introduce artifacts [31]. Figure 3.6 shows an example of the two types of artifacts.

3.2.3 4D-CT IMAGE SORTING

The two general categories of breathing cycle descriptions are phase-angle and amplitude based. The phase-angle description assumes that the breathing cycle can be reproducibly subdivided in time. A specific breathing phase (e.g., peak inhalation) is selected as the start of the breathing cycle. The time at which this breathing

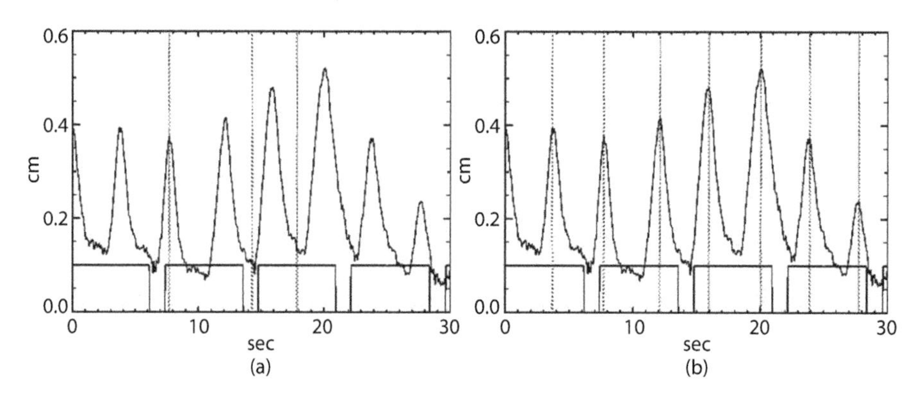

Figure 3.5 Example of a respiratory signal over 30 s with an inaccurate identification of the end-inspiration phases in (a), marked by dotted vertical lines. Accurate identification of the end-inspiration phase is in (b).

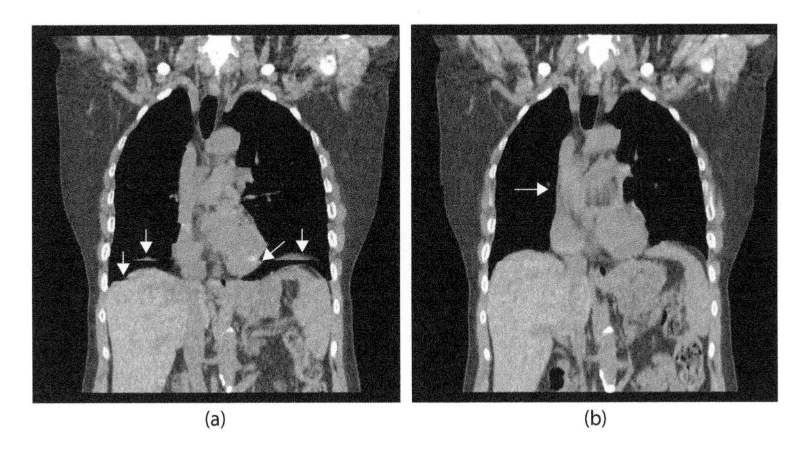

Figure 3.6 4D-CT artifacts due to (a) an irregular respiration and (b) insufficient sampling from a prolonged breath cycle.

phase repeats is identified and the breathing cycle is defined as the fraction of time from that time to the next time the same phase occurs. For example, if the breathing cycle starts at peak inhalation, the relative time between successive peak inhalations corresponds to a single breath. Phases in between are usually defined by the fraction of time between successive peaks, often described in terms of angles, with 360° between successive peaks. Additionally, the breathing cycle is further subdivided between inhalation and exhalation. Peak inhalation and exhalation are designated 0° and 180°, with linear interpolation of phase-angles in time between these extremes.

Phase-angle sorting is effective when the patient's breathing cycle, especially his breathing amplitude, is consistent. If breathing is irregular, the algorithm breaks down. Due to the regularity of the cardiac cycle, this algorithm was the first to be commercially introduced into the CT workflow because of the ease with which the CT imaging companies could transfer cardiac image gating algorithms to respiratory gating.

The second commonly used breathing cycle description category is based on the breathing amplitude. Amplitude-based sorting assumes that the internal anatomic positions are related to the depth of breathing rather than the fraction of time between breaths. In cases where the patient breathes irregularly, amplitude-based sorting results in images with fewer motion-based artifacts than phase-angle-based sorting. The main drawback for amplitude-based sorting is that it does not distinguish between the period during inhalation relative to the period during exhalation. Lung tissue motion is often known to be different during inhalation and exhalation, a phenomenon known as hysteresis.

Phase-angle-based approaches rely on the reproducibility of the breathing pattern in the time domain. Likewise, amplitude based image reconstruction assumes the anatomical position is repeatable with respect to the breathing depth. While phase- and amplitude-based sorting methods can characterize patient breathing motion, they are not without their shortcomings. Most notably, phase-based approaches are susceptible to irregular breathing patterns that violate the periodicity assumption of the breathing cycle. In amplitude-based techniques, missing image data at the desired breathing amplitudes cause problems in the sorting process.

Lu et al. [21], studied the impact of breathing cycle variation on phase-angle- and amplitude-based sorting. They reconstructed 3D image datasets for 12 breathing phases for 40 patients. They computed the air content, defined the amount of air in the lungs based on the CT scan, and used air content as a surrogate for tumor position. They correlated breathing phase and amplitude to air content and determined the residual for the correlation. In most cases, the residual for amplitude gating was smaller than the residual for phase-angle gating. When tidal volume was used as the comparator, the variation was always less for amplitude than phase-angle gating. As an example, Figure 3.7 shows the definition of mid-inspiration for amplitude and phase-angle sorting algorithms. The tidal volume for the points in time where amplitude sorting has determined the patient is at mid-inspiration are shown in Figure 3.7a, and would very likely correspond to consistent internal anatomy positions. The tidal volume for the points in time where phase-angle sorting has determined the patient is at

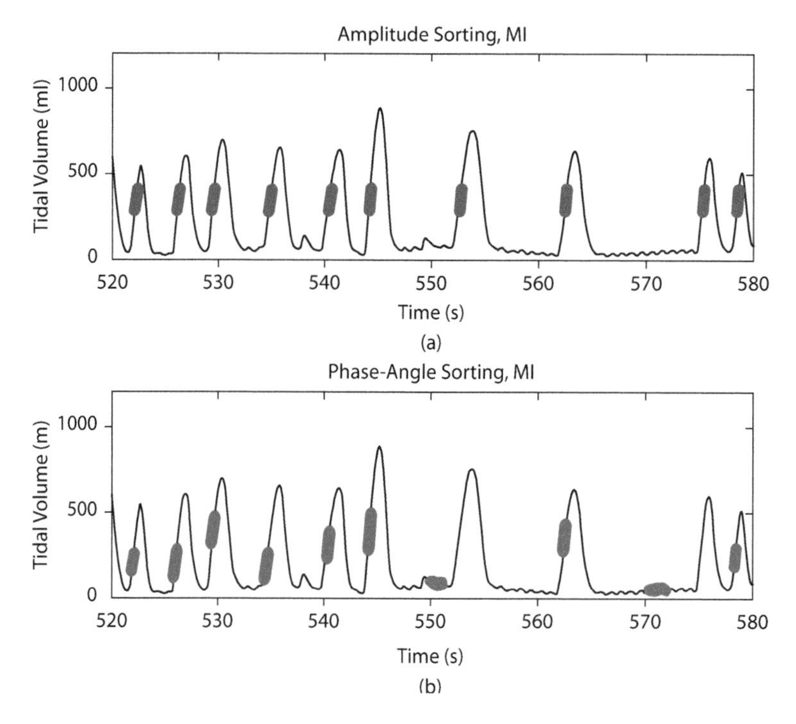

Figure 3.7 Example of the definition of mid-inspiration using (a) amplitude sorting and (b) phase-angle sorting. The thicker lines indicate the times at which each algorithm has identified that the patient is at mid-inspiration. (From Lu, W. et al., *Med Phys.*, 33, 2964–74, 2006.)

mid-inspiration are shown in Figure 3.7b. While there were many points in time where the patient's anatomy would have been in a consistent location, there were three times when the patient's breathing was paused. At these times, mid-inspiration was less clear for phase-angle sorting and the algorithm failed twice to identify a time at which the tidal volume was at mid-inspiration.

3.3 MOTION MANAGEMENT CONSIDERATIONS

Respiratory motion can be managed either actively or passively during imaging simulation. Breath-hold, respiratory gating using an external or internal marker and motion encompassing technique such as 4D-CT are the most common methods to manage respiratory motion [16,32–35]. It is important to evaluate during the simulation whether the patient can comply with breath-hold techniques or if the patient's breathing is regular enough for respiratory gating. The motion management and correction methods used in simulation will also influence the treatment planning, localization, and delivery techniques, thus any decisions should consider all aspects of the treatment chain. American Association of Physicists in Medicine (AAPM) Task Group Report No. 76 recommends patient-specific assessment of target motion and management for motion exceeding 5 mm in any direction [4].

3.3.1 Free breathing

Respiratory motion increases the apparent size of the tumor, necessitating the definition of internal target volume margins, leading to the irradiation of normal lung tissues. The size of the margin must be carefully chosen; it should be large enough to ensure the delivery of the prescribed dose to a moving target and small enough to keep the normal tissue complications to an acceptable level. In the following, we review several strategies for treatment delivery under free-breathing condition.

3.3.1.1 INTERNAL TARGET VOLUME

Accounting for tumor motion is crucial in patients undergoing radiation therapy under free-breathing conditions. To account for the uncertainties in the size, shape, and position of the clinical target volume, the International Commission on Radiation Units and Measurements (ICRU) has devised the concept of an internal target volume (ITV) to provide an envelope for target motion in Report 83 [36]. More specifically, ITV was defined to encompass the geometrical locations of the gross tumor volume (GTV) during all of the breathing phases. The ITV delineation can be performed by manually or automatically contouring of the GTV in each phase of the 4D-CT image set. An alternative method was proposed that creates an image of maximal intensity projection through combining the set of 4D-CT images from the whole breathing cycle [37–39]. Such an approach was found to be equivalent to the composite contour generated from the individual breathing phases [40].

ITV delineation errors can lead to geometric misses and irradiation of healthy tissues. Multiple studies have investigated the uncertainties in ITV quantification due to different imaging and post-processing techniques [41–43]. In [39], the authors reported that the median and range of the ITV for 20 stage I stereotactic body radiation therapy (SBRT) patients were 7.6 (1.1–35.6), 10.2 (1.9–43.7), and 9.0 (1.3–37.3) cm^3 from helical-, maximum intensity projection (MIP)-, and average intensity projection (AIP)-defined ITV. These studies found that MIP-based ITV can most effectively capture the tumor excursion [39,44]. However, caution needs to be exercised as commercial clinical 4D-CT imaging might not capture the full extent of tumor motion since the axial scanning in CT imaging takes much longer than the breathing cycle and each image slice contains breathing information from only one or two breathing cycles.

3.3.1.2 MID-INSPIRATION

An alternative approach to reducing the target margin is through the construction of mid-ventilation scans. Wolthaus et al. [45,46] proposed the mid-ventilation scan, which represents the mean position of the target in its motion trajectory. The construction of the mid-ventilation scan involves the calculation of the time-averaged scan and identifying the image in the 4D-CT dataset that most closely matches this phase. If the beam is positioned in the middle of the tumor trajectory, the required additional margin to correct for breathing motion is small. This is because the tissues spend most of their time in phases other than the extremes of inhalation and exhalation. For example, the superior portion of the tumor might be in the beam penumbra only during maximum exhalation, when it would momentarily receive somewhat less than the prescribed dose. Sonke et al. advocate using only small margins that provide sufficient dosimetric coverage, coupled with quantitative daily position verification to align the radiation treatment to the tumor's mid-position to be certain that the treatment is delivered as planned daily [47]. Such an approach would not require margins as large as the ITV approach since the time spent by the tumors at the extreme spatial positions in the ITV is relatively small and the beam penumbra extends beyond the field edges. The limitations of the mid-ventilation method include difficulties managing tumor motion patterns with large hysteresis and irregular breathing patterns. In addition, since the mid-ventilation approach typically involves planning using breathing phases where tissue motion velocity is large, planning images are susceptible to motion artifacts.

3.3.2 Breath-hold

3.3.2.1 VOLUNTARY

Controlling tumor motion can potentially remove the motion uncertainty, which was observed to be larger than setup uncertainties [48]. Moreover, lung tissues are susceptible to late radiation response, such as pneumonitis and fibrosis [49], and these effects are related to the irradiated lung volume [50,51]. In [52–54], the authors at Memorial Sloan Kettering Cancer Center (MSKCC) presented a deep inhalation breath-hold (DIBH) technique where the patients were coached into deep inspiration and breath-holding, with the lung inflation level monitored by spirometer and the diaphragm position recorded by fluoroscopy. The DIBH technique was motivated by the benefits of decreased lung density and the potential for treatment margin reduction, both of which facilitated target dose escalation and normal tissue sparing. In the five patients of this study, the range of comfortable breath-hold duration was reported to be 12–16 s. The average centroid position of the GTV was found to be 0.2 ± 1.4 mm for diaphragm displacements of −1.0 ± 4.0 mm from CT scans. Barnes et al. [55] showed a significant reduction in the percent lung volume receiving ≥20 Gy at DIBH compared to free breathing condition. Disadvantages to the DIBH technique included patient noncompliance with the maneuver and poor reproducibility leading to residual tumor movement.

3.3.2.2 ACTIVE BREATHING CONTROL

Active breathing control (ABC) was designed to facilitate the reproducibility of breath-hold. It is an approach that was first described by Wong et al. in 1999 [56] and later marketed as the Active Breathing Coordinator (Elekta, Stockholm, Sweden). The ABC system can manage a patient's breathing to a specified lung volume through an apparatus consisting of scissor valves, a flow monitor, and multimedia glasses for flow-time curve visualization. A ventilator apparatus is used to block the patient's airflow at a predetermined lung volume threshold, thereby initiating a breath-hold to immobilize the lung and tumor position [56–60]. A nose clip is generally used to prevent nasal breathing. Verbal instructions to the patients are usually very helpful to maintain a steady breathing pattern. In an ABC procedure, the patient breathes normally through the apparatus. The operator determines the specific tidal volume and the breathing phase and activates the system, at which point the balloon valve closes. The ABC apparatus can suspend breathing at any pre-determined amplitude and is often used at moderate to deep inhalation levels. The breath-hold duration varies from patient to patient, typically 15–30 s and is well tolerated by the patients to allow for breath-hold repetition.

Breath-hold can also be performed by the patient voluntarily holding breath, and this can be done with or without external breathing monitoring. In self-held breath-hold, the patient voluntarily holds his/her breath at a point in the breathing cycle and simultaneously presses a hand-held switch to clear the therapy machine interlock, allowing for the radiation beam to be delivered. The interlock can be re-established when the switch is released. This technique has been implemented by Varian C-Series accelerator, which uses the Customer Minor (CMNR) Interlock system.

A study found that ~60% of lung cancer patients at one institution were not able to perform breath-holds reproducibly enough to be treated with ABC [4], often due to compromised lung function and other toxicities such as chemotherapy. To improve patient compliance, Kashani et al. found good tumor short- and long-term stability under moderate deep inspiration (i.e., 75–80% of vital capacity) [58]. Glide-Hurst et al. also improved patient compliance by instituting short (10–12 s) breath-holds to reduce fatigue at ~80% of the normal tidal volume on inhalation [60]. Similarly, Murphy et al. designed breath-hold levels to follow normal patient respiration [61].

Another device that facilitates DIBH is SpiroDynX (SDX, Dyn'R, Toulouse, France). SDX uses a spirometer to monitor patient breathing and displays the waveform for patients to view and voluntarily hold their breath. In a large, multi-institutional clinical trial of ~400 lung cancer patients, total lung volume was found significantly greater on acquisitions using a DIBH system (ABC and SDX) than those obtained using an inspiration-synchronized system (i.e., Varian's Real-Time Position Management system) [62]. While DIBH leads to more favorable lung geometry and thus reduces the total volume of lung receiving certain tolerance values, patient compliance and ability to complete treatment under these conditions is an important consideration. Nevertheless, only 21 patients out of ~400 were not able to use breath-hold systems (either ABC or SDX) for their treatment due to poor performance status, poor comprehension of breath-hold, or functional capacity [62].

3.3.3 Abdominal compression

The use of abdominal compression reduces tumor excursion by forcing conditions of shallow breathing via limited diaphragmatic excursion [4]. Abdominal compression plates (ACPs) can be placed between the costal margin of the ribs and inferior to the xiphoid process and have been shown to reduce average lung tumor movement 5–6 mm depending on the amount of compression applied [63,64]. ACPs can be indexed for reproducibility (i.e., to regulate the amount of pressure) and are often used when lung tumor motion exceeds a certain threshold [65] (e.g., 10 mm [64,66] or 15 mm of excursion [67]). Pneumatic compression belts with inflatable bags placed in between the patient and the belt can also be used [68]. These belts can be indexed for more accurate repositioning and a hand pump is used to inflate the bag to a known amount of pressure. A vacuum bag restriction system coupled with a vacuum pump that removes the air in between the patient, a vacuum cushion, and a plastic cover sheet can also be used to apply uniform pressure [69]. In a direct comparison of ACP and the vacuum bag restriction system for 16 lung cancer patients, both approaches reduced lung tumor motion although ACP reduced the superior-inferior and overall tumor motion more than the vacuum bag restriction system [69].

3.3.4 Respiratory gating

Respiratory gated radiation delivery aims at target motion reduction during irradiation. A radiation beam gating methodology was first presented by Ohara et al. [70], where the signal from an implanted gold marker was used to control the linear accelerator in real-time. Later, at the University of California, Davis, signals from a video camera were used to switch the radiation beam on and off [26,71]. The respiratory gating device has since been made commercially available as the real-time position management respiratory gating system (RPM), for which clinical studies can be found in [33,72]. Compared to breath-hold techniques, respiratory gated treatments require reduced patient compliance.

When considering employing a respiratory gated treatment, the gating window is typically determined based on 4D-CT and patient's breathing signal. It is selected to be near the full exhalation phase, which reflects the most reproducible portion of the breathing cycle. The internal margin is determined using the target displacement within the gating window (e.g., 50% phase ± 10%). Gating can be performed using a specific amplitude level of the breathing signal and a pre-defined gating window. It was found that tumor motion correlated well with the external fiducial markers in the thorax and abdomen [73,74]. Despite generally good external-to-internal correlation, large residual tumor motion can occur relative to the measured surrogate signal [73,74]. In addition, in gating for an irregular breathing patient, phase gating is susceptible to larger residual error due to significant cycle-to-cycle variability or slow drift in target position or breathing signals. To improve treatment efficiency, more robust gating techniques have been proposed, including a hybrid gating method involving high-frequency external surrogate sampling and intermittent internal marker update [75], and marker-less template matching techniques using fluoroscopic imaging [76–79]. In addition, irregular breathing patterns compromise gated treatment accuracy, as was found by Cai et al. [80] in a simulation study comparing phase-binned 4D-CT and dynamic MRI. The problems in gated radiation therapy led to the development of treatment delivery systems that integrate real-time imaging devices.

3.3.5 Tumor tracking

The next level of target motion compensation can be performed by synchronizing the radiation beam to the motion of the target. Such techniques afford the benefit of margin reduction like beam gating methods, but with continuous irradiation, they can do so without prolonging treatment times. Beam tracking was first proposed by Keall et al. for motion adaptive photon therapy [81]. As a commercial solution, a dynamic tracking technique has been implemented in CyberKnife® Synchrony® [82], where the correlation between the LED markers placed on the patient chest wall and internal tumor position (based on the position of implanted markers) were used to construct a correspondence model. During the therapy session, the LED markers monitored the patient breathing, and the signal was fed into the correspondence model for predicting the tumor position. The tumor position prediction is verified from time to time using x-ray imaging. The Synchrony technology can either update or completely reconstruct the correspondence model.

3.3.6 Respiratory surrogate

Respiratory gated treatment and tumor tracking treatment can account for tumor motion under normal breathing conditions during treatment and have dosimetric advantages by reducing lung toxicity. They use an external respiration signal, internal land markers, or fiducial markers as surrogates to infer tumor motion.

3.3.6.1 EXTERNAL SURROGATE

The most widely implemented external respiration gating system is the Real-Time Position Management (RPM) system (Varian Medical Systems, Palo Alto, CA). The system tracks a reflective marker placed on the patient's abdomen using an infrared tracking camera to record the patient's respiratory cycle. Radiation beams are activated when the maker moves to the gated threshold preset on the gating system monitor [83,84] using either amplitude or phase sorting. The phase position in the phase sorting could be affected by inhale and exhale slopes, and breathing amplitude, etc. Whereas amplitude sorting is relatively more reliable, it is also susceptible to irregularities in amplitude [21,85]. End of exhalation (EOE) is usually selected as the gating window since it is more reproducible. End of inhalation (EOI) might be beneficial for gating treatment since the expanded lungs can limit dose to the normal lung. Proper breath-coaching is needed for EOI to achieve the same residual motion as EOE [86]. The gate width should be chosen to achieve a balance between treatment efficiency and residual tumor motion. The duty cycle, defined as the ratio of beam on time to the total treatment time, should be less than 30% for gated IMRT and 30%–50% for Three-Dimensional Conformal Radiotherapy (3D-CRT).

3.3.6.2 INTERNAL SURROGATE

The accuracy of predicting the internal tumor position using external surrogates is limited since the correlation can vary in time [87,88]. Tumor motion can be directly measured using implanted fiducial markers. Fiducials can be implanted in or near the lung tumor for gated radiation delivery. Gold seeds are commonly used for lung tumor tracking due to their good contrast and small size (0.8 mm in diameter and 4 mm in length). For example, in Shirato [89], a radio-opaque seed was surgically implanted in or near the tumor, and the seed positions were tracked using fluoroscopy throughout the treatment session. Tumor tracking was performed using pattern recognition software that ran in real-time. The shortcomings of such an approach included the migration or loss of the implanted marker and the risks of the patient developing pneumothorax during implantation. Several groups have been developing marker-less tracking techniques based on image analysis of the features in x-ray images so that marker implementation can be avoided [90–95].

An alternative form of target tracking had been developed using electromagnetic tracking systems. This approach has been investigated by several researchers [96–98]. As a commercial system, the Calypso® system uses an implanted Beacon transponder, a radiofrequency antenna array, and three infrared cameras for position monitoring. The advantage of the Calypso system is that it provides continuous imaging of the mobile tumor without ionizing radiation. It monitors tumor position at great accuracy and high temporal resolution, but this technique only provides the position of a single point per beacon and does not consider organ deformation. In addition, the beacons are relatively large (diameter ~2 mm and length 8.5 mm) and are not suitable for implantation in all tumors.

3.4 IMMOBILIZATION

Immobilization devices are an important factor to be considered in the treatment process. Sio et al. investigated the impact of pulmonary function, body habitus, and immobilization on the setup and reproducibility for upper lung tumors and confirmed that the immobilization device could significantly impact couch shift errors [99]. Alpha-cradles and evacuated cushions do not themselves assist in breathing motion mitigation. Abdominal compression was shown to effectively reduce the respiratory tumor movement from a range of 8–20 mm to a range of 2–11 mm [64]. However, it is mainly effective for tumors close to the diaphragm. The benefit in upper or middle lobe tumors is very limited [100]. The BodyFIX (SBF, Elekta AB, Stockholm, Sweden) was also shown to effectively reduce tumor movement during free breathing conditions [69,101]. However, it was prone to setup errors compared to 9-point thermoplastic frames for immobilization of the upper thoracic region [99]. A variety of devices are available to immobilize lung cancer patients for simulation and treatment. The decision of which system to use should be made based on the intensity of respiration motion control, patient comfort, and tumor location. For patient setup, plastic or solid sponge headrests can be used to support the patient's head. Patients should be set up with arms above the head if possible, to allow for better beam placement. When forming evacuated cushions or alpha cradles, it is important to ensure good arm support and obtain good arm/shoulder and feet impressions for reproducibility.

3.5 SUMMARY

Respiratory motion imaging and management is challenging in IGRT of lung cancer due to its magnitude and breathing irregularity. Tools such as 4D-CT are improving our ability to image respiratory motion more accurately than before and subsequently improve the quality of respiratory motion management. Understanding the pros and cons of different 4D-CT imaging techniques and motion management strategies are crucial for successful implementation of IGRT for lung cancer. Future improvements in 4D imaging and treatment will enable more clinics to employ accurate breathing motion management strategies.

REFERENCES

1. Yamamoto, T. et al., Retrospective analysis of artifacts in four-dimensional CT images of 50 abdominal and thoracic radiotherapy patients. *Int J Radiat Oncol Biol Phys*, 2008. **72**(4): 1250–8.
2. Bortfeld, T., S.B. Jiang, and E. Rietzel, Effects of motion on the total dose distribution. *Semin Radiat Oncol*, 2004. **14**(1): 41–51.
3. Beckham, W.A., P.J. Keall, and J.V. Siebers, A fluence-convolution method to calculate radiation therapy dose distributions that incorporate random set-up error. *Phys Med Biol*, 2002. **47**(19): 3465–73.
4. Keall, P.J. et al., The management of respiratory motion in radiation oncology report of AAPM Task Group 76. *Med Phys*, 2006. **33**(10): 3874–900.
5. Suh, Y. et al., An analysis of thoracic and abdominal tumour motion for stereotactic body radiotherapy patients. *Phys Med Biol*, 2008. **53**(13): 3623–40.
6. Kalender, W.A. et al., Spiral volumetric CT with single-breath-hold technique, continuous transport, and continuous scanner rotation. *Radiology*, 1990. **176**(1): 181–3.
7. Conway, J. and M.H. Robinson, CT virtual simulation. *Br J Radiol*, 1997. **70 Spec No:** S106–18.
8. Flohr, T.G. et al., First performance evaluation of a dual-source CT (DSCT) system. *Eur Radiol*, 2006. **16**(2): 256–68.
9. Klingebiel, R. et al., 4-D Imaging in cerebrovascular disorders by using 320-slice CT: Feasibility and preliminary clinical experience. *Acad Radiol*, 2009. **16**(2): 123–9.
10. PMBVedam, S.S. et al., Acquiring a four-dimensional computed tomography dataset using an external respiratory signal. *Phys Med Biol*, 2003. **48**(1): 45–62.
11. Dewey, M. et al., Three-vessel coronary artery disease examined with 320-slice computed tomography coronary angiography. *Eur Heart J*, 2008. **29**(13): 1669.
12. Siebert, E. et al., 320-slice CT neuroimaging: Initial clinical experience and image quality evaluation. *Br J Radiol*, 2009. **82**(979): 561–70.
13. Coolens, C. et al., Dynamic volume vs respiratory correlated 4DCT for motion assessment in radiation therapy simulation. *Med Phys*, 2012. **39**(5): 2669–81.
14. Ford, E.C. et al., Respiration-correlated spiral CT: A method of measuring respiratory-induced anatomic motion for radiation treatment planning. *Med Phys*, 2003. **30**(1): 88–97.
15. Pan, T. et al., 4D-CT imaging of a volume influenced by respiratory motion on multi-slice CT. *Med Phys*, 2004. **31**(2): 333–40.
16. Keall, P.J. et al., Acquiring 4D thoracic CT scans using a multislice helical method. *Phys Med Biol*, 2004. **49**(10): 2053–67.
17. Low, D.A. et al., A method for the reconstruction of four-dimensional synchronized CT scans acquired during free breathing. *Med Phys*, 2003. **30**(6): 1254–63.

18. Cai, J. et al., Four-dimensional magnetic resonance imaging (4D-MRI) using image-based respiratory surrogate: A feasibility study. *Med Phys*, 2011. **38**(12): 6384–94.
19. Li, R.J. et al., 4D CT sorting based on patient internal anatomy. *Phys Med Biol*, 2009. **54**(15): 4821–33.
20. Sonke, J.J. et al., Respiratory correlated cone beam CT. *Med Phys*, 2005. **32**(4): 1176–86.
21. Lu, W. et al., A comparison between amplitude sorting and phase-angle sorting using external respiratory measurement for 4D CT. *Med Phys*, 2006. **33**(8): 2964–74.
22. Pan, T., Comparison of helical and cine acquisitions for 4D-CT imaging with multislice CT. *Med Phys*, 2005. **32**(2): 627–34.
23. Rietzel, E. and G.T.Y. Chen, Improving retrospective sorting of 4D computed tomography data. *Med Phys*, 2006. **33**(2): 377–9.
24. Rietzel, E., T.S. Pan, and G.T.Y. Chen, Four-dimensional computed tomography: Image formation and clinical protocol. *Med Phys*, 2005. **32**(4): 874–89.
25. Parker, D.L., Optimal short scan convolution reconstruction for fanbeam CT. *Med Phys*, 1982. **9**(2): 254–7.
26. Kubo, H.D. and B.C. Hill, Respiration gated radiotherapy treatment: A technical study. *Phys Med Biol*, 1996. **41**(1): 83–91.
27. Quick Steps for Retrospective Spiral Respiratory Correlated Imaging with Varian RPM for the Brilliance CT Big Bore v2.2.2 system and the Brilliance 16–64 v2.2.5, 2007.
28. Somatom Sensation Open Reference Manual. pp. 159–177.
29. Hurkmans, C.W. et al., Quality assurance of 4D-CT scan techniques in multicenter phase III trial of surgery versus stereotactic radiotherapy (radiosurgery or surgery for operable early stage (stage 1A) non-small-cell lung cancer [ROSEL] study). *Int J Radiat Oncol Biol Phys*, 2011. **80**(3): 918–27.
30. Klein, E.E. et al., Task Group 142 report: Quality assurance of medical accelerators. *Med Phys*, 2009. **36**(9): 4197–212.
31. Han, D. et al., Characterization and identification of spatial artifacts during 4D-CT imaging. *Med Phys*, 2011. **38**(4): 2074–87.
32. Lu, W. et al., Quantitation of the reconstruction quality of a four-dimensional computed tomography process for lung cancer patients. *Med Phys*, 2005. **32**(4): 890–901.
33. Vedam, S.S. et al., Quantifying the predictability of diaphragm motion during respiration with a noninvasive external marker. *Med Phys*, 2003. **30**(4): 505–13.
34. Mageras, G.S. and E. Yorke, Deep inspiration breath-hold and respiratory gating strategies for reducing organ motion in radiation treatment. *Semin Radiat Oncol*, 2004. **14**(1): 65–75.
35. Remouchamps, V.M. et al., Initial clinical experience with moderate deep-inspiration breath-hold using an active breathing control device in the treatment of patients with left-sided breast cancer using external beam radiation therapy. *Int J Radiat Oncol Biol Phys*, 2003. **56**(3): 704–15.
36. 4. Definition of Volumes. *J ICRU*, 2010. **10**(1): 41–53.
37. Rietzel, E. et al., Maximum-intensity volumes for fast contouring of lung tumors including respiratory motion in 4DCT planning. *Int J Radiat Oncol Biol Phys*, 2008. **71**(4): 1245–52.
38. Rietzel, E. et al., Four-dimensional image-based treatment planning: Target volume segmentation and dose calculation in the presence of respiratory motion. *Int J Radiat Oncol Biol Phys*, 2005. **61**(5): 1535–50.
39. Bradley, J.D. et al., Comparison of helical, maximum intensity projection (MIP), and averaged intensity (AI) 4D CT imaging for stereotactic body radiation therapy (SBRT) planning in lung cancer. *Radiother Oncol*, 2006. **81**(3): 264–8.
40. Underberg, R.W.M. et al., Use of maximum intensity projections (MIP) for target volume generation in 4DCT scans for lung cancer. *Int J Radiat Oncol Biol Phys*, 2005. **63**(1): 253–60.
41. St James, S. et al., Quantifying ITV instabilities arising from 4DCT: A simulation study using patient data. *Phys Med Biol*, 2012. **57**(5): L1–7.
42. Muirhead, R. et al., Use of maximum intensity projections (MIPs) for target outlining in 4DCT radiotherapy planning. *J Thorac Oncol*, 2008. **3**(12): 1433–8.
43. Cai, J. et al., Estimation of error in maximal intensity projection-based internal target volume of lung tumors: A simulation and comparison study using dynamic magnetic resonance imaging. *Int J Radiat Oncol Biol Phys*, 2007. **69**(3): 895–902.

44. Ge, H. et al., Quantification and minimization of uncertainties of internal target volume for stereotactic body radiation therapy of lung cancer. *Int J Radiat Oncol Biol Phys*, 2013. **85**(2): 438–43.
45. Wolthaus, J.W.H. et al., Mid-ventilation CT scan construction from four-dimensional respiration-correlated CT scans for radiotherapy planning of lung cancer patients. *Int J Radiat Oncol Biol Phys*, 2006. **65**(5): 1560–71.
46. Wolthaus, J.W.H. et al., Comparison of different strategies to use four-dimensional computed tomography in treatment planning for lung cancer patients. *Int J Radiat Oncol Biol Phys*, 2008. **70**(4): 1229–38.
47. Sonke, J.J. et al., Frameless stereotactic body radiotherapy for lung cancer using four-dimensional cone beam CT guidance. *Int J Radiat Oncol Biol Phys*, 2009. **74**(2): 567–74.
48. Van de Steene, J. et al., Electronic portal imaging with on-line correction of setup error in thoracic irradiation: Clinical evaluation. *Int J Radiat Oncol Biol Phys*, 1998. **40**(4): 967–76.
49. Coggle, J.E., B.E. Lambert, and S.R. Moores, Radiation effects in the lung. *Environ Health Perspect*, 1986. 70: 261–91.
50. Martel, M.K. et al., Dose-volume histogram and 3-D/CT treatment planning evaluation of patients with radiation pneumonitis. *Int J Radiat Oncol Biol Phys*. **24**: 173–4.
51. Emami, B. et al., Tolerance of normal tissue to therapeutic irradiation. *Int J Radiat Oncol Biol Phys*, 1991. **21**(1): 109–22.
52. Hanley, J. et al., Deep inspiration breath-hold technique for lung tumors: The potential value of target immobilization and reduced lung density in dose escalation. *Int J Radiat Oncol Biol Phys*, 1999. **45**(3): 603–11.
53. Mah, D. et al., Technical aspects of the deep inspiration breath-hold technique in the treatment of thoracic cancer. *Int J Radiat Oncol Biol Phys*, 2000. **48**(4): 1175–85.
54. Rosenzweig, K.E. et al., The deep inspiration breath-hold technique in the treatment of inoperable non-small-cell lung cancer. *Int J Radiat Oncol Biol Phys*, 2000. **48**(1): 81–7.
55. Barnes, E.I.A. et al., Dosimetric evaluation of lung tumor immobilization using breath-hold at deep inspiration. *Int J Radiat Oncol Biol Phys*, 2001. **50**(4): 1091–8.
56. Wong, J.W. et al., The use of active breathing control (ABC) to reduce margin for breathing motion. *Int J Radiat Oncol Biol Phys*, 1999. **44**(4): 911–19.
57. Cheung, P.C. et al., Reproducibility of lung tumor position and reduction of lung mass within the planning target volume using active breathing control (ABC). *Int J Radiat Oncol Biol Phys*, 2003. **57**(5): 1437–42.
58. Koshani, R. et al., Short-term and long-term reproducibility of lung tumor position using active breathing control (ABC). *Int J Radiat Oncol Biol Phys*, 2006. **65**(5): 1553–9.
59. Gagel, B. et al., Active breathing control (ABC): Determination and reduction of breathing-induced organ motion in the chest. *Int J Radiat Oncol Biol Phys*, 2007. **67**(3): 742–19.
60. Glide-Hurst, C.K., E. Gopan, and G.D. Hugo, Anatomic and pathologic variability during radiotherapy for a hybrid active breath-hold gating technique. *Int J Radiat Oncol Biol Phys*, 2010. **77**(3): 910–17.
61. Murphy, M.J. et al., The effectiveness of breath-holding to stabilize lung and pancreas tumors during radiosurgery. *Int J Radiat Oncol Biol Phys*, 2002. **53**(2): 475–82.
62. Giraud, P. et al., Respiratory gating techniques for optimization of lung cancer radiotherapy. *J Thorac Oncol*, 2011. **6**(12): 2058–68.
63. Heinzerling, J.H. et al., Four-dimensional computed tomography scan analysis of tumor and organ motion at varying levels of abdominal compression during stereotactic treatment of lung and liver. *Int J Radiat Oncol Biol Phys*, 2008. **70**(5): 1571–8.
64. Negoro, Y. et al., The effectiveness of an immobilization device in conformal radiotherapy for lung tumor: Reduction of respiratory tumor movement and evaluation of the daily setup accuracy. *Int J Radiat Oncol Biol Phys*, 2001. 50(4): 889–98.
65. Foster, R. et al., Localization accuracy and immobilization effectiveness of a stereotactic body frame for a variety of treatment sites. *Int J Radiat Oncol Biol Phys*, 2013. **87**(5): 911–16.
66. Purdie, T.G. et al., Cone-beam computed tomography for on-line image guidance of lung stereotactic radiotherapy: Localization, verification, and intrafraction tumor position. *Int J Radiat Oncol Biol Phys*, 2007. **68**(1): 243–52.

67. RTOG 1106/ACRIN 6697, Randomized Phase II Trial of Individualized Adaptive Radiotherapy Using During-Treatment FDG-PET/CT and Modern Technology in Locally Advanced Non-Small Cell Lung Cancer (NSCLC). Available at: http://www.rtog.org/ClinicalTrials/, 2012.
68. Uematsu, M. et al., Computed tomography-guided frameless stereotactic radiotherapy for stage I non-small cell lung cancer: A 5-year experience. *Int J Radiat Oncol Biol Phys*, 2001. **51**(3): 666–70.
69. Han, K. et al., A comparison of two immobilization systems for stereotactic body radiation therapy of lung tumors. *Radiother Oncol*, 2010. **95**(1): 103–8.
70. Ohara, K. et al., Irradiation synchronized with respiration gate. *Int J Radiat Oncol Biol Phys*, 1989. **17**(4): 853–7.
71. Kubo, H.D. et al., Breathing-synchronized radiotherapy program at the University of California Davis Cancer Center. *Med Phys*, 2000. **27**(2): 346–53.
72. Wagman, R. et al., Respiratory gating for liver tumors: Use in dose escalation. *Int J Radiat Oncol Biol Phys*, 2003. **55**(3): 659–68.
73. Gierga, D.P. et al., The correlation between internal and external markers for abdominal tumors: Implications for respiratory gating (vol 61, pg 1551, 2005). Int J Radiat Oncol Biol Phys, 2005. **62**(4): 1257.
74. Berbeco, R.I. et al., Residual motion of lung tumours in gated radiotherapy with external respiratory surrogates. *Phys Med Biol*, 2005. **50**(16): 3655–67.
75. Wu, H. et al., Gating based on internal/external signals with dynamic correlation updates. *Phys Med Biol*, 2008. **53**(24): 7137–50.
76. Cui, Y. et al., Robust fluoroscopic respiratory gating for lung cancer radiotherapy without implanted fiducial markers. *Phys Med Biol*, 2007. **52**(3): 741–55.
77. Berbeco, R.I. et al., Towards fluoroscopic respiratory gating for lung tumours without radiopaque markers. *Phys Med Biol*, 2005. **50**(19): 4481–90.
78. Cui, Y. et al., Fluoroscopic gating without implanted fiducial markers for lung cancer radiotherapy based on support vector machines. *Phys Med Biol*, 2008. **53**(16): N315–27.
79. Li, R. et al., A feasibility study of markerless fluoroscopic gating for lung cancer radiotherapy using 4DCT templates. *Phys Med Biol*, 2009. **54**(20): N489–500.
80. Cai, J. et al., Effects of breathing variation on gating window internal target volume in respiratory gated radiation therapy. *Med Phys*, 2010. **37**(8): 3927–34.
81. Keall, P.J. et al., Motion adaptive x-ray therapy: A feasibility study. *Phys Med Biol*, 2001. **46**(1): 1–10.
82. Ozhasoglu, C. et al., Synchrony—CyberKnife respiratory compensation technology. *Med Dosim*, 2008. **33**(2): 117–23.
83. Keall, P., 4-dimensional computed tomography imaging and treatment planning. *Semin Radiat Oncol*, 2004. **14**(1): 81–90.
84. Giraud, P. et al., Respiratory gated radiotherapy: The 4D radiotherapy. *Bull Cancer*, 2005. **92**(1): 83–9.
85. Wink, N., C. Panknin, and T.D. Solberg, Phase versus amplitude sorting of 4D-CT data. *J Appl Clin Med Phys*, 2006. 7(1): 77–85.
86. Berbeco, R.I. et al., Residual motion of lung tumors in end-of-inhale respiratory gated radiotherapy based on external surrogates. *Med Phys*, 2006. **33**(11): 4149–56.
87. Lu, X.Q. et al., Organ deformation and dose coverage in robotic respiratory-tracking radiotherapy. *Int J Radiat Oncol Biol Phys*, 2008. **71**(1): 281–9.
88. Tsunashima, Y. et al., Correlation between the respiratory waveform measured using a respiratory sensor and 3D tumor motion in gated radiotherapy. *Int J Radiat Oncol Biol Phys*, 2004. **60**(3): 951–8.
89. Shirato, H. et al., Four-dimensional treatment planning and fluoroscopic real-time tumor tracking radiotherapy for moving tumor. *Int J Radiat Oncol Biol Phys*, 2000. **48**(2): 435–42.
90. Korreman, S. et al., Comparison of respiratory surrogates for gated lung radiotherapy without internal fiducials. *Acta Oncol*, 2006. **45**(7): 935–42.
91. Li, R. et al., Real-time 3D tumor localization and volumetric image reconstruction using a single X-ray projection image for lung cancer radiotherapy. *Int J Radiat Oncol Biol Phys*, 2010. **78**(3): S23.
92. Lin, T. et al., Fluoroscopic tumor tracking for image-guided lung cancer radiotherapy. *Phys Med Biol*, 2009. **54**(4): 981–92.

93. Richter, A. et al., Feasibility study for markerless tracking of lung tumors in stereotactic body radiotherapy. *Int J Radiat Oncol Biol Phys*, 2010. **78**(2): 618–27.
94. Rottmann, J. et al., A multi-region algorithm for markerless beam's-eye view lung tumor tracking. *Phys Med Biol*, 2010. **55**(18): 5585–98.
95. Xu, Q.Y. et al., Lung tumor tracking in fluoroscopic video based on optical flow. *Med Phys*, 2008. **35**(12): 5351–9.
96. Houdek, P.V. et al., Computer-controlled stereotaxic radiotherapy system. *Int J Radiat Oncol Biol Phys*, 1992. **22**(1): 175–80.
97. Balter, J.M. et al., Accuracy of a wireless localization system for radiotherapy. *Int J Radiat Oncol Biol Phys*, 2005. **61**(3): 933–7.
98. Seiler, P.G. et al., A novel tracking technique for the continuous precise measurement of tumour positions in conformal radiotherapy. *Phys Med Biol*, 2000. **45**(9): N103–10.
99. Sio, T.T. et al., Influence of patient's physiologic factors and immobilization choice with stereotactic body radiotherapy for upper lung tumors. *J Appl Clin Med Phys*, 2014. **15**(5): 4931.
100. Bouilhol, G. et al., Is abdominal compression useful in lung stereotactic body radiation therapy? A 4DCT and dosimetric lobe-dependent study. *Phys Med*, 2013. **29**(4): 333–40.
101. Baba, F. et al., Stereotactic body radiotherapy for stage I lung cancer and small lung metastasis: Evaluation of an immobilization system for suppression of respiratory tumor movement and preliminary results. *Radiat Oncol*, 2009. **4**: 15.

4 Treatment planning

YAN YU, KAMILA NOWAK CHOI, AND VIRGINIA LOCKAMY

4.1 INTRODUCTION

One of the main goals of image-guided radiation therapy (IGRT) is to reduce treatment uncertainties. These uncertainties can arise from inter- and intrafractional motion [1]. Previous to treatment or even during, the imaging provides direct confirmation that the beams are targeting the exact location of the tumor. Any shifts or corrections detected by the imaging can be made to ensure the proper treatment. The other main goal of IGRT is to improve tumor control while limiting dose to normal tissues [2]. Highly conformal, highly modulated, and escalated dosing schemes are being used more routinely. If slight errors are not detected prior to the execution of treatment, there is a possibility of under- or overdosing not only the intended area but critical structures as well. IGRT provides the ability to ensure that the tumor is being properly targeted while limiting toxicities to normal structures.

4.2 CONTOURING/DELINEATION OF TARGET VOLUMES AND CRITICAL STRUCTURES

4.2.1 Target volumes

Computed tomography (CT) continues to be the main diagnostic tool for detecting lung cancer. The first step in treatment planning following acquisition of appropriate planning images is target volume delineation. The standard of care in radiation oncology is to use CT to delineate the tumor volumes and critical structures [3]. CT imaging can distinguish the difference between non-uniform densities, such as bone and lung. It also provides the CT-to-ED data to use heterogeneity corrections. It is easy to define the sensitive structures (spinal cord, heart, lungs, etc.) on CT images. However, it can be difficult to delineate the extent of the gross disease, potential microscopic extent such as metastatic regional lymph nodes (mediastinal, hilar), and potential setup errors.

The overall quality of a conventional CT scan depends on the amount of motion—whether it is from breathing, peristalsis, or other internal motion. Images can appear blurred or distorted based on the amount of motion during a scan. This could result in a tumor volume that is of limited use [4]. Applying a simple uniform expansion for the planning target volume (PTV) would lead to excessive irradiation of normal tissue and treatment related complications. To best characterize the tumor motion, it is recommended to perform four-dimensional computed tomography (4D-CT). Studies have shown that individualized margins are essential to account for the variation and unpredictable motion of lung tumors [5–8]. The regularity (or irregularity) of the patient's breathing drastically affects the quality of the 4DCT images. If the patient has an irregular breathing pattern, the subsequent images could have artifacts. Abnormally deep or shallow breaths during the scan acquisition can also lead to errors in image reconstruction. The severity of these artifacts varies and could result in tumors or organs appearing split, distorted, or even with incorrect location and volume of the tumors [9–14]. The artifacts are shown in Figure 4.1. The arrows point to examples of where organs appear split, which is attributed to the patient's irregular breathing pattern as indicated by the error bars in each phase of breathing. Motion artifacts

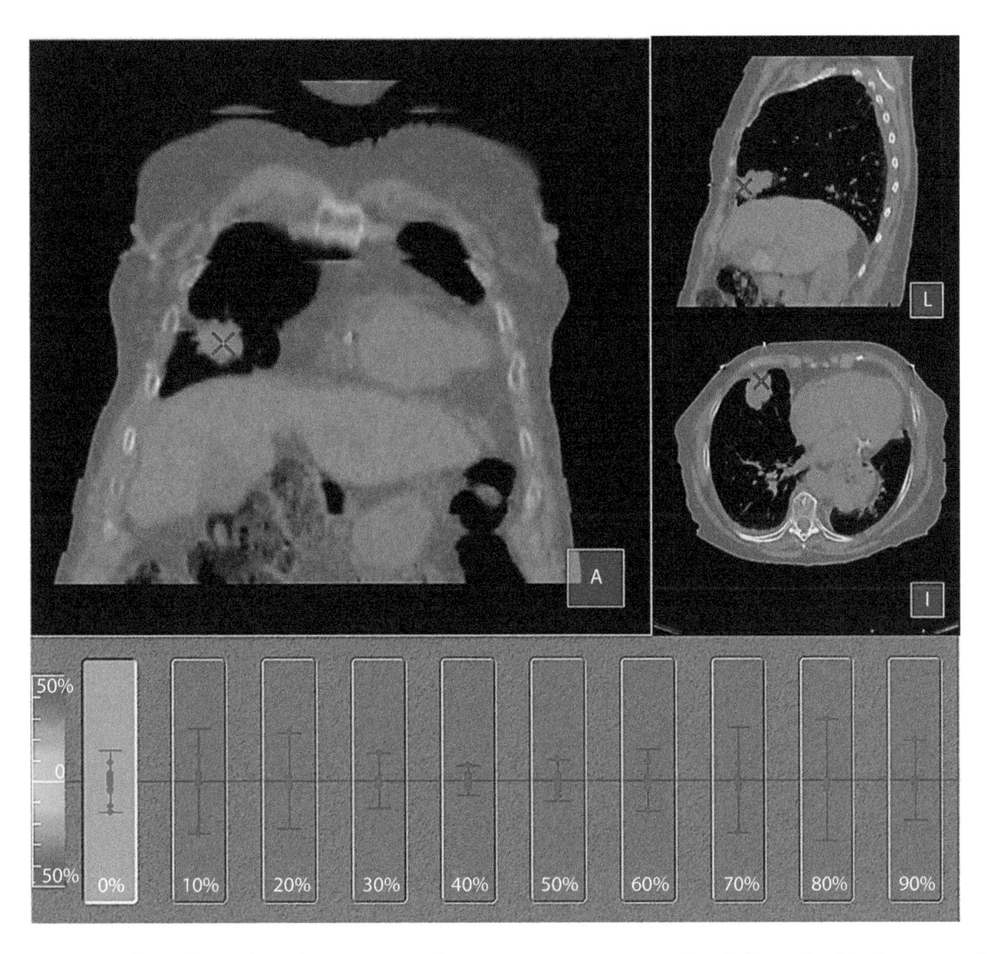

Figure 4.1 Artifacts due to breathing motion. The arrows point to examples of discontinuities in organs due to motion. The error bars indicate that the patient's breathing is irregular and does not follow the predicted breathing pattern.

are typically seen in three-dimensional computed tomography (4D-CT) of the lung and therefore 4DCT should be used to reduce the artifacts due to motion as well as understand the motion of the lung tumor.

To accurately encompass the tumor motion, an internal target volume (ITV) is contoured based on the movement seen on the different phases of the 4DCT, as seen in Figure 4.2. There are two approaches to account for the motion, maximum intensity projection (MIP) and average intensity projection (Ave-IP). The MIP is defined as the maximum value of a pixel over all phases and indicates any location where the tumor is present during any of the phases [15]. The Ave-IP is the average pixel value over all the phases [16]. A comparison is shown in Figure 4.3 of the ITV and PTV contours displayed on both the Ave-IP and MIP scans. This figure also demonstrates the higher pixel display of the tumor for the MIP versus Ave-IP scans. It has been shown that the ITV contoured on the MIP shows excellent agreement with the ITV generated by contouring the tumor on all 10 phases of the 4DCT [15]. Figure 4.4 demonstrates the agreement of the tumor being contoured on all 10 phases as compared to the ITV being generated on just the MIP. There are a few limitations to using the MIP for contouring. One possible limitation is if the 4DCT images are distorted due to the patient's erratic breathing. This could affect the visualization of the tumor and lead to an incorrect volume. Another limitation is if the tumor and/or nodal volumes are located near a major bronchial structure, the diaphragm, or if the tumor is surrounded by atelectasis, it may be hard to distinguish the borders of the gross tumor volume (GTV).

Most contouring software automatically propagates the tumor volume to all 10 phases once it is drawn on the initial phase, which saves clinicians time when contouring on all phases. Only one set of contours needs

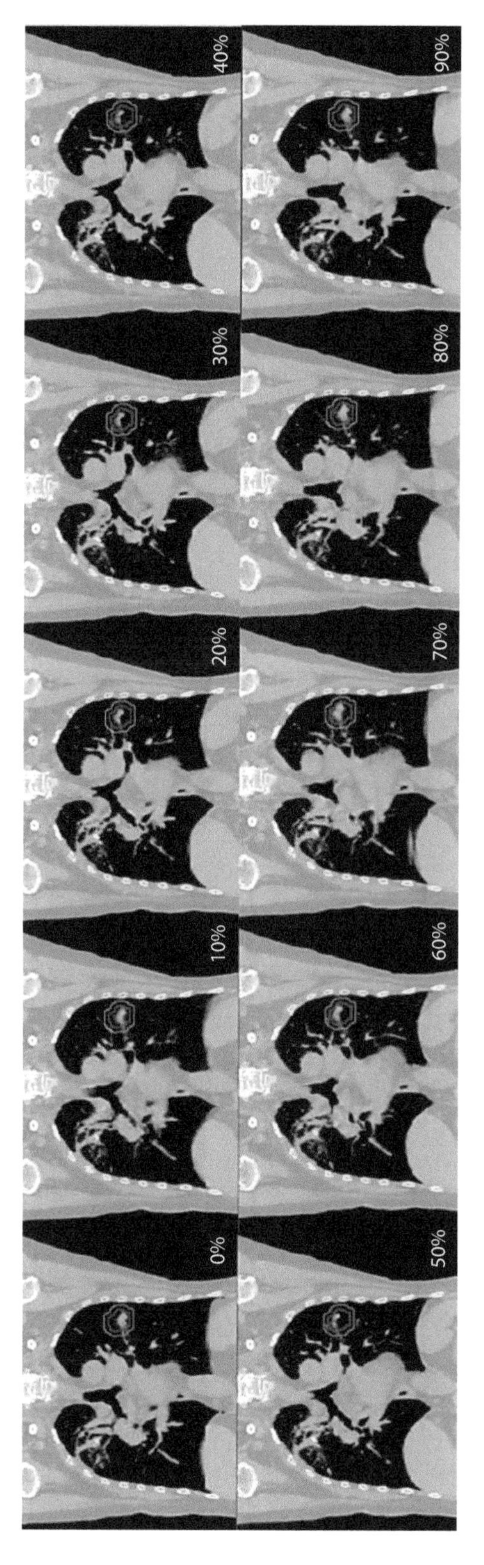

Figure 4.2 The internal target volume (ITV) (magenta line) and PTV contours are displayed on all 10 phases. The extent of the tumor motion stays within the ITV on each of the phases.

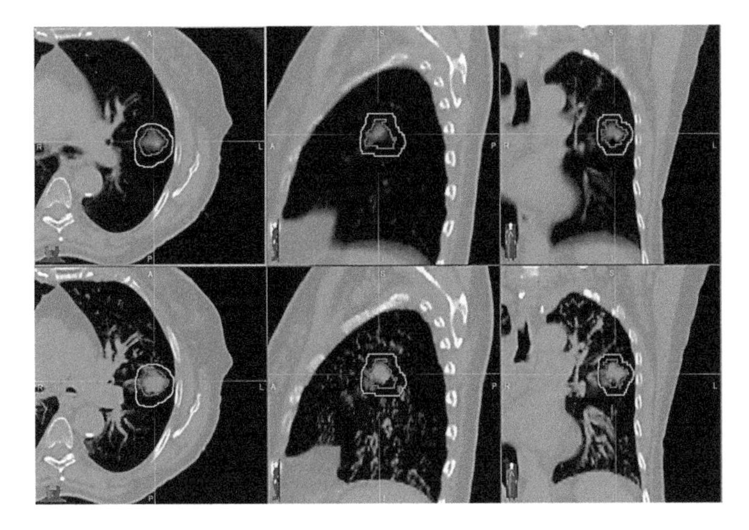

Figure 4.3 ITV and PTV contours displayed on the (a) Ave-IP (top row) and (b) MIP scans (bottom row).

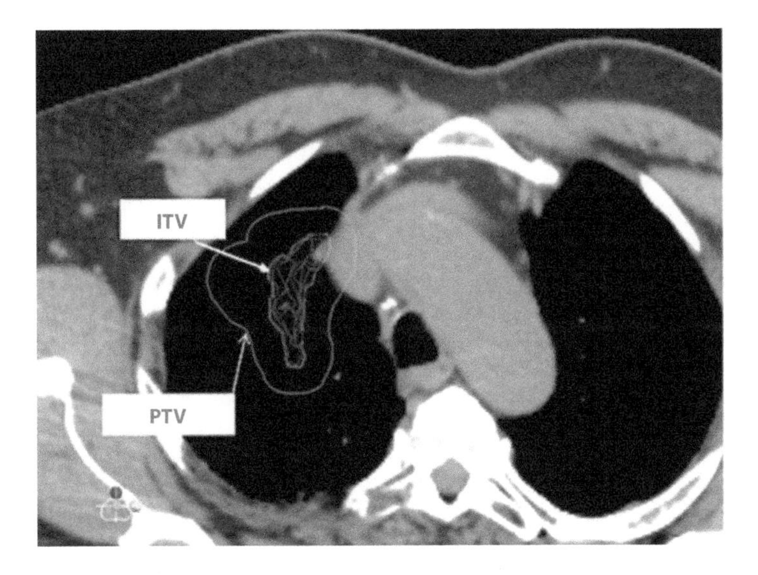

Figure 4.4 The red lines indicate the tumor hand contoured on all 10 phases of the 4DCT. The green line represents the ITV, which was contoured on the MIP. This shows excellent agreements between the overall tumor volume contoured on the 10 phases and the ITV contoured on the MIP.

to be drawn on either the MIP or the Ave-IP. A study by Bradley et al. showed that the tumor volumes contoured on the MIP were slightly larger than ones contoured on either the helical CT scan or the Ave-IP [16]. The difference in tumor volume between the MIP and Ave-IP is demonstrated in Figure 4.5. For planning purposes, the Ave-IP provides actual CT numbers and can be used for dose calculation [17,18]. Regardless of where the contours are generated, the image sets can be fused and the contours can be transferred to the Ave-IP for planning purposes.

While target volume delineation itself is done on the planning scan, it requires the integration of a variety of clinical information, including diagnostic imaging as well as pathological information. In the case of lung cancer, this pathological information is often obtained from invasive procedures such as mediastrinoscopy or endobronchial ultrasound (EBUS), which are necessary for accurate nodal staging.

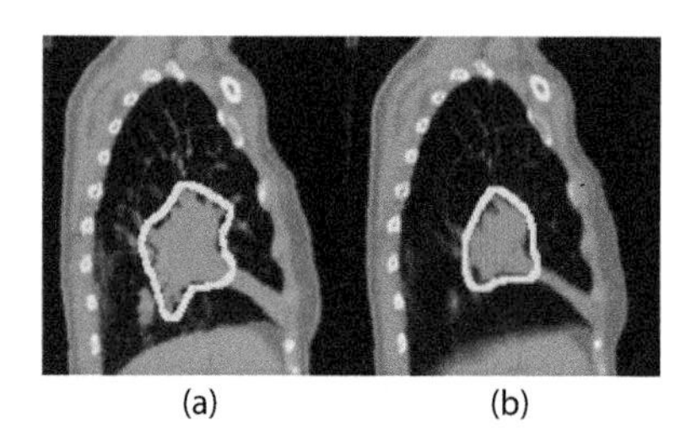

Figure 4.5 Tumor contour based on (a) MIP and (b) Ave-IP. The contour on the Ave-IP slightly underestimates the extent of the tumor as seen on the MIP.

The amount of technology available has drastically increased over the years to help clinicians determine the extent of the disease versus normal tissues. While CT is always necessary for treatment planning, positron emission tomography (PET) and magnetic resonance imaging (MRI) are two of the techniques used to help distinguish the tumor and nodal volumes from normal tissues. All three modalities complement one another and provide anatomical localization when delineating normal and cancerous tissues.

^{18}F-fluorodeoxyglucose (^{18}F-FDG) is the most common tracer used in PET scanning. PET images are based on metabolic activity, not anatomy. PET is commonly used to distinguish suspicious lesions, more accurately define tumor volume and lymph node involvement, detect distant metastases, and aid in treatment planning [19–25]. Both CT and PET are part of the standard workup for all newly diagnosed cases of lung cancer (NCCN). While PET is considered a more accurate imaging modality in clinical staging of lung cancer, a combined PET/CT approach leads to an increased accuracy in the staging of lung cancer [26–28]. By using integrated PET/CT scanners, one can obtain information on abnormal uptake and anatomy since they share DICOM coordinates, as seen in Figure 4.6. In a study performed by Ciernik et al. using an integrated PET/CT scanner, 56% of the cases had significantly altered GTV contours based on the PET images [29]. In another 2003 study published in the *New England Journal of Medicine*, for two years of patients from a tertiary teaching institution in Switzerland diagnosed with NSCLC underwent integrated whole body PET-CT as part of their staging. The PET-CT provided additional information in 41% of patients, leading to improved staging accuracy [30]. However, when PET scans are performed separately from CT scans, image fusion becomes more challenging since the PET images are based on metabolic activity instead of anatomy.

In addition to being a powerful diagnostic tool, PET-CT also has a positive impact on radiation treatment planning. It is used for accurate identification of mediastinal involvement for target delineation in selective nodal radiation. In a 2005 prospective phase I/II study from The Netherlands, patients with non-metastatic NSCLC were treated with RT to the primary tumor and positive lymph nodes as defined by CT and FDG-PET. At a median follow-up time of 16 months, there was a 2% rate of isolated nodal recurrence [31]. The additional information provided by PET can be useful in delineating target volumes in patients with atelectasis secondary to tumor obstruction. In a 2004 study from Washington University School of Medicine, patients underwent sequential CT and FDG-PET simulation. Subsequently, separate contours were drawn for each patient on PET-CT planning scan and CT planning scan. In 58% of the patients, the PET images significantly altered the areas to be treated. In addition to detection of unknown nodal disease, information obtained from PET-CT helped distinguish tumor from atelectasis [32]. Overall, the utilization of PET-CT information during radiation treatment planning leads to decreased inter-observer contouring variability [33]. PET-CT may overestimate the lymph node (LN) involvement and, whenever possible, LN involvement should be pathologically confirmed.

It has been shown that the data obtained from PET scans influenced the radiation delivery of 65% of patients receiving definitive radiation therapy [34]. Other studies using PET in conjunction with radiation treatment planning have shown a reduction in the variability of tumor delineation among radiation oncologists and allow automatic tumor delineation that can be manually edited if needed [33,35,36]. PET scans supplement CT scans by being able to discriminate between malignant and benign lesions; identify metastases in normal sized lymph nodes; and exclude enlarged lymph nodes that do not have any uptake [37]. Therefore,

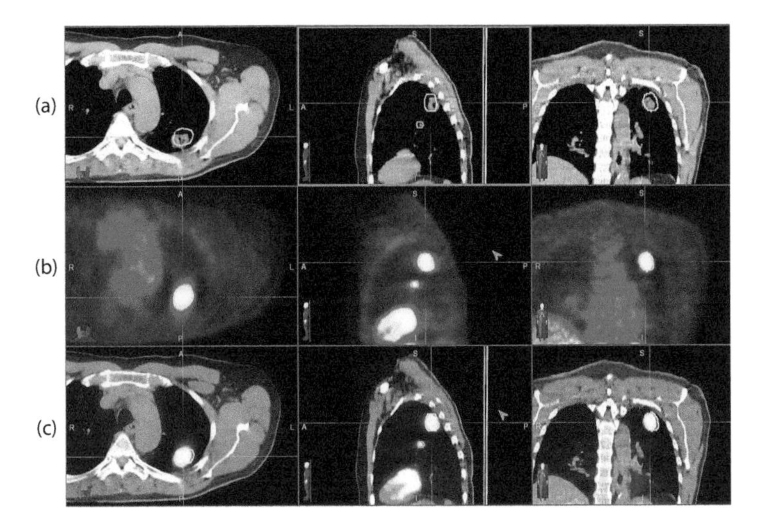

Figure 4.6 Lung tumor as detected by (a) CT and (b) PET using a PET/CT scanner. Since the two sets of images share DICOM coordinates, the images are easily fused, as seen in (c), and the tumor volume contoured (displayed in yellow) on the PET is transposed to the CT images.

PET is a useful imaging modality to supplement the contours of the GTV and clinical tumor volume (CTV) as well as to determine the expansion needed for the PTV.

Magnetic resonance imaging (MRI) is advantageous in comparison to CT as it can provide both structural and physiologic information [19,38]. MRI provides superior soft tissue contrast as compared to other imaging modalities. The treatment planning CT can be fused with the MRI to better delineate the gross tumor volume as well as any lymph nodes detected. Another advantage of MRI is that high-resolution images can be obtained without the use of ionizing radiation. Multiple studies have been performed to study the accuracy of CT and MRI to stage lung cancer [39–44]. While both CT and MRI provide anatomic information, the accuracy for both modalities differs in these studies and there is no clear advantage to using one modality versus the other when it comes to staging the disease. In a study performed by the Radiologic Diagnostic Oncology Group comparing CT and MRI in staging of non-small-cell bronchogenic carcinoma (NSCBC) [45], it was reported that both modalities are equally accurate in tumor classification and detecting mediastinal node metastases but MRI detects mediastinal invasion more accurately. The use of MRI is helpful in determining the extent of invasion into the chest wall, neural foramen, brachial plexus, subclavian vessels or vertebral body from superior sulcus carcinomas [19,46–49] or peripheral carcinomas [45]. Figure 4.7 [50] shows PET/CT and MRI images of a lung tumor in the mediastinum as well as post-obstructive atelectasis. The use of PET and/or MRI versus CT alone helps delineate the soft tissue extension (if any) as well as distinguishing between tumor and atelectasis. Therefore, MRI is a useful tool when determining the GTV (tumor and/or nodes) as well as the extent of tumor invasion into soft tissues.

As described by Kauczor and Kreitner, there are three main issues when considering MRI for lung: (1) signal loss due to physiological motion (cardiac pulsation and respiration); (2) susceptibility artifacts caused by multiple air-tissue interfaces; and (3) low proton density and low signal-to-noise ratio (SNR) [51]. Standard sequences used for MRI are too long as compared to a patient's breathing cycle and cardiac motion. Multiple approaches have been proposed to reduce the first two pitfalls, which include breath-hold and various pulse sequences [52,53]. To reduce the susceptibility artifacts due to the multiple air-tissue interfaces, different paramagnetic contrast agents, such as oxygen enhancement or hyperpolarized noble gases, have been studied [51,54–59]. A study by Ireland et al. demonstrated that the information provided by fusing the hyperpolarized ^{3}He-MRI to treatment planning CT led to the development of treatment plans with significantly lower V_{20} for the total and functional lung, as well as lower mean dose to the functional lung [54]. Work is ongoing to study various hyperpolarized noble gases for functional MRI, which can be of great use when trying to distinguish functional lung.

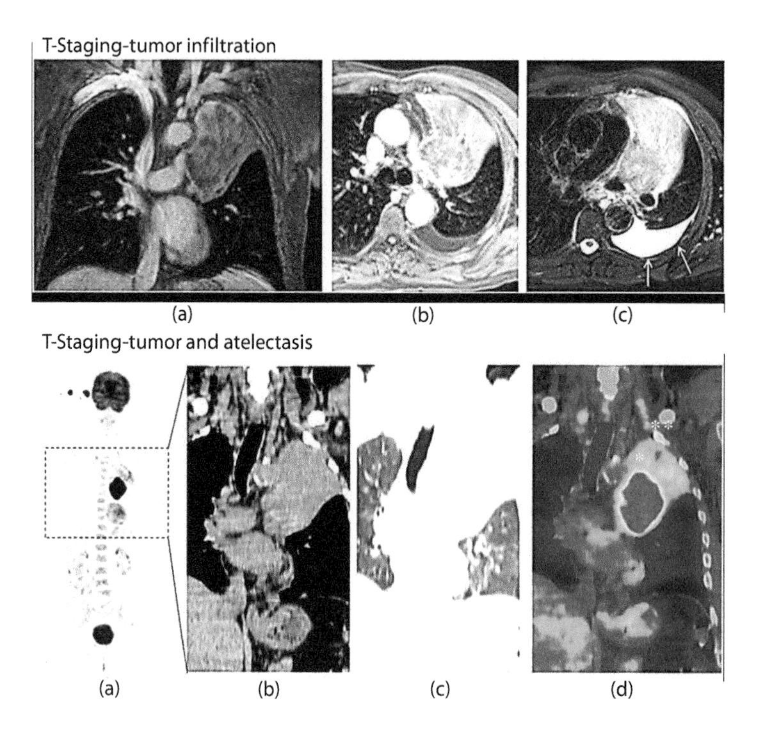

Figure 4.7 Different imaging modalities of primary tumor in the mediastinum. The upper panel of images represents different MRI imaging sequences of the tumor infiltrating the vessels and hilar region. Upper panel: (a) T1 weighted contrast-enhanced MRI; (b) T1 weighted arterial-phase MRI of the lung; (c) T2 weighted MRI. The arrows point to an area of pleural effusion. The lower panel of images represents CT and PET/CT images of the same patient. Lower panel: (a) Maximum intensity projection of PET; (b) CT scan using soft tissue window; (c) CT scan using lung window; (d) Fusion of PET/CT. The (*) represents the primary tumor based on the high-level FDG uptake while (**) indicates region of postobstructuve atelectasis based on lower FDG uptake. (Reprinted from Semin Nucl Med, 45, Flechsig, P. et al., PET/MRI and PET/CT in lung lesions and thoracic malignancies, 268–281. Copyright (2015), with permission from Elsevier.)

4.2.1.1 GROSS TUMOR VOLUME (GTV)

The gross tumor volume (GTV) represents the visible extent of the malignant tumor. In the case of lung cancer, it is constituted by the primary lesions and clinically involved lymph nodes as well as any metastatic disease that is included in the treatment plan. If radiotherapy is done in the adjuvant setting and a gross total resection has been achieved, there is no definable GTV as the clinically visible tumor has been removed.

The GTV is to be defined prior to treatment planning. The determination of its extent is done based on previously obtained clinical, radiographic, and pathologic information, including the techniques used in staging as per AJCC guidelines (see previous section).

4.2.1.2 CLINICAL TARGET VOLUME (CTV)

The clinical target volume (CTV) includes the GTV as well as the volume of subclinical disease surrounding the GTV where tumor cells are likely present but cannot be appreciated with currently available technology. Figure 4.8 shows a schematic of the expansion of the GTV to form the CTV. Pathologically involved nodes (with EBUS/mediastinoscopy) that are not suspicious on staging imaging are included in the CTV. Just as with the GTV, the CTV is defined prior to treatment planning.

The different nodal stations of the chest are illustrated in Figure 4.9 [60]. This diagram provides regional lymph node classification and mapping for staging lung cancer. In the setting of definitive treatment, only the primary tumor and involved lymph nodes are included in the CTV, and generally elective nodal irradiation (ENI) is not done, as elective nodal failure (defined as recurrence in an uninvolved lymph node in the absence of local failure) is seen rarely [61] and ENI has not shown to lead to a clinical benefit in NSCLC [62] or SCLC [63].

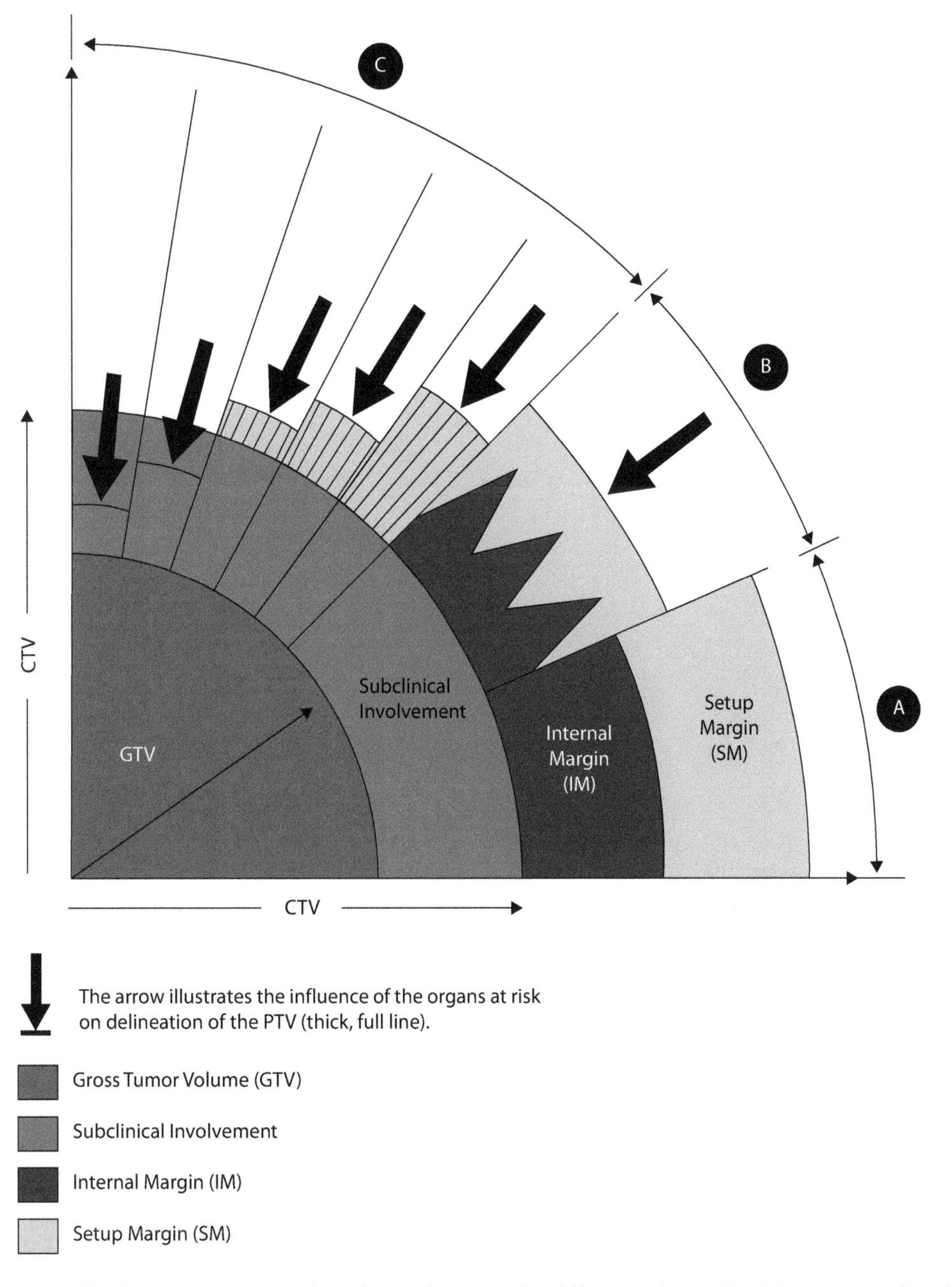

Figure 4.8 This diagram represents the relations between the different volumes (GTV, CTV, PTV, and PRV) in different clinical scenarios. (Reprinted with permission from International Commission on Radiation Units and Measurements: Prescribing, recording, and reporting photon beam therapy (ICRU Report 62), Bethesda, 1993.)

The role of radiation therapy in the post-operative setting for patients with NSCLC remains a controversial topic. Whereas a 1998 meta-analysis examining nine randomized trials of surgery with or without post-operative radiation therapy (PORT) indicated that PORT was detrimental and led to an increased risk of death [64], the study has been subject to many criticisms, among which the use of antiquated radiation techniques and large fraction size, which makes the study not applicable to modern radiation techniques. Subsequently published studies suggest a potential benefit of PORT. A post-hoc analysis from the ANITA trial (which randomized patients with completely resected stage IB-IIIA NSCLC to either observation or cisplatin and vinorelbine) published in 2008 of patients who received PORT showed improved survival for

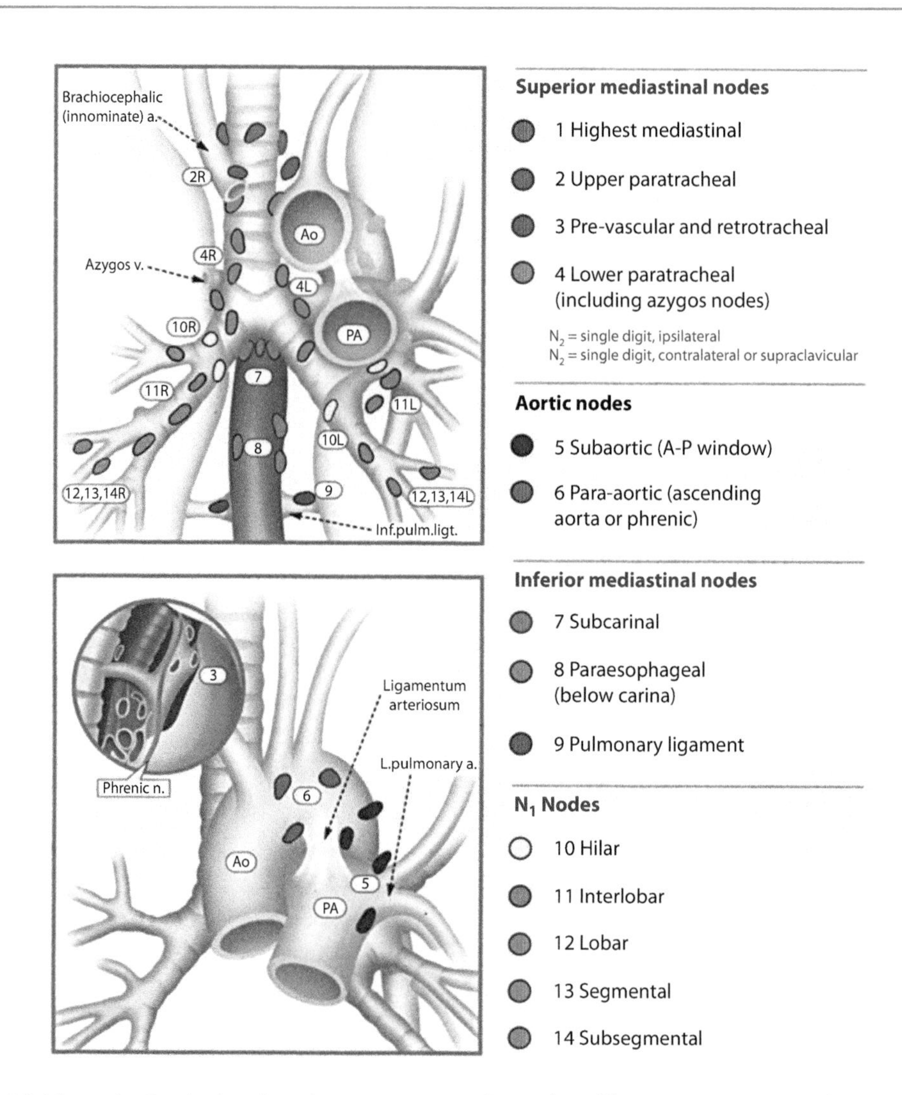

Figure 4.9 Mountain–Dresler lymph node staging system. (Reproduced from Mountain, C.F. and C.M. Dresler, *Chest*, 111, 1718–1723, 1997. With permission.)

patients with N1 disease in the observation arm (MS 50.2 versus 25.9 months with and without PORT). Patients with N1 disease receiving post-operative chemotherapy had worse survival with the addition of PORT (MS 46.6 versus 93.6 with and without PORT). A survival benefit was shown for all patients with N2 disease regardless of whether they received chemotherapy (MS 47.4 versus 23.8 months with and without PORT in the chemotherapy arm and 22.7 versus 12.7 months with and without PORT in the observation arm) [65].

The current NCCN guidelines recommend PORT in the setting of positive margins and N2 disease. PORT CTV includes the bronchial stump and high-risk draining lymph node stations. Typical PORT doses range from 50–54 Gy in 1.8–2 Gy daily fractions. A boost may be added to high risk areas such as positive margins or lymph node levels with ECE [66–68].

The benefit of PORT in the setting of NSCLC remains an open question. The ongoing European LungART trial is a phase III trial randomizing patients with completely resected NSCLC and pathologically proven mediastinal N2 involvement to post-operative conformal RT or no PORT, with a primary endpoint of DFS and secondary endpoints such as OS, LC, and toxicity. Chemotherapy concurrent with RT is not allowed, however patients can receive sequential chemotherapy. The CTV in this trial includes the bronchial stump,

Table 4.1 Lymph node contouring guidelines for PORT based on mediastinal lymph node involvement

Surgically involved mediastinal nodes	LN stations to be included in the CTV
1–2R	1–2R, 4R, 7, 10R Maximal upper limit: 1 cm above sternal notch but homolateral subclavicular node station may be treated if needed Maximal lower limit: 4 cm below the carina[a]
1–2L	1–2L, 4L, 7, 10L Maximal upper limit: 1 cm above the sternal notch but homolateral subclavicular node station may be treated if needed Maximal lower limit: 4 cm below the carina[a]
3 (Right-sided tumor)	3, 4R, 7, 10R Maximal upper limit: 1 cm above the sternal notch Maximal lower limit: 4 cm below the carina[a]
3 (Left-sided tumor)	3, 4L, 7, 10L Maximal upper limit: 1 cm above the sternal notch Maximal lower limit: 4 cm below the carina[a]
4R	2R, 4R, 7, 10R Maximal upper limit: sternal notch Maximal lower limit: 4 cm below the carina[a]
4L	2L, 4L, 7, 10L Maximal upper limit: sternal notch Maximal lower limit: 4 cm below the carina[a]
5	2L, 4L, 5, 6, 7 Maximal upper limit: top of aortic arch Maximal lower limit: 4 cm below the carina[a]
6	2L, 4L, 5, 6, 7 Maximal upper limit: sternal notch Maximal lower limit: 4 cm below the carina[a]
7 (Right-sided tumor)	4R, Maximal upper limit: top of aortic arch Maximal lower limit: 5 cm below the carina[a]
7 (Left-sided tumor)	4L, 5, 6, 7 Maximal upper limit: top of aortic arch Maximal lower limit: 5 cm below the carina[a]
8 (Right-sided tumor)	4R, 7, 8 Maximal upper limit: top of aortic arch The lower limit should be the gastroesophageal junction
8 (Left-sided tumor)	4L, 5, 6, 7 8 Maximal upper limit: top of aortic arch The lower limit should be the gastroesophageal junction

Source: Reprinted from *Int J Radiat Oncol Biol Phys*, 76, Spoelstra, F.O.B. et al., Variations in target volume definition for post-operative radiotherapy in stage III non-small-cell lung cancer: Analysis of an international contouring study, 1106–113. Copyright (2010), with permission from Elsevier.
Abbreviations: LN = lymph node; CTV = Clinical target volume.
[a] Unless other nodes are involved.

the ipsilateral hilar lymph node region and the lymph nodes considered at high risk based on positive lymph nodes (see Table 4.1 [69]).

4.2.1.3 INTERNAL MARGIN (IM)

Intrathoracic tumors are subject to changes in location, secondary to movement of the ribcage and the diaphragm during the respiratory cycle. These must be accounted for to ensure adequate target coverage throughout the respiratory cycle. The internal margin (IM) is added to the CTV to account for projected variations in size, shape, and position relative to the internal reference point as described in ICRU Report 62 [70]. Due to the different magnitude of displacement in different directions, the IM is often an asymmetric margin around the CTV.

4.2.1.4 INTERNAL TARGET VOLUME (ITV)

The internal target volume (ITV) represents the CTV with the addition of the IM to account for movement. In the case of intrathoracic lesions, the movement is most commonly from respiratory motion [70].

4.2.1.5 SETUP MARGIN (SM)

The setup margin (SM) is added to account for uncertainties in day-to-day patient positioning, dosimetric uncertainties, mechanical uncertainties, and beam alignment. These factors may differ across institutions, and within an institution they may vary across treatment machines. Choice of immobilization devices must also be accounted for when choosing the SM [70].

4.2.1.6 PLANNING TARGET VOLUME (PTV)

Unlike the GTV and CTV, which are defined based on clinical information, the planning target volume (PTV) is a geometrical concept and it is dependent on the technique used. The PTV is meant to account for setup uncertainties, day-to-day variation in the size and shape of the tissues surrounding the CTV as well as potential variation in beam geometry characteristics, as seen in Figure 4.8 [71].

4.2.2 Normal structures/organs-at-risk (OARs)

In addition to appropriate delineation of the target volumes, it is also critical to delineate organs at risk (OARs) in the treatment field for tracking dose and avoiding overdose to those structures. The Quantitative Analyses of Normal Tissue Effects in the Clinic (QUANTEC) publications review studies looking at normal tissue tolerances and potential toxicities. Whenever thinking about potential risk to OARs it is also important to consider any concurrent therapies such as systemic treatment or pre-existing conditions that might predispose to development of toxicity.

4.2.2.1 LUNGS

One of the most commonly seen toxicities following thoracic RT is radiation pneumonitis (RP), an inflammatory state of the lung parenchyma that can range in severity from asymptomatic and only seen on imaging to life-threatening or lethal respiratory compromise. The incidence of RP ranges anywhere from 5–50% depending on the reported series. Most clinically symptomatic cases manifest themselves within 10 months from RT. When contouring the lungs for the purposes of treatment planning, the GTV volume should be excluded from the total lung volume. Excluding PTV is discouraged as it leads to underestimation of the apparent lung exposure. Several different V_x values (percent lung volume receiving ≥x Gy) have been associated with risk of RP, indicating that there is not a dose threshold below which pneumonitis is unlikely. Dosimetric parameters that have shown a correlation with risk of pneumonitis include V_{20}, V_5, and mean lung dose (MLD). Recommended QUANTEC lung constraints for conventional fractionation in 2 Gy fractions include limiting V_{20} to ≤30–35%, V_5≤65% and MLD to ≤20–23 Gy, to keep the risk of RP below 20% (Marks et al., 2010). Constraints are inevitably different for SBRT. In SBRT, the utilization of several beams or arcs leads to high conformity and steep dose gradients; however, this also leads to a bigger area of lung exposed to a low dose. Lung SBRT constraints from recent RTOG trials use a lung V_{20} of 10–15% [72,73].

4.2.2.2 SPINAL CORD

Unlike the lungs, which are a structure in parallel, which implies that each functional subunit can work independently of others and that radiation-induced damage in a subunit does not affect function of surrounding subunits not exposed to radiation damage, the spinal cord is a structure in series. As such, its subunits are organized serially, and damage to a subunit may lead to functional damage of adjacent subunits that were not subject to radiation damage. Radiation-induced spinal cord injury or myelopathy is a rare but devastating late toxicity which may result in paralysis, paresthesia, pain, and bowel/bladder incontinence. Radiation myelopathy seldom manifests in the first 6 months following completion of treatment, with most cases occurring within 3 years of treatment completion [74]. Because of its devastating consequences, the goal of spinal cord dose constraints is to keep the risk of myelopathy to <1%. In the setting of conventional fractionation at 2 Gy per fraction, a maximum dose of 50 Gy is associated with a risk of myelitis of 0.2% based on QUANTEC modeling. For lung SBRT, a maximum

point dose of 14 Gy for a single fraction regimen and maximum of 6 Gy per fraction for 3–5 fraction regimens are recommended [75].

4.2.2.3 HEART

Acute heart injury in the form of pericarditis is not common. Late injury can present as coronary artery disease (CAD) and subsequent myocardial infarction, congestive heart failure (CHF), or chronic pericarditis. The latency period varies from months (for pericarditis) to several years following completion of treatment (for CAD). Delineation of cardiac structures itself can be challenging and subject to significant inter-observer variability, secondary to uncertainties in border definition and inclusion of muscle only versus the whole pericardium [76]. Given the variability, an anatomically correct cardiac atlas was developed based on imaging and cadaveric anatomy [77]. (See Figure 4.10).

Heart constraints for conventional fractionation in 2 Gy fractions include a V_{30} of ≤50–55% and V_{45} of ≤35–40% (NRG Oncology, 2015). For SBRT the maximum heart point dose constraint is 22 Gy for single fraction treatment, 30 Gy for 3-fraction regimens (10 Gy/fx), 34 Gy for a 4-fraction regimen (6.8 Gy/fx), and no more than 105% of the PTV prescription for a 5-fraction regimen [66].

4.2.2.4 GREAT VESSELS

When contouring the great vessels, the aorta is contoured for left-sided tumors and the vena cava is contoured for right-sided tumors; it is recommended to contour the great vessels 10 cm above and 10 cm below the extent of the PTV. The pulmonary artery and pulmonary vein are not included in the great vessel contours. It is recommended to use the mediastinal window for contouring the great vessels, as it allows visualization of all the layers of the vessels [73]. Maximum dose constraints for SBRT include 37 Gy for a single fraction, 49 Gy for a 4-fraction regimen, and no more than 105% of PTV prescription for a 5-fraction regimen [66].

4.2.2.5 ESOPHAGUS

Radiation dose to the esophagus is associated with both acute and chronic toxicities. Acutely, esophagitis is commonly experienced by patients undergoing thoracic RT; symptoms generally start during treatment and may persist for a few weeks following completion of treatment. Delayed esophageal injury, such as esophageal stricture, is less commonly reported, and fatal esophageal injury, such as tracheoesophageal (TE) fistula or perforation, is reported in the literature in ≤1% of patients [78]. The esophagus should be delineated on

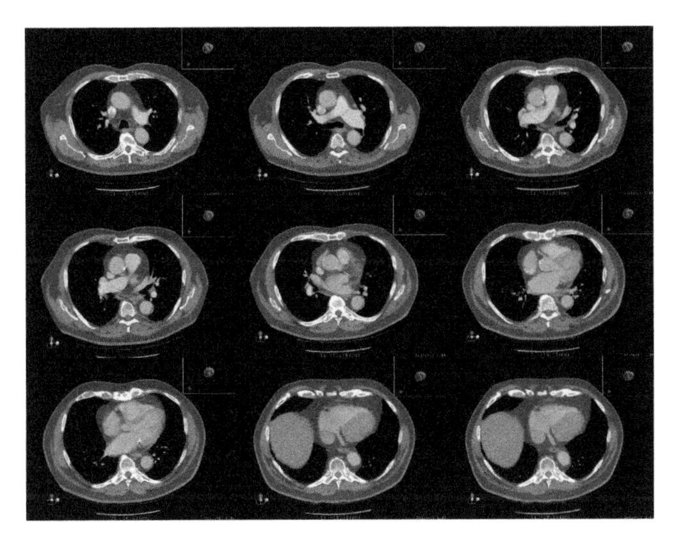

Figure 4.10 Cardiac contouring atlas. Red: pericardium; Green: ventricles; Blue: atria. (Reprinted with permission from Wheatley, M.D. et al. *Int J Radiat Oncol Biol Phys.*, 90, S658, 2014.)

the CT in the mediastinal window, which allows for better identification of all its layers. Several dosimetric parameters reported in the literature appear to correlate with an increased risk of esophagitis; it is therefore challenging to establish which dose constraints are most useful in decreasing risk of esophageal toxicity. The currently ongoing NRG LU001 recommends a V_{35} ≤50–55 Gy, V_{70} ≤20–25 Gy and a mean dose ≤34–37 Gy. For SBRT the NCCN guidelines recommend a maximum dose of 15.4 Gy with a single fraction regimen, 27 Gy (9 Gy/fx) for a 3-fraction regimen, 30 Gy (7.5 Gy/fx) for a 4-fraction regimen, and no more than 105% of PTV prescription for a 5-fraction regimen [79].

4.2.2.6 PROXIMAL BRONCHIAL TREE

The phase II SBRT trial from Indiana showed a higher incidence of grade 3–5 toxicity for patients with central tumors treated with SBRT, defined as within 2 cm of the proximal bronchial tree (see Figure 4.11 [80]). Toxicities included pneumonia, pleural effusion, hemoptysis, and respiratory failure [81]. Central airway

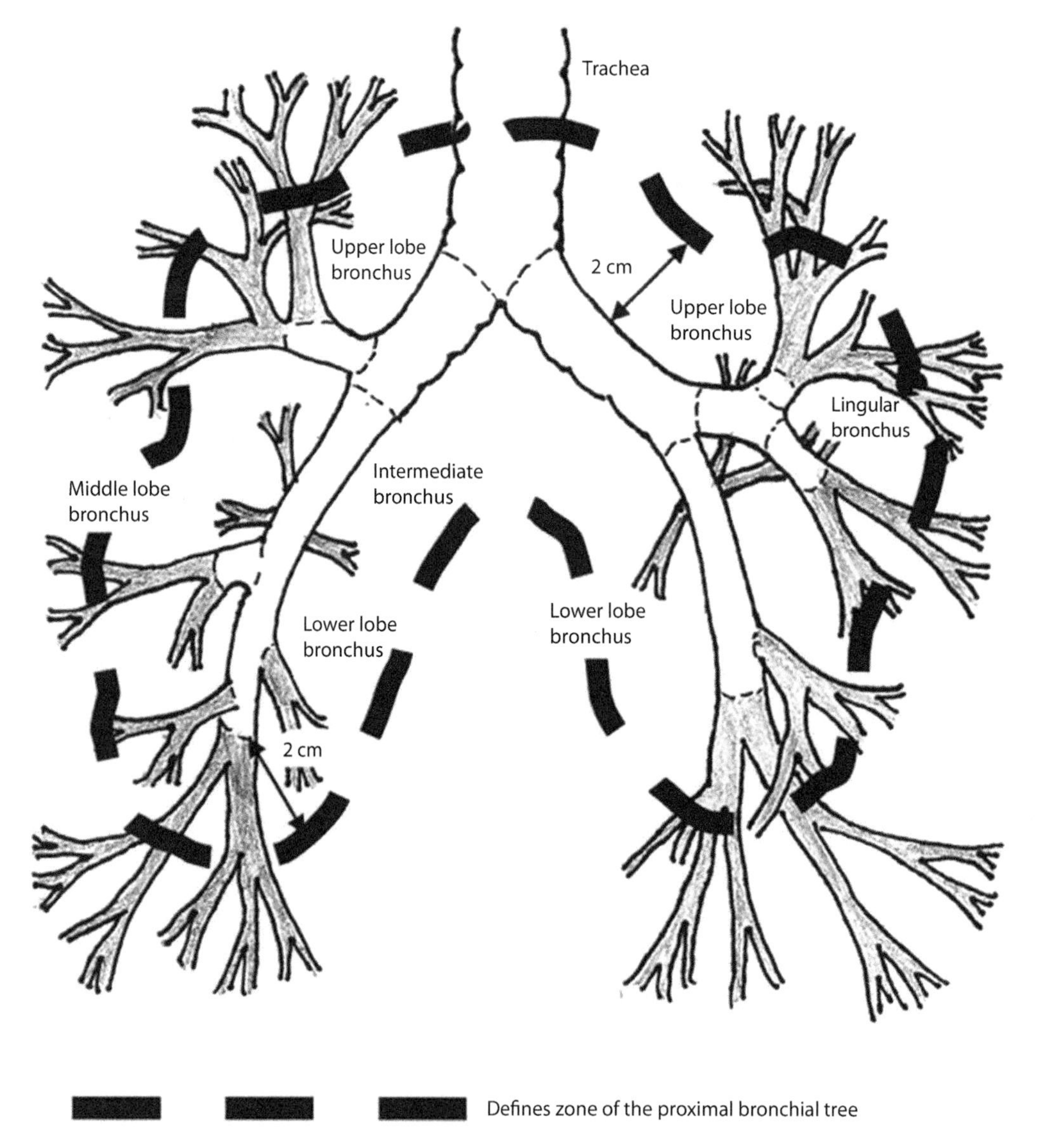

Figure 4.11 Proximal bronchial. (Reprinted with permission from Timmerman, R. et al., *J Clin Oncol.*, 24, 4833–4839, © 2006 by American Society of Clinical Oncology. All rights reserved.)

necrosis was also reported [82]. Patients with central tumors were subsequently excluded from RTOG 0236 and a separate trial, RTOG 0813, was run to address the question of dose in patients with centrally located tumors. The proximal bronchial tree contour includes the last 2 cm of the distal trachea, the carina, bilateral main stem bronchi, bilateral upper and lower lobe bronchi, the bronchus intermedius, the right middle lobe bronchus, and the lingular bronchus. A separate volume should be drawn for the trachea that is further than 2 cm from the carina and continues to 5 cm above the carina or 10 cm above the topmost aspect of the PTV, whichever is more superior [73].

4.2.2.7 RIBS AND CHEST WALL

Exposure of ribs and chest wall to radiation is associated with a risk of fracture and development of chest wall pain. Rib fracture risks may be increased with underlying conditions such as osteoporosis [83]. The RTOG 0915 protocol recommends contouring the ribs within 5 cm of the PTV by outlining the bone and the marrow; adjacent ribs should not be contoured in contiguous fashion in the contour. For single-fraction regimen, maximum recommended dose is 30 Gy and less than 1 cc should receive 22 Gy or more. For the 4-fraction regimen, maximum recommended rib dose is 40 Gy (10 Gy/fx), and less than 1 cc should receive 32 Gy or more [72].

4.2.2.8 BRACHIAL PLEXUS

The brachial plexus is a nervous network that arises from the four lower-most cervical nerves and the first thoracic nerves. This network controls the sensation and motor function of the upper extremities. Radiation injury of the brachial plexus, or brachial plexopathy, may manifest as pain, paresthesia, or motor weakness. A 2012 retrospective study of patients with NSCLC undergoing conventionally fractionated RT with concurrent chemotherapy examining rates of brachial plexopathy found a strong association and higher rates of brachial plexopathy with median brachial plexus doses greater than 69 Gy and doses to 0.1 cm^3 of brachial plexus greater than 75 Gy [84]. In a retrospective study from Indiana University looking at apical lung lesions treated with SBRT, a maximum brachial plexus dose of 26 Gy or greater was associated with significantly higher rates of brachial plexopathy. Current clinical trials recommend a maximum dose ≤63–66 Gy [79] with conventional fractionation. For SBRT, brachial plexus dose constraints include 17.5 Gy if single fraction, 24 Gy (8 Gy/fx) max with 3-fraction regimens, 27.2 Gy (6.8 Gy per fraction with 4-fraction regimens, and 32 Gy max (6.4 Gy/fx) with 5-fraction regimens [66].

4.2.2.9 CARINA

The carina is the point where the trachea bifurcates into the right and left main stem bronchi. It is a useful landmark that can be used for CBCT registration, and carina matching has been shown to identify setup errors and provide superior nodal coverage and combined target coverage as compared to spine matching [85].

4.2.2.10 STOMACH

Acute toxicity to the stomach includes nausea and vomiting. Later potential effects include ulceration, bleeding, and perforation, which can be life threatening. A dose of 45 Gy to the whole stomach with conventional fractionation is associated with a 5–7% risk of ulceration. For SBRT it is recommended to limit the volume of the stomach receiving >22.5 Gy to <4% of the organ volume or 5 cc [86], and for maximum dose 12.4 Gy for single-fraction regimens, and 27.2 Gy for 4-fraction regimens [66].

4.2.2.11 SKIN

When looking at skin doses, the greatest concern is the potential for ulceration. In RTOG 0618 skin is defined as the outer 0.5 cm of the body surface, and as such it is to be contoured as a uniformly thick 0.5-cm rind of the outer surface. The maximum recommended dose is 26 Gy for single-fraction SBRT, 24 Gy for 3-fraction regimens (8 Gy/fx), 36 Gy for 4-fraction regimens (9 Gy/fx), and 32 Gy for 5-fraction regimens (6.4 Gy/fx) [70].

4.2.3 Planning organ at risk volume (PRV)

Just as for the PTV, where movement might add a degree of uncertainty that must be accounted for, the same might happen in OARs. At times, it is beneficial to add a margin to an OAR structure to account for this degree of uncertainty, leading to the creation of the planning organ at risk volume (PRV) structure. A PTV and a PRV may overlap. PRVs are more important in structures that are in series rather than structures in parallel, as the former is at higher risk of significant irreparable damage [87].

4.3 DOSE FRACTIONATION AND CONSTRAINTS

4.3.1 Conventional fractionation

4.3.1.1 PRESCRIBED DOSE

Concurrent chemoradiation is the standard of care treatment for inoperable locally advanced NSCLC. The optimal dose and fractionation of radiation for NSCLC has been the subject of much research throughout the years. Prior to the integration of chemotherapy and radiation, unresectable patients were treated with radiation only. RTOG 7301 and 7302 were two parallel randomized clinical trials run in the 1970s which explored dose escalation in patients with unresectable or medically inoperable tumors. Patients in RTOG 7301 included less advanced disease (medically inoperable stage I and II, unresectable stage III excluding T4 or N3 disease) and they were randomized to 40 Gy split course, 40 Gy continuous, 50 Gy, or 60 Gy, all delivered in 2 Gy fractions. Patients in RTOG 7302 had more advanced disease without distant metastases, including T4 disease and N3 nodes, and they were randomized to 30 Gy in 10 3-Gy fractions, 40 Gy split course or 40 Gy continuous course in 2 Gy fractions. The groups receiving 50 and 60 Gy showed fewer infield failures. The 60 Gy group also showed a longer median time to failure (19 months, as compared to 12 months for 50 Gy and 8 months for 40 Gy) as well as a small improvement in 3-year overall survival (15% for the 60-Gy group versus 10% in the 50-Gy group and 6% in the 40-Gy group). This trial established 60-Gy as the standard radiation dose in NSCLC [88,89]. Given the dismal survival rates, subsequent trials were attempted.

The CALGB 8433 showed that addition of chemotherapy led to an improvement in survival. Patients with stage III NSCLC were randomized to 60 Gy in 2-Gy fractions alone or with induction chemotherapy with cisplatin and vinblastine. Median OS was 13.8 months in the combination arm, versus 9.7 months in the radiation alone (RT) arm, and 3-year OS was 23% in combination arm versus 11% in the RT alone arm. This established combination treatment as superior to RT alone for unresectable patients. Subsequently, RTOG 94–10 asked the question of concurrent versus sequential treatment as well as exploring a hyperfractionation alternative. In this trial 610 patients were randomized to one of three arms: a sequential arm with induction cisplatin and vinblastine followed by radiation therapy to a total dose of 63 Gy, starting at day 50 of treatment; a concurrent chemoRT arm with the same chemotherapy and RT regiment as in the first arm, but starting on day 1 of treatment; a concurrent arm utilizing oral etoposide and cisplatin and hyperfractionated RT with a total dose of 69.6 Gy at 1.2 Gy twice daily fractions. At a median follow-up of 11 years, the median OS was significantly better in the concurrent, daily radiation arm, with a median OS of 17.1 months, compared to 14.6 months in the sequential arm and 15.6 months in the hyperfractionated arm [90]. Meta-analysis of concurrent versus sequential chemo RT confirmed benefit to concurrent approach [91].

The goal of RTOG 0617 was to explore radiation therapy dose escalation as a different strategy to improve patient survival. This was a randomized multi-institutional study that randomized patients with unresectable stage III NSCLC to either 60-Gy or 74-Gy in 2-Gy fractions with concurrent weekly paclitaxel and carboplatin with or without cetuximab. Unexpectedly, at a median follow-up time of 22.9 months, patients in the 74-Gy group were found to have no improvement in survival, with a median survival of 20.3 months in the dose escalation group and a survival of 28.7 months in the standard dose group [92]. Preoperative concurrent chemo RT is a treatment option for select patients with resectable locally advanced disease, such as stage

IIIA patients with minimal N2 disease (limited to one station). It is also the standard of care for resectable superior sulcus tumors [66].

The Intergroup 0139 trial randomized patients with NSCLC stage IIIA to concurrent chemotherapy and radiation therapy alone or followed by resection. There was no difference in overall survival for the two groups in all-comers. However, an unplanned exploratory analysis showed improved survival in the patients in the surgery group who underwent lobectomy as compared to matched patients in the definitive chemo RT group. Decreased survival in overall surgical groups was thought to be driven by perioperative mortality in the pneumonectomy patients [93].

4.3.1.1.1 Post-operative RT

Radiation in the postoperative setting is a controversial topic. A meta-analysis of 10 trials published initially in 1998 and updated in 2005 showed a significant detriment to the addition of post-operative RT. The pooled analysis showed a 2-year OS of 53% for patients treated with postoperative RT, as compared to 58% for patients who did not receive adjuvant RT, corresponding to an 18% relative increase in death. Subgroup analysis showed PORT to be most detrimental for patients with stage I and II disease and patients with lower nodal status [67]. However, the results of this meta-analysis have been the subject of much criticism, specifically that many of the centers used antiquated techniques and high dose per fraction, which would not be acceptable for today's standards.

While the publication of the PORT meta-analysis significantly dampened the use of RT in the postoperative settings, other studies have suggested a potential benefit of PORT for certain patient subsets. A 2006 SEER database analysis of 7465 patients, with a median follow-up time of 3.5 years, did not show an overall impact on survival. However, subset analysis revealed a survival benefit for patients with N2 disease, with a 5-year OS rate of 27% for patients receiving PORT versus 20% for observation patients. In patients with N0-N1 disease PORT was detrimental to survival [94].

The ANITA trial was a randomized trial initially published in 2006 that randomized completely resected patients with stage IB-IIIA to adjuvant chemotherapy with vinorelbine and cisplatin or no chemotherapy. PORT was recommended for node-positive patients; however, it was not required. Subsequent post hoc analysis of the impact of PORT showed a significant benefit for patients with pN2 disease regardless of whether they received adjuvant chemotherapy (MS 23.8 for no PORT versus 47.4 months for PORT) or not (MS 12.7 months for no PORT versus 22.7 months for PORT). Patients with pN1 disease benefited from PORT only if they did not receive adjuvant chemotherapy (MS 25.9 months for no PORT versus 50.2 for PORT), while in the chemotherapy arm PORT led to decreased survival (MS 93.6 for no PORT versus 46.6 for PORT) [65].

While none of the data suggesting a benefit to PORT for the N2 subset of patients is prospective, it certainly suggests a strong benefit for the subset of patients with N2 disease. The current NCCN guidelines recommend PORT after adjuvant chemotherapy for patients with pN2 disease. For patients with positive surgical margins, NCCN guidelines recommend PORT with concurrent chemotherapy. PORT is not recommended for patients with N0 or N1 disease [66].

The LungART trial is an ongoing phase III randomized EORTC trial that investigates the role of PORT in patients with completely resected NSCLC with pN2 disease. Following resection, patients are randomized to PORT or no PORT. PORT consists of 54 Gy in 27 2-Gy or 30 1.8-Gy daily fractions, with no concurrent chemotherapy allowed. Pre-operative and post-operative chemotherapy is allowed but not mandated. Use of conformal techniques is mandatory, and the trial mandates the use of beam energies equal to or greater than 6MV but no greater than 10 MV to avoid electron transfer in lung tissues associated with higher energy beams. Use of heterogeneity correction in planning is mandatory. The primary endpoint is DFS, and secondary endpoints include OS, local control, toxicity, and patterns of recurrence. This trial will hopefully shed more light on PORT in patients with stage IIIA disease [95].

Small cell lung cancer (SCLC) is a completely different entity with a different clinical course compared to NSCLC. In addition to the AJCC staging, in common with NSCLC, SCLC patients are classically divided into limited stage, which includes patients whose disease can safely be encompassed in a tolerable radiation plan, and extensive stage patients. The treatment paradigm for SCLC differs from that of NSCLC and it is dependent on the extent of disease [96].

For patients with limited stage disease, concurrent chemotherapy and radiation is the accepted standard of care treatment. The randomized clinical trial Intergroup 0096 randomized patients with LS-SCLC to 45-Gy delivered either daily (in 1.8-Gy fractions) or twice daily (in 1.5-Gy fractions) with concurrent cisplatin and etoposide. Patients in the twice daily regimen group had a significant improvement in average survival, which was 23 months, compared to 19 months in the daily RT group. Five-year OS was 26% in the twice daily group and 16% in the daily group. Twice daily radiation was associated with significantly higher rates of esophagitis. Given the overwhelming improvement in survival associated with the twice daily regimen, this is considered standard of care for patients with LS-SCLC [97].

One of the criticisms of Intergroup 0096 is that the dose in the once daily regimen is not biologically equivalent to the BID regimen, and while considered an appropriate dose, for current standard it would be considered inadequately low. The phase II CALGB 39808 aimed to investigate prospectively the feasibility of delivering 70 Gy concurrent with chemotherapy to patients with LS-SCLC. Chemotherapy consisted of two cycles of induction topotecan and paclitaxel, while concurrent chemotherapy consisted of three cycles of carboplatin and etoposide. Patients with a partial or complete responses were subsequently offered PCI. Median overall survival was 22.4 months, which is comparable to the results in the BID arm of Intergroup 0096.

While the results of CALGB 39808 are very promising, without a head-to-head comparison it is unclear whether conventional daily fractionation can be equivalent to the twice daily regimen. There are two ongoing clinical trials comparing twice daily RT with conventional fractionation. The CALGB 30610 is a randomized trial comparing the Intergroup 0096 twice daily regimen to 70 Gy in 35 daily fractions. Both arms receive concurrent cisplatin or carboplatin and etoposide. This study is open and still accruing subjects. The CONVERT trial is a UK trial that randomized patients to either the Intergroup 0096 twice daily regimen on 66 Gy in 33 daily fractions, with both arms receiving concurrent cisplatin and etoposide. The trial has completed accrual; however, results are not yet available.

The treatment paradigm for patients with extensive stage (ES) SCLC focuses initially on the delivery of systemic treatment. For patients with a response to initial systemic treatment, the use of consolidation thoracic radiation is beneficial [96].

In a 1999 trial, patients with a distant complete response and a local partial or complete response were randomized to one of two groups: accelerated hyperfractionated consolidation RT, for a dose of 54 Gy in 36 1.5-Gy BID fractions with concurrent carboplatin and etoposide followed by two additional cycles of cisplatin and etoposide. Patients in the comparison arm received four additional cycles of cisplatin and etoposide. All patients were offered PCI. Patients who received thoracic RT had improved mean survival (17 months versus 11 months) and 5-year OS (9.1% versus 3.7%) [98].

Table 4.2 OAR dose constraints for standard fractionation

OAR	Constraints for 30–35 fractions
Spinal cord	Max ≤50Gy
Lung	V_{20} ≤35%; V_5 ≤65%; MLD ≤20Gy
Heart	V_{40} ≤80%; V_{45} ≤60%; V_{60} ≤30%; mean ≤35Gy
Esophagus	Mean ≤34 Gy; max ≤105% of prescription dose
Brachial plexus	Max ≤66Gy

Source: Ettinger, D.S. et al., *NCCN Guidelines (R) Non-Small Cell Lung Cancer*. Version 7.2015, National Comprehensive Cancer Network, Fort Washington, 2015. (Adapted with permission from the NCCN Clinical Practice Guidelines in Oncology (NCCN Guidelines®) for Non-Small Cell Lung Cancer V.7.2015. To view the most recent and complete version of the NCCN Guidelines, go online to NCCN.org. NATIONAL COMPREHENSIVE CANCER NETWORK®, NCCN®, NCCN GUIDELINES®, and all other NCCN content are trademarks owned by the National Comprehensive Cancer Network, Inc.)

A recent randomized trial studied patients with ES-SCLC with any response after 4–6 cycles of chemotherapy to thoracic radiotherapy (consisting of 30 Gy in 10 daily fractions) followed by PCI or PCI alone. While the primary endpoint, which was survival at one year, did not show any statistical difference (33% in the thoracic RT group versus 28 in the PCI only group), the thoracic RT group had improved 2-year OS (13% versus 3%) and 6 months PFS (24% versus 7%) [99].

4.3.1.2 DOSE CONSTRAINTS

The dose constraints for each organ at risk have been discussed in the previous sections and are summarized in Table 4.2 [66] for standard fractionation.

4.3.2 STEREOTACTIC BODY RADIATION THERAPY (SBRT) FRACTIONATION

4.3.2.1 PRESCRIBED DOSE

RTOG 0236 is a 2010 clinical trial that examined the role of SBRT in patients with early stage (T1-T2 N0 M0) inoperable NSCLC. Patients were treated to a total dose of 54 Gy in 3 18-Gy fractions, with fractions separated by at least 40 hours. Due to significant toxicity observed for patients with central tumors treated with SBRT, phase I/II dose escalation trial RTOG 0813 explored the use of SBRT in medically inoperable patients

Table 4.3 OAR dose constraints for SBRT

OAR	Single fraction	3 fractions	4 fractions	5 fractions
Spinal cord	14 Gy	18 Gy (6 Gy/fraction)	26 Gy (6.5 Gy/fraction)	30 Gy (6 Gy/fraction)
Esophagus	15.4 Gy	27 Gy (9 Gy/fraction)	30 Gy (7.5 Gy/fraction)	105% of PTV prescription
Brachial plexus	17.5 Gy	24 Gy (8 Gy/fraction)	27.2 Gy (6.8 Gy/fraction)	32 Gy (6.4 Gy/fraction)
Heart/pericardium	22 Gy	30 Gy (10 Gy/fraction)	34 Gy (8.5 Gy/fraction)	105% of PTV prescription
Great vessels	37 Gy	NS	49 Gy (12.25 Gy/fraction)	105% of PTV prescription
Trachea and proximal bronchi	20.2 Gy	30 Gy (10 Gy/fraction)	34.8 Gy (8.7 Gy/fraction)	105% of PTV prescription
Rib	30 Gy	30 Gy (10 Gy/fraction)	40 Gy (10 Gy/fraction)	NS
Skin	26 Gy	24 Gy (8 Gy/fraction)	36 Gy (9 Gy/fraction)	32 Gy (6.4 Gy/fraction)
Stomach	12.4 Gy	NS	27.2 Gy (6.8 Gy/fraction)	NS

Source: Ettinger, D.S. et al., *NCCN Guidelines (R) Non-Small Cell Lung Cancer.* Version 7.2015, National Comprehensive Cancer Network, Fort Washington, 2015. (Adapted with permission from the NCCN Clinical Practice Guidelines in Oncology (NCCN Guidelines®) for Non-Small Cell Lung Cancer V.7. 2015. To view the most recent and complete version of the NCCN Guidelines, go online to NCCN.org. NATIONAL COMPREHENSIVE CANCER NETWORK®, NCCN®, NCCN GUIDELINES®, and all other NCCN Content are trademarks owned by the National Comprehensive Cancer Network, Inc.)

NS: not specified.

with central tumors. The initial dose cohort was 50 Gy in 5 10-Gy fractions, with escalation up to 60 Gy in 5 12-Gy fractions. The trial is currently closed and we are awaiting results.

4.3.2.2 DOSE CONSTRAINTS

The dose constraints for each organ at risk have been discussed in the previous sections and are summarized in Table 4.3 [66] for SBRT fractionation.

4.3.2.3 CONFORMITY INDEX

The conformity index is the quotient of the treated volume and the PTV. It is a useful concept that can be used as part of plan optimization, if the PTV is fully enclosed by the treated volume.

4.4 PLANNING TECHNIQUES

For any of the planning techniques described below, the selected photon beam energy should be between 4 and 10 MV [100–102]. Lower energy beams are preferred over higher energy (greater than 10 MV) because of the loss of lateral scatter equilibrium of the beam in the lung [103]. Multiple studies have reported on the effects of the loss of lateral scatter equilibrium [101,104–107]. One way to overcome such a loss is to add a larger margin for the PTV, which defeats one of the advantages of IGRT—the ability to reduce margins since more sophisticated imaging techniques are included during daily treatments. The larger margin would also lead to more normal tissue receiving unnecessarily higher doses. Another issue that can arise with high energy beams is that electronic equilibrium can also be lost along the central axis of the beam if the field size is too small. This can lead to a significant decrease in the percent depth dose of the beam [101,108]. Since small field sizes are typically used for SBRT, this can lead to underdosing of the tumor and a higher probability of recurrence. Prior studies have shown that a small decrease in dose (7–15%) to the tumor can drastically diminish tumor control [109–111]. Therefore, it is recommended that the photon energy selected for lung plans should be in the range of 4–10 MV.

Any form of IGRT, whether it is kV or MV based, can be used with any of the treatment techniques listed below. Depending on the capabilities of the treatment machine, imaging can be performed prior, during, or after treatment to assess inter- and intrafraction motion of the target.

4.4.1 3D

For standard fractionation dose schemes, there are no set numbers of beams recommended. The beam arrangement may consist of a combination of coplanar and non-coplanar beams. Arrangements can be as simple as AP/PA, parallel opposed beams to more complex arrangements with multiple non-coplanar ones. AP/PA beam arrangement is classically used for more extensive disease that is centrally located. By using this beam arrangement, the dose to the unaffected lung tissue is minimized. However, this plan can only be delivered to 45–50 Gy (1.8–2 Gy per fraction) due to spinal cord tolerance. To deliver a higher dose to the PTV, an "off-cord" plan must be developed to spare the spinal cord.

Beams are chosen to provide the best tumor volume coverage while limiting the dose to the normal structures. Multileaf collimators (MLCs), compensators, and blocks (though not widely used) are just some of the tools used to conform the port of the field to the tumor while reducing dose to critical structures. The ability to spare normal tissues is limited by the need to provide adequate dose to the target. If a large portion of the lung is to be irradiated, the plan must be designed to adhere to normal lung tolerance doses. To avoid radiation pneumonitis or other complications, certain dose indices, such as V_{20}, V_5, and mean lung dose, should be reviewed prior to treatment initiation [112,113]. As seen in Figure 4.12, the use of an anterior-superior oblique, posterior, and left-posterior oblique beam provide adequate coverage for the centrally located tumor while sparing the spinal cord and lungs as best as possible.

Based on multiple RTOG protocols (0236, 0813, 0915) for 3D SBRT plans, it is recommended to use greater than or equal to 10 beams, at least 7 of which should be non-opposing. The reason for choosing so many beams is to minimize the entrance dose and the toxicity to the skin and chest wall [100]. The use of non-coplanar beams is also preferable. The beams are typically equally weighted. The size of the tumor being treated also determines the number of beams used—the larger the tumor, the more beams necessary to provide adequate coverage [72,73,80]. Figure 4.13 demonstrates a 3D SBRT lung plan, which used 7 beams, 2 of which

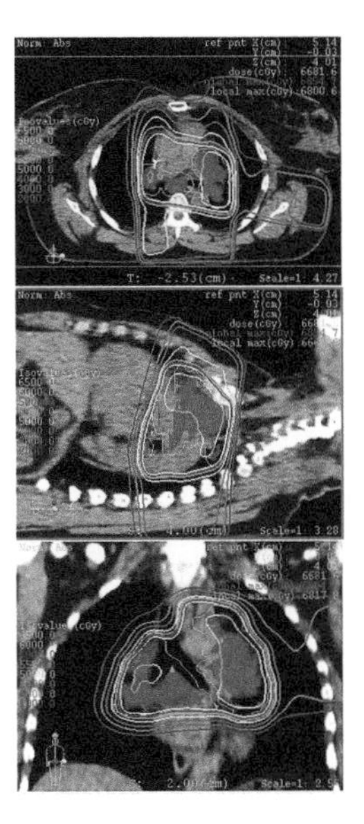

Figure 4.12 3D conventional plan using anterior-superior oblique, posterior, and left-posterior oblique beams. Beam arrangement was chosen to adequately cover the PTV while sparing critical structures, such as the spinal cord, heart, and lungs.

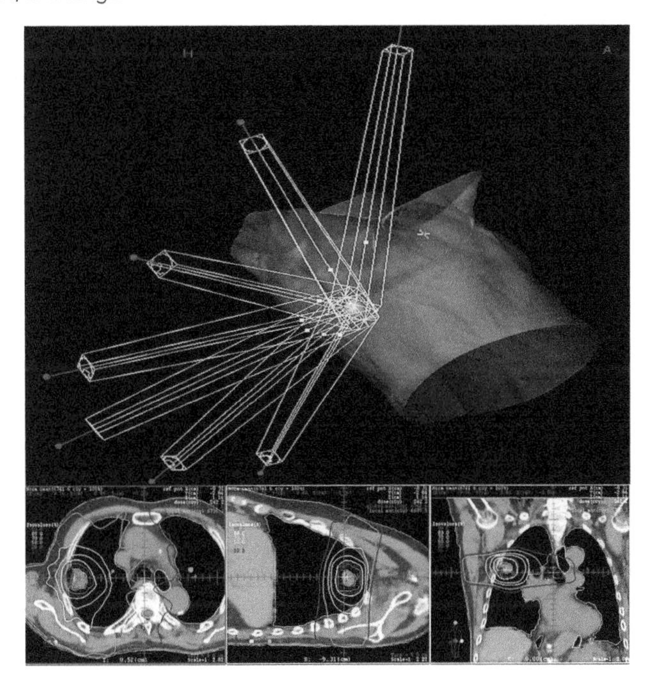

Figure 4.13 3D plan for SBRT lung. A total of seven beams were used in this plan in order to meet RTOG 0813 protocol guidelines.

were non-coplanar. These beam angles were selected based on tumor location as well as the critical structures as per RTOG 0813 (see Table 4.3). Again, the MLCs are used to conform the port to the shape of the PTV. 3D plans are still the most common and standard form of treatment available for lung tumors.

4.4.2 IMRT

Intensity modulated radiation therapy (IMRT) is a type of radiation therapy that is used to modulate the photon or proton beams to deliver a more conformal dose to the tumor. Depending on the capability of the linear accelerator and treatment planning system, the movement of the MLCs is either classified as "step-and-shoot" or "sliding window." In the step-and-shoot delivery, the MLCs are stationary while the beam is on, and then the beam is halted while the MLCs move to the next control point until all positions have been treated for that field. For the sliding window technique, the beam is continuously on while the MLCs sweep across the field. The MUs for the sliding window method tend to be higher than the step-and-shoot technique since the beam is constantly on.

IMRT is currently used to treat a multitude of different cancers in various areas of the body. The use of IMRT for the treatment of lung cancer has proven to be a useful tool for tumors that are large and located in critical areas of the body with difficult geometry to overcome [114,115]. A case where IMRT was necessary to treat a lesion, which included the right middle lobe, mediastinum, and right supraclavicular region, with the issues of size and location, is shown in Figure 4.14. Dosimetrists initially started with a 3D plan but were unable to meet the constraints on critical structures. There is no set number of beams for IMRT field arrangements. The separation of the beams is typically based on the number of beams being used. However, opposing beams tend to be avoided. Constraints are added as needed for all critical structures listed in the previous section during the inverse optimization process to limit the risk of toxicities to normal tissues.

Numerous studies have been performed to investigate the optimal number of beams for IMRT lung plans [116–120]. A retrospective planning study performed by Christian et al. compared five different IMRT plans that used multiple beam arrangements (3, 5, 7, and 9 coplanar fields and 6 non-coplanar fields) to a 3D that used 6 non-coplanar beams for 10 patients with NSCLC. They discovered that the normal lung volume receiving 20 Gy (V_{20}) was lower for the IMRT plans that used more than 3 fields as compared to the 3D plans. They also found that there was a relationship between the number of coplanar beams and the dose to normal lungs being reduced, where the plan with 9 beams was better than the ones using fewer beams [118]. The study performed by Liu et al. shows that IMRT plans not only reduce the V_{20}, V_{30}, and mean lung dose, but they also could maintain or improve the V_{45} to the heart and esophagus when compared to 3D plans [116].

While IMRT plans have shown some benefits in dose reduction to the lungs (V_{20} and V_{30}), the volume of lung receiving low dose (V_5) has greatly increased, which can lead to both acute and late pulmonary toxicity [19,121,122]. More clinical data are needed to better understand the complications (both early and late) that may arise from having more integral low dose to a larger volume of the lungs.

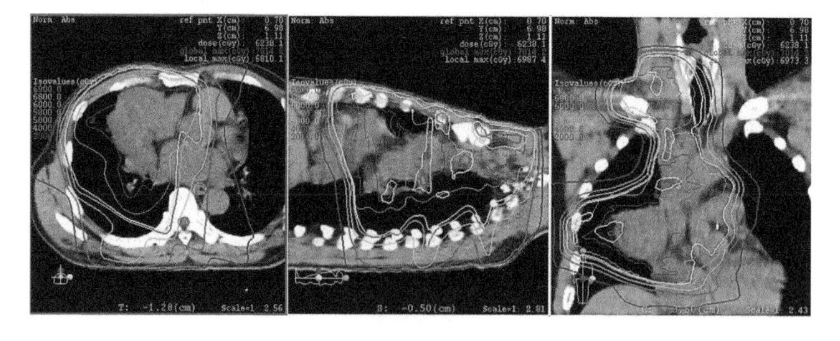

Figure 4.14 Example of IMRT lung plan to treat right middle lobe, mediastinum, and right supraclavicular region.

4.4.3 VMAT

Volumetric modulated arc therapy (VMAT) is also a type of radiation treatment that involves the modulation of the multileaf collimators (MLCs) speed and positions while the dose rate and gantry rotation speed are also varied. This technique can deliver a highly conformal dose to the tumor while sparing normal tissue. Potential advantages of VMAT over 3D and IMRT are that there is improved dose distribution since there are more angles available for treatment as well as a reduction in treatment times. VMAT is still a relatively new procedure and not all linear accelerators can deliver this type of treatment.

Most VMAT cases are planned with at least two coplanar arcs with variable collimators. The size and location of the tumor tend to influence the length of the arcs—some arcs are the full 360°, while others are only a fraction of this. The sum of the degrees in all the arcs should be greater than 340° for SBRT dose fractionations [72,73,80]. Non-coplanar arcs can also be used if warranted to develop a better plan. Careful consideration must be taken when choosing the angles of the gantry rotation and the couch not to cause a collision with the linear accelerator and the patient. VMAT has more degrees of freedom compared to IMRT plans during the inverse optimization since the gantry is free to rotate around the patient. As with inverse optimization for IMRT, it is also necessary to add constraints to critical structures when executing VMAT planning.

Various studies have found that VMAT plans yield a reduction in dose to critical structures while increasing the conformity of dose to the lung tumor as compared to highly conformal 3D plans [123,124]. The comparison of these plans also resulted in a significant reduction in mean lung dose values, including V_{20}, $V_{12.5}$, V_{10}, and V_5 [124]. On initial glance, VMAT plans would deliver a greater amount of low dose to the lungs. If the arcs are limited during the selection of the gantry angles, then the low dose spread to the lungs

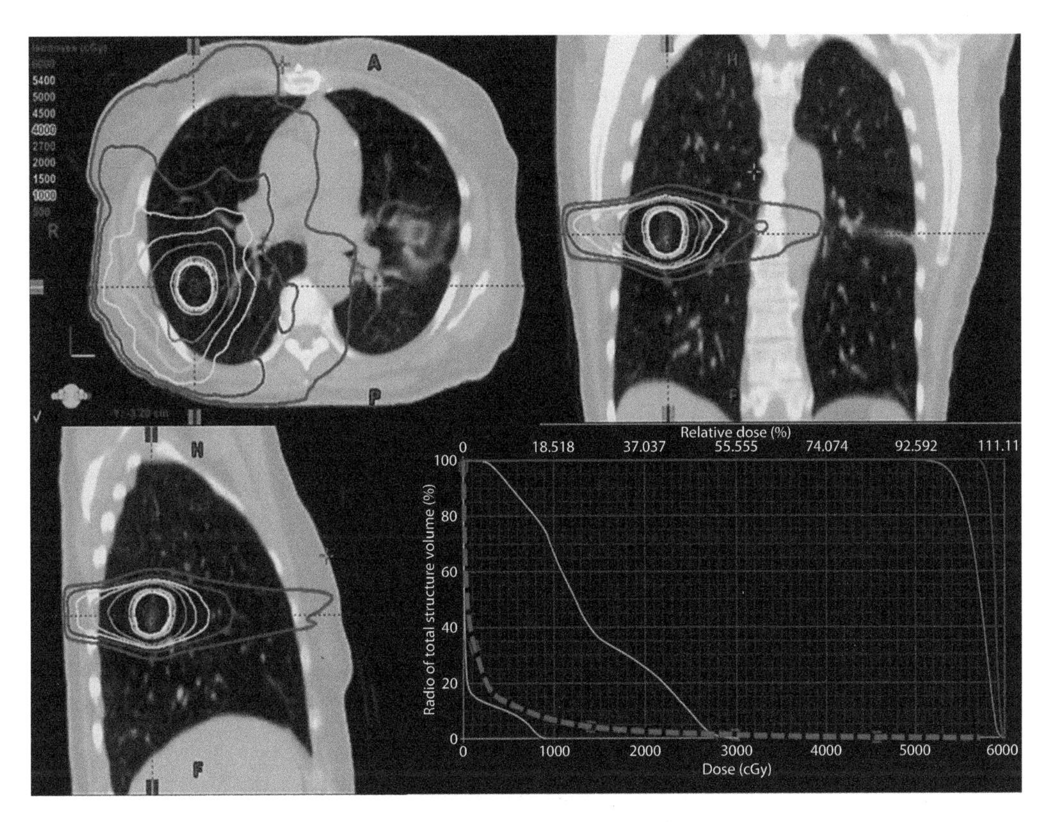

Figure 4.15 Right lung mass SBRT plan. On the DVH display, the red line represents the tumor, pink is PTV, yellow is ribs, cyan is spinal cord, and the dashed blue line is the lung-GTV. Even with using three full arcs, the low dose to the lungs is limited.

can be minimized. As seen in Figure 4.15 the low dose to the lungs is limited even with a plan that utilizes three full arcs. The reduction in dose to the lungs reduces the risk of radiation-induced pneumonitis for patients already with compromised lung function. Another benefit of VMAT is the decreased risk of skin and soft tissue toxicity since the dose is distributed over a greater surface area as compared to 3D and IMRT plans [125].

4.4.4 Dynamic conformal arc

Arc therapy was initially introduced to address limitations from fixed field treatments, such as 3D and IMRT. Dynamic conformal arc therapy allowed the target to be treated from all angles [126]. Other advantages of using arc therapy are the improvement of treatment times and the decrease in monitor units (MUs). A study comparing MU factors between IMRT and dynamic arc therapy by Morales-Paliza et al. found that there was significant decrease in MUs for the arc plans [127]. This would be beneficial in terms of treatment times and the comfort of the patient. There is also less chance of deviation from the prescribed dose due to setup errors and/or internal motion for dynamic arc therapy since the treatment times are shorter [127].

In both VMAT and dynamic conformal arc therapy, the shape of the field is constantly changing. However, the MLCs in VMAT modulate such that the PTV is partially blocked as the gantry rotates around the patient. For dynamic conformal arc therapy, the field-shape changes such that it fits the beam's eye view (BEV) of the target volume as it rotates around the patient. If a critical structure is within the BEV, the MLCs can be adjusted such that the OAR is blocked as the arc is delivered. Dynamic conformal arc plans tend to have 3–4 non-coplanar arcs, but the number can vary based on location and size of the target. The number of arcs, their length, and their arrangement are all determined during the planning process such that the PTV is adequately covered.

4.4.5 Dose calculation and heterogeneity correction

Complications may arise during computation of radiation treatment plans due to the volume of low-density lung present in the fields for lung tumors. The loss of charged-particle equilibrium (CPE) is cause for concern in low-density volumes such as the lung. This deficiency occurs when the field size is decreased to a small enough size that the lateral ranges of secondary electrons become comparable or even larger than the field size [128]. Since the range of electrons is greater in lung versus water, this effect occurs for larger field sizes in lungs. When irradiating lung tumors with small field sizes, most of the dose to the tumor is from secondary electron interactions and dose deposition. As the beam traverses from tissue to the lower density lung, the dose is reduced due to electron scattering in the lungs. Once the beam enters the tumor (tissue equivalent) from the lower density lung, the dose must build back up at the surface of the lung/tumor interface prior to the dose being deposited in the tumor. These reductions in dose can lead to significant underdosage at the tumor periphery. The loss of peripheral tumor coverage is also worsened using higher energy beams, due to the increased electron range.

The accuracy of the dose calculation algorithm is of the utmost importance, especially when calculating plans involving lung tumors. Certain dose calculation algorithms do not account for secondary electron interactions and therefore the displayed dose is inaccurate. According to Report Number 85 from the American Association of Physicists in Medicine (AAPM), a difference in dose as small as 5% may result in a 10–20% variation in tumor control probability (TCP) at 50% as well as a 20–30% change on normal tissue complication probabilities (NTCP) [129]. When planning lung cancer cases, the calculation algorithm that is selected should include three-dimensional (3D) scatter integration such as convolution/superposition or Monte Carlo (MC), which accounts explicitly for electron transport [130]. The algorithm selection is of extreme importance when designing a plan for small tumors with small field sizes (less than 5×5 cm^2) and should use one of the previously mentioned ones.

Based on recommendations from AAPM Task Group Report Number 101 and other articles, pencil beam algorithms should not be used for dose calculation of SBRT lung plans [130]. Another recommendation from the Task Group is that MC calculations should be the algorithm of choice for the most complex geometry

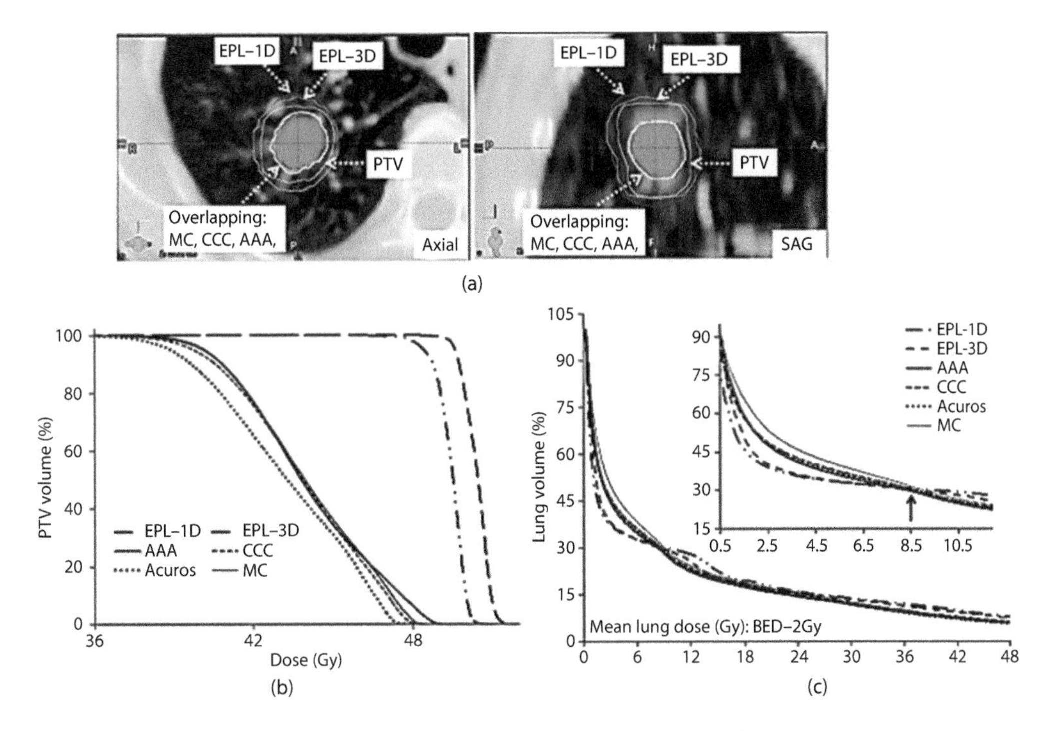

Figure 4.16 Comparison of PTV coverage using multiple dose calculation algorithms. (a) Axial and sagittal images of peripheral tumor and PTV. The 90% isodose lines (IDLs) for each algorithm are displayed. The 1D and 3D pencil beam algorithms overestimate the coverage of the PTV, which is 95% in this case, whereas all of the model-based algorithms show a drastic reduction in PTV coverage. (b) PTV DVH for all algorithms, which also demonstrates the reduction in PTV coverage by the model based algorithms. All of the model based algorithms agree within a few percent of one another. (c) DVH of lungs for all algorithms. (Reprinted from *Radiother Oncol*, 109, Chetty, I.J. et al., Correleation of dose computed using different algorithms with local control following stereotactic ablative radiotherapy (SABR)-based treatment of non-small-cell lung cancer, 498–504. Copyright [2013], with permission from Elsevier.)

encountered in SBRT lung cases, which include small, peripherally located lung tumors that are surrounded by lung tissue [130]. A study performed by Chetty et al. comparing multiple dose calculation algorithms, which included pencil beam (1D equivalent path-length and 3D equivalent path-length) and model based (anisotropic analytical algorithm (AAA), collapsed cone convolution-superposition (CCC), Acuros XB, and Monte Carlo), showed that the pencil beam-based algorithms provide good coverage of the PTV but the model-based algorithms show a substantial reduction in coverage of the PTV as seen in Figure 4.16 [131]. This demonstrates how insensitive pencil beam algorithms are to low density regions and how they do not incorporate electron scattering within the lung into the model. Hence, the use of a pencil beam algorithm would lead to an overestimate of the tumor dose versus the more accurate model-based algorithms, which calculates a considerably lower dose to the tumor.

4.5 SUMMARY

The incorporation of IGRT into radiation treatments has led to the reduction of uncertainty of lung tumor motion, whether it is inter- or intrafraction motion. Visualization of the tumor using IGRT can be performed at any point—before, during, or after treatment. By utilizing IGRT, margins to lung tumors can be personalized to everyone based on the motion of the tumor. This leads to smaller expansions for PTVs as well as reducing the amount of normal tissue irradiated. IGRT is a useful tool regardless of the complexity of the plan. Integrating IGRT with treatment helps ensure that the delivered dose is what was intended by the treatment plan [132].

REFERENCES

1. Wu, Q.J. et al., Adaptive radiation therapy: Technical components and clinical applications. *Cancer J*, 2011. **17**(3): 182–9.
2. Kim, J., J.L. Meyer, and L.A. Dawson, Image guidance and the new practice of radiotherapy: What to know and use from a decade of investigation, in *IMRT, IGRT, SBRT—Advances in the Treatment Planning and Delivery of Radiotherapy*, J.L. Meyer, Editor. 2011, Basel: Karger. pp. 196–216.
3. Mutic, S. et al., The simulation process in the determination and definition of the treatment volume and treatment planning, in *Technical Basis of Radiation Therapy*, S.H. Levitt, et al., Editors. 2006, Berlin Heidelberg New York: Springer. pp. 107–33.
4. Wolthaus, J.W.H. et al., Comparison of different strategies to use four-dimensional computed tomography in treatment planning for lung cancer patients. *Int J Radiat Oncol Biol Phys*, 2008. **70**(4): 1229–38.
5. Stevens, C.W. et al., Respiratory-driven lung tumor motion is independent of tumor size, tumor location, and pulmonary function. *Int J Radiat Oncol Biol Phys*, 2001. **51**(1): 62–8.
6. Koste, J.R.v.S.d. et al., Tumor location cannot predict the mobility of lung tumors: A 3D analysis of data generated from multiple CT scans. *Int J Radiat Oncol Biol Phys*, 2003. **56**(2): 348–54.
7. Sixel, K.E. et al., Digital fluoroscopy to quantify lung tumor motion: Potential for patient-specific planning target volumes. *Int J Radiat Oncol Biol Phys*, 2003. **57**(3): 717–23.
8. Plathow, C. et al., Analysis of intrathoracic tumor mobility during whole breathing cycle by dynamic MRI. *Int J Radiat Oncol Biol Phys*, 2004. **59**(4): 952–9.
9. Mayo, J.R., N.L. Muller, and R.M. Henkelman, The double-fissure sign: A motion artifact on thin-section CT scans. *Radiology*, 1987. **165**(2): 580–1.
10. Ritchie, C.J. et al., Predictive respiratory gating: A new method to reduce motion artifacts on CT scans. *Radiology*, 1994. **190**(3): 847–52.
11. Shepp, L.A., S.K. Hilal, and R.A. Schulz, The tuning fork artifact in computerized tomography. *Comput Graph Image Process*, 1979. **10**(3): 246–55.
12. Tarver, R.D., D.J. Conces. Jr., and J.D. Godwin, Motion artifacts on CT simulate bronchiectasis. *AJR Am J Roentgenol*, 1988. **151**(6): 1117–9.
13. Shimizu, S. et al., Detection of lung tumor movement in real-time tumor-tracking radiotherapy. *Int J Radiat Oncol Biol Phys*, 2001. **51**(2): 304–10.
14. Keall, P.J. et al., Potential radiotherapy improvements with respiratory gating. *Australas Phys Eng Sci Med*, 2002. **25**(1): 1–6.
15. Underberg, R.W.M. et al., Use of maximum intensity projections (MIP) for target volume generation in 4DCT scans for lung cancer. *Int J Radiat Oncol Biol Phys*, 2005. **63**(1): 253–60.
16. Bradley, J.D. et al., Comparison of helical, maximum intensity projection (MIP), and averaged intensity (AI) 4D CT imaging for stereotactic body radiation therapy (SBRT) planning in lung cancer. *Radiother Oncol*, 2006. **81**(3): 264–8.
17. Cai, J., P.W. Read, and K. Sheng, The effect of respiratory motion variability and tumor size on the accuracy of average intensity projection from four-dimensional computed tomography: An investigation based on dynamic MRI. *Med Phys*, 2008. **35**(11): 4974–81.
18. Guckenberger, M. et al., Four-dimensional treatment planning for stereotactic body radiotherapy. *Int J Radiat Oncol Biol Phys*, 2007. **69**(1): 276–85.
19. Cheng, S.K. et al., Lung cancer, in *Practical Essentials of Intensity Modulated Radiation Therapy*, K.S.C. Chao, Editor. 2014, Philadelphia, PA: Lippincott Williams & Wilkins. pp. 295–314.
20. Farrell, M.A. et al., Non-small cell lung cancer: FDG PET for nodal staging in patients with stage I disease 1. *Radiology*, 2000. **215**(3): 886–90.
21. Lowe, V.J. and K.S. Naunheim, Positron emission tomography in lung cancer. *Ann Thorac Surg*, 1998. **65**(6): 1821–9.
22. Marom, E.M. et al., Staging non-small cell lung cancer with whole-body PET I. *Radiology*, 1999. **212**(3): 803–9.

23. Vanuytsel, L.J. et al., The impact of 18 F-fluoro-2-deoxy-D-glucose positron emission tomography (FDG-PET) lymph node staging on the radiation treatment volumes in patients with non-small cell lung cancer. *Radiother Oncol*, 2000. **55**(3): 317–24.
24. Munley, M.T. et al., Multimodality nuclear medicine imaging in three-dimensional radiation treatment planning for lung cancer: Challenges and prospects. *Lung Cancer*, 1999. **23**(2): 105–14.
25. Silvestri, G.A. et al., The noninvasive staging of non-small cell lung cancer: The guidelines. *Chest*, 2003. **123**(Suppl. 1): 147S–56.
26. Gould, M.K. et al., Test performance of positron emission tomography and computed tomography for mediastinal staging in patients with non-small-cell lung cancer: A meta-analysis. *Ann Intern Med*, 2003. **139**(11): 879–92.
27. Antoch, G. et al., Non-Samll cell lung cancer: Dual-modality PET/CT in preoperative staging 1. *Radiology*, 2003. **229**(2): 526–33.
28. Cerfolio, R.J. et al., The accuracy of integrated PET-CT compared with dedicated PET alone for the staging of patients with nonsmall cell lung cancer. *Ann Thorac Surg*, 2004. **78**(3): 1017–23.
29. Ciernik, I.F. et al., Radiation treatment planning with an integrated positron emission and computer tomography (PET/CT): A feasibility study. *Int J Radiat Oncol Biol Phys*, 2003. **57**(3): 853–63.
30. Lardinois, D. et al., Staging of non–small-cell lung cancer with integrated positron-emission tomography and computed tomography. *N Engl J Med*, 2003. **348**(25): 2500–7.
31. Ruysscher, D.D. et al., Selective mediastinal node irradiation based on FDG-PET scan data in patients with non–small-cell lung cancer: A prospective clinical study. *Int J Radiat Oncol Biol Phys*, 2005. **62**(4): 988–94.
32. Bradley, J. et al., Impact of FDG-PET on radiation therapy volume delineation in non–small-cell lung cancer. *Int J Radiat Oncol Biol Phys*, 2004. **59**(1): 78–86.
33. Caldwell, C.B. et al., Observer variation in contouring gross tumor volume in patients with poorly defined non-small-cell lung tumors on CT: The impact of 18 FDG-hybrid PET fusion. *Int J Radiat Oncol Biol Phys*, 2001. **51**(4): 923–31.
34. Kalff, V. et al., Clinical impact of (18)F fluorodeoxyglucose positron emission tomography in patients with non-small-cell lung cancer: A prospective study. *J Clin Oncol*, 2001. 19(1): 111–8.
35. Steenbakkers, R.J.H.M. et al., Observer variation in target volume delineation of lung cancer related to radiation oncologist-computer interaction: A "Big Brother" evaluation. *Radiother Oncol*, 2005. **77**(2): 182–90.
36. Werner-Wasik, M. et al., What is the best way to contour lung tumors on PET scans? multiobserver validation of a gradient-based method using a NSCLC digital PET phantom. *Int J Radiat Oncol Biol Phys*, 2012. **82**(3): 1164–71.
37. Macapinlac, H.A. et al., PET imaging for target determination and delineation, in *Practical Essentials of Intensity Modulated Radiation Therapy*, K.S.C. Chao, Editor. 2005, Philadelphia, PA: Lippincott Williams & Wilkins. pp. 62–81.
38. Bradbury, M. and H. Hricak, Molecular MR imaging in oncology. *Magn Reson Imaging Clin N Am*, 2005. **13**(2): 225–40.
39. Martini, N. et al., Comparative merits of conventional, computed tomographic, and magnetic resonance imaging in assessing mediastinal involvement in surgically confirmed lung carcinoma. *J Thorac Cardiovasc Surg*, 1985. **90**(5): 639–48.
40. Musset, D. et al., Primary lung cancer staging: Prospective comparative study of MR imaging with CT. *Radiology*, 1986. **160**(3): 607–11.
41. Patterson, G.A. et al., A prospective evaluation of magnetic resonance imaging, computed tomography, and mediastinoscopy in the preoperative assessment of mediastinal node status in bronchogenic carcinoma. *J Thorac Cardiovasc Surg*, 1987. **94**(5): 679–84.
42. Poon, P.Y. et al., Mediastinal lymph node metastases from bronchogenic carcinoma: Detection with MR imaging and CT. *Radiology*, 1987. **162**(3): 651–6.
43. Laurent, F. et al., Bronchogenic carcinoma staging: CT versus MR imaging. Assessment with surgery. *Eur J Cardiothorac Surg*, 1988. **2**(1): 31–6.

44. Grenier, P.H. et al., Preoperative thoracic staging of lung cancer: CT and MR evaluation. *Diagn Intervent Radiol*, 1989. **1**: 23–8.
45. Webb, W.R. et al., CT and MR imaging in staging non-small cell bronchogenic carcinoma: Report of the radiologic diagnostic oncology group. *Radiology*, 1991. **178**(3): 705–13.
46. Heelan, R.T. et al., Superior sulcus tumors: CT and MR imaging. *Radiology*, 1989. **10**(3 Pt 1): 637–41.
47. Rapoport, S. et al., Brachial plexus: Correlation of MR imaging with CT and pathologic findings. *Radiology*, 1988. **167**(1): 161–5.
48. Castagno, A.A. and W.P. Shuman, MR imaging in clinically suspected brachial plexus tumor. *AJR Am J Roentgenol*, 1987. **149**(6): 1219–22.
49. McLoud, T.C. et al., MR imaging of superior sulcus carcinoma. *J Comput Assist Tomogr*, 1989. **13**(2): 233–9.
50. Flechsig, P. et al., PET/MRI and PET/CT in lung lesions and thoracic malignancies. *Semin Nucl Med*, 2015. **45**(4): 268–81.
51. Kauczor, H.-U. and K.-F. Kreitner, Contrast-enhanced MRI of the lung. *Eur J Radiol*, 2000. **34**(3): 196–207.
52. Bergin, C.J., J.M. Pauly, and A. Macovski, Lung parenchyma: Projection reconstruction MR imaging. *Radiology*, 1991. **179**(3): 777–81.
53. Lutterbey, G. et al., Ein neuer Ansatz in der Magnetresonanztomographie der Lunge mit einer ultrakurzen Turbo-Spin-Echo-Sequenz (UTSE). *RöFo*, 1996. 164: 388–93.
54. Ireland, R.H. et al., Feasibility of image registration and intensity-modulated radiotherapy planning with hyperpolarized helium-3 magnetic resonance imaging for Non-Small-cell lung cancer. *Int J Radiat Oncol Biol Phys*, 2007. **68**(1): 273–81.
55. Beek, E.J.R.v. et al., Functional MRI of the lung using hyperpolarized 3-helium gas. *J Magn Reson Imaging*, 2004. **20**(4): 540–54.
56. Wild, J.M. et al., Comparison between 2D and 3D gradient-echo sequences for MRI of human lung ventilation with hyperpolarized 3He. *Magn Reson Med*, 2004. **52**(3): 673–8.
57. Wild, J.M. et al., 3D volume-localized pO2 measurement in the human lung with 3He MRI. *Magn Reson Med*, 2005. **53**(5): 1055–64.
58. Möller, H.E. et al., MRI of the lungs using hyperpolarized noble gases. *Magn Reson Med*, 2002. **47**(6): 1029–51.
59. Mirsadraee, S. and E.J.R. v. Beek, Functional imaging: Computed tomography and MRI. *Clin Chest Med*, 2015. **36**(2): 349–63.
60. Mountain, C.F. and C.M. Dresler, American College of Chest Physicians. *Chest*, 1997. **111**(6): 1718–23.
61. Rosenzweig, K.E. et al., Involved-field radiation therapy for inoperable non small-cell lung cancer. *J Clin Oncol*, 2007. **25**(35): 5557–61.
62. Yuan, S. et al., A randomized study of involved-field irradiation versus elective nodal irradiation in combination with concurrent chemotherapy for inoperable stage III nonsmall cell lung cancer. *Am J Clin Oncol*, 2007. **30**(3): 239–44.
63. Kies, M.S. et al., Multimodal therapy for limited small-cell lung cancer: A randomized study of induction combination chemotherapy with or without thoracic radiation in complete responders; and with wide-field versus reduced-field radiation in partial responders: A southwest oncology group study. *J Clin Oncol*, 1987. **5**(4): 592–600.
64. Group, P.M.-a.T., Postoperative radiotherapy in non-small-cell lung cancer: Systematic review and meta-analysis of individual patient data from nine randomised controlled trials. *Lancet*, 1998. **352**(9124): 257–63.
65. Douillard, J.-Y. et al., Impact of postoperative radiation therapy on survival in patients with complete resection and stage I, II, or IIIa non-small-cell lung cancer treated with adjuvant chemotherapy: The adjuvant navelbine international trialist association (ANITA) randomized trial. *Int J Radiat Oncol Biol Phys*, 2008. **72**(3): 695–701.
66. Ettinger, D.S. et al., *NCCN Guidlines (R) Non-Small Cell Lung Cancer.* Version 7.2015. 2015, National Comprehensive Cancer Network: Fort Washington, PA.

67. Bradley, J.D. et al., Phase II trial of postoperative adjuvant paclitaxel/carboplatin and thoracic radiotherapy in resected stage II and IIIA non-small-cell lung cancer: Promising long-term results of the radiation therapy oncology group—RTOG 9705. *J Clin Oncol*, 2005. **23**(15): 3480–7.
68. Feigenberg, S.J. et al., A phase II study of concurrent carboplatin and paclitaxel and thoracic radiotherapy for completely resected stage II and IIIA non-small cell lung cancer. *J Thorac Oncol*, 2007. **2**(4): 287–92.
69. Spoelstra, F.O.B. et al., Variations in target volume definition for postoperative radiotherapy in stage III non-small-cell lung cancer: Analysis of an international contouring study. *Int J Radiat Oncol Biol Phys*, 2010. **76**(4): 1106–13.
70. ICRU, International Commission on Radiation Units and Measurements: Prescribing, recording, and reporting photon beam therapy, supplement to ICRU report no. 50. 1999: Bethesda, MD.
71. ICRU, International Commission on Radiation Units and Measurements: Prescribing, recording, and reporting photon beam therapy. 1993: Bethesda, MD.
72. Group, R.T.O., RTOG 0915: A randomized phase II study comparing 2 stereotactic body radiation therapy (SBRT) schedules for medically inoperable patients with stage I peripheral non-small cell lung cancer. 2009, RTOG: Philadelphia, PA.
73. Group, R.T.O., RTOG 0813: Seamless phase I/II study of stereotactic lung radiotherapy (SBRT) for early stage, centrally located, non-small cell lung cancer (NSCLC) in medically inoperable patients. 2010, RTOG: Philadelphia, PA.
74. Abbatucci, J.S. et al., Radiation myelopathy of the cervical spinal cord: Time, dose and volume factors. *Int J Radiat Oncol Biol Phys 1978*. **4**(3): 239–48.
75. Kirkpatrick, J.P., A.J.v.d. Kogel, and T.E. Schultheiss, Radiation dose-volume effects in the spinal cord. *Int J Radiat Oncol Biol Phys*, 2010. **76**(3): S42–9.
76. Gagliardi, G. et al., Radiation dose-volume effects in the heart. *Int J Radiat Oncol Biol Phys*, 2010. **76**(3): S77–85.
77. Wheatley, M.D. et al., Defining a novel cardiac contouring atlas for NSCLC using cadaveric anatomy. *Int J Radiat Oncol Biol Phys*, 2014. **90**(1): S658.
78. Qiao, W.B. et al., Clinical and dosimetric factors of radiation-induced esophageal injury: Radiation-induced esophageal toxicity. *World J Gastroenterol*, 2005. **11**(17): 2626–9.
79. Oncology, N., NRG-LU001: Randomized phase II trial of concurrent chemoradiotherapy +/- metformin HCL in locally advanced NSCLC. 2015, NRG Oncology: Philadelphia, PA.
80. Timmerman, R.D. et al., RTOG 0236: A phase II trial of stereotactic body radiation therapy (SBRT) in the treatment of patients with medically inoperable stage I/II non-small cell lung cancer, in *Proceedings of the 13th World Conference on Lung Cancer*. 2007, San Francisco, CA: IASLC.
81. Fakiris, A.J. et al., Stereotactic body radiation therapy for early-stage non-small-cell lung carcinoma: Four-year results of a prospective phase II study. *Int J Radiat Oncol Biol Phys*, 2009. **75**(3): 677–82.
82. Corradetti, M.N., A.R. Haas, and R. Rengan, Central-airway necrosis after stereotactic body-radiation therapy. *N Engl J Med*, 2012. **366**(24): 2327–9.
83. Thibault, I. et al., Predictors of chest wall toxicity after lung stereotactic ablative radiotherapy. *Clin Oncol*, 2016. **28**(1): 28–35.
84. Amini, A. et al., Dose constraints to prevent radiation-induced brachial plexopathy in patients treated for lung cancer. *Int J Radiat Oncol Biol Phys*, 2012. **82**(3): e391–8.
85. Lavoie, C. et al., Volumetric image guidance using carina vs spine as registration landmarks for conventionally fractionated lung radiotherapy. *Int J Radiat Oncol Biol Phys*, 2012. **84**(5): 1086–92.
86. Kavanagh, B.D. et al., Radiation dose-volume effects in the stomach and small bowel. *Int J Radiat Oncol Biol Phys*, 2010. **76**(3): S101–7.
87. ICRU, International commission on radiation units and measurements: Prescribing, recording, and reporting photon-beam intensity-modulated radiation therapy (IMRT). *J ICRU*, 2010. 10(1): 41–53.
88. Perez, C.A. et al., A prospective randomized study of various irradiation doses and fractionation schedules in the treatment of inoperable non-oat-cell carcinoma of the lung. preliminary report by the radiation therapy oncology group. *Cancer*, 1980. **45**(11): 2744–53.

89. Perez, C.A. et al., Long-term observations of the patterns of failure in patients with unresectable non-oat cell carcinoma of the lung treated with definitive radiotherapy report by the radiation therapy oncology group. *Cancer*, 1987. **59**(11): 1874–81.
90. W. J. Curran, et al., Sequential vs. concurrent chemoradiation for stage III non-small cell lung cancer: Randomized phase III trial RTOG 9410. *J Natl Cancer Inst*, 2011. **103**(19): 1452–60.
91. Auperin, A. et al., Meta-analysis of concomitant versus sequential radiochemotherapy in locally advanced non-small-cell lung cancer. *J Clin Oncol*, 2010. **28**(13): 2182–90.
92. Bradley, J.D. et al., Standard-dose versus high-dose conformal radiotherapy with concurrent and consolidation carboplatin plus paclitaxel with or without cetuximab for patients with stage IIIA or IIIB non-small-cell lung cancer (RTOG 0617): A randomised, two-by-two factorial phase 3 study. *Lancet Oncol*, 2015. **16**(2): 187–99.
93. Albain, K.S. et al., Radiotherapy plus chemotherapy with or without surgical resection for stage III non-small-cell lung cancer: A phase III randomised controlled trial. *Lancet*, 2009. **374**(9687): 379–86.
94. Lally, B.E. et al., Postoperative radiotherapy for stage II or III non-small-cell lung cancer using the surveillance, epidemiology, and end results database. *J Clin Oncol*, 2006. **24**(19): 2998–3006.
95. Dunant, A. et al., Phase III study comparing post-operative conformal radiotherapy to no post-operative radiotherapy in patients with completely resected non-small cell lung cancer and mediastinal N2 involvement(LungART). 2010. Available at: HYPERLINK "https://na01.safelinks.protection.outlook.com/?url=http%3A%2F%2Fwww.ifct.fr%2Fimages%2Fstories%2FProtocoles%2FDocsPratiques%2FIFCT-0503-LungArt%2FProtocole_LungART_v8.pdf&data=02%7C01%7CYan.Yu%40jefferson.edu%7C570adaa89b7a478d931708d4cfbec833%7C55a89906c710436bbc444c590cb67c4a%7C0%7C1%7C636361865685470558&sdata=ZHzKoEMrJGP6966MV%2FBMn9kWycqujsOzis0lZsTSKuA%3D&reserved=0" http://www.ifct.fr/images/stories/Protocoles/DocsPratiques/IFCT-0503-LungArt/Protocole_LungART_v8.pdf. Accessed March 4, 2016.
96. Kalemkerian, G.P. et al., NCCN clinical practice guidelines in oncology. *Small Cell Lung Cancer*, version 1.2016. Available at: http://www.nccn.org/professionals/physician_gls/pdf/sclc.pdf. Accessed March 4, 2016.
97. Turrisi, A.T. et al., Twice-daily compared with once-daily thoracic radiotherapy in limited small-cell lung cancer treated concurrently with cisplatin and etoposide. *N Engl J Med*, 1999. **340**(4): 265–71.
98. Jeremic, B. et al., Role of radiation therapy in the combined-modality treatment of patients with extensive disease small-cell lung cancer: A randomized study. *J Clin Oncol*, 1999. **17**(7): 2092–9.
99. Slotman, B.J. et al., Use of thoracic radiotherapy for extensive stage small-cell lung cancer: A phase 3 randomised controlled trial. *Lancet*, 2015. **385**(9982): 36–42.
100. Buyyounouski, M.K. et al., Stereotactic body radiotherapy for early-stage non-small-cell lung cancer: Report of the ASTRO emerging technology committee. *Int J Radiat Oncol Biol Phys*, 2010. **78**(1): 3–10.
101. Ekstrand, K.E. and W.H. Barnes, Pitfalls in use of high energy X rays to treat tumors in the lung. *Int J Radiat Oncol Biol Phys*, 1990. **18**(1): 249–52.
102. Wang, L. et al., Dosimetric advantage of using 6 MV over 15 MV photons in conformal therapy of lung cancer: Monte carlo studies in patient geometries. *J Appl Clin Med Phys*, 2002. **3**(1): 51–9.
103. Khan, F.M. and J.P. Gibbons. *Khan's the Physics of Radiation Therapy*. 2014, Philadelphia, PA: Lippincott Williams & Wilkins.
104. Kornelsen, R.O. and M.E.J. Young, Changes in the dose-profile of a 10 MV x-ray beam within and beyond low density material. *Med Phys*, 1982. **9**(1): 114–6.
105. White, P.J., R.D. Zwicker, and D.T. Huang, Comparison of dose homogeneity effects due to electron equilibrium loss in lung for 6 MV and 18 MV photons. *Int J Radiat Oncol Biol Phys*, 1996. **34**(5): 1141–6.
106. Young, M.E.J. and R.O. Kornelsen, Dose corrections for low-density tissue inhomogeneities and air channels for 10-MV x rays. *Med Phys*, 1983. **10**(4): 450–5.
107. Klein, E.E. et al., A volumetric study of measurements and calculations of lung density corrections for 6 and 18 MV photons. *Int J Radiat Oncol Biol Phys*, 1997. **37**(5): 1163–70.

108. Mackie, T.R. et al., Lung dose corrections for 6- and 15-MV x rays. *Med Phys*, 1985. **12**: 327–32.
109. Dutreix, A., When and how can we improve precision in radiotherapy? *Radiother Oncol*, 1984. **2**(4): 275–92.
110. Goitein, M. and J. Busse, Immobilization error: Some theoretical considerations 1. *Radiology*, 1975. **117**(2): 407–12.
111. Stewart, J.G. and A.W. Jackson, The steepness of the dose response curve both for tumor cure and normal tissue injury. *The Laryngoscope*, 1975. **85**(7): 1107–11.
112. Allen, A.M. et al., Fatal pneumonitis associated with intensity-modulated radiation therapy for mesothelioma. *Int J Radiat Oncol Biol Phys*, 2006. **65**(3): 640–5.
113. Marks, L.B. et al., Radiation dose-volume effects in the lung. *Int J Radiat Oncol Biol Phys*, 2010. **76**(3): S70–6.
114. Sura, S. et al., Intensity-modulated radiation therapy (IMRT) for inoperable non-small cell lung cancer: The memorial sloan-kettering cancer center (MSKCC) experience. *Radiother Oncol*, 2008. **97**(1): 17–23.
115. Yom, S. et al., Analysis of acute toxicity reults of intensity modulated radiation therapy. *Lung Cancer*, 2005. **49**(Suppl. 2): S52.
116. Liu, H.H. et al., Feasibility of sparing lung and other thoracic structures with intensity-modulated radiotherapy for non–small-cell lung cancer. *Int J Radiat Oncol Biol Phys*, 2004. **58**(4): 1268–79.
117. Murshed, H. et al., Dose and volume reduction for normal lung using intensity-modulated radiotherapy for advanced-stage non–small-cell lung cancer. *Int J Radiat Oncol Biol Phys*, 2004. **58**(4): 1258–67.
118. Christian, J.A. et al., Comparison of inverse-planned three-dimensional conformal radiotherapy and intensity-modulated radiotherapy for non–small-cell lung cancer. *Int J Radiat Oncol Biol Phys*, 2007. **67**(3): 735–41.
119. Grills, I.S. et al., Potential for reduced toxicity and dose escalation in the treatment of inoperable non–small-cell lung cancer: A comparison of intensity-modulated radiation therapy (IMRT), 3D conformal radiation, and elective nodal irradiation. *Int J Radiat Oncol Biol Phys*, 2003. **57**(3): 875–90.
120. Schwarz, M. et al., Dose heterogeneity in the target volume and intensity-modulated radiotherapy to escalate the dose in the treatment of non–small-cell lung cancer. *Int J Radiat Oncol Biol Phys*, 2005. **62**(2): 561–70.
121. Stevens, C., T. Guerrero, and K. Forster, Lung cancer radiotherapy, in *Intensity-Modulated Radiation Therapy: The State of the Art*, J.R. Palta and T.R. Mackie, Editors. 2003, Madison, WI: Medical Physics Publishing. pp. 645–62.
122. Seppenwoolde, Y. et al., Comparing different NTCP models that predict the incidence of radiation pneumonitis. *Int J Radiat Oncol Biol Phys*, 2003. **55**(3): 724–35.
123. Merrow, C.E., I.Z. Wang, and M.B. Podgorsak, A dosimetric evaluation of VMAT for the treatment of non-small cell lung cancer. *J Appl Clin Med Phys*, 2012. **14**(1): 4110.
124. McGrath, S.D. et al., Volumetric modulated arc therapy for delivery of hypofractionated stereotactic lung radiotherapy: A dosimetric and treatment efficiency analysis. *Radiother Oncol*, 2010. **95**(2): 153–7.
125. Brock, J. et al., Optimising stereotactic body radiotherapy for non-small cell lung cancer with volumetric intensity-modulated arc therapy—A planning study. *Clin Oncol*, 2012. **24**(1): 68–75.
126. Palma, D.A. et al., New developments in arc radiation therapy: A review. *Cancer Treat Rev*, 2010. **36**(5): 393–9.
127. Morales-Paliza, M.A., C.W. Coffey, and G.X. Ding, Evaluation of the dynamic conformal arc therapy in comparison to intensity-modulated radiation therapy in prostate, brain, head-and-neck and spine tumors. *J Appl Clin Med Phys*, 2011. **12**(2): 5–19.
128. Glide-Hurst, C.K. and I.J. Chetty, Improving radiotherapy planning, delivery accuracy, and normal tissue sparing using cutting edge technologies. *J Thorac Dis*, 2014. **6**(4): 303.
129. Papanikolaou, N. et al., Tissue inhomogeneity corrections for megavoltage photon beams—Report of Task Group No. 65 of the Radiation Therapy Committee of the American Association of Physicists in Medicine. 2004, Madison, WI: American Association of Physicists in Medicine.

130. Benedict, S.H. et al., Stereotactic body radiation therapy: The report of AAPM task group 101. *Med Phys*, 2010. **37**(8): 4078–101.
131. Chetty, I.J. et al., Correleation of dose computed using different algorithms with local control following stereotactic ablative radiotherapy (SABR)-based treatment of non-small-cell lung cancer. *Radiother Oncol*, 2013. **109**: 498–504.
132. De Los Santos, J. et al., Image guided radiation therapy (IGRT) technologies for radiation therapy localization and delivery. *Int J Radiat Oncol Biol Phys*, 2013. **87**(1): 33–45.

5

Treatment verification and delivery

NING WEN, CARRI GLIDE-HURST, KAREN CHIN SNYDER, MISCHA HOOGEMAN, MARTINA DESCOVICH, LEI REN, AND INDRIN CHETTY

5.1 INTRODUCTION

The goal of radiotherapy is to control tumor progression or ablate the tumor with minimal harm to the patient. It requires high precision to localize the tumors accurately and deliver highly conformal doses to targets while sparing the surrounding radiosensitive healthy organs. For lung tumors, motion is exaggerated due to respiration, which is a serious challenge in the lung cancer radiotherapy. Historically, a large margin is applied to account for the setup uncertainties. The systematic errors could be up to 3 cm for lung cancer treatments if less intense immobilization and no imaging are applied for patient localization [1,2]. Even with active motion control, the required margin may still need be up to 1.5 cm if patients are aligned only to skin tattoos [3]. Large margins increase lung toxicity which can induce severe complications, especially for lung cancer patients with compromised lung function.

Image-guided radiation therapy (IGRT) is used to monitor tumor motion and minimize setup errors. The development of IGRT has significantly improved the precision of radiotherapy, along with customized immobilization devices and advanced radiation delivery techniques such as intensity modulated radiation therapy (IMRT) [4–7]. By utilizing IGRT in lung cancer treatments, setup errors can be further reduced and thus smaller margins can be implemented. Not only can it spare normal lung dose, but it can also allow for further dose escalation, which can improve local control in patients with non-small-cell lung cancer.

In this chapter, we will focus on the principles and theories of IGRT-based treatment verification and delivery for lung cancer. It includes an overview of principles and clinical workflow of image guidance, practices of inter- and intrafractional motion management, treatment delivery techniques, and clinical impacts of IGRT on the lung cancer treatment.

5.2 PRINCIPLES FOR VERIFICATION AND DELIVERY

5.2.1 Principles for target verification

Target verification can be classified into interfraction verification, which localizes the target before the start of the treatment for each fraction, and intra-fraction verification, which localizes the target during the actual treatment. Interfraction verification addresses the patient's anatomical and positional changes between different fractions, and intrafraction verification addresses the misalignment of the target due to changes of respiratory motion and patient position during the treatment. While interfraction verification has been commonly performed in lung radiation therapy treatments, intrafraction verification has been largely overlooked in the past. However, several clinical studies suggested that intra-fraction can be as important as interfraction verification, especially for hypo-fractionated lung stereotactic body radiation therapy (SBRT) due to its long treatment time (30–60 min), tight planning target volume (PTV) margin (5–10 mm), and high fractional dose (10–34 Gy) [8,9]. Purdie et al. showed that lung tumor intrafraction motion increases with treatment time to over 1 cm for long SBRT treatments [1]. Zhao et al. reported a maximal drop of PTV coverage from 95% to 78% in gated lung SBRT using 5-mm margin due to intrafraction motion [10]. Therefore, the usage of intrafraction verification needs to be carefully considered for lung radiation therapy treatments. Different techniques have been developed for inter- and intrafraction target verification. These techniques can be classified into the following categories:

1. X-ray-based imaging techniques: X-ray-based imaging techniques include 2D kilo voltage (kV) or mega-voltage (MV) imaging and 3D/4D cone beam CT (CBCT). 2D kV/MV imaging has the advantages of high imaging efficiency and low imaging dose, which makes it suitable for real-time target verification and delivery tracking. However, because it does not provide 3D volumetric information of the patient, the target localization accuracy in 2D imaging can be limited by the availability of traceable features, low contrast of the target, and overlaying high contrast features (e.g., spine, chest wall), as reported by Rottmann et al. [11,12]. Implanting markers in the tumor can improve the localization accuracy in 2D imaging, but this approach may not be applicable for all patients as it requires the invasive procedure of marker implantation. In addition, the locations of the markers may not accurately reflect the location of the tumor owing to soft-tissue deformation, tumor size change, and marker migration [13]. 3D/4D CBCT generates 3D/4D images of the patient by acquiring 2D kV projections all around the patient. CBCT has been used as the gold standard among x-ray-based techniques for interfraction verification due to the volumetric information it provides [14,15]. However, it has limited applications for intra-fraction verification due to long scanning time, high imaging dose, and limited mechanical clearance. It takes around 1 min for a 3D-CBCT scan and 4–5 min for a 4D-CBCT scan. Taking multiple CBCTs for intrafraction verification will increase the total treatment time substantially, leading to more intrafraction motion [1], which defeats the purpose of intrafraction verification. CBCT imaging dose can be up to 1–2 cGy, much higher than 2D kV/MV imaging due to the large number of projections acquired [16]. This prevents CBCT from being acquired multiple times intrafractionally over different fractions as the accumulated imaging dose is not negligible and may cause concerns for secondary cancer induction especially for young patients. In addition, CBCT requires scan angles of 200° or 360° which may not always be mechanically feasible especially when the imaging target is in the peripheral region of the body.
2. On-board MRI imaging: MRI integrated with radiotherapy unit has been proposed for both inter- and intrafraction verification [17,18]. Compared to CT, MRI has no radiation dose and better soft tissue contrast, which is useful for localizing low-contrast tumors in the soft tissue such as liver and prostate cancer. Currently, commercial on-board MRI systems can generate 2D cine MRI and 3D volumetric MRI images. 2D cine MRI provides real-time images of the patient in a 2D plane, which can be used for either gated treatment or target tracking in lung cancer radiation therapy [19]. However, 2D cine MRI does not provide volumetric information of the patient for 3D verification. In contrast, 3D MRI provides high quality volumetric images of the patient for target verification, but it does not capture the information along the time domain, which is important for tracking the respiratory motion of the lung tumor. 4D-MRI is being developed to address the limitations of both 2D cine and 3D MRI. Compared to x-ray-based imaging, on-board MRI imaging is less widely available in clinics, due in part to the high cost of the system. Besides, MRI is not applicable for imaging patients with pacemaker, metal implants, or claustrophobia. The accuracy and clinical significance of using MRI imaging for target verification remains to be understood.
3. Verification using electromagnetic transponders: The Calypso® System (Varian Medical Systems, Inc., Palo Alto, CA) has been developed to localize the tumor by tracking the locations of multiple electro-magnetic transponders implanted in the tumor [20]. The system consists of wireless transponders, an in-room 4D electromagnetic array housing the excitation and receiver coils and corresponding control console, a system of three infrared cameras mounted on the ceiling, and a tracking station located in the therapy control room [21,22]. The 4D electromagnetic array is placed over the patient and tracks the relative position of the implanted transponder. The infrared cameras detect the position of the array relative to the treatment machine. This information is used to determine the offset between the tumor

center and the machine isocenter. Calypso can provide real-time localization of the target for gated treatment or target tracking. Similar to the marker-based 2D x-ray imaging, the localization accuracy of Calypso could be affected by beacon migration, tumor deformation, and size changes. The invasive and permanent implantation of beacons also makes it not applicable for some lung cancer patients.

The pros and cons of each technique need to be weighed carefully when selecting the appropriate verification technique for lung cancer treatment. The key aspects that need to be considered include: (1) Efficiency: The imaging efficiency needs to be considered, especially for intrafraction verification, to minimize interruption to the treatment. (2) Imaging dose: Imaging dose to the patient needs to be minimized when using x-ray-based techniques. This needs to be considered together with the frequency of the imaging technique used throughout the treatment course to minimize the total accumulated imaging dose. (3) Image quality and localization accuracy: The localization accuracy of the verification technique is the key for the success of radiation therapy treatments. It's also an important factor when designing the PTV margin used in planning. (4) Patient-specific condition: Patient-specific conditions, such as suitability for marker implantation or being claustrophobia, need to be considered when choosing the appropriate verification technique. Note that the above factors can be weighed differently based on the types of treatments and applications of the verification techniques. SBRT treatments weigh more heavily on image quality and localization accuracy than imaging dose due to the high demand of treatment precision and small number of fractions. In contrast, fractionated treatments generally are less sensitive to localization errors due to the larger PTV margin used, but are more susceptible to accumulated imaging dose due to the large number of fractions employed. Therefore, imaging dose may be weighed more heavily than localization accuracy in fractionated lung cancer treatments when selecting an efficient low-dose imaging technique for daily verification. The verification technique selected will vary, based on its application for interfraction, intrafraction verification, or target tracking. Intrafraction verification demands high imaging efficiency of the technique to minimize delay of the treatment. Target tracking requires a verification technique with high temporal resolution to provide real-time localization of the target.

5.2.2 Principles for delivery

Respiration-induced target motion during lung cancer treatment can be managed either at the treatment planning stage or during radiation delivery. In the first approach, the target can move relative to the radiation beam, and the full motion envelope of the target is included in the planning target volume. In the second approach, the tumor is static in the reference frame of the radiation beam. This can be achieved by controlling tumor motion (breath-hold, forced shallow breading, abdominal compression), or by controlling the delivery equipment to deliver radiation only when the target is in a fixed position relative to the treatment beam (respiratory gating, beam tracking). Gating and tracking techniques enable control to reduce motion-induced errors and allow for margin reductions and dose escalation, while limiting the dose received by adjacent normal tissues [23,24]. A complete description of motion management strategies can be found in Chapter 3. In this section, we focus on the treatment delivery aspects of respiratory gating and real-time tracking techniques.

5.2.2.1 Respiratory gating

In a respiratory-gated treatment, the patient breathes normally and radiation is delivered intermittently. A breathing signal is used to trigger the beam delivery only during a predetermined portion of the breathing cycle, when the tumor lies inside the radiation field [25–27]. Internal or external surrogates of the tumor motion provide the breathing/gating signal. External surrogates consist of infrared markers placed on the patient torso (RPM, Varian), 3D surface imaging derived from infrared cameras (VisionRT), or measurement of air flow (spirometry). The position of infrared markers is detected by a video camera and used to create a representation of the breathing cycle. Internal surrogates consist of gold fiducial markers or electromagnetic transponders implanted in or near the tumor. Their positions are detected by orthogonal fluoroscopic images or an electromagnetic array to determine the offset between the tumor center and the machine isocenter.

Advancements in treatment verification techniques also enable direct visualization of the target and generate a breathing signal from the target motion itself. Fiducial-less tracking methods are highly desirable to eliminate the risk associated with marker implantation procedures such as pneumothorax [28] and marker migration.

In respiratory gating, the beam is turned on when the breathing signal is within a predefined range relative to the reference position. This range is called a gating window and is established at the time of simulation. The amplitude of the gating window determines the duty cycle (the ratio of the beam-on time to the total treatment time) and the residual target motion within the gating window. The smaller the gating window, the smaller the residual target motion, and the longer the treatment time. Typical duty cycles for gated treatment are 30–50% [25]. Residual target motion is accounted for by extending the radiation field to encompass the motion envelope of the target. Gukenberger et al. have shown that the treatment efficiency can be further increased by introducing the concept of mean target position [29]. In this case, the isocenter is placed at the time-weighted mean target position, and the residual target motion is compensated by applying safety margins based on 4D dose calculations.

Patient cooperation is important to maintain a reproducible breathing signal and an efficient treatment delivery. Coaching the patient and using visual and audio-respiratory feedback have been shown to improve breathing consistency and delivery efficiency in some studies [30–33]. Gating based on external markers assumes that the relationship between the position of the surrogate marker and the internal target position is constant. It is, however, well known that patients experience changes in breathing patterns and tumor motion trajectory during treatment (interfraction) and during a single treatment session (intrafraction) [34]. Therefore, it is important to verify the internal target anatomy during treatment using verification techniques such as x-ray-based imaging techniques [35].

5.2.2.2 REAL-TIME TRACKING

The term real-time tracking refers to techniques that enable following the target trajectory synchronizing the radiation delivery with the moving target. For this, the position of the target must be monitored continuously during treatment. The position of the target can be determined from x-ray images or from the signal emitted by electromagnetic transponders. Based on this information, the radiation beam is re-targeted by robotically repositioning the linear accelerator [36], by reshaping the multileaf (MLC) collimator [37], or by moving the patient positioning system [38]. In the case of charged particle radiation, the beam can also be steered using an electromagnetic system.

The advantages of dynamic tracking are several:

1. More comfortable to the patient than breath-holding techniques as the patient can breathe normally during treatment
2. More efficient than gating, as there are no interruptions in radiation delivery
3. Compared to motion encompassing methods (ITV-approach), target tracking enables us to reduce the normal tissues included in the radiation field
4. Moreover, changes in respiratory pattern and tumor motion trajectory are accounted for during treatment. Dynamic tracking, however, poses technical challenges, as it relies on sophisticated imaging and delivery techniques. It is important to understand its full functionality and the corresponding uncertainties (Chapter 12).

For 2D discrete image acquisition, a model of target motion must be built to enable dynamic tracking. The model is built by correlating the target position and the simultaneous position of external surrogate markers placed on the patient's chest prior to each treatment session. Models can be linear, quadratic, or polynomial. Studies have shown that higher-order polynomial fits (dual quadratic model) are required to provide an accurate representation of target motion during the respiratory cycle [39]. For 2D continuous image acquisition (keV images in fluoroscopic mode or 2D MRI in cine mode) a correlation model might not be necessary. Studies have shown that model-less dynamic tracking can achieve accuracy of 1.5 mm [40]. Model-less dynamic tracking also can be achieved using the continuous signal from small electromagnetic transponders implanted in the tissue (Calypso, Varian).

5.3 CLINICAL IMPLEMENTATION OF IGRT FOR LUNG CANCER

Online IGRT has been shown to be an effective tool to reduce systematic and random errors in the radiotherapy process and thus impact clinical endpoints [5,41,42] as shown in Figure 5.1. The reduction of the variation in the process can lead to margin reduction and dosimetric improvement, which could impact clinical endpoints [43]. It is particularly important to overhaul the whole chain of treatments when implementing IGRT to fully utilize its advantages. This section presents an overview of the clinical flow of IGRT for lung cancer, including considerations of immobilization devices and proper positioning during the simulation, intravenous (IV) contrast consideration, computed tomography (CT) / four-dimensional CT (4D-CT) simulation, patient localization and verification, and the basic principles of online image registration.

The typical online IGRT workflow has been described by several institutions [44–46]. Figure 5.2 shows the flowchart of a typical online IGRT process using volumetric imaging technique for localization. The CBCT and AVG-CT images are first registered based on bony anatomy (vertebral bodies and other rigid landmarks) using an automatic registration algorithm. Then, soft-tissue match is performed manually to shift the tumor visualized in the CBCT into the planning target volume (PTV) using a lung window. After the CBCT localization, an MV/kV orthogonal pair or second CBCT scan should be acquired to quantify the residual errors. If the residual alignment is within the tolerance, treatment proceeds as a conventional beam delivery method considering the PTV as a static target.

5.3.1 IMAGE REGISTRATION METHODS

There are two different objects in the image registration, the fixed image and the moving image. The purpose of image registration is to maximize the similar metrics between the fixed image and the moving image through transformation. In the registration process, image metrics measure similarity distance between images, the optimizer aligns the images based on the measures, and the moving image is transformed toward the fixed image based on the optimization results.

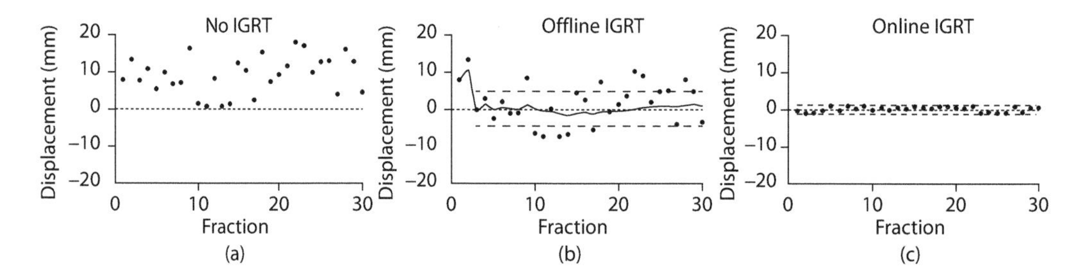

Figure 5.1 "Runtime" charts for the position of a single patient showing daily position (filled circles), running mean (solid line), and control limits (dashed lines). (a) The daily position without image guidance shows a large systematic error (10 mm) and large random uncertainty. (b) The application of an offline correction protocol results in small systematic error but does not reduce large random uncertainties, which manifests as daily positions that are "out of control." (c) Using daily online corrections results in small systematic and random uncertainties, indicating a process that is "in control." (Courtesy of Alexis, B. et al., *Sem Radiat Oncol.*, 22, 50–61, 2012.)

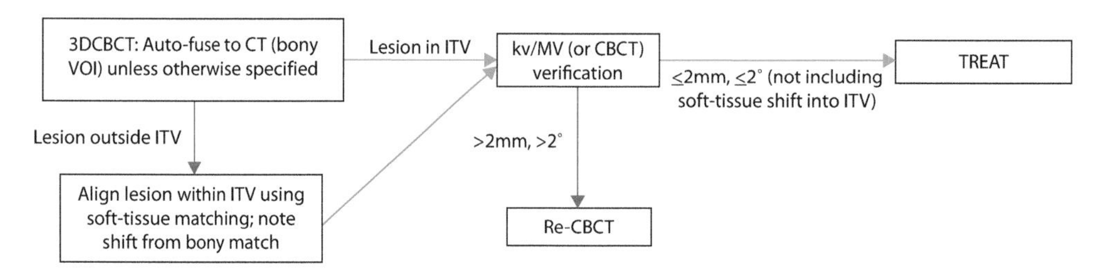

Figure 5.2 Online IGRT flowchart for lung cancer treatment.

5.3.1.1 2D/2D IMAGE REGISTRATION

Two orthogonal portal images are commonly taken after patient leveling and positioning in the treatment room. The images can be registered to the corresponding digital reconstructed radiographs (DRRs). Only planar transformations can be determined by superimposing the anatomical structures of the portal image and DRR. Three translational and one rotational degree of freedom (DOF) can be achieved for patient correction.

5.3.1.2 2D/3D IMAGE REGISTRATION

2D/3D image registration can register an orthogonal pair of kV or MV x-ray images acquired prior or during treatment to DRRs rendered from the original CT set. DRRs are rendered iteratively from the CT data set until the optimal similarity measure is achieved [47]. Various methods have been proposed to expedite the rendering process, such as the ray casting method and the shear warp method [48]. Six DOF corrections can be applied for patient setup from the 2D/3D image registration. 2D/3D image registration has proven to be an accurate and reliable target localization method on various platforms including ExacTrac® [49], CyberKnife® [50], or On-Board Imager [51].

5.3.1.3 3D/3D IMAGE REGISTRATION

CBCT provides online patient setup information to correct for interfraction motion with volumetric information. Rigid image registration is used to match CBCT to simulation CT with six DOF (three translational and three rotational). Common information is generally used as the similarity measure for 3D/3D image registration, especially between different image modalities. The image intensities are stochastically sampled using linear partial volume interpolation. The number of sampling points and noise and scatter from the CBCT could affect the accuracy of registration. The use of CBCT for localization has been proved to reduce the magnitude of setup errors and the variation in setup uncertainty between tumors undergoing respiratory motion of varying magnitude.

5.4 INTERFRACTIONAL MOTION LOCALIZATION AND VERIFICATION

Interfractional motion localization and the application of setup correction protocols is key for safe and accurate delivery of a curative dose to tumors in the lung. It can reduce systematic errors that arise from changes in average (mid-ventilation) [52] tumor location or the respiratory motion trajectory between the preparation phase (localization and treatment planning) and execution phase (treatment delivery). In terms of margins, (from clinical-target-volume to planning-target-volume) the contribution of systematic errors is the largest [53]. Interfractional motion localization can be used not only to compensate for systematic errors in an offline patient setup correction protocol [54], but also to compensate for day-to-day changes in the position of the target volume if the correction protocol is executed online, just prior to the delivery of the treatment fractions [55]. The latter is recommended strongly by the AAPM task group 101 on SBRT to guarantee an accurate dose delivery in hypofractionated treatment schedules. The following sections describe various methods for interfractional localization of the tumors in the lung. The methods can be divided into volumetric imaging techniques, planar imaging techniques, often combined with implanted fiducial markers, and techniques that use implanted electromagnetic beacons. Volumetric imaging techniques comprise kilo voltage (kV) cone beam computed tomography (CBCT), kV CT on-rails, megavoltage (MV) CT, and integrated Magnetic Resonance Imaging (MRI).

5.4.1 VOLUMETRIC IMAGING TECHNIQUES

5.4.1.1 kV CONE BEAM CT

The feasibility of a CBCT system integrated with a medical linear accelerator (Linac) was first demonstrated by Jaffray et al. [56]. CBCT uses a flat-panel detector to acquire projection images of the whole volume of interest in one rotation (Figures 5.3 and 5.4). Feldkamp reconstruction techniques are used to reconstruct a

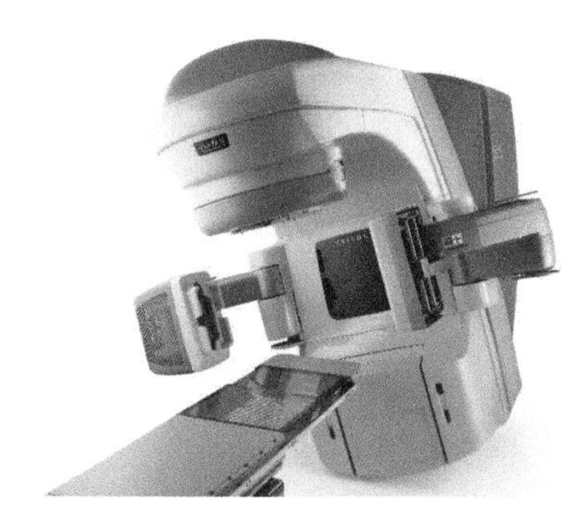

Figure 5.3 Varian Trilogy® linear accelerator with On-Board Imager® device for image-guided radiation therapy. (Image courtesy of Varian Medical Systems. All rights reserved.)

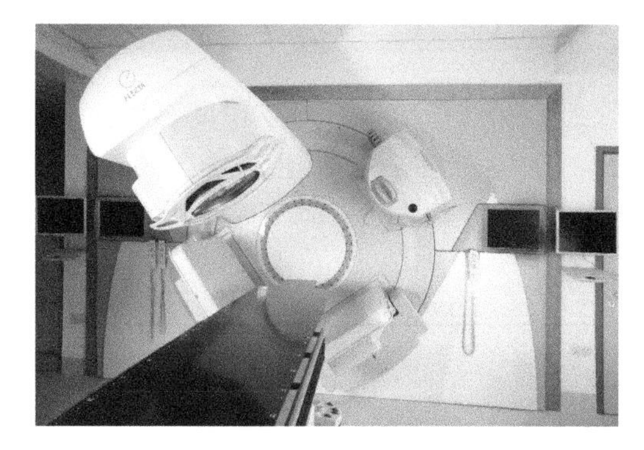

Figure 5.4 Elekta Synergy® 3 linear accelerator with cone beam CT scanner for image-guided radiation therapy.

three-dimensional (3D) volume from the two-dimensional (2D) projection images [57]. The high-spatial resolution in the z-direction of the flat-panel detectors makes it possible to reconstruct volumes with a high resolution in all three directions. The major advantage of integrated CBCT systems is that they provide volumetric images with soft-tissue contrast taken at isocenter position enabling in-room verification of the target position just prior to dose delivery. On the other hand, soft-tissue contrast is lower than for diagnostic CT scanners due to respiratory motion blurring and scatter radiation contributions originating from the patient. The latter can be reduced by collimating the cone beam in the z-direction, the use of a bow-tie filter, iterative reconstruction techniques, or an anti-scatter grid [58–60].

Respiration correlated CBCT (4D-CBCT) takes advantage of the slow acquisition time of a CBCT by retrospectively sorting and binning the projection images to the breathing phase and subsequently reconstructing the volumetric images for distinct phases of the breathing cycle into a 4D-CBCT dataset [61]. In this way, not only can the mean position of the target can be verified, but also the trajectory and target shape. Sweeney et al. demonstrated that—compared to 3D or motion-blurred CBCT—respiratory-correlated 4D-CBCT improved the accuracy of target localization of tumors that move with respiration and reduced interobserver variability in the image-guidance workflow [62]. Despite technological advances in image quality, soft-tissue contrast in CBCT scans remains limited. For tumors centrally located and for involved nodes, CBCT scans often do not provide sufficient contrast for image guidance. Alternatively, implanted fiducial markers or the injection of radiopaque contrast agents can be used to improve target localization in the CBCT images. Other in-room imaging techniques, e.g., diagnostic CT-on-rails or in-room MRI, provide better soft-tissue contrast.

The center of the CBCT imaging system, often referred as the imaging (or kV) isocenter, is mechanically connected to the treatment (or MV) isocenter. For safe application of CBCT-based image guidance the imaging isocenter needs to be calibrated to the treatment isocenter and this calibration should be tested periodically. The test frequency depends on the clinical application. For example, in lung SBRT patient positioning, daily quality assurance checks of the geometric accuracy are highly recommended. For calibration, a ball bearing is centered at the treatment isocenter using portal imaging. The portal images are acquired at four gantry angles (0, 90, 180, and 270 degrees) and at two collimator angles (0 and 180 degrees) each, to eliminate the gantry angle dependence of the radiation center and to eliminate variation in the positioning of the jaws. After a careful alignment of the ball bearing, which is usually an iterative process of correction and verification based on the portal images, CBCT projection images of the ball bearing are acquired. The projection images yield the position of the ball bearing as a function of the gantry angle on the imaging panel. This position is not fixed due to the flex of the gantry and its components due to gravity. The position data are stored as a flex map and can be used for correction either by a software shift, comparing the projection images before reconstruction, or by a real-time adjustment of the position of the imaging panel. Both techniques also calibrate the imaging center to the radiation center.

5.4.1.2 CT-ON-RAILS

A CT-on-rails system combines a diagnostic CT scanner with a medical linac. The CT scanner is positioned inside the treatment room and the treatment couch is shared with the CT scanner. Uematsu et al. were the first to develop such a system for frameless, fractionated stereotactic treatments of tumors in the brain and in the lung. In contrast to a conventional CT scan where the patient moves, the gantry of the CT moves over the patient, acquiring a volumetric data set. To this end, the CT scanner gantry is mounted on rails and is also referred to as sliding CT. The most salient advantage is the ability to acquire images with diagnostic CT quality just prior to dose delivery. Additional advantages are the ability to use intravenous contrast agents and a lower dose, compared with CBCT scanning [63]. The disadvantage of this process is that the imaging does not take place at the treatment isocenter. In the setup of Uematsu et al. the couch must rotate by 180 degrees to go from the imaging position to the treatment position. During rotation, the patient remains immobilized on the treatment couch. Figure 5.5 shows a CT-on-rails combined with a CyberKnife system (Accuray, Sunnyvale, US).

In this setup, a robotic couch transports the patient by a 90-degree rotation from the imaging to the treatment location. Similar to CBCT imaging, accurate image guidance needs a fixed relationship between the imaging and treatment isocenter. Compared to CBCT systems, this is less trivial for CT-on-rails systems as this relationship depends on the mechanical accuracy of two devices and the precision of the table couch. Court et al. demonstrated that for a CT-on-rails setup at 180 degrees with respect to the linac a submillimeter precision (1 standard deviation) could be achieved [64]. Alternatively, radiopaque markers on the patient can be used to transfer the imaging isocenter to the treatment isocenter [64]. Compared to CBCT imaging the adoption of CT-on-rails systems was slow. However, there is renewed interest from the field of particle therapy. For particle therapy, daily monitoring of the patient anatomy and accurate conversion of CT numbers to relative stopping power is crucial to mitigate uncertainties in the range of the particles [65–67].

5.4.1.3 MV CT

Instead of using a separate kV radiation source, the therapeutic MV beam can also be used to acquire a volumetric image of a patient. This has been implemented clinically in the TomoTherapy® system (Accuray, Sunnyvale, US) [68,69]. The system can produce fan-beam helical CT images using the collimated treatment beam. The use of the treatment beam makes the alignment of the imaging and the treatment center straightforward. The collimated fan beam produces less scatter and fewer beam hardening effects and is also

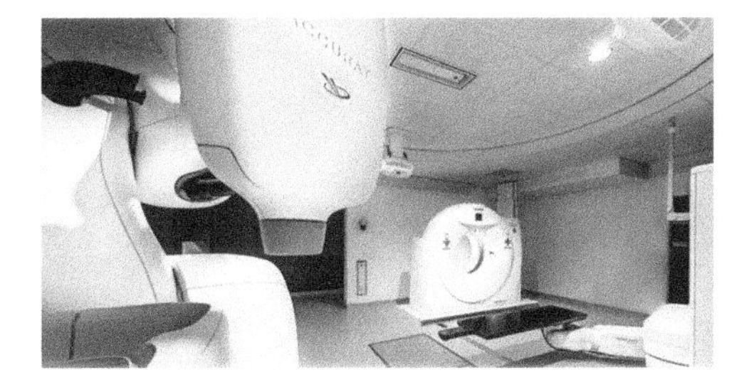

Figure 5.5 CyberKnife® system combined with a CT scanner on rails as installed at Erasmus MC, Rotterdam, The Netherlands.

less sensitive to high-Z materials compared to kV CT and CBCT solutions. Another advantage here is that the beam can be modeled in the treatment planning system such that the imaging dose can be calculated and incorporated in the treatment plan. However, MV CT imaging suffers from reduced soft-tissue contrast compared to kV CT imaging, even though the energy of the imaging beam is reduced from 6 MV to 3.5 MV.

5.4.1.4 INTEGRATED MRI

Obviously, the highest soft-tissue contrast can be achieved by integrating MR imaging with a radiation therapy unit. Various groups are developing such a system but currently, only one system (MRIdian®, ViewRay®, Cleveland, US) is commercially available. This system combines a 0.35 Tesla MR scanner with a radiation therapy unit using three Cobalt-60 heads as the radiation source. Apart from the improved soft-tissue contrast, an additional advantage is that no ionization radiation is used to acquire volumetric images of the patient and volumetric imaging can be performed while the beam is on.

The University Medical Center (UMC) Utrecht together with Elekta and Philips Healthcare are developing a system that integrates a linac with an MRI system. The system comprises a 6 MV linac which is combined with a modified 1.5 T MRI scanner [70]. The accelerator rotates on a ring-shaped gantry around the MRI scanner. Other projects integrating real-time MR imaging and treatment are the linac-MR system under development at Cross Cancer Institute, Edmonton, Canada [71] and the MRI-LINAC project of the University of Sydney, Australia [72].

5.4.2 Planar imaging techniques

5.4.2.1 STEREOSCOPIC kV-BASED SYSTEMS

Acquisition of two orthogonal x-ray kV images can be used to reconstruct the location of common features in the 2D images to 3D coordinates. The advantage is a fast acquisition in tenths of a second and the low dose needed. An obvious disadvantage of planar imaging is the lack of volumetric image information and low soft-tissue contrast. Therefore, the stereoscopic planar imaging techniques are predominantly used to align the bony anatomy to the planning CT scan using Digital Reconstructed Radiographs (DRRs) as reference or for localizing fiducial markers implanted inside or near the tumor. In the latter case, the 2D positions of the markers are manually or automatically extracted from the x-ray images and back projected to reconstruct their 3D coordinates in the imaging center of the treatment unit. Like the volumetric image-guidance systems, the imaging center and the treatment center should be accurately aligned and checked periodically. For tumors in the lung that are of sufficient size, and that are peripherally located, the kV planar images may provide adequate contrast to localize the tumor directly in the images (Figure 5.6) [73].

By repeated acquisition of the stereoscopic x-ray images across the different phases of the respiratory cycle, the planar imaging system can be used to build a correlation model that relates the implanted markers with an external breathing signal. Subsequently, this correlation model can be used to track the tumor that moves respiration in real time by adjusting the position of the treatment beam. Examples of systems that feature real-time respiratory motion tracking are the CyberKnife [74] and the Vero system (Brainlab, Feldkirchen, Germany) [75].

5.4.2.2 FIDUCIAL MARKERS

Metallic markers, for example, made of gold, are often used as surrogates for tumor locations in the lung. In particular, in the thorax, those markers are clearly visible using kV planar imaging and can be detected automatically by the image-guidance or tracking system. Various techniques exist to implant fiducial markers in or around the tumor. The standard technique to implant markers is the percutaneous transthoracic puncture under CT guidance. However, the risk of a pneumothorax after marker placement may be unacceptably high [76]. An alternative is the use of vascular embolization coils [77]. Those coils are inserted through the femoral vein and placed in small subsegmental pulmonary artery branches surrounding the tumor. A third method is ultrasound-guided bronchoscopy marker implantation.

It is important that the positions of the implanted markers relative to the tumor remain stable to accurately align the treatment beams to the tumor. However, markers may migrate from their positions that were localized

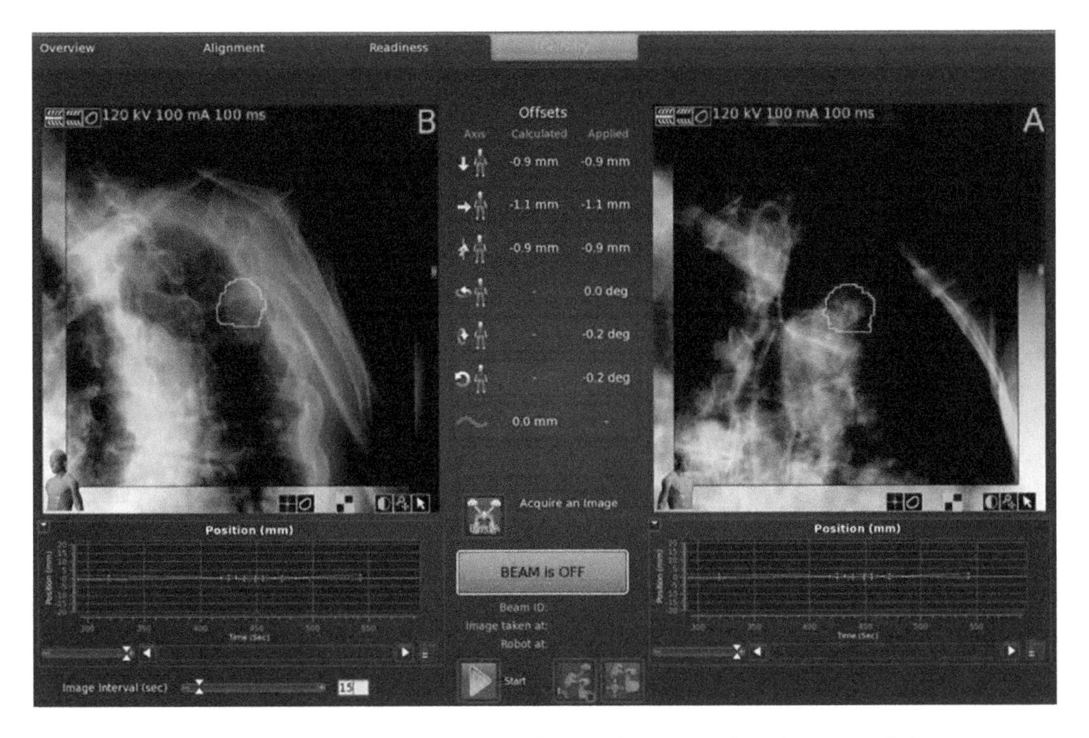

Figure 5.6 Screen capture of the tracking console software. The images show the acquired planar image in a blue overlay on top of the DRR. Images A and B each correspond to an orthogonal imager. The solid blue line outlines the tracking target volume and is positioned at the location the automatic tracking algorithm found the tumor.

in the planning CT scanning before and during the radiation therapy course [78]. Van der Voort van Zyp et al. studied the stability of markers placed using the percutaneous intrapulmonary method [79]. Repeat CT scans were used to detect marker displacements relative to the tumor. Although the authors found that the median marker displacement was small, marker displacement exceeded 5 mm in 12% of the implanted markers and 10 mm in 5% of the implanted markers. Considering the risk of displacement, it was recommended to implant multiple markers instead of a single marker. The use of multiple markers enables an easy check of marker displacements by calculating the change in the mutual marker distances. This check was considered reliable as it was found to detect targeting errors equal to or greater than 2 mm in 97% of the treatment fractions in lung SBRT. Alternatively, the position of an implanted marker relative to the tumor may be checked using volumetric imaging.

5.5 INTRAFRACTIONAL MOTION LOCALIZATION AND VERIFICATIONS

5.5.1 Monoscopic, stereoscopic, and hybrid planar X-ray imaging

Monoscopic imaging—or the acquisition of data using a single source/imager—includes single-modality on-board MV and kV imaging. However, single-imager systems are not adequate for intrafraction motion localization due to lung tumor complex 3D motion patterns [80]. Berbeco et al. hypothesized that using a single gantry-mounted source and *a priori* knowledge of tumor target trajectory, monoscopic imaging would be sufficient for real-time tumor tracking [81]. However, in a feasibility study of seven lung cancer patients with tumor excursion >1 cm, five cases had mean localization errors >2 mm and two cases had mean errors >3 mm. Thus, they recommended the use of stereoscopic localization—or two source/imager pairs—for robust 3D

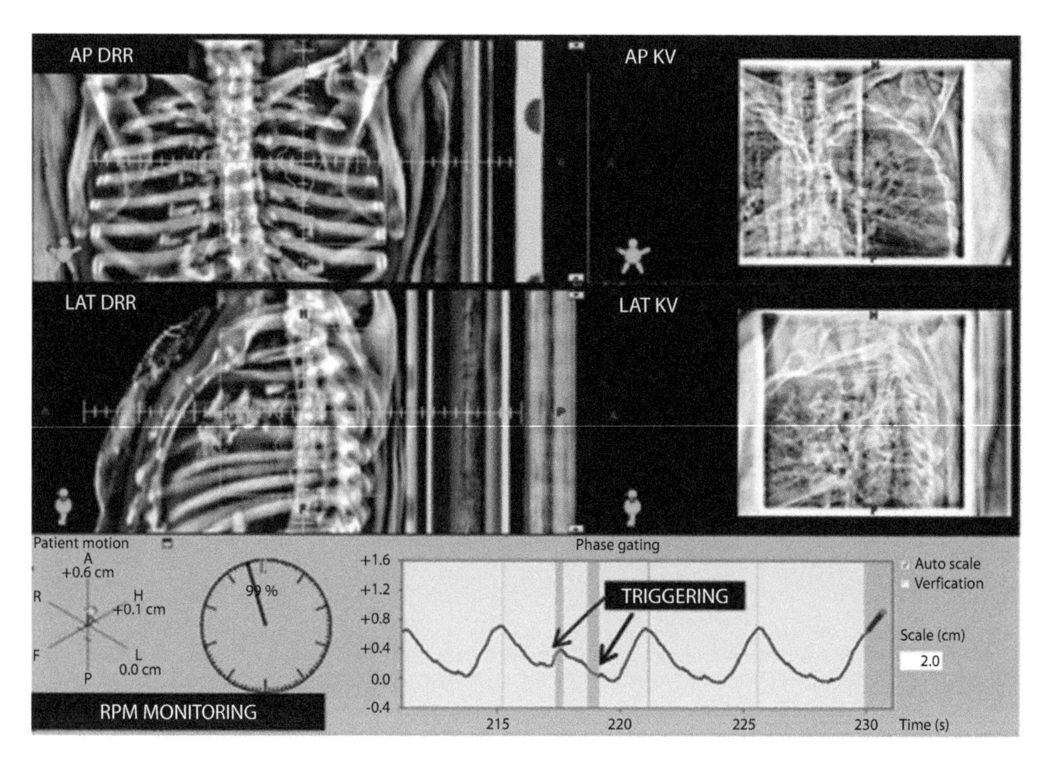

Figure 5.7 Screen capture of the treatment console for online setup. The images show the acquired orthogonal planar images (right) and the corresponding DRRs (left). Varian RPM is used to trigger the imaging acquisition.

target localization. Stereoscopic imaging involves taking images from two different angles in a fixed geometry to reconstruct 3D information via triangulation of corresponding features.

The Exactrac gating system (BrainLAB AG, Feldkirchen, Germany) combines infrared, optical, and stereoscopic kV imaging. Two amorphous silicon detectors are mounted to the ceiling while the corresponding kV x-ray sources are floor mounted to enable 3D localization of implanted fiducials at or near lung tumors [82,83]. During treatment, monoscopic intrafraction "snapshot" images Snap Verification (BrainlAB AG, Feldkirchen, Germany) can also be acquired using one of the oblique digital radio graphics to monitor patient motion [84]. The infrared and optical systems can also be used to detect patient motion and monitor patient respiration for gating of the treatment beam while stereoscopic KV images verify target position within the gating window. A cohort of 11 patients with upper lobe lung lesions were treated using gating with implanted fiducials and localization accuracy using the stereoscopic imaging system was 1.7 mm [82].

While not simultaneous, Figure 5.7 shows how on-board AP and lateral KV images can be used together to generate a 3D couch shift. Also, note how Varian RPM is used to trigger the imaging acquisition. In this case, no gating is implemented for this patient and thus images are triggered at arbitrary time points in the breathing cycle.

Hybrid methods have also been described, for example, where monoscopic imaging is used for real-time tumor tracking combined with instances of internal target monitoring and continuous external surrogate tracking [85]. While this hybrid model was found to have ~10% higher error as compared to stereoscopic localization, the imaging dose was halved.

5.5.2 X-RAY FLUOROSCOPY

Historically, x-ray fluoroscopy was implemented in conventional simulators to assess lung tumor motion for treatment planning [2]. With the advent of 4D-CT, more common applications of fluoroscopy are via on-board x-ray imaging. Like monoscopic imaging, on-board fluoroscopy using standard linacs is limited to assessing intrafraction lung tumor motions in two of three dimensions [80,86] unless two subsequent orthogonal portals are used. From the anterior or posterior direction, the apex of the diaphragm, tumor, or other nearby area of interest can be identified in a frame and then tracked in subsequent frames via a template-matching technique to track motion trajectories [86]. Other specialized systems, such as the integrated radiotherapy imaging system (IRIS) [81], consists of two pairs of gantry-mounted diagnostic x-ray tubes and flat-panel imagers that can acquire real-time orthogonal fluoroscopic images for lung tumor tracking. In the seminal work by Seppenwoolde et al. real-time fluoroscopic imaging was made possible by measuring 3D trajectories of fiducial markers located at or near the tumor using the real-time tumor-tracking system (RTRT system) (Mitsubishi Electronics Co. Ltd., Tokyo, Japan). The RTRT system uses four sets of diagnostic x-ray systems oriented with the central axis at the isocenter from several oblique angles for marker tracking [26,78,80,87,88]. In practice, TG-76 recommends a minimum of 30 seconds of fluoroscopy imaging data to characterize motion of the gross tumor volume or nearby anatomic surrogate while ensuring <0.5 second latency between external surrogates [2].

5.5.3 Cine imaging using electronic portal imaging devices (EPIDs)

Several investigators have explored the use of the EPID in cine mode that acquires data in the beam's eye view while the treatment beam is on [89–91]. Images are passively acquired, but may be limited when the beam is obscured by the multi-leaf collimators (i.e., with IMRT). Using the EPID in such a manner can enable verification of the tumor's presence within the treatment portal with no extra imaging dose and equipment needed. Acquisition frame rates on the order of <1 fps for older models [89,92] and ~9 fps for more modern EPIDs [93] have been reported. Recent efforts have suggested a minimum frame rate of ~4.3 fps is necessary for marking less tumor tracking [94].

5.5.4 Fiducial marker

In a similar manner to Exactrac, the Synchrony® Respiratory Tracking System, which is part of the CyberKnife® Robotic Radiosurgery System (Accuray Inc., Sunnyvale, CA) [34,95] that can make real-time adjustments to changes in tumor position, uses a stereotactic localization positioning system with two ceiling-mounted kV x-ray tubes and accompanying orthogonally flat-panel imagers on the floor. Two to four markers are implanted at or near the tumor and tracked with the kV imaging system. Their position is then back-projected, to derive the 3D coordinates while the external surface is being tracked by three optical markers affixed to the patient's chest to develop an external-internal correlation model [74]. The correspondence model predicts the tumor position, sends feedback to the robotic linac, and then the robot realigns the beam with the tumor. Correlation errors have been reported to be <0.3 mm with time lag to prediction ranging from 115 to 192.5 ms, depending on which prediction model is being implemented [74]. Another real-time tumor-tracking system (RTRT system) (Mitsubishi Electronics Co. Ltd., Tokyo, Japan) uses four sets of diagnostic x-ray systems oriented with the central axis at the isocenter from several oblique angles to track gold markers implanted at or near moving tumors [26,78,80,87,88].

5.5.5 Optical surface

AlignRT®, also known as the Optical Surface Monitoring System (OSMS) (Vision RT, London, UK), is a video-based, 3D imaging system that uses a projected speckled-light pattern to derive 3D surface images using three ceiling-mounted camera units (one central and two lateral) for surface rendering. For intrafraction motion monitoring, a reference surface image is taken, and a region of interest (ROI) on the abdomen surface is selected (Figure 5.8 (right)). The intersection point between the normal between the reference surface and the real-time surface patch reconstructed is used to compute the "normal displacement" for each subsequent frame [96]. In the example case shown in Figure 5.8, the initial patient setup using OSMS is shown on the left, while a tracking surface and resultant breathing amplitude is shown on the right. 3D optical surface tracking has been shown to be strongly associated with tumor and diaphragm motion as determined by on-board fluoroscopy [86], with the added advantage of being non-invasive, tracking online, in near real-time, with no associated imaging dose. However, the approach may need to be combined with other imaging

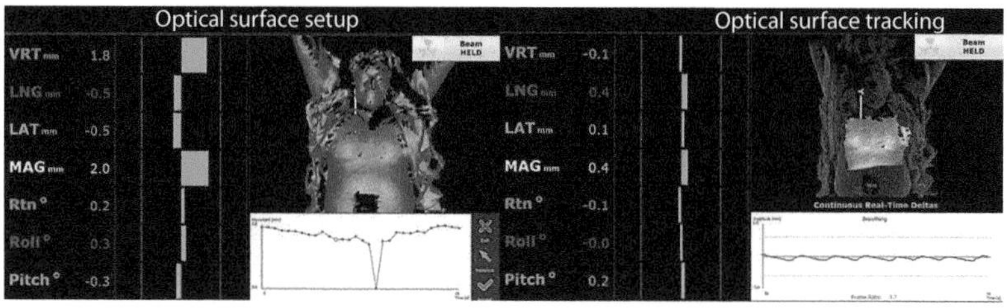

Figure 5.8 Screen capture of the OSMS console. The initial patient setup using OSMS is shown on the left, while a tracking surface and resultant breathing amplitude is shown on the right.

such as planar images (MV/KV) or CBCT to visualize alignment with internal anatomy or to ascertain the relationship between internal and external anatomy.

5.5.6 Electromagnetic beacons

The Calypso Electromagnetic Transponder system (Varian Medical Systems, Palo Alto, CA) was developed to track tumors in real time. Review articles by D'Ambrosio et al. [97] and Shah et al. [98] provide detailed information about technical aspects of this technology, how it is used clinically, and benefits and limitations, based on early clinical studies. As described by Balter et al. [21], the Calypso system uses an array of AC magnetic coils to generate a resonant response in implanted transponders, which is subsequently detected using a separate array of receiver coils. The transponders are approximately 8 mm in length and 2 mm in diameter. Typically, three beacons are implanted, though the system can use as few as two [99]. The beacon coordinates are identified on a treatment planning CT, and the offset between the centroid and the intended (treatment planning) isocenter is reported at a frequency of 10 Hz (or every 0.1 s). The location of the array relative to the linac isocenter is defined through a calibration procedure, and the array itself is tracked in the room using the three ceiling-mounted infra-red cameras.

The Calypso system is used in the clinic as follows:

1. The patient is first localized using the skin marks and room lasers.
2. The Calypso system is subsequently used in localization mode by moving the couch in three dimensions until the offset between the beacon-defined centroid and the treatment planning isocenter is noted to be zero. This process establishes the patient's initial treatment position.
3. During treatment, the system continuously monitors and reports the offset (in the three dimensions) between the actual and the desired isocenter locations. Centers may then choose to re-localize the patient or interrupt treatment based on the observed intrafraction motion if the motion exceeds a specified threshold (e.g., a threshold of 3 mm for a duration of 30 s continuously) [100].

Clinically, the Calypso transponder system has been cleared by the U.S. Food and Drug Administration (FDA) for use in prostate cancers, where it has been used successfully to track intrafraction prostate motion [97,100]. Using the criterion that 90% of patients receive 95% of the prescribed dose within the PTV, Litzenberg et al. [101] showed that planning margins required to accommodate intrafraction motions were approximately 2 mm in all directions. In the absence of Calypso-based localization, these margins are approximately 10 mm, indicating that a substantial reduction in margins is possible when daily alignment is performed using the Calypso system, in the context of prostate cancer [101]. To assess the accuracy of motion prediction using Calypso, investigators have performed 4D phantom studies using arbitrary multidimensional motion traces and have shown errors with Calypso tracking to be within 1 mm, which compared favorably to continuous fluoroscopic tracking methods, without the ionizing radiation burden [102].

Although Calypso transponders are not currently approved for implantation within lung tumors, an animal study involving implantation of the FDA-approved transponders within canine lungs has been carried out. This study (performed in five canines) analyzed transponder migration over 57 days [103] and demonstrated that measurements taken on the first day post-implant varied significantly from later measurements (up to day 9), presumably due to local tissue trauma. The inter-transponder distances were stable up to 30 days post-implant with mean values ranging from 0.9 to 1.9 mm from days 9–29 [103]. In one animal, the geometric relationship between the transponders changed after 30 days [103]. Furthermore, retention of the transponders was problematic, as only one animal retained all three transponders for the full duration of the study and two of four others lost all three transponders [103]. There has been one clinical study involving the insertion of FDA-approved Calypso transponders in human lungs. Shah et al. [20] performed an Institutional Review Board (IRB)-approved clinical trial (with off-label use of the transponders for lung cancer cleared by the FDA per protocol) in which Calypso transponders were implanted in the lungs of seven lung cancer patients to assess real-time tumor tracking. The aims of their study were to investigate the safety of bronchoscopic transponder implantations and the stability and retention rate of the transponders, in addition to acquiring 4D motion information [20]. The authors could implant at least one transponder for each of the seven patients, but noted that for three patients, insertion into the lung proved difficult, with only one transponder remaining fixed during implantation [20]. They further reported that 13 of 14 transponders remained stable within the lung and were successfully tracked with the Calypso system. Of note, one patient developed a pneumothorax after implantation of a transponder [20]. The authors concluded that, in using the Calypso system to track the motion of lung tumors in real time, lung tumor motion was found to exhibit large interfraction variations within a given patient [20]. They cautioned that improvements to both the transponder and tracking system are still necessary to create a clinically feasible system for routine use in radiation therapy [20].

In summary, the Calypso electromagnetic transponder system has been shown to be clinically useful for tracking real-time motion of the prostate. Challenges associated with the use of Calypso include the invasiveness and morbidity associated with implantation of transponders within lung tumors [20], artifacts and contradictions related to the use of MRI for patients with implanted transponders [104], and limitations to reimbursement to cover implantation of the transponders and other technical costs in radiation therapy [98]. While the technology shows promise for use in lung cancer patients, optimization of the tools, as well as additional clinical investigations, are warranted before the technology can be applied routinely in the clinical setting.

5.6 DELIVERY TECHNIQUES AND CONSIDERATIONS

Techniques used to deliver treatments to lung cancer patients may vary depending on the specific treatment platform. Linacs are used in radiotherapy to achieve photon energies able to penetrate tumors located within the body. Common delivery platforms include c-arm Linacs as well as Linacs mounted on robotic arms and slip ring gantries. The goal of any delivery technique is to deliver the correct dose accurately to the tumor volume. These can be categorized into two major subgroups, 3D-CRT and IMRT.

5.6.1 3D CONFORMAL RADIOTHERAPY

In 3D-CRT, the aperture of the beam is shaped to the target volume from the beam's-eye-view [105] of each field. The beam is then shaped using multi-leaf collimators (MLCs), which consist of multiple leaves of high Z material which attenuate and shape the radiation to the target volume. With the 3D-CRT delivery technique, beams can either be static fields or move dynamically during treatment. In static field 3D-CRT, 7–10 beams are spread out evenly, either in a coplanar or non-coplanar fashion, using a combination of gantry and couch angles. Beam weights and aperture shapes are manually modified by the treatment planner to create a conformal dose distribution.

Dynamic conformal arc (DCA) is a common 3D-CRT delivery method in which the gantry moves around a fixed isocenter. An arc is split into multiple control points which are used to direct the machine delivery. The MLCs conform to the target in the BEV at each control point, and as the gantry rotates, the MLCs move dynamically to reach the position at the next control point. The MLCs move to change the shape of the beam aperture, but are not used to modulate the intensity beam. The weight of each arc can be manually modified to provide more conformal coverage. Due to the ellipsoidal dose distributions resulting from this delivery technique, it is often used in cranial stereotactic radiosurgery to treat small circular lesions [106]. However, because the weighting cannot be modified within an arc and the choice of gantry angles and pedestal rotations are often limited in the thorax due to machine clearance, the hot spot typically occurs laterally in the target with poorer coverage medially. This difference is accentuated for larger targets; therefore, the DCA technique is typically used for SBRT of small spherical lesions.

5.6.2 Intensity-modulated radiotherapy

In IMRT, the beam is modulated using MLCs to create a desired dose distribution. Unlike 3D-CRT, IMRT beams are modulated to minimize dose to organs-at-risk (OARs) that are in close proximity to the target. This is accomplished by using inverse optimization. The optimization uses a cost function to achieve the desired target dose while minimizing the dose to the OARs. Each beam has a unique fluency map made up of small beamlets that are delivered by the MLCs using either of two techniques: sliding window or step-and-shoot. In sliding window IMRT delivery, the MLCs are continuously moving while the beam is on. The amount of radiation that passes through the leaves is dictated by the speed of and distance between the leaves. In step-and-shoot IMRT delivery, the MLCs form multiple static field shapes, and a set amount of radiation is delivered before moving to the next MLC shape.

5.6.2.1 Volumetric modulated arc therapy

Like the 3D-CRT technique, IMRT can be delivered using a fixed-beam or rotational technique. One common rotational IMRT technique is volumetric modulated arc therapy (VMAT), based on the work by Otto et al. [107]. In VMAT, the beam is delivered in a continuous arc while the gantry speed, MLCs, and dose rate are all modulated to achieve the desired dose distribution. In lung treatment delivery, partial arcs are often used to avoid collisions with the gantry and the couch and to avoid beams entering through the contralateral lung.

5.6.2.2 Tomotherapy

Another common form of rotational IMRT is TomoTherapy. In TomoTherapy, a linac is mounted on a slip ring gantry. The beam is delivered by a beam collimated slit beam, which is further modulated with a binary MLC. While the linac rotates, the patient is translated longitudinally through the machine, like a CT imaging machine where the longitudinal motion can either be in a stepwise or continuous fashion.

5.6.3 Normal lung dose

While IMRT has proved to be effective in treating prostate and head and neck cancers with conformal, concave dose distributions that reduce dose to the OARs [108]. The advantages of IMRT in treating lung cancer are still debatable due to uncertainties in delivered dose distributions introduced by respiratory motion.

Before the introduction of IMRT, lung cancer patients were treated using 3D-CRT techniques with simple field arrangements such as opposed anterior-to-posterior (AP-PA) fields or three to four fields, avoiding the cord and the contralateral lung. Several studies have shown that IMRT can decrease dose to the surrounding organs at risk as well as lower the volume of lung receiving 20 Gy (V20) and mean lung dose [108–111]. However, for IMRT, the spread of low doses to normal lung tissues has been shown to increase. This low dose spread is often evaluated by the volume of lung receiving 5Gy (V5), which is thought to correlate with increased risk of radiation pneumonitis. This increase in low dose may be due to the increase in the number of fields and complexity of the plan, which further increases the number of monitor units, beam on time, and leakage through the MLCs. The low dose spread is further increased in arc techniques such as VMAT where the beam is continuously delivering radiation. Figure 5.9 shows an example of a target planned with equivalent target coverage using four different treatment techniques.

5.6.4 MLC interplay effect

Although IMRT can be a powerful tool used to minimize and shape dose to OARs, the complexity of an IMRT delivery can be a factor in accurately delivering doses. One of the concerns in IMRT delivery of lung cancer is the interplay between the motion of the tumor volume due to respiratory motion and the motion of

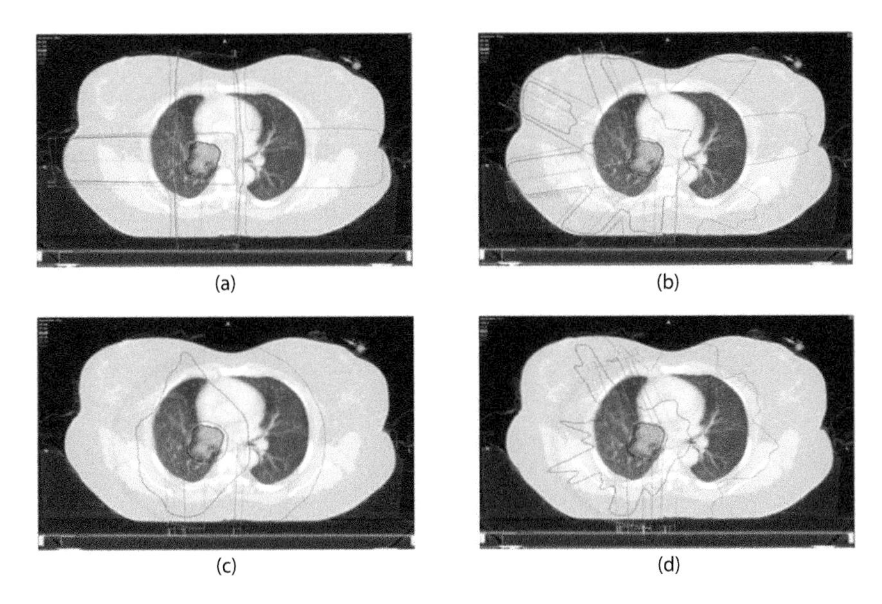

Figure 5.9 Example of a target planned with equivalent target coverage using four different treatment techniques: a 3-field 3D plan (a), a 5-field IMRT plan (b), a dynamic conformal arc (DCA) plan (c), and a 2-arc VMAT plan (d). Note the larger spread of the 5Gy isodose line (dark green) in the rotation techniques (DCA (c) and VMAT (d)) compared to the techniques (3D-CRT (a) and IMRT (b)). Also, note the increase in conformality of the 90% isodose line (dark blue) from the intensity modulated techniques (IMRT (b) and VMAT (d)) compared to the 3D-CRT techniques (3D-CRT (a) and DCA (c)).

the MLCs as illustrated in Figure 5.10. The discrepancy between planned and delivered doses increases with the amount of modulation and delivery complexity, which is dependent on the combination of MLC speed and segment size.

Other factors that can exacerbate the interplay effect include large amplitude tumor motion, high breathing frequency, high dose gradients, insufficient margins, and areas of high heterogeneity such as at the tumor/lung interface. Several studies have been performed to quantify the interplay effect [112–115] using either simulations or phantom measurements. Jiang et al. showed that in one fraction, dose discrepancies up to 18% are possible. Due to arbitrary position and phases the tumor is located in during the start of treatment, when the treatment is fractionated and delivered over 30 fractions the difference is reduced to 1–2% [113]. Furthermore, by minimizing the MLC modulation by decreasing the maximum leaf speed and minimizing the number of small segments, the dose discrepancy can be kept to a minimum [112]. A trade-off may exist with the use of fewer segments and slower leaf speed, between a more modulated plan with a better dose distribution and a compromised dose distribution with a more robust delivery.

Interplay studies have also been performed looking at VMAT delivery for lung treatments. Several studies have found that the interplay effect is minimal and comparable to IMRT delivery [116]. One reason is that VMAT delivery differs from IMRT delivery in that the collimator is typically rotated at 30–45 degrees for optimization purposes and the MLCs move both in and out of the field, not only in one direction as in sliding window IMRT. The combination of collimator angle and MLC movements should theoretically help minimize the effect; however, VMAT plans that are highly modulated and contain many small MLC segments which may offset any of the benefits of the MLC/collimator geometry.

Yang et al. also studied the interplay effect in TomoTherapy delivery, where the interplay effect occurs between the superior-to-inferior motion of the target and the simultaneous movement of the patient longitudinally through the machine [117]. At a point in time, only a small area of the target volume is being irradiated by a narrow slit of radiation. Thus, depending on the position of the couch and the movement of the target, areas within the target may be over- or underdosed. Larger dose discrepancies occurred when the target speed was closest to the longitudinal couch speed, but this could be mitigated by decreasing the gantry rotation and using a larger field size. Greater discrepancies also occurred for sequential segmented delivery,

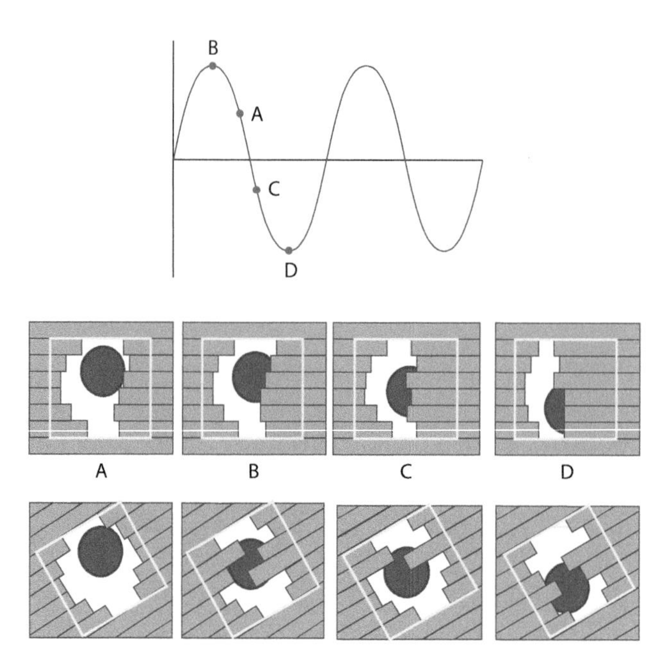

Figure 5.10 Example of the motion interplay for IMRT an VMAT techniques. Breathing trace (top) shown with four highlighted areas: (A) End inhale, (B) Mid inhale, (C) Mid exhale, (D) End exhale. Corresponding tumor location from the beam's eye view of the treatment field with examples of the MLC leaf postions for an IMRT plan (middle row) and VMAT plan (bottom row). Note differences in shapes of MLCs, where in IMRT, the target becomes more and more occluded as the MLCs move in one direction (right to left), in VMAT, the MLCs move in and out, blocking small areas of the target at one time.

where the couch is translated in a stepwise fashion, compared to helical delivery, where the couch moves continuously through the machine.

In 3D-CRT, the interplay effect is usually not an issue because the field is not modulated; thus for more mobile tumors with large motion amplitudes, 3D-CRT may be preferable. However, adequate margins must still be given to provide any underdosage at the edge of the beam aperture [118].

5.6.5 Dose rate and treatment time

Another method that has been suggested to minimize the interplay effect is to decrease the dose rate. Several studies have shown that the maximum interplay occurs when the tumor motion and leaf speeds are similar [114,115,119]. Thus, by lowering the dose rate, the leaf speed will decrease to create a greater difference between the tumor and leaf speeds. However, by decreasing the dose rate and increasing delivery time, the comfort of the patient must also be considered. Prolonged treatment times may cause the patient to move voluntarily or involuntarily on the treatment table, creating even larger unplanned dose discrepancies [120].

High dose rate beams are often used for SBRT in the treatment of early stage non-small-cell lung cancer. SBRT treatments are typically longer because a larger amount of dose is delivered in one fraction compared to conventional treatments. High dose rate beams without flattening filters have dose rates up to 2400 MU/min, which have been shown to decrease treatment times by up to 50% [121]. However, because SBRT treatments are delivered in fewer fractions the interplay effect can have a greater effect when not dispersed over a larger number of fractions. Studies have shown that the interplay effect in SBRT treatments using high dose rates is insignificant. This is partly because the MLCs move much slower at the very high dose rates; however, the amount of modulation and small segments should be kept to a minimum.

Studies have also shown a decrease in treatment time in VMAT compared to IMRT technique without any degradation in the target dose distribution [122]. VMAT delivery uses the treatment beam more efficiently by modulating the beam while continuously delivering the dose. However, the number of beams in both VMAT and IMRT plans is an important factor when comparing the two techniques. IMRT delivery time increases as more beams are used, and as the modulation increases the monitor units increase. The amount of modulation in VMAT is constrained by the MLC leaf position between control points in an arc. Thus, if more modulation is required additional arcs should be used, but as the number of VMAT arcs increases the treatment time increases. For a difficult plan that needs significant modulation, an IMRT plan may be more efficient, allowing for greater modulation within one beam without requiring additional beams and multiple arc passes.

5.7 SUMMARY

Accurate treatment of lung cancers is confounded by many technical factors, the two most important being associated with tumor motion and tissue heterogeneity. Considering the generally poor tumor control and survival rates associated with locally advanced stage non-small-cell lung cancers (NSCLC), ~15% five-year overall survival, and the relatively high incidence of normal tissue toxicity [123], the need for proper margin design and accurate planning and target accuracy is of paramount consideration. In the context of early stage NSCLC, where stereotactic ablative radiotherapy (SABR) is becoming a more mainstream treatment approach [124], technical factors arguably became even more important, as these patients are treated with five or less fractions and with doses ranging from 10 to 18 Gy per fraction.

5.7.1 Margin reduction

Van Herk et al. [53] proposed the theoretical framework for proper planning margin design. They defined the concepts of systematic and random errors, and showed that systematic errors have the potential to significantly impact target dose distributions; since for these errors, the potential to miss the target due to a systematic shift in the isocenter position, for instance, can lead to significant dosimetric consequences [53]. Respiratory-induced motion, if not properly managed, can result in large systematic differences between planned and delivered doses, potentially impacting accurate targeting and normal tissue sparing [2]. The most common approach for managing respiratory-induced motion at the time of simulation involves the use of a 4D-CT which is acquired by correlating the respiration trace (using an external surrogate of the motion) with time of acquisition. One is then able to sort the CT dataset into phases corresponding to the various states of respiration, from end inhale to end exhale. Information about the tumor motion is extracted from the 4D-CT dataset for design of the planning margins to form an ITV [125]. The ITV is further expanded to account for setup errors to specify the PTV. The design of the PTV is of utmost importance. A PTV designed with a small margin is likely to lead to a geometric miss of the target, while too large of a margin will lead to excessive doses to surrounding normal organs. In the context of lung cancer, where respiratory-induced motion confounds proper margin design, it is imperative that margins be assessed for individual patients during treatment, ultimately for optimization of the margin design for each patient.

IGRT has played a central role in reducing planning margins, ultimately to improve the therapeutic ratio for lung cancer patients. Online IGRT has been shown to regulate margin process control by enabling reduction of both systematic and random errors to within control limits [42]. Investigators have shown that planning margins can be reduced using many different online IGRT techniques [126,127], such as CBCT imaging [5,44,128–132], ultrasound-based IGRT [133], ABC [134], gating [135], and tracking [135,136].

5.7.2 Clinical outcome of IGRT for lung cancer

The dosimetric benefits associated with online IGRT, improved targeting accuracy, and better sparing of normal tissues have likely led to improvement in outcomes for patients with lung cancer, although first-level evidence (based on clinical trials) of impact of daily image guidance on outcomes is limited. Indeed, it has been reported in a detailed review of the impact of IGRT that the evidence "...supports that higher-quality dose delivery enabled by IGRT results in higher clinical control rates, reduced toxicity, and new treatment options for patients that previously were without viable options" [42]. The working group Extracranial Stereotactic

Radiotherapy of the German Society for Radiation Oncology performed a retrospective multicenter analysis of practice and outcome after SBRT for 582 patients with stage I NSCLC [137]. They found that the type of patient setup had a significant impact on 3-year freedom from local progression (FFLP). Daily in room IGRT showed an FFLP of 83%, which was significantly higher ($p = 0.006$) than that of daily pre-SBRT CT resimulation performed outside the treatment room (FFLP of 77%) [137]. Moreover, when patients were set up using stereotactic immobilization only, without IGRT, FFLP was significantly lower at 67% ($p = 0.006$) [137].

The ability to capture systematic drifts between simulation and treatment (baseline shifts) [138], as well as large magnitude excursions [139], emphasizes the importance of daily IGRT for lung cancer treatments. For locally advanced NSCLC, dose-volume-effect relationships have been published for normal organs, such as healthy lung tissue, and show clearly that increased dose to healthy lung tissue (for instance, due to excessively large planning margins) compromises parenchymal reserve, potentially resulting in dose-limiting toxicity, such as radiation pneumonitis [140]. Increased risk of radiation pneumonitis, resulting from violation of normal lung dose tolerances, has also been observed for early stage lung tumors treated with stereotactic ablative radiotherapy (SABR) [141]. The use of SABR has expanded to early stage, centrally located tumors, where other organs (e.g., the bronchial trees), are subject to dose-limiting toxicity, such as bronchial airway collapse [142]. For such tumors, careful attention must be given to motion and planning margin design, with the goal of reducing the dose to centrally located critical organs. Finally, one could argue that assessment of tumor response by daily volumetric IGRT during treatment for locally advanced lung tumors may show reduction in tumor volumes, leading to the potential for isotoxic dose escalation, which may well lead to improved outcomes. The Radiation Therapy Oncology Group (RTOG No. 1106) has initiated a cooperative group clinical trial to evaluate whether isotoxic dose escalation for locally advanced stage NSCLC, and enabled by mid-treatment CT and PET imaging, has an impact on outcomes [143].

In summary, IGRT for lung cancer treatments has been shown to provide more accurate targeting of the tumor and better sparing of normal tissues. IGRT has enabled reduction of planning margins, and therefore reduced dose to surrounding healthy tissues, making treatments safer. Moreover, reduction of planning margins afforded by IGRT may facilitate isotoxic dose escalation, and therefore potentially improve outcomes for patients with locally advanced NSCLC.

ACKNOWLEDGMENT

This work was supported in part by the American Cancer Society under a Research Scholar Grant RSG-15-137-01-CCE and the National Cancer Institute of the National Institutes of Health under Award Number R01CA204189.

REFERENCES

1. Purdie, T.G. et al., Cone-beam computed tomography for on-line image guidance of lung stereotactic radiotherapy: Localization, verification, and intrafraction tumor position. *Int J Radiat Oncol Biol Phys*, 2007. **68**(1): 243–52.
2. Keall, P.J. et al., The management of respiratory motion in radiation oncology report of AAPM Task Group 76. *Med Phys*, 2006. **33**(10): 3874–900.
3. Yeung, A.R. et al., Tumor localization using cone-beam CT reduces setup margins in conventionally fractionated radiotherapy for lung tumors. *Int J Radiat Oncol Biol Phys*, 2009. **74**(4): 1100–7.
4. Hof, H. et al., The use of the multislice CT for the determination of respiratory lung tumor movement in stereotactic single-dose irradiation. *Strahlenther Onkol*, 2003. **179**(8): 542–7.
5. Bissonnette, J.P. et al., Cone-beam computed tomographic image guidance for lung cancer radiation therapy. *Int J Radiat Oncol Biol Phys*, 2009. **73**(3): 927–34.
6. Borst, G.R. et al., Kilo-voltage cone-beam computed tomography setup measurements for lung cancer patients; first clinical results and comparison with electronic portal-imaging device. *Int J Radiat Oncol Biol Phys*, 2007. **68**(2): 555–61.

7. Imura, M. et al., Insertion and fixation of fiducial markers for setup and tracking of lung tumors in radiotherapy. *Int J Radiat Oncol Biol Phys*, 2005. **63**(5): 1442–7.
8. Timmerman, R.D. et al., A phase II trial of stereotactic body radiation therapy (SBRT) in the treatment of patients with operable stage I/II non-small cell lung cancer. RTOG 0618, 2012. https://www.rtog.org/ClinicalTrials/ProtocolTable/StudyDetails.aspx?study=0618.
9. Videtic, G. et al., A randomized phase II study comparing 2 stereotactic body radiation therapy (SBRT) schedules for medically inoperable patients with stage I peripheral non-small cell lung cancer. RTOG 0915, 2012. https://www.rtog.org/ClinicalTrials/ProtocolTable/StudyDetails.aspx?study=0915.
10. Zhao, B. et al., Dosimetric effect of intrafraction tumor motion in phase gated lung stereotactic body radiotherapy. *Med Phys*, 2012. **39**(11): 6629–37.
11. Rottmann, J. et al., A multi-region algorithm for markerless beam's-eye view lung tumor tracking. *Phys Med Biol*, 2010. **55**(18): 5585–98.
12. Rottmann, J., P. Keall, and R. Berbeco, Markerless EPID image guided dynamic multi-leaf collimator tracking for lung tumors. *Phys Med Biol*, 2013. **58**(12): 4195–204.
13. Murphy, M.J., Fiducial-based targeting accuracy for external-beam radiotherapy. *Med Phys*, 2002. **29**(3): 334–44.
14. Jaffray, D.A. and J.H. Siewerdsen, Cone-beam computed tomography with a flat-panel imager: Initial performance characterization. *Med Phys*, 2000. **27**(6): 1311–23.
15. Siewerdsen, J.H. and D.A. Jaffray, Cone-beam computed tomography with a flat-panel imager: Magnitude and effects of x-ray scatter. *Med Phys*, 2001. **28**(2): 220–31.
16. Ding, G.X. et al., Reducing radiation exposure to patients from kV-CBCT imaging. *Radiother Oncol*, 2010. **97**(3): 585–92.
17. Dempsey, J. et al., A real-time MRI guided external beam radiotherapy delivery system. *Med Phys*, 2006. **33**(6): 2254.
18. Lagendijk, J.J. et al., MRI/linac integration. *Radiother Oncol*, 2008. **86**(1): 25–9.
19. Cervino, L.I., J. Du, and S.B. Jiang, MRI-guided tumor tracking in lung cancer radiotherapy. *Phys Med Biol*, 2011. **56**(13): 3773–85.
20. Shah, A.P. et al., Real-time tumor tracking in the lung using an electromagnetic tracking system. *Int J Radiat Oncol Biol Phys*, 2013. **86**(3): 477–83.
21. Balter, J.M. et al., Accuracy of a wireless localization system for radiotherapy. *Int J Radiat Oncol Biol Phys*, 2005. **61**(3): 933–7.
22. Willoughby, T.R. et al., Target localization and real-time tracking using the Calypso 4D localization system in patients with localized prostate cancer. *Int J Radiat Oncol Biol Phys*, 2006. **65**(2): 528–34.
23. Wagman, R. et al., Respiratory gating for liver tumors: Use in dose escalation. *Int J Radiat Oncol Biol Phys*, 2003. **55**(3): 659–68.
24. Hugo, G.D., N. Agazaryan, and T.D. Solberg, The effects of tumor motion on planning and delivery of respiratory-gated IMRT. *Med Phys*, 2003. **30**(6): 1052–66.
25. Jiang, S.B., Technical aspects of image-guided respiration-gated radiation therapy. *Med Dosim*, 2006. **31**(2): 141–51.
26. Shirato, H. et al., Physical aspects of a real-time tumor-tracking system for gated radiotherapy. *Int J Radiat Oncol Biol Phys*, 2000. **48**(4): 1187–95.
27. Kubo, H.D. et al., Breathing-synchronized radiotherapy program at the University of California Davis Cancer Center. *Med Phys*, 2000. **27**(2): 346–53.
28. Geraghty, P.R. et al., CT-guided transthoracic needle aspiration biopsy of pulmonary nodules: Needle size and pneumothorax rate. *Radiology*, 2003. **229**(2): 475–81.
29. Guckenberger, M. et al., A novel respiratory motion compensation strategy combining gated beam delivery and mean target position concept a compromise between small safety margins and long duty cycles. *Radiother Oncol*, 2011. **98**(3): 317–22.
30. Kini, V.R. et al., Patient training in respiratory-gated radiotherapy. *Med Dosim*, 2003. **28**(1): 7–11.
31. Nelson, C. et al., Respiration-correlated treatment delivery using feedback-guided breath hold: A technical study. *Med Phys*, 2005. **32**(1): 175–81.

32. He, P. et al., Respiratory motion management using audio-visual biofeedback for respiratory-gated radiotherapy of synchrotron-based pulsed heavy-ion beam delivery. *Med Phys*, 2014. **41**(11): 111708.
33. George, R. et al., Audio-visual biofeedback for respiratory-gated radiotherapy: Impact of audio instruction and audio-visual biofeedback on respiratory-gated radiotherapy. *Int J Radiat Oncol Biol Phys*, 2006. **65**(3): 924–33.
34. Seppenwoolde, Y. et al., Accuracy of tumor motion compensation algorithm from a robotic respiratory tracking system: A simulation study. *Med Phys*, 2007. **34**(7): 2774–84.
35. Korreman, S.S., T. Juhler-Nottrup, and A.L. Boyer, Respiratory gated beam delivery cannot facilitate margin reduction, unless combined with respiratory correlated image guidance. *Radiother Oncol*, 2008. **86**(1): 61–8.
36. Kilby, W. et al., The CyberKnife® Robotic Radiosurgery System in 2010. *Technol Cancer Res Treat*, 2010. **9**(5): 433–52.
37. Keall, P.J. et al., The first clinical implementation of electromagnetic transponder-guided MLC tracking. *Med Phys*, 2014. **41**(2): 020702.
38. D'Souza, W.D., S.A. Naqvi, and C.X. Yu, Real-time intra-fraction-motion tracking using the treatment couch: A feasibility study. *Phys Med Biol*, 2005. **50**(17): 4021–33.
39. Poels, K. et al., A comparison of two clinical correlation models used for real-time tumor tracking of semi-periodic motion: A focus on geometrical accuracy in lung and liver cancer patients. *Radiother Oncol*, 2015. **115**(3): 419–24.
40. Tang, X., G.C. Sharp, and S.B. Jiang, Fluoroscopic tracking of multiple implanted fiducial markers using multiple object tracking. *Phys Med Biol*, 2007. **52**(14): 4081–98.
41. Guckenberger, M. et al., Intra-fractional uncertainties in cone-beam CT based image-guided radiotherapy (IGRT) of pulmonary tumors. *Radiother Oncol*, 2007. **83**(1): 57–64.
42. Bujold, A. et al., Image-guided radiotherapy: Has it influenced patient outcomes? *Semin Radiat Oncol*, 2012. **22**(1): 50–61.
43. Velec, M. et al., Effect of breathing motion on radiotherapy dose accumulation in the abdomen using deformable registration. *Int J Radiat Oncol Biol Phys*, 2011. **80**(1): 265–72.
44. Grills, I.S. et al., Image-guided radiotherapy via daily online cone-beam CT substantially reduces margin requirements for stereotactic lung radiotherapy. *Int J Radiat Oncol Biol Phys*, 2008. **70**(4): 1045–56.
45. Worm, E.S. et al., Inter- and intrafractional localisation errors in cone-beam CT guided stereotactic radiation therapy of tumours in the liver and lung. *Acta Oncol*, 2010. **49**(7): 1177–83.
46. Glide-Hurst, C.K. and I.J. Chetty, Improving radiotherapy planning, delivery accuracy, and normal tissue sparing using cutting edge technologies. *J Thorac Dis*, 2014. **6**(4): 303–18.
47. Khamene, A. et al., Automatic registration of portal images and volumetric CT for patient positioning in radiation therapy. *Med Image Anal*, 2006. **10**(1): 96–112.
48. Russakoff, D.B. et al., Fast generation of digitally reconstructed radiographs using attenuation fields with application to 2D-3D image registration. *IEEE Trans Med Imaging*, 2005. **24**(11): 1441–54.
49. Jin, J.Y. et al., 2D/3D image fusion for accurate target localization and evaluation of a mask based stereotactic system in fractionated stereotactic radiotherapy of cranial lesions. *Med Phys*, 2006. **33**(12): 4557–66.
50. Rohlfing, T. et al., Markerless real-time 3-D target region tracking by motion backprojection from projection images. *IEEE Trans Med Imaging*, 2005. **24**(11): 1455–68.
51. Li, G. et al., Clinical assessment of 2D/3D registration accuracy in 4 major anatomic sites using on-board 2D kilovoltage images for 6D patient setup. *Technol Cancer Res Treat*, 2015. **14**(3): 305–14.
52. Wolthaus, J.W. et al., Reconstruction of a time-averaged midposition CT scan for radiotherapy planning of lung cancer patients using deformable registration. *Med Phys*, 2008: 3998–4011.
53. van Herk, M. et al., The probability of correct target dosage: Dose-population histograms for deriving treatment margins in radiotherapy. *Int J Radiat Oncol Biol Phys*, 2000. **47**(4): 1121–35.
54. de Boer, H.C. and B.J. Heijmen, A protocol for the reduction of systematic patient setup errors with minimal portal imaging workload. *Int J Radiat Oncol Biol Phys*, 2001. **50**(5): 1350–65.
55. Sonke, J.J. et al., Frameless stereotactic body radiotherapy for lung cancer using four-dimensional cone beam CT guidance. *Int J Radiat Oncol Biol Phys*, 2009. **74**(2): 567–74.

56. Jaffray, D.A. et al., Flat-panel cone-beam computed tomography for image-guided radiation therapy. *Int J Radiat Oncol Biol Phys*, 2002. **53**(5): 1337–49.
57. Feldkamp, L.A., L.C. Davis, and S. Webb, Comments, with reply, on "Tomographic reconstruction from experimentally obtained cone-beam projections" by S. Webb, et al. *IEEE Trans Med Imaging*, 1988. **7**(1): 73–4.
58. Mail, N. et al., The influence of bowtie filtration on cone-beam CT image quality. *Med Phys*, 2009. **36**(1): 22–32.
59. Stankovic, U. et al., Improved image quality of cone beam CT scans for radiotherapy image guidance using fiber-interspaced antiscatter grid. *Med Phys*, 2014. **41**(6): 061910.
60. Yan, H. et al., Towards the clinical implementation of iterative low-dose cone-beam CT reconstruction in image-guided radiation therapy: Cone/ring artifact correction and multiple GPU implementation. *Med Phys*, 2014. **41**(11): 111912.
61. Sonke, J.J. et al., Respiratory correlated cone beam CT. *Med Phys*, 2005. **32**(4): 1176–86.
62. Sweeney, R.A. et al., Accuracy and inter-observer variability of 3D versus 4D cone-beam CT based image-guidance in SBRT for lung tumors. *Radiat Oncol*, 2012. **7**: 81.
63. Steiner, E. et al., Imaging dose assessment for IGRT in particle beam therapy. *Radiother Oncol*, 2013. **109**(3): 409–13.
64. Court, L. et al., Evaluation of mechanical precision and alignment uncertainties for an integrated CT/LINAC system. *Med Phys*, 2003. **30**(6): 1198–210.
65. Kraan, A.C. et al., Dose uncertainties in IMPT for oropharyngeal cancer in the presence of anatomical, range, and setup errors. *Int J Radiat Oncol Biol Phys*, 2013. **87**(5): 888–96.
66. Lomax, A.J., Intensity modulated proton therapy and its sensitivity to treatment uncertainties 2: The potential effects of inter-fraction and inter-field motions. *Phys Med Biol*, 2008. **53**(4): 1043–56.
67. Lomax, A.J., Intensity modulated proton therapy and its sensitivity to treatment uncertainties 1: The potential effects of calculational uncertainties. *Phys Med Biol*, 2008. **53**(4): 1027–42.
68. Meeks, S.L. et al., Performance characterization of megavoltage computed tomography imaging on a helical tomotherapy unit. *Med Phys*, 2005. **32**(8): 2673–81.
69. Woodford, C., S. Yartsev, and J. Van Dyk, Optimization of megavoltage CT scan registration settings for thoracic cases on helical tomotherapy. *Phys Med Biol*, 2007. **52**(15): N345–54.
70. Raaymakers, B.W. et al., Integrating a 1.5 T MRI scanner with a 6 MV accelerator: Proof of concept. *Phys Med Biol*, 2009. **54**(12): N229–37.
71. Yun, J. et al., First demonstration of intrafractional tumor-tracked irradiation using 2D phantom MR images on a prototype linac-MR. *Med Phys*, 2013. **40**(5): 051718.
72. Keall, P.J. et al., The Australian magnetic resonance imaging-linac program. *Semin Radiat Oncol*, 2014. **24**(3): 203–6.
73. Bahig, H. et al., Predictive parameters of CyberKnife fiducial-less (XSight Lung) applicability for treatment of early non-small cell lung cancer: A single-center experience. *Int J Radiat Oncol Biol Phys*, 2013. **87**(3): 583–9.
74. Hoogeman, M. et al., Clinical accuracy of the respiratory tumor tracking system of the CyberKnife: Assessment by analysis of log files. *Int J Radiat Oncol Biol Phys*, 2009. **74**(1): 297–303.
75. Depuydt, T. et al., Geometric accuracy of a novel gimbals based radiation therapy tumor tracking system. *Radiother Oncol*, 2011. **98**(3): 365–72.
76. Kupelian, P.A. et al., Implantation and stability of metallic fiducials within pulmonary lesions. *Int J Radiat Oncol Biol Phys*, 2007. **69**(3): 777–85.
77. Prevost, J.B. et al., Endovascular coils as lung tumour markers in real-time tumour tracking stereotactic radiotherapy: Preliminary results. *Eur Radiol*, 2008. **18**(8): 1569–76.
78. Harada, T. et al., Real-time tumor-tracking radiation therapy for lung carcinoma by the aid of insertion of a gold marker using bronchofiberscopy. *Cancer*, 2002. **95**(8): 1720–7.
79. van der Voort van Zyp, N.C. et al., Stability of markers used for real-time tumor tracking after percutaneous intrapulmonary placement. *Int J Radiat Oncol Biol Phys*, 2011. **81**(3): e75–81.
80. Seppenwoolde, Y. et al., Precise and real-time measurement of 3D tumor motion in lung due to breathing and heartbeat, measured during radiotherapy. *Int J Radiat Oncol Biol Phys*, 2002. **53**(4): 822–34.

81. Berbeco, R.I. et al., Integrated radiotherapy imaging system (IRIS): Design considerations of tumour tracking with linac gantry-mounted diagnostic x-ray systems with flat-panel detectors. *Phys Med Biol*, 2004. **49**(2): 243–55.
82. Willoughby, T.R. et al., Evaluation of an infrared camera and X-ray system using implanted fiducials in patients with lung tumors for gated radiation therapy. *Int J Radiat Oncol Biol Phys*, 2006. **66**(2): 568–75.
83. Siddiqui, F. et al., Image-guided radiation therapy for lung cancer, In *Image-Guided Cancer Therapy*, Dupuy, D.E., McMullen, W.N. (Eds.). 2013, New York, NY: Springer. pp. 585–606.
84. De Los Santos, J. et al., Image guided radiation therapy (IGRT) technologies for radiation therapy localization and delivery. *Int J Radiat Oncol Biol Phys*, 2013. **87**(1): 33–45.
85. Cho, B. et al., A monoscopic method for real-time tumour tracking using combined occasional x-ray imaging and continuous respiratory monitoring. *Phys Med Biol*, 2008. **53**(11): 2837–55.
86. Glide-Hurst, C.K. et al., Coupling surface cameras with on-board fluoroscopy: A feasibility study. *Med Phys*, 2011. **38**: 2937.
87. Shimizu, S. et al., Detection of lung tumor movement in real-time tumor-tracking radiotherapy. *Int J Radiat Oncol Biol Phys*, 2001. **51**(2): 304–10.
88. Shirato, H. et al., Four-dimensional treatment planning and fluoroscopic real-time tumor tracking radiotherapy for moving tumor. *Int J Radiat Oncol Biol Phys*, 2000. **48**(2): 435–42.
89. Berbeco, R.I. et al., Clinical feasibility of using an EPID in CINE mode for image-guided verification of stereotactic body radiotherapy. *Int J Radiat Oncol Biol Phys*, 2007. **69**(1): 258–66.
90. Berbeco, R.I. et al., A novel method for estimating SBRT delivered dose with beam's-eye-view images. *Med Phys*, 2008. **35**(7): 3225–31.
91. Park, S.-J. et al., Automatic marker detection and 3D position reconstruction using cine EPID images for SBRT verification. *Med Phys*, 2009. **36**(10): 4536–46.
92. Murphy, M.J. et al., The management of imaging dose during image-guided radiotherapy: Report of the AAPM Task Group 75. *Med Phys*, 2007. **34**(10): 4041–63.
93. Stanley, D.N., N. Papanikolaou, and A.N. Gutierrez, An evaluation of the stability of image-quality parameters of Varian on-board imaging (OBI) and EPID imaging systems. *J Appl Clin Med Phys*, 2015. **16**(2): 87–98.
94. Yip, S., J. Rottmann, and R. Berbeco, The impact of cine EPID image acquisition frame rate on markerless soft-tissue tracking. *Med Phys*, 2014. **41**(6): 061702.
95. Sayeh, S. et al., Respiratory motion tracking for robotic radiosurgery, in *Treating Tumors That Move with Respiration*. 2007, Berlin: Springer. 15–29.
96. Cervino, L.I. et al., Frame-less and mask-less cranial stereotactic radiosurgery: A feasibility study. *Phys Med Biol*, 2010. **55**(7): 1863–73.
97. D'Ambrosio, D.J. et al., Continuous localization technologies for radiotherapy delivery: Report of the American Society for Radiation Oncology Emerging Technology Committee. *Pract Radiat Oncol*, 2012. **2**(2): 145–50.
98. Shah, A.P. et al., Expanding the use of real-time electromagnetic tracking in radiation oncology. *J Appl Clin Med Phys*, 2011. **12**(4): 3590.
99. Litzenberg, D.W. et al., Positional stability of electromagnetic transponders used for prostate localization and continuous, real-time tracking. *Int J Radiat Oncol Biol Phys*, 2007. **68**(4): 1199–206.
100. Kupelian, P. et al., Multi-institutional clinical experience with the Calypso System in localization and continuous, real-time monitoring of the prostate gland during external radiotherapy. *Int J Radiat Oncol Biol Phys*, 2007. **67**(4): 1088–98.
101. Litzenberg, D.W. et al., Influence of intrafraction motion on margins for prostate radiotherapy. *Int J Radiat Oncol Biol Phys*, 2006. **65**(2): 548–53.
102. Parikh, P. et al., Dynamic accuracy of an implanted wireless AC electromagnetic sensor for guided radiation therapy; Implications for real-time tumor position tracking. *Med Phys* (abstract), 2005. **32**: 2112.
103. Lechleiter, K. et al., The effect of time on inter-transponder distance implanted in lung: An initial study in a canine model. *Med Phys* (abstract), 2007. **34**: 2385.

104. Turrisi, A.T., 3rd, et al., Twice-daily compared with once-daily thoracic radiotherapy in limited small-cell lung cancer treated concurrently with cisplatin and etoposide. *N Engl J Med*, 1999. **340**(4): 265–71.
105. Bevington, P.R., *Data Reduction and Error Analysis for the Physical Sciences*, 1st edition. 1969, New York, NY: McGraw-Hill Book Co.
106. Jin J, W.N., Ren L et al, Advances in treatment techniques: Arc-based and other intensity modulated therapies. *Cancer J*, 2011. **17**: 166–76.
107. Otto, K., Volumetric modulated arc therapy: IMRT in a single gantry arc. *Med Phys*, 2008. **35**(1): 310–7.
108. Grills, I.S. et al., Potential for reduced toxicity and dose escalation in the treatment of inoperable non-small-cell lung cancer: A comparison of intensity-modulated radiation therapy (IMRT), 3D conformal radiation, and elective nodal irradiation. *Int J Radiat Oncol Biol Phys*, 2003. **57**(3): 875–90.
109. Liu, H.H. et al., Feasibility of sparing lung and other thoracic structures with intensity-modulated radiotherapy for non-small-cell lung cancer. *Int J Radiat Oncol Biol Phys*, 2004. **58**(4): 1268–79.
110. Yom, S.S. et al., Initial evaluation of treatment-related pneumonitis in advanced-stage non-small-cell lung cancer patients treated with concurrent chemotherapy and intensity-modulated radiotherapy. *Int J Radiat Oncol Biol Phys*, 2007. **68**(1): 94–102.
111. Allen, A.M. et al., Fatal pneumonitis associated with intensity-modulated radiation therapy for mesothelioma. *Int J Radiat Oncol Biol Phys*, 2006. **65**(3): 640–5.
112. Bortfeld, T. et al., Effects of intra-fraction motion on IMRT dose delivery: Statistical analysis and simulation. *Phys Med Biol*, 2002. **47**(13): 2203–20.
113. Jiang, S.B. et al., An experimental investigation on intra-fractional organ motion effects in lung IMRT treatments. *Phys Med Biol*, 2003. **48**(12): 1773–84.
114. Court, L.E. et al., Management of the interplay effect when using dynamic MLC sequences to treat moving targets. *Med Phys*, 2008. **35**(5): 1926–31.
115. Yu, C.X., D.A. Jaffray, and J.W. Wong, The effects of intra-fraction organ motion on the delivery of dynamic intensity modulation. *Phys Med Biol*, 1998. **43**(1): 91–104.
116. Ong, C. et al., Dosimetric impact of interplay effect on RapidArc lung stereotactic treatment delivery. *Int J Radiat Oncol Biol Phys*, 2011. **79**(1): 305–11.
117. Yang, J.N. et al., An investigation of tomotherapy beam delivery. *Med Phys*, 1997. **24**(3): 425–36.
118. Li, X. et al., Dosimetric effect of respiratory motion on volumetric-modulated arc therapy-based lung SBRT treatment delivered by TrueBeam machine with flattening filter-free beam. *J Appl Clin Med Phys*, 2013. **14**(6): 4370.
119. Jiang, S.B., A.L. Boyer, and C.M. Ma, Modeling the extrafocal radiation and monitor chamber backscatter for photon beam dose calculation. *Med Phys*, 2001. **28**(1): 55–66.
120. Ong, C.L. et al., Dosimetric impact of intrafraction motion during RapidArc stereotactic vertebral radiation therapy using flattened and flattening filter-free beams. *Int J Radiat Oncol Biol Phys*, 2013. **86**(3): 420–5.
121. Prendergast, B.M. et al., Flattening filter-free linac improves treatment delivery efficiency in stereotactic body radiation therapy. *J Appl Clin Med Phys*, 2013. **14**(3): 4126.
122. Abbas, A.S. et al., Volumetric-modulated arc therapy for the treatment of a large planning target volume in thoracic esophageal cancer. *J Appl Clin Med Phys*, 2013. **14**(3): 4269.
123. Bradley, J. et al., Toxicity and outcome results of RTOG 9311: A phase I-II dose-escalation study using three-dimensional conformal radiotherapy in patients with inoperable non-small-cell lung carcinoma. *Int J Radiat Oncol Biol Phys, 2005.* **61**(2): 318–28.
124. Timmerman, R.D. et al., Stereotactic body radiation therapy for medically inoperable early-stage lung cancer patients: Analysis of RTOG 0236. *Int J Radiat Oncol Biol Phys*, 2009. **75**(3): S3.
125. ICRU report 62: Prescribing, recording, and reporting photon beam therapy (Supplement to ICRU Report 50). 1999, International Commission on Radiation Units and Measurements: Bethesda, MD.
126. Dawson, L.A. and M.B. Sharpe, Image-guided radiotherapy: Rationale, benefits, and limitations. *Lancet Oncol*, 2006. **7**(10): 848–58.
127. Verellen, D. et al., An overview of volumetric imaging technologies and their quality assurance for IGRT. *Acta Oncol*, 2008. **47**(7): 1271–8.

128. Chang, J.Y. et al., Image-guided radiation therapy for non-small cell lung cancer. *J Thorac Oncol*, 2008. **3**(2): 177–86.
129. Guckenberger, M. et al., Cone-beam CT based image-guidance for extracranial stereotactic radiotherapy of intrapulmonary tumors. *Acta Oncol*, 2006. **45**(7): 897–906.
130. Mageras, G.S. and J. Mechalakos, Planning in the IGRT context: Closing the loop. *Semin Radiat Oncol*, 2007. **17**(4): 268–77.
131. Mayyas, E. et al., Analysis of CBCT-based image guidance for a large cohort of lung cancer patients treated with SABR. *Biomed Phys Eng Express*, 2015. **1**: 035203.
132. Sonke, J.J. et al., Frameless stereotactic body radiotherapy for lung cancer using four-dimensional cone beam CT guidance. *Int J Radiat Oncol Biol Phys*, 2009. **74**: 567–74.
133. Fuss, M. et al., Daily ultrasound-based image-guided targeting for radiotherapy of upper abdominal malignancies. *Int J Radiat Oncol Biol Phys*, 2004. **59**(4): 1245–56.
134. Wong, J.W. et al., The use of active breathing control (ABC) to reduce margin for breathing motion. *Int J Radiat Oncol Biol Phys*, 1999. **44**(4): 911–19.
135. Verellen, D. et al., Gating and tracking, 4D in thoracic tumours. *Cancer Radiother*, 2010. **14**(6–7): 446–54.
136. Shirato, H. et al., Real-time tumour-tracking radiotherapy. *Lancet*, 1999. **353**(9161): 1331–2.
137. Guckenberger, M. et al., Safety and efficacy of stereotactic body radiotherapy for stage 1 non-small-cell lung cancer in routine clinical practice: A patterns-of-care and outcome analysis. *J Thorac Oncol*, 2013. **8**(8): 1050–8.
138. Shah, C. et al., Required target margins for image-guided lung SBRT: Assessment of target position intrafraction and correction residuals. *Pract Radiat Oncol*, 2013. **3**(1): 67–73.
139. Bortfeld, T., S.B. Jiang, and E. Rietzel, Effects of motion on the total dose distribution. *Semin Radiat Oncol*, 2004. **14**(1): 41–51.
140. Marks, L.B. et al., Radiation dose-volume effects in the lung. *Int J Radiat Oncol Biol Phys*, 2010. **76**(3): S70–6.
141. Guckenberger, M. et al., Dose-response relationship for radiation-induced pneumonitis after pulmonary stereotactic body radiotherapy. *Radiother Oncol*, 2010. **97**(1): 65–70.
142. Timmerman, R. et al., Excessive toxicity when treating central tumors in a phase II study of stereotactic body radiation therapy for medically inoperable early-stage lung cancer. *J Clin Oncol*, 2006. **24**(30): 4833–9.
143. Kong, F.M., RTOG 1106/ACRIN 6697: Randomized Phase II Trial of Individualized Adaptive Radiotherapy Using During-Treatment FDG-PET/CT and Modern Technology in Locally Advanced Non-Small Cell Lung Cancer (NSCLC). Available at: https://www.rtog.org/ClinicalTrials/ProtocolTable/StudyDetails.aspx?study=1106. 2014, 2014.

6 Quality assurance of IGRT

KRISHNI WIJESOORIYA, TAEHO KIM, JOSH EVANS, AND QUAN CHEN

6.1 INTRODUCTION

The objective of radiation therapy is to treat the defined tumor region and spare the surrounding normal tissue from radiation damage. Reducing the positioning uncertainty of the target region will lead to smaller planning target volume (PTV) margins and lower normal tissue toxicity. Image-guided radiation therapy (IGRT) utilizes knowledge of the target location and change in anatomy during treatment obtained through various imaging techniques to guide the radiation delivery. Particularly with advanced treatment delivery techniques such as intensity-modulated radiation therapy (IMRT) leads to high-precision dose sculpting with sharp dose gradients; it is critical to ensure the precision of the IGRT through carefully designed quality assurance (QA) procedures.

6.2 QA OF IMAGING MODALITIES USED IN IGRT

6.2.1 Major components of IGRT QA

Various imaging techniques have been used for IGRT. These techniques can be categorized as radiological approaches, which include kilovoltage (kV)/megavoltage (MV) planar imagers (on-board or in-room) [1–3], kVCT [4], MVCT [5], MV/kV cone beam CT (CBCT) [6,7], and non-radiological approaches, such as magnetic resonance imaging (MRI) [8–10], ultrasound [11], optical imaging [12], and radio-frequency system [13]. Most of these practices have been in clinical use for a long time. There are task group reports recommending the QA practice, such as the American Association of Physicists in Medicine (AAPM) Task Group 58 (TG-58) report on electronic portal imaging [14], TG-104 on in-room kV planar imaging [15], TG-154 on IGRT using ultrasound [16], TG-179 on CT-based technologies in IGRT [17], and TG-147 on non-radiographic localization and positioning systems [18]. In addition, for those imaging systems that are integrated to specific machines, the QA was covered in TG-40 [19] and TG-142 [20] as well as in TG-148 for TomoTherapy® MVCT [21] and TG-135 for the CyberKnife® imaging system [22].

While the specifics of the QA procedure vary with imaging techniques, the principles of the QA are similar. In general, the QA of imaging modalities should include the following key components: imaging system performance, repositioning accuracy, and geometric accuracy. These components cover the three important aspects in the IGRT workflow, namely, the identification of the target, the correction of positioning offsets, and the accurate irradiation to the desired target.

6.2.1.1 IMAGING SYSTEM PERFORMANCE

The QA of imaging system performance typically includes the spatial integrity, image uniformity, noise, contrast, and high/low contrast resolution. Spatial integrity checks whether the imaging system correctly reports the dimensions of the patient anatomy without obvious distortion. The accuracy of spatial integrity is the fundamental requirement of the imaging system used in IGRT. The QA procedure commonly involves imaging a phantom with known dimensions and verifying through measurement on the image. For some imaging systems, the QA procedure also includes the measurements with multiple detector positions to verify system scaling integrity.

In IGRT, the purpose of the imaging system is to locate the target and organs at risk (OARs) so that the treatment can be directed correctly. Therefore, it is important for the imaging system to maintain sufficient image quality (uniformity, noise, contrast, resolution, etc.) for the task. Studies have shown that image quality impacts the registration accuracy [23–26]. There are many factors that can impact image quality, such as detector sensitivity changes due to radiation [27] and imaging spectrum changes due to target wearing [28,29]. In extreme cases, severe image artifacts can arise that severely cripple the image-guidance ability. In this regard, the image quality of the imaging system needs to be monitored regularly. Typically, a baseline was obtained through the system acceptance tests. Deviations from the baseline during the future routine QA should be investigated. Many commercially available phantoms that include well-designed structures to test various aspects of image quality have been employed for QA of the imaging system. These phantoms were designed to streamline the image quality QA process. For instance, in Figure 6.1, the imager QA module of PIPSpro software and QC phantoms can be used for the tests. Readers are encouraged to explore those offerings and identify a solution best suited to the needs of their individual clinics.

6.2.1.2 REPOSITIONING ACCURACY

The patient positioning device is an important part of any image-guidance system. It usually exists in the format of a motorized, remote-controlled couch. Most systems, including conventional linac and MRIdian® (ViewRay Inc., Oakwood Village, OH) come with a couch capable of translation along three axes [30]. There

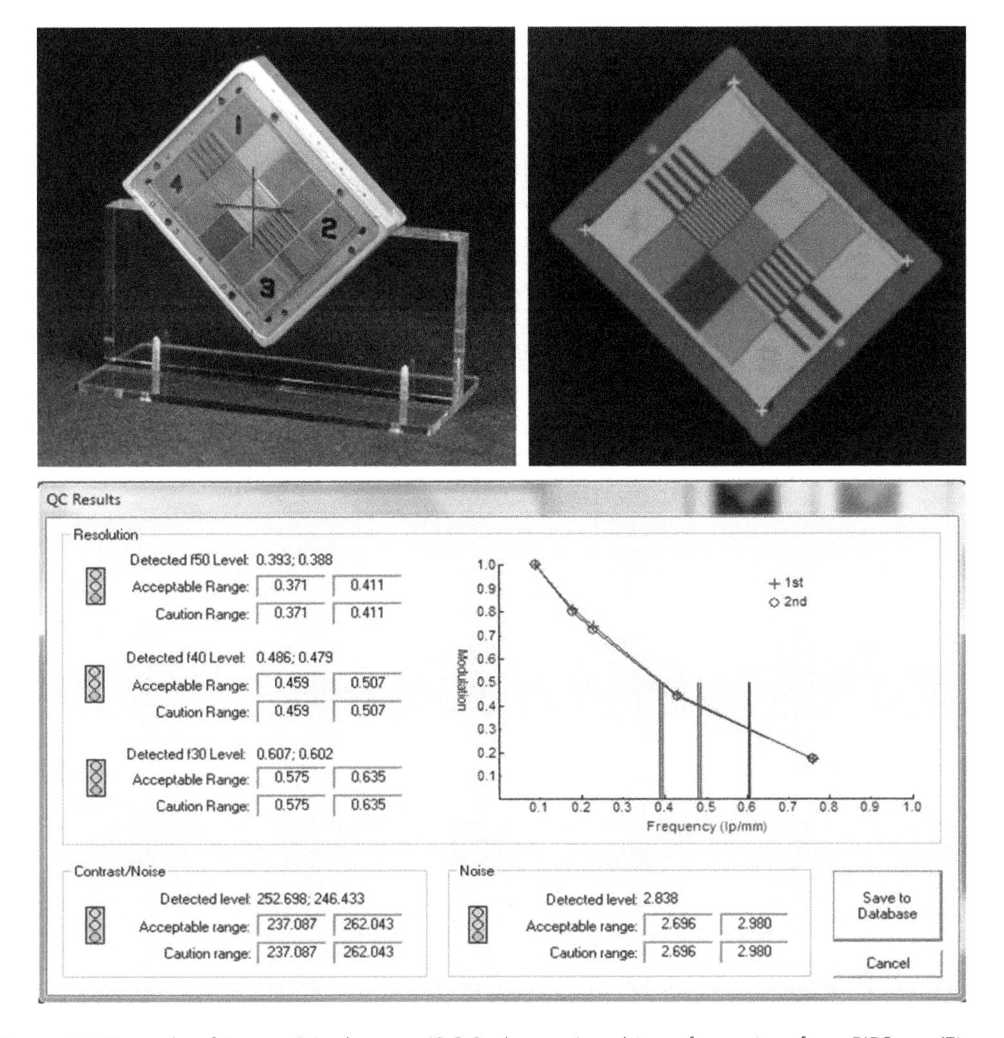

Figure 6.1 Example of image QA phantom (QC-3 phantom) and its software interface, PIPSpro. (Figures extracted from PIPSpro user manual.)

are also commercial solutions that provide movement with 6 degrees of freedom. [31,32]. Some systems come with the capability of correcting patient positioning error by moving linac instead. The CyberKnife system (Accuray Inc., Sunnyvale, CA) is capable in moving its robotic arm to follow the three-dimensional (3D) respiratory motion [33]. The Vero system (Brainlab AG, Munich, Germany) has the capability of correcting the yaw angle offset (rotation about vertical axis) through the rotation of the gantry ring [34–36]. The TomoTherapy system (Accuray Inc., Madison, WI) has the roll angle correction (rotation about the longitudinal axis) achieved through changing the initial angle of the delivery plan [37]. For IGRT to be successful, the accuracy and precision of the correction movements must be ensured. Studies have demonstrated positioning accuracy in the submillimeter range for several commercial couches using various verification methods [30–32,38–41]. However, it is still recommended that users perform such verification during their regular QA activities. One such recommended practice by TG-179 is to perform the check through daily end-to-end QA testing [17].

6.2.1.3 GEOMETRIC ACCURACY

With IGRT, patients can be repositioned for treatment based on the locations of targets and OARs as determined via imaging. It is very important to ensure that the geometry obtained with imaging systems is accurately related to the radiation beam geometry. Commonly, a Winston-Lutz [42–44] type of test is performed

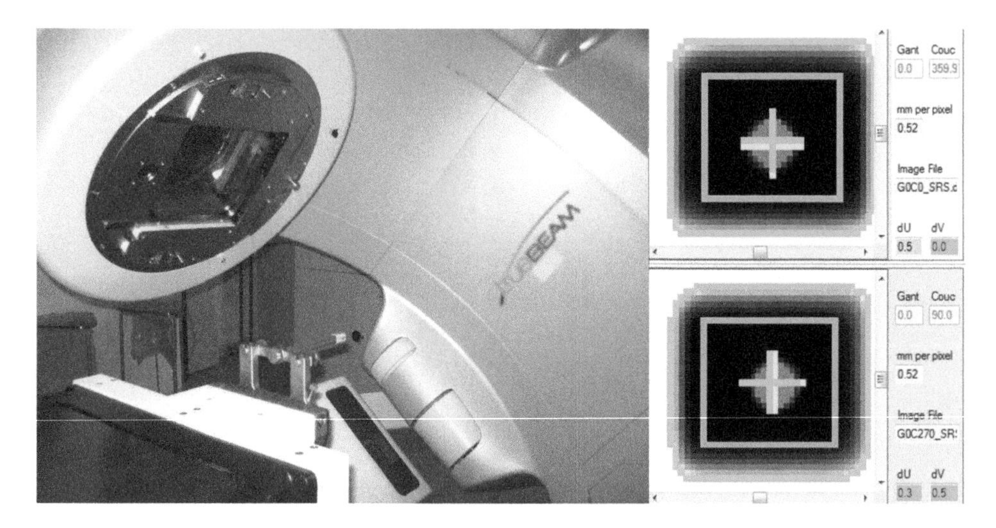

Figure 6.2 Winston–Lutz setup and analysis of the EPID images.

for this purpose, as shown in Figure 6.2. One such test can be briefly described as follows: A small radiopaque ball is imaged and moved to the isocenter based on the image guidance. The ball is then irradiated with a 2- × -2-cm^2 field onto the electronic portal imaging device (EPID) or film stripe. The degree of agreement between the image guidance and irradiating systems can be established from the relative position between the centroid of the ball image and the field edges.

Alternative methods can also be used for the geometric accuracy verification. One approach is to first establish the agreement between the room laser system and the treatment isocenter, then by imaging phantom with markers align to the laser, the agreement between the imaging isocenter and treatment isocenter can be inferred [45]. This alternative method is more applicable to the MRIdian system because the MRI system is not capable of finding the treatment isocenter. In addition, end-to-end tests that include imaging, registration, reposition, and treatment have also been recommended as a test for the geometric accuracy [18,22,46].

6.2.2 QA FREQUENCY AND ACTION LEVELS

The QA frequencies and action levels for the imaging modalities in an IGRT system have been recommended by multiple task groups. The distributions of the tests among daily, monthly, and annual QA have been carefully considered to balance cost and effort with accuracy. TG-142 [20] allows deviations from their recommendations if they are well justified. The upcoming TG-100 [47] encourages individual departments to develop their unique QA programs based on the procedures and resources performed at their institutions. Failure modes and effects analysis should be performed to study the effects of those deviations. Test frequency can be reduced if it is supported by the statistical analysis of historical data. TG-179 has recommended reducing the image quality tests from monthly to semi-annually after the parameter stability had been demonstrated by the users [17]. In addition, while TG-142 recommends that daily tests of the IGRT system should demonstrate an accuracy of within 1 mm for stereotactic body radiation therapy (SBRT) techniques, TG-179 states that 2-mm tolerance should be more appropriate given the cost and effort of the daily QA procedure. It is recommended to have a simple end-to-end procedure in daily QA that involves phantom setup using room lasers, performs predefined shift, and image guidance capability to move it back. This procedure can be performed quickly while achieving 2mm accuracy to 95% confidence [48]. On the other hand, if less than 1-mm accuracy is required, more sophisticated tests must be performed and they could be prohibitive to run on a daily basis in a busy clinic. Readers are therefore recommended to examine those TG reports and adopt the most appropriate approach for their own institutions.

6.3 QA OF IGRT WITH MOTION MANAGEMENT

Various techniques, including breath-holding, respiratory gating, and beam tracking, have been introduced to the clinic to address the organ motion issue during treatment delivery. For treatment simulation, four-dimensional computed tomography (4D-CT) is implemented in many cancer centers to acquire tumor location and geometry at various breathing phases. As always, when new technology is introduced to the clinic, appropriate QA measures should be established. When new motion management hardware and software arrive at the clinic, the interfacing of these with the existing technology and individual equipment performance must be quantifiably verified. This section provides such QA measures with specific examples.

6.3.1 4D QA

AAPM TG-76 on motion management [49] and others [50,51] describe three phases of 4D QA:

1. Typical QA measures
2. Initial testing of equipment and clinical procedures
3. Frequent QA examination during early stage of implementation

Most of these QA procedures would require the institutions to own some type of a motion platform and a lung phantom with a lung phantom tumor. The QUASAR™ phantom (Modus Medical Devices Inc., London, Canada), shown in Figure 6.3, is one such phantom. This could be used with a cylinder of lung density material, embedded with a lung tumor closer to the density of actual patient tumor.

Prior to initiation of a lung SBRT program in a clinic, it is recommended that the certified medical physicist get access to a motion phantom and verify all aspects of a motion management program. 4D-CT imaging, image sorting, and motion amplitude verification would be the first on the list. To perform QA for the 4D-CT scanner, for instance, one could set the motion range to be 10 mm in the S/I direction of the QUASAR phantom and acquire an image using the CT scanner in the 4D-CT mode, with a slice thickness of 2 mm. Synchronizing the image acquisition with the external surrogate allows one to use the external surrogate to perform the retrospective image sorting to create the ten or so 4D-CT image sets. Figure 6.4 shows an example of axial and coronal images of a 4D-CT at the end of inhalation phase with the tumor contoured in red showing the position of the tumor at the end of the exhalation phase. This example shows an inferior displacement of 9.87 mm, for known motion amplitude of 10 mm, resulting in a deviation of 0.13 mm.

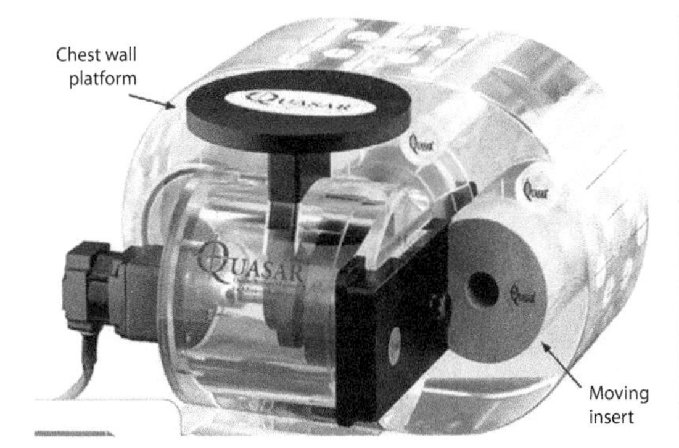

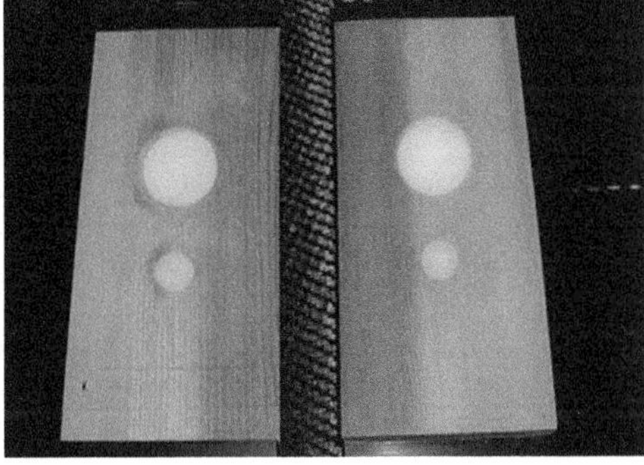

Figure 6.3 Left: Motion phantom with thorax phantom, and moving platform. An external surrogate could be placed on the chest wall platform to simulate patient's AP motion of thorax, and the lung phantom shown by the moving insert simulates the patient's lung tumor motion that is primarily S/I dimension. Right: An insert showing lung density and two embedded tumors of different sizes.

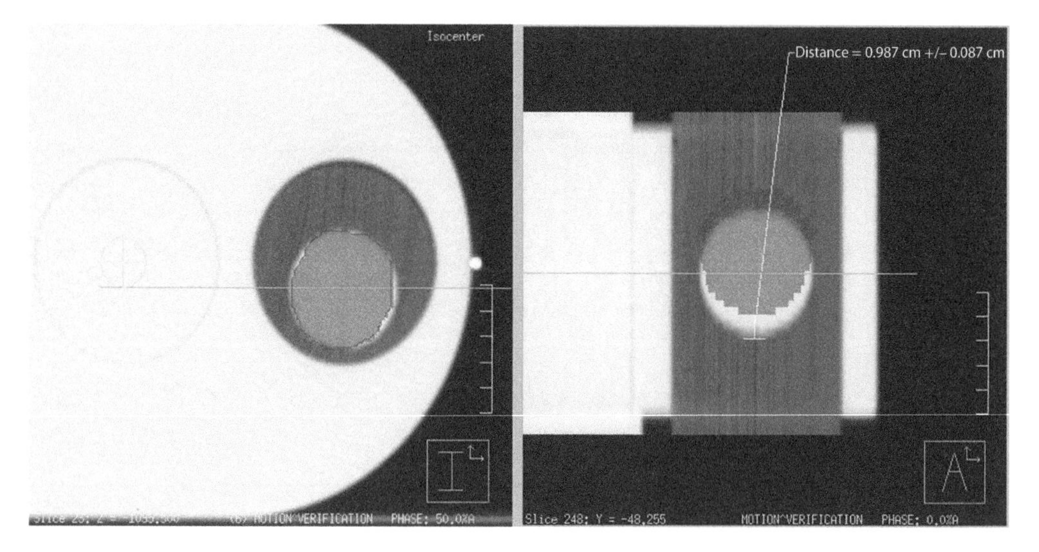

Figure 6.4 Image shows a motion amplitude between end inhalation (0% phase) and the end exhalation (50% phase, shown in red). The left-hand side shows an axial-plane image and the right-hand side shows a coronal-plane image.

6.3.2 Image registration with CBCT for motion

A dynamic phantom that simulates respiratory correlated organ motion should also be used to test the target localization during lung cancer treatments. This phantom ideally should have typical lung density type materials for the lung volume, and tumor density type material for the tumor, as described above. This would allow the user to verify and establish the window and level parameters that should be used during CBCT/MVCT pre-treatment verification image registration with the time-averaged 4D-CT-based planning CT.

4D-CT created time-averaged images from the previous sections should be sent to the treatment planning system (TPS), the necessary contours should be drawn, and an isocenter should be positioned in the middle of the tumor that aligns with the external BBs. This planning CT image with the structure set could be exported to the clinic's record and verify (RV) system, and then imported into the imaging platform of the treatment machine. The motion phantom should be set up at the treatment delivery machine, with the treatment isocenter aligning to the external BBs. Upon performing a volumetric CT with the phantom moving identical to the motion at the CT simulator, one could perform an image registration using the tools available with the on-board-imager software, and try to establish the window/level that best suit the image obtained at the treatment machine and the planning CT. This typically should be very close to the lung window/level. Isocenter shifts should be within the tolerance given by AAPM TG-142. This should be verified for a larger and a smaller tumor to validate there are no distortion artifacts. An example of such a study is shown in Figure 6.5.

6.3.3 QA program for a treatment delivery machine with gating

AAPM TG-142, quality assurance of medical accelerators, recommends that users perform certain QA measures for a treatment machine with respiratory gating. Table 6.1 summarizes these requirements. Although there are many different techniques for implementing respiratory gating, these techniques require the synchronization of the radiation beam with the patient's respiratory signal. Therefore, it is very important that not only the localization of the treatment target during gating should be verified, but also that the beam characteristics such as beam energy and output are not modified during gated treatments. It is equally important

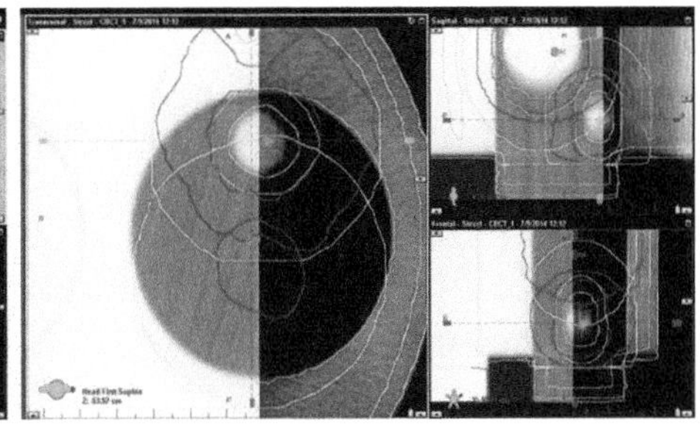

Figure 6.5 ITV comparison of 4D-CT-created time-averaged image and pre-treatment CBCT-created image. Two tumor volumes (96.9 cc and 8.1cc) have been compared between CBCT- and 4D-CT-created time-averaged image.

Table 6.1 TG-142 recommended QA procedures for a treatment machine with respiratory gating

Frequency	Procedure	Tolerance
Monthly	Beam output constancy	2%
	Phase, amplitude beam control	Functional
	In-room respiratory monitoring system	Functional
	Gating interlock	Functional
Annually	Beam energy constancy	2%
	Temporal accuracy of phase/amplitude gate on	100 ms of expected
	Calibration of surrogate for respiratory phase/amplitude	100 ms of expected
	Interlock testing	Functional

to verify the temporal accuracy of the gated window, whether treatments are amplitude or phase based. Actual examples and techniques that users could employ to achieve these are rare in the literature. Reference [52] describes one way of performing these measurements.

To verify the stability of beam output and the energy with and without gating, one could use the monthly output/energy verification system and measure the output and energy with and without the motion phantom and gated treatment. Even though the tolerances for these are given as 2%, our measurements show very much smaller deviations using a depth difference of 5 cm for energy verification for a Varian accelerator, as shown in Table 6.2.

Calibration of the respiratory sensor for amplitude and phase (Table 6.1) is to validate the constancy between a known location/movement of the surrogate and its response. As an example, for an optical system, this can be accomplished by placing a fiducial block at a series of known locations within the field of view and comparing the reported displacements to the known values. Once you verify the spatial accuracy, the second step would be to verify the phase accuracy using a motion phantom.

To verify the temporal accuracy of the gating window, one could deliver a patient plan with the respiratory system ON, hence the beam will be ON, only during the gated parts of the respiratory signal. One could employ a dose-measuring device that records the snapshots and has a temporal resolution of better than 50 ms. After the plan is delivered, one could obtain the average time for delivery of only the beam ON snap shots, and compare that to the respiratory motion signal-based beam ON time in gating. During this process, the motion phantom moving velocity should be kept less than 20 mm/s. The example given in Figure 6.6, during the gating window, shows the motion amplitude is only 4.1 mm, and the time of the gating window is 43% of the respiratory cycle of 5.5 s. The example of average temporal accuracy of the gating window was obtained from both the analysis of the Varian Real-time Position Management (RPM) software and dosimetry measurement software compared to the motion phantom predicted gating window accuracy. Both techniques produced a temporal accuracy of better than 100 ms, the AAPM TG-142 recommended limit.

Table 6.2 Results for treatment machine output and energy variation with and without gating

Energy/status	Output/energy – percentage difference
6MV gating	Output: 0%
6MV gating	Energy: 0%
15 MV gating	Output: 0.1%
15 MV gating	Energy: –0.2%

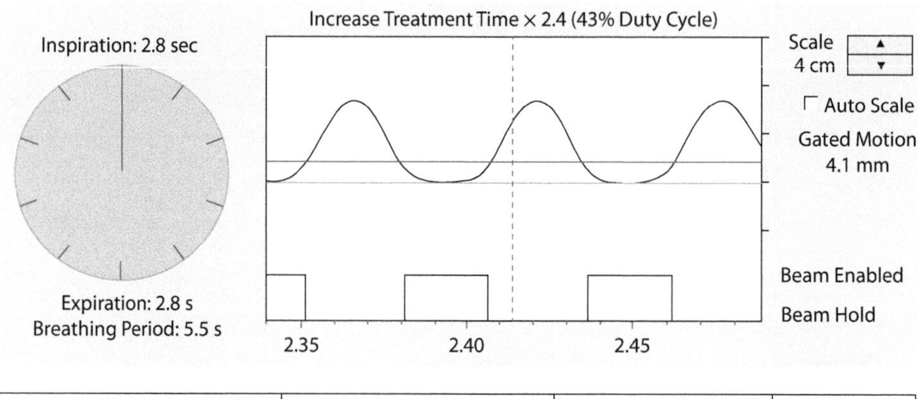

	Period	Gating time (s)	Diff (ms)
Motion phantom	5.4	2.48	
Imaging		2.55	–60
RPM		2.50	20

Figure 6.6 Top: Varian RPM signal gated window with amplitude gating used during verification of temporal accuracy. Bottom: Results of gating window temporal accuracy using two techniques compared to the motion phantom expected value.

6.3.4 Patient-specific QA for gated/breath-hold imaging

When using the two external and internal gating/breath-hold surrogates, the user needs to be extra careful when external surrogates are used, and special QA measures need to be implemented in the clinical practice to avoid major errors such as desynchronization of the internal target motion with the external surrogate [53–55]. To ensure accurate tumor targeting during gating and breath-hold treatments, when external surrogates are used to predict the internal target position, one could follow five QA steps:

1. During CT simulation, the reference position should be accurately measured. Some form of appropriate imaging such as 4D-CT, fluoroscopy should be used to evaluate the tumor motion and to establish the reference position, typically closer to the end exhalation, during which the treatment delivery would occur. Figure 6.7 shows an example. Here, the tumor is attached to the chest wall and moving in both inferior/superior dimensions as well as anterior/posterior dimensions.
2. During the treatment planning process, patient and tumor geometry corresponding to the gating window or breath-hold amplitude should be used. During the planning process, in addition to ITV definition on the correct set of 4D images, if the gated treatment is used, maximum intensity projection (MIP) image corresponding to the gated phases should be used to contour the gated ITV. If the non-gated treatment is used, the full MIP encompassing all respiratory phases should be used to

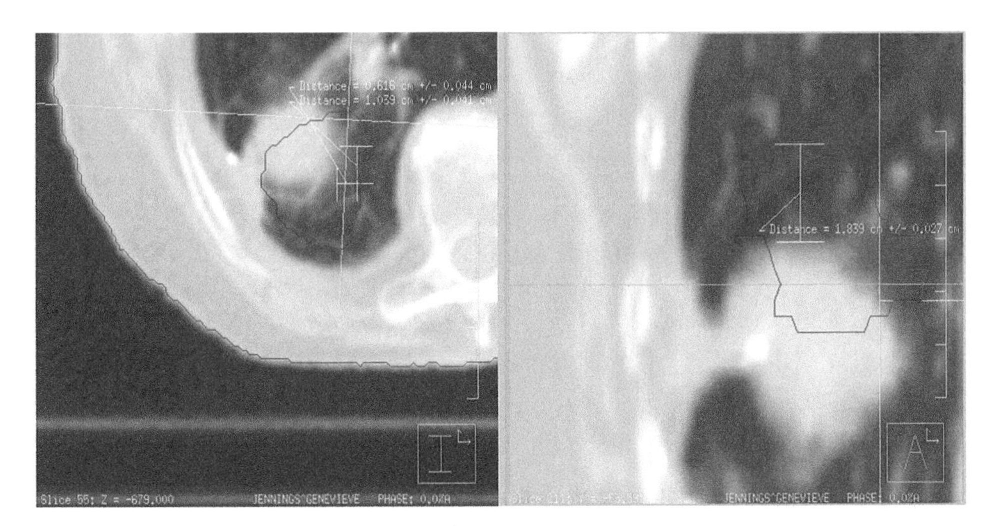

Figure 6.7 Axial and coronal slices of a 4D-CT through a tumor. Red contour is the tumor at the end-exhalation phase (50%), and the image is at the end-inhalation phase (0%).

create the ITV. However, planning should take place on the time-averaged image set that has a higher statistical accuracy of voxel-based attenuation coefficients for non-moving structures. Additionally, this is the image that is exported to the treatment delivery unit for IGRT verification with a cone beam CT, or an MVCT, which are also in principle time-averaged images that encompass the full motion envelopes.

3. During patient setup, the pre-treatment imaging tumor position at each fractionation should be matched to the reference position. During the planning process, gated DRRs should be created either using the 50% phase image set or using the MIP corresponding to the gated phases. Figure 6.8a is gated digitally reconstructed radiograph (DRR) showing a left lower lobe lung tumor and multileaf collimator (MLC)s in the treatment position for an AP beam. One could use the implanted markers, ipsilateral diaphragm location, or the tumor location, and use the electronic graticule for position verification at the treatment machine, as shown by Figure 6.8b. Displacements up to 5 mm are allowed between the DRR tumor location and the pre-treatment image tumor location if the motion allowed in the gating window is 5 mm.
4. During treatment delivery, measures should be taken to ensure constant tumor position so that the tumor is at the planned position when the beam is on. This could be achieved with the aid of visual and audio coaching techniques. Figure 6.9 (left) shows a visual aid used during breath-hold technique. The patient could visualize his/her breath-hold signal with the allowed margins for variation (shown in blue and orange) via the visual aid. Figure 6.9 (right), taken from reference [56], shows the improvements to irregular breathing (c to d) and baseline shift (a to b) via audio-visual coaching.
5. During treatment delivery, tumor positions corresponding to the gating window should be measured and compared with the reference position via either on- or offline review. EPID in cine mode could be utilized for small patients and non-IMRT treatments [57], and on-board kV images for others. During breath-hold treatment delivery, one could use kV orthogonal images to verify the internal anatomy-based breath-hold amplitude and compare them to treatment planning DRR images taken with the breath-hold CT scans [58]. Since the ribs and sternum bony anatomy expand with the patient's deep breath with respect to the spine, the co-registration of the planning deep inspiration breath-hold (DIBH) image DRR pair and the kV image pair is the best measure of the patient's breath-hold displacement reproducibility. Such a registration for the full bony anatomy of the thorax is shown in Figure 6.10. A vector originating at the spine and ending at the sternum across the isocenter in the lateral image co-registration was measured to quantify chest wall position and therefore reproducibility of DIBH displacement.

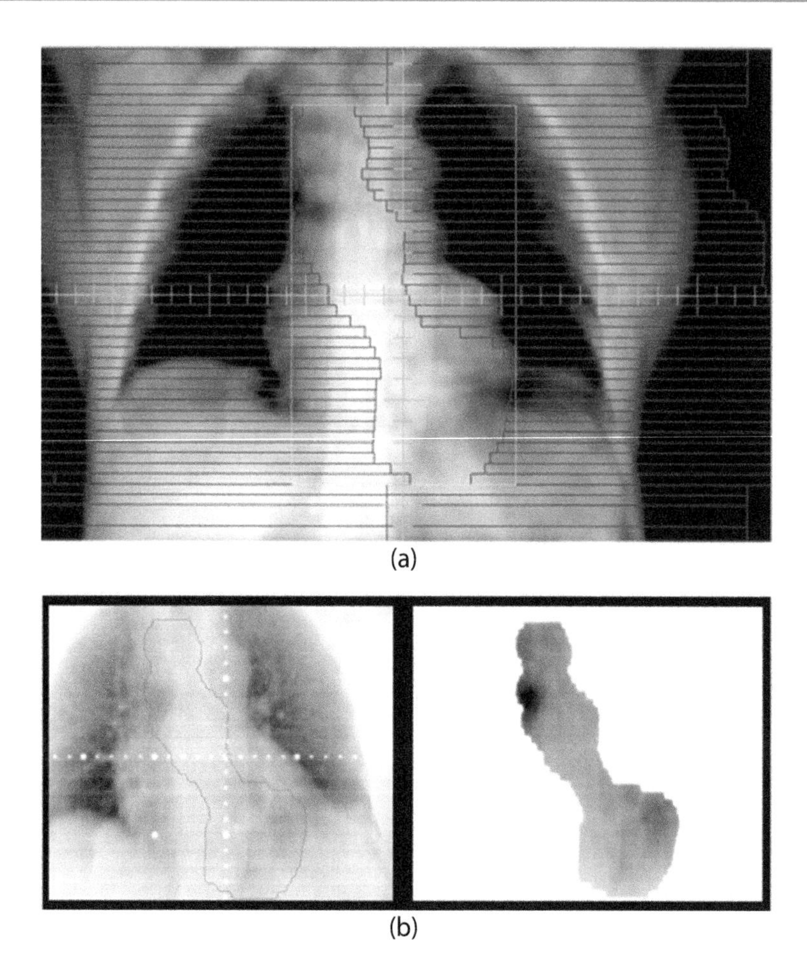

Figure 6.8 (a) DRR for a 50% phase image of a left lower lobe tumor with the MLCs in position for an AP image. (b) At the treatment machine, pre-treatment, gated AP portal images, open and with the MLCs in the treatment position showing the tumor location.

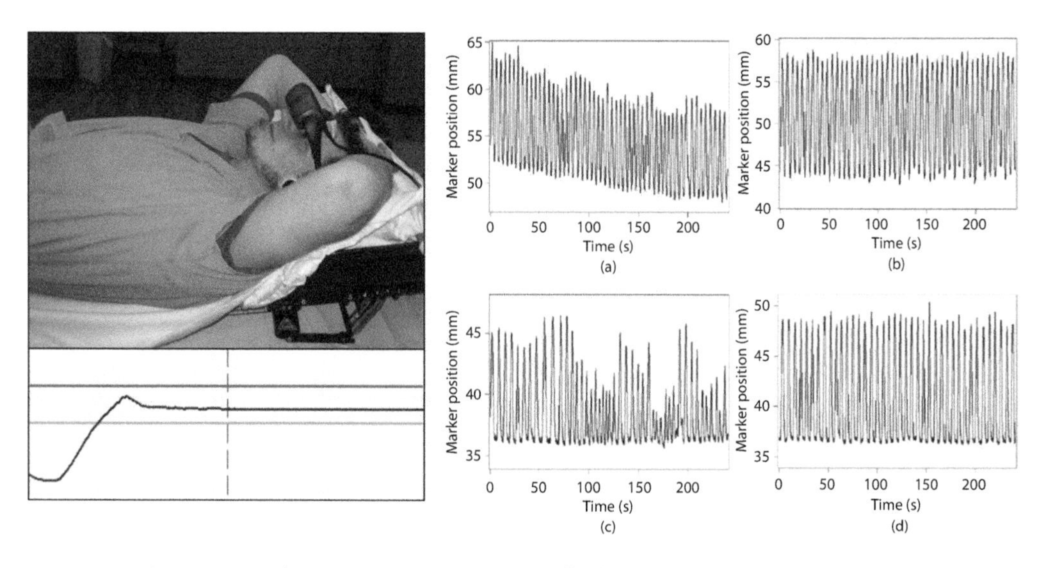

Figure 6.9 Left: Using visual monitoring devices as a biofeedback to keep breath hold amplitude stable, Right: (a) and (c) - free breathing – baseline shift & irregular breathing; (b) and (d) - audio-visual coaching.

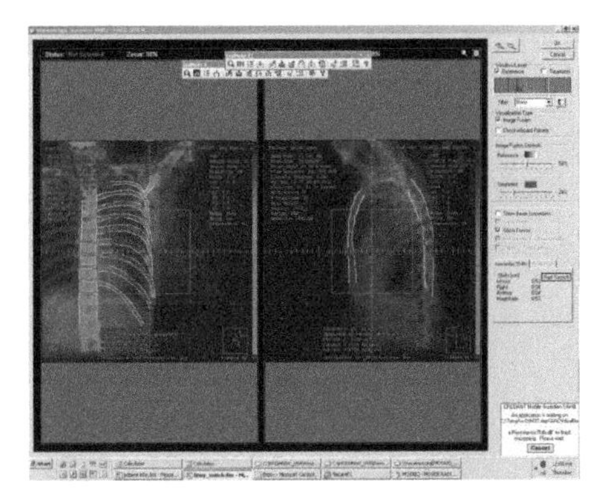

Figure 6.10 The registration results for the bony anatomy of planning CT DRR and pre-treatment kV orthogonal images during deep inspiratory breath-hold treatment. Note the excellent agreement of the fine features of the two images.

6.4 QA FOR MOTION-ADAPTIVE IMAGE GUIDANCE (IGART)

Motion-adaptive image-guided radiation therapy, or IGART, is an exciting and promising technique for reducing the margins needed to treat moving tumors, potentially reducing normal tissue doses and associated treatment toxicities. The technique is also referred to as real-time tumor tracking or respiratory-synchronized therapy. To summarize, motion-adaptive IGART is a technique in which a radiation beam that tightly conforms to the GTV is moved dynamically in response to tumor motion, which is a conceptually different way of dealing with target motion than motion-encompassing margin or gating methods.

Before working to implement a QA program for motion-adaptive IGART, you must first step back and identify the specific details of the motion-adaptive IGART technique that you are aiming to implement. Only once you understand the specifics of your proposed motion-adaptive IGART procedure, the details of which are discussed elsewhere in this book, can you design a reasonable suite of QA processes and tests to ensure that the highest risk uncertainties are addressed. Most of these systems and techniques are cutting-edge, and thus rigorous QA standards have not yet been established. The goal of this section is to identify the major characteristics of currently implemented or proposed motion-adaptive IGART procedures that would reasonably need to be QA-ed and to communicate efforts already published in the literature that have begun working toward that goal.

The first specific to understand is how your target could potentially move. There will be different tumor-motion uncertainties for different anatomical sites. This book focuses on lung tumors, which generally move in a semi-periodic pattern due to respiration. However, it is known that lung tumor motion due to respiration can be irregular, location dependent, vary from simulation and treatment sessions, and can exhibit hysteresis within a session. TG-76 presents an excellent graph that shows representative average tumor motion paths for various tumor locations within the lung (Figure 6.11) [49]. But remember, an individual's motion can differ greatly from the average population and patients can move or breathe very differently during treatment than they did at the time of simulation, so time and effort will also need to be devoted to designing intra-fraction image verification schemes with specific considerations for each treatment site. This section is devoted to QA of the hardware and software components of the motion-adaptive IGART system, not the patient.

6.4.1 Main components of motion-adaptive IGART systems

The next step is to understand the major components of motion-adaptive IGART systems and how they are used to track moving lung tumors. As identified in TG-76 [49], there are four broad tasks needed to achieve accurate lung tumor tracking and real time-beam re-alignment:

1. *Identify* the tumor position in real time.
2. *Anticipate* the tumor position to account for time delays in system response.

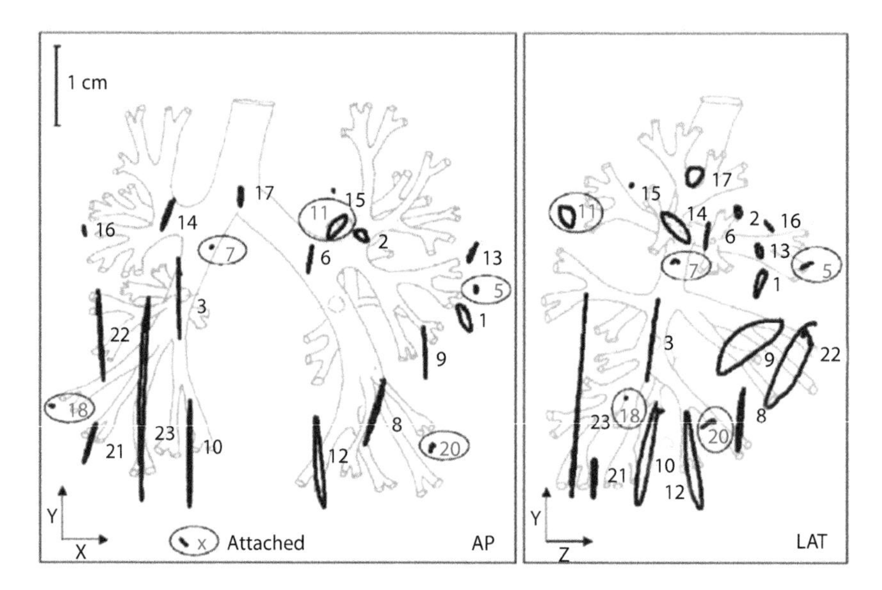

Figure 6.11 Lung tumor trajectories from 23 patients assessed by observing implanted fiducial markers with real-time fluoroscopy. The image highlights the wide range of tumor motion trajectories in lung cancer patients. (Taken from Keall, P.J. et al., *Med Phys.*, 33, 3874–900, 2006. Permission granted from Medical Physics.)

3. *Reposition* the treatment beam to align with the tumor position.
4. *Adapt* the dosimetry for the non-static patient geometry.

Different motion-adaptive IGART systems will all use different techniques and systems to address the first three of these four major tasks. The last task of adapting the dosimetry is the least developed now and most of the work, especially in terms of QA, has been done in regard to tasks 1, 2, and 3. Understanding how your motion-adaptive IGART system addresses each of these tasks will inform what type of QA to implement to ensure the overall system performance is operating within tolerances to meet your clinical goals.

6.4.1.1 IDENTIFY

The method of target identification is paramount for the accuracy and reliability of motion-adaptive IGART. Some systems will identify the target directly, some will identify high-contrast fiducial markers inside the target, and some systems will rely on surrogates external to the target itself. The different identification methods will create different uncertainties and risk priorities. If your system relies on tracking a surrogate in real time, some method of updating the surrogate-target model periodically will be an important component to ensure the correlation between the target and the surrogate remains relevant. If your system relies on imaging the tumor directly, image contrast will be an important quality metric to check.

Motion platforms or phantoms with known two-dimensional (2D) trajectories can be used to assess a system's accuracy of tracking a moving target. Both static known-shift and dynamic known-trajectory tests are commonly employed to assess basic system tracking performance [22,59,60]. Choosing phantoms with appropriate characteristics such as noise and contrast to represent lung patients is important. If your system will always be using high-contrast fiducial markers, then it is appropriate to use a phantom with similar fiducials. If your system will be tracking soft tissue alone, more anatomically accurate lung body phantoms should be considered. The use of 3d printing is an exciting technological development that is allowing clinicians to design phantoms for motion-adaptive IGART QA that more closely mimic real patient characteristics. For example, Jung et al. designed a 3D-printed lung insert that can be used with the QUASAR motion platform to compare the overall tracking accuracy of the CyberKnife's marker-less tracking system, Xsight, in comparison to CyberKnife's marker-based tracking system [61]. Tests for system-specific fault modes should also be included in routine QA, for example, making sure that swapped or migrating electromagnetic (EM) transponders in the Calypso® system correctly identified [60]. While assessing tracking accuracy with phantoms can never ensure accurate tracking for individual patient cases, these phantom assessments are still useful to establishing a baseline of tracking accuracy for a given system which can be used to ensure that the accuracy is not degrading over time.

It is intuitive that good tracking results in a simple phantom with a well-defined target and trajectory do not necessarily mean the same system will track well for all patient cases in which the target may be smaller, have lower contrast, or exhibit a very irregular breathing pattern. While no phantom test will be able to test the full range of conditions presented in real patient cases and guidance on tracking algorithm accuracy as a function of imaging parameters is currently sparse and will be system specific, rigorous image-quality QA should still be included to ensure that image quality does not degrade significantly from the time of system commissioning. TG-135 for robotic radiosurgery using the CyberKnife system provides a table describing imaging system-specific QA tests to be performed routinely, for example, checking kVp, filtration, contrast-to-noise ratio (CNR), and signal-to-noise ratio (SNR) annually and recommends comparing to baseline values acquired at the time of commissioning [22]. TG-135 also provides advice on how to test the limits of your system's tracking algorithm by purposefully degrading the image quality to assess when the tracking accuracy of known shifts begins to degrade, which may be a useful process during commissioning to inform clinical action limits on these more basic image-quality tests.

It is crucial for all team members to be aware of the potential for tracking accuracy to be reduced from poor image quality because of patient-specific factors like large body habitus or metal implants. Visualization of the real-time tracking images with appropriate overlaid information, such as an outline of the "tracked" fiducial marker location on top of the live fluoroscopic image as in the CyberKnife system [22], can provide an excellent method for team members to monitor algorithm tracking performance during patient treatments, allowing them to stop treatment as soon as possible if a deviation arises.

6.4.1.1.1 Imaging and treatment isocenter alignment and imaging dose

After considering the many technical factors involved in "tracking" the lung tumor, it is natural to immediately jump to considering how the system is going to re-align the MV treatment beam to the target's current position, but there are other steps to consider first. Whatever the method of tracking the target and re-aligning the beam, ensuring that the imaging and treatment coordinate systems are aligned with each other is of paramount importance. The need for this system alignment is well appreciated and vendor-provided phantoms and routines are often provided to facilitate this. However, the authors would like to note that some vendor-provided calibration routines assume the initial phantom setup as ground truth and the in-built verification checks can be internally consistent. That is, in some cases, if the imaging system's calibration phantom was aligned to lasers, and the lasers were 2 mm off from the true radiation isocenter, then the imaging system is now calibrated 2 mm off from the true radiation isocenter, and the in-built vendor routines may not be designed to catch that. In these scenarios, an independent end-to-end QA test that uses the MV radiation beam itself will need to be used to verify that the imaging system accurately repositions a phantom to the true radiation isocenter.

Furthermore, the imaging dose from near-real time x-ray imaging must be considered. An excellent example of a dose evaluation from x-ray tracking is presented by Depuydt et al., who determined that using the Vero kV imaging at a frequency of 1 Hz to deliver an average skin dose of 1.8 mGy/min [62].

6.4.1.2 ANTICIPATE

As the lung tumor targets we are aiming to track dynamically can move relatively quickly, and these systems will have some finite amount of lag time, most of these systems will need to perform some sort of forward target position prediction to position the beam where the target is going to be, not where it just was. Working from studies like Krauss et al. [63], which compared four motion prediction models for breathing motion and found root-mean-square error (RMSE) prediction errors on the order of approximately 1 mm for 0.2-s system latency to 2 mm for 0.6-s latency, AAPM TG-76 recommends overall tracking system lag time should not exceed 0.5s [49]. Lag time is a major component of how well your system will respond to sudden, unpredictable non-periodic movements, and thus should be known and QAed periodically. Lag time should be quantified and system response to anomalous conditions should be understood and checked periodically as well.

Santanam et al. present a method for assessing lag time for the tracking component of motion-adaptive IGART using the Calypso EM-transponder system [60]. They used a 4D motion platform driven in a sine-wave pattern. Then, the team uses a video camera system to simultaneously record the phantom motion and the Calypso workstation's tracking results. By analyzing the video file offline, they could determine the phase shift between the two sine-wave patterns, and thus quantify the latency of their Calypso real-time tracking system. Note that this is the lag time for only the target identification and tracking portion of the motion-adaptive IGART process; the time needed to re-align the radiation beam will also need to be factored in. Depuydt et al. described using a similar sinusoidal phase shift method and video tracking using the radiation light field to determine the beam re-alignment lag time for the Vero system using IR marker surface tracking [64], as shown in Figures 6.12 and 6.13. Performing the test with the system's motion prediction turned off

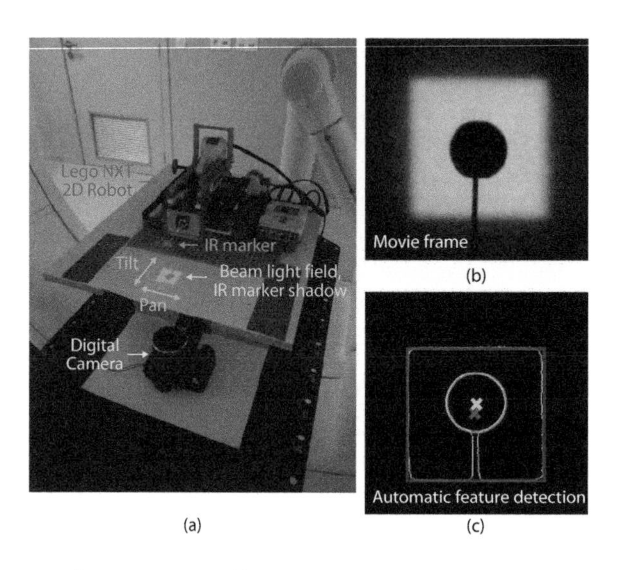

Figure 6.12 The experimental setup presented by Depuydt et al. 2011 to assess their gimbaled linac's tracking accuracy. The top panel shows the 2D motion platform with the infrared marker target and the digital camera for independent verification of the target centroid and light field edge. (From Depuydt, T., et al, *Radiother Oncol.*, 98, 365–72. Copyright [2011], with permission from Elsevier.)

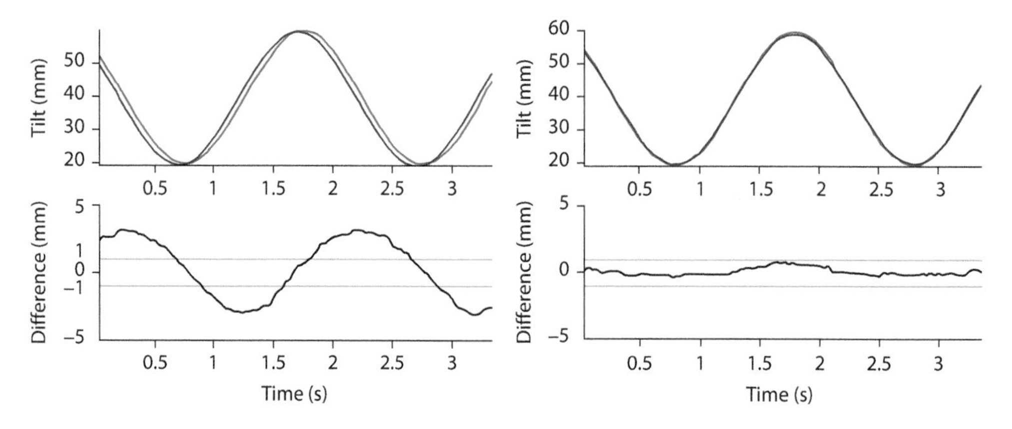

Figure 6.13 Real-time object position (blue) and the beam position (red) for the marker tracing a simple sinusoidal motion path. The bottom left shows the position with the lag compensation forward prediction turned off, which can be utilized to assess the system lag time, and the bottom right shows the positions with the forward prediction turned on, which illustrates that the system's lag time compensation algorithm is working appropriately. It is also important to utilize representative patient motion trajectories as well to assess the system's accuracy in tracking irregular motion. (From Depuydt, T. et al., *Radiother Oncol.*, 98, 365–72, 2011.)

allows assessment of the system's native lag time, and then performing the test again with the motion predictive algorithm turned on allows verification that the prediction algorithm is working appropriately.

If your system is using a surrogate-target correlation model, the correlation can feasibly be tested at system commissioning and periodically thereafter. Depuydt et al. presented retrospective patient tracking data acquired on the Vero system showing that the quality of the correlation model between the surrogate and the target directly impacts the residual error of the tracking [65]. For their patient workflow, they include a dry run session a few days before treatment, in which the patient is imaged on the Vero machine and a target-surrogate correlation model is made. This allows them to better identify patients in which the correlation-model may have a poor fit that may limit the utility of real-time tumor tracking. The correlation-model updates could then be checked using breathing traces exhibiting baseline shifts.

6.4.1.3 BEAM RE-ALIGNMENT

How the various beam-target realignment methods differ is important to understand because of potential synchrony effects with the target motion, and the specifics of your system will need to be appreciated to design relevant QA tests. For example, while the Vero's gimbaled linac system has been shown to track motion in two dimensions with almost equal lag time and accuracy [64], the dynamic MLC tracking method has a much slower system response to motions that are perpendicular to the leaf motion due to finite leaf speed [66]. In some cases, the beam may need to be interrupted due to the speed of target motion exceeding the speed of beam adjustment. QA tests that use motions beyond the system's physical limits should be incorporated to ensure the system turns off the MV beam at the appropriate time, and knowledge of the system's response time and any directional or other dependencies is crucial in designing these tests.

6.4.1.4 ADAPT AND ASSESS

The final piece of the puzzle is how to adapt and/or assess the dosimetry of the dynamic tracking treatments. Poulsen [67] showed a treatment planning system (TPS) calculation of time-resolved dosimetry validated in a dynamic thorax phantom using film dosimetry. However, the study is limited by simple one-dimensional motion trajectories implemented as rigid shifts of the whole patient with no anatomical deformations. Deformable phantoms like the one recently presented by Graves et al. [68] for head and neck radiotherapy could potentially be used to assess the efficacy of dose calculation and deformable image registration (DIR) algorithms used in conjunction with motion-adaptive IGART delivery systems. Due to complexity and cost, these types of phantoms will likely be used for new system investigations, or at most at commissioning of a new system installation. Long-term development in auditing post-treatment patient tracking traces will likely be a realistic compromise of cost and effort for monitoring motion-adaptive IGART patient treatments.

6.5 IGRT CREDENTIALING PROCESS FOR CLINICAL TRIALS

IGRT can detect, evaluate, reduce the interfraction setup errors, and minimize intra-fraction motion. With lung SBRT, data support an improvement in the required PTV margin and dose distribution from a variety of IGRT techniques [69–74]. Because IGRT allows a better understanding of the uncertainty involved at the outset than if IGRT were not used, it is highly unlikely that protocols without in-treatment/online imaging and registration will be used in the future. To the contrary, the trend is toward an intensification of imaging to further reduce treatment margins such as tracking techniques. Some of the RTOG protocols related to lung SBRT are listed in Table 6.3.

Despite this valuable tool, there are still significant variations in IGRT tools and procedures used by different sites, and inter-operator variations. This variation may lead to different clinical trial outcomes. Therefore, it is imperative that there be a QA process of IGRT for the credentialing process of clinical trials to ensure consistency in treatment delivery across the institutions that participate in a given clinical trial [74–77].

Image-guided radiation therapy is a complex process [78,79], and the quality assurance of 3D IGRT is especially challenging. The issues include large variations in image quality among different modalities of imaging systems, complex anatomy in the images, and complex processes for the image registration. It is

Table 6.3 A description of RTOG clinical trials for lung SBRT

Protocol number	Trial name
0813	Seamless phase I/II study of stereotactic body radiation therapy (SBRT) for early-stage, centrally located, non-small-cell lung cancer (NSCLC) in medically inoperable patients
0618	A phase II trial of SBRT in the treatment of patients with operable stage I/II NSCLC
0915	A randomized phase II study comparing two SBRT schedules for medically inoperable patients with stage I peripheral NSCLC

important to develop a uniform QA procedure for 3D IGRT data from different sources. In addition, to adapt to large-scale clinical trials such as the trials conducted by the Radiation Therapy Oncology Group (RTOG), an efficient remote review approach to evaluate these IGRT data from many institutions is essential.

Multiple steps of the treatment process such as 4D-CT scanning (with or without motion management), ITV definition process, treatment planning process, pre-treatment imaging process to identify and shift to the tumor isocenter, and finally the accurate treatment delivery process need to be verified for accuracy. In this section, we will discuss credentialing processes that address all of the above.

6.5.1 IGRT PROTOCOLS

At least three or more fractions of daily IGRT data from a single patient (off protocol) are required for credentialing purposes. The IGRT data to be included are: the planning computed tomography (CT), radiation therapy plan (RT PLAN), contoured structures (RTSTRUCT), dose (RT DOSE), and the daily in-room image datasets in Digital Imaging and Communications in Medicine (DICOM) format. An IGRT data spreadsheet is also required, which includes the information specific to IGRT, such as daily shifts made, IGRT timing, imaging mode, imaging technique, image registration process, and the instructions to complete the form. All the above information should be submitted to the Imaging and Radiation Oncology Core (IROC) via digital data export.

6.5.1.1 INDEPENDENT VERIFICATION OF INDIVIDUAL INSTITUTION SPECIFIC IMAGE REGISTRATION SHIFTS

The goal of this process is to independently verify and reproduce the registration shifts obtained by the person at the credentialing institution. Figure 6.14 gives a flowchart of the overall workflow of credentialing for IGRT taken from ref [80]. Reference [80] shows results for IGRT registration shifts submitted for an institution and an independent reviewer verification of shifts of a 3D dataset such as CBCT. For a combination of lung SBRT cases from RTOG 0813 (for centrally located lung tumors) and RTOG 0915 (for peripheral lung tumors) protocols they give a mean ± SD of 1.80 ± 1.06 mm, 2.05 ± 1.05 mm, and 2.01 ± 0.93 mm (mean ± SD, in left-right, superior-inferior, and anterior-posterior directions, respectively).

6.5.2 MOTION MANAGEMENT PROTOCOLS

In accruing lung cancer patients for clinical trials, one needs to pay attention to the process of minimizing organ motion due to respiration, or treating during free-breathing, while accounting for the full motion envelope of the tumor.

To obtain credentialing status for such clinical trials one need to establish the accuracy of the full process by performing an end-to-end test (from 4D simulation to treatment delivery). Institutions could request a heterogeneous thorax phantom with the motion platform from Radiological Physics Center (RPC). The RPC's lung phantom includes two lungs with density 0.33 g/cm^3, a heart, and a spinal cord with densities near 1.2 g/cm^3. A target of density 1.2 g/cm^3 is centrally located in the left lung as shown in Figure 6.15. Thermoluminescent dosimeters (TLDs) are used for dose determination and are embedded near the center of

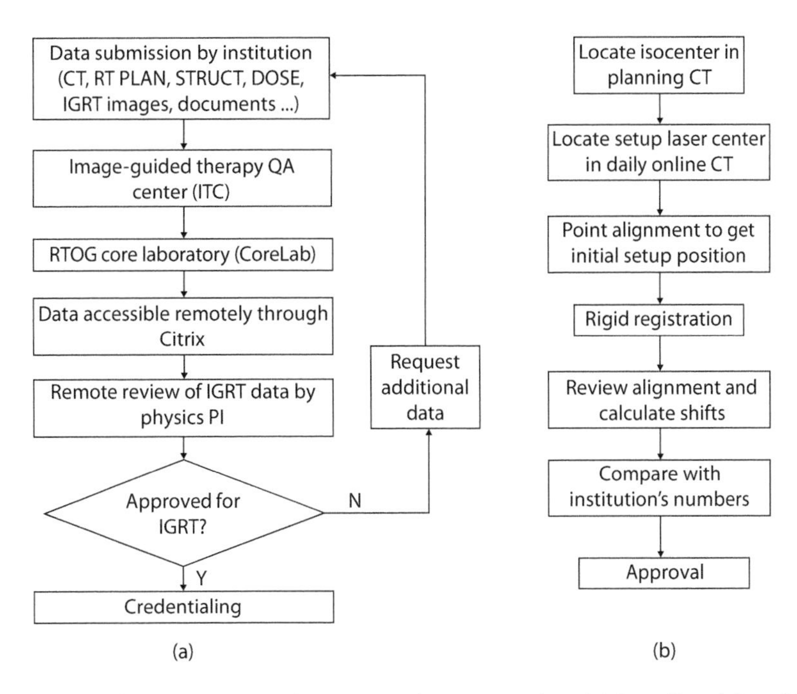

Figure 6.14 Workflow of remote credentialing process for 3D IGRT data. (a) Overall workflow. (b) Verification of image registration with third-party software system.

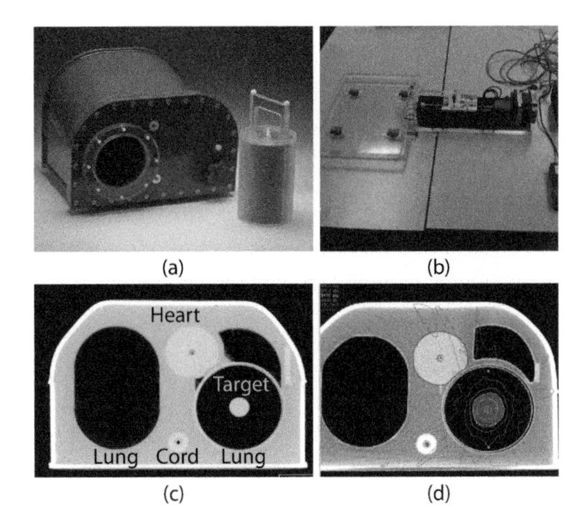

Figure 6.15 RPC lung phantom (a) with the motion platform (b), inserts representing target and critical structures (c), and isodose map for a 600 cGy prescription (d).

the target. Radio chromic films are located on the axial, coronal, and sagittal planes for relative dose measurements. Film doses are normalized to the TLD dose.

Institutions could use breath-hold, gating, and ITV tracking techniques to account for respiratory motion. Upon receiving the phantom, physicists could fill the phantom with water, set up the motion platform to move with known amplitude, and acquire a 4D-CT scan. This allows the institution to independently verify the accuracy of motion amplitude via the 4D-CT image technique.

Using the 4D-CT images, create the ITV and the motion phases that one wishes to perform gated treatment with. Prepare the treatment plan, prior to delivery, at the treatment machine, obtain the kV orthogonal

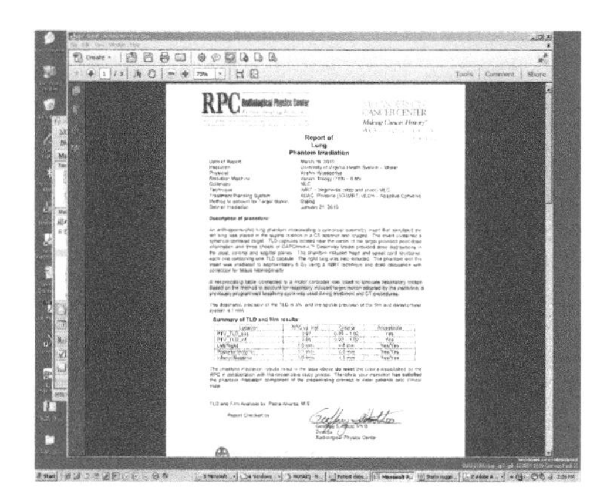
RPC Radiological Physics Center

CANCER CENTER

Report of
Lung
Phantom Irradiation

Description of procedure:

Summary of TLD and film results

Figure 6.16 RPC lung phantom irradiation results for a gated treatment.

Table 6.4 How different motion management systems perform in the credentialing process compared to free breathing

Motion management	Pass rate (%)	Attempts	Criteria failed		
			Dose	Film	Dose and film
Breath-hold	100	4	0	0	0
Gating	79	68	2	7	5
ITV	70	61	0	13	5
Tracking	96	24	1	0	0
Static	87	270	8	24	4
All		427	11	44	14

images during gated window, and shift accordingly. Finally, deliver the plan with or without gating with <5 mm motion. Results from an RPC lung phantom irradiation with gating is shown in Figure 6.16.

The TLD passing criteria used by the RPC include ±5% for a ratio of 0.97. Film criterion used is ≥80% of the pixels in the ROI must pass a 5%/5-mm gamma threshold per each plane. An average for all three planes should be ≥85%. A study performed by the RPC on institutions submitting credentialing data on the moving lung phantom [81] shows that 79% of the irradiation using the motion phantom met or exceeded the RPC criteria, and 30% of the moving phantom failures were in the film dosimetry. Table 6.4, taken from Reference [81], shows the pass rates for the different motion management systems and the static irradiations.

6.6 CURRENT DEVELOPMENTS IN IGRT QA

This area of research is currently under development and is very active in the literature. There are some excellent examples of QA programs for motion-adaptive IGART systems or subsystems. The CyberKnife system was the first widespread clinical system to treat moving lung tumors by mounting a compact linac to an industrial robot. The experience gained from that system is a great starting point for anyone tasked with developing a QA program for his or her institution's new motion-adaptive treatment system. The report of AAPM TG-135 [22] concerning the robotic CyberKnife system is a must read and represents some of the trade-offs that need to be made in terms of cost, time, and ability to detect meaningful system errors. The ViewRay® integrated MRI-Co-60 unit that was recently brought to market has garnered much excitement as it holds the promise of non-ionizing MRI tumor tracking [82,83]. Green et al. reported on their

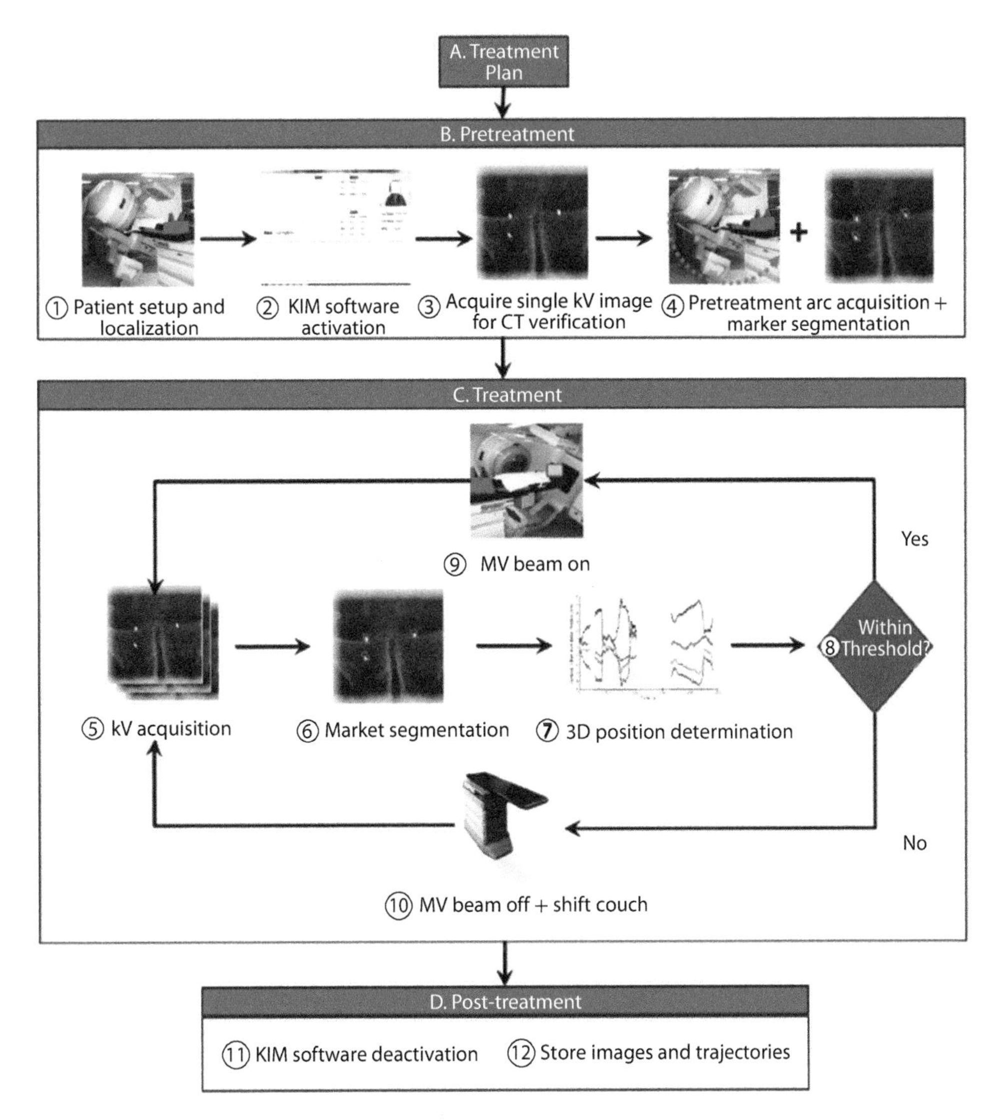

Figure 6.17 The clinical process workflow for the kilovoltage intrafraction monitoring (KIM) system. This type of clinical process map is a crucial first step to performing a failure mode and effects analysis (FMEA), which is a method to quantify a risk priority number that can help prioritize high-risk systems and processes in the development of a QA program. (Taken from Ng, J.A. et al., *Med Phys.*, 41, 111712, 2014. Permission granted from Medical Physics.)

efforts to commission synchronized tumor-tracking and beam control for the ViewRay MRIdian system at the 2015 AAPM Annual Meeting [84]. Ng et al. presented their clinical processes and QA development for their real-time kilovoltage intrafraction monitoring (KIM) system that uses gantry-mounted x-ray imaging systems to track tumor motion [59], as shown in Figure 6.17. Santanam et al. reported on the QA developed for clinical implementation of the Calypso electromagnetic fiducial system for use in prostate intrafraction motion tracking [60]. This report displays the different tests that are needed to utilize the system for dynamic tracking, not just initial target localization. Sawant et al. employed FEMA to inform the development of a QA program for their dynamic MLC tracking system [85]. They presented a detailed process map and, based on the relative RPNs, designed QA checks for the highest-scoring items. The FMEA methodology will certainly play an increasing role in informing the design of effective QA programs for the rapidly evolving area of motion-adaptive IGART techniques and technologies.

REFERENCES

1. Murphy, M.J. and R.S. Cox, The accuracy of dose localization for an image-guided frameless radiosurgery system. *Med Phys*, 1996. **23**: 2043–9.
2. Schewe, J.E. et al., A room-based diagnostic imaging system for measurement of patient setup. *Med Phys*, 1998. **25**: 2385–7.
3. Shirato, H. et al., Physical aspects of a real-time tumor-tracking system for gated radiotherapy. *Int J Radiat Oncol Biol Phys*, 2000. **48**: 1187–95.
4. Lattanzi, J. et al., Daily CT localization for correcting portal errors in the treatment of prostate cancer. *Int J Radiat Oncol Biol Phys*, 1998. **41**: 1079–86.
5. Mackie, T.R. et al., Image guidance for precise conformal radiotherapy. *Int J Radiat Oncol Biol Phys*, 2003. **56**: 89–105.
6. Pouliot, J. et al., Low-dose megavoltage cone-beam CT for radiation therapy. *Int J Radiat Oncol Biol Phys*, 2005. **61**: 552–60.
7. Jaffray, D.A. et al., A radiographic and tomographic imaging system integrated into a medical linear accelerator for localization of bone and soft-tissue targets. *Int J Radiat Oncol Biol Phys*, 1999. **45**: 773–89.
8. Lagendijk, J.J. et al., MRI/linac integration. *Radiother Oncol*, 2008. **86**: 25–9.
9. Jaffray, D.A. et al., A facility for magnetic resonance-guided radiation therapy. *Semin Radiat Oncol*, 2014. **24**: 193–5.
10. Mutic, S. and J.F. Dempsey, The ViewRay system: Magnetic resonance-guided and controlled radiotherapy. *Semin Radiat Oncol*, 2014. **24**: 196–9.
11. Lattanzi, J. et al., Ultrasound-based stereotactic guidance of precision conformal external beam radiation therapy in clinically localized prostate cancer. *Urology*, 2000. **55**: 73–8.
12. Schoffel, P.J. et al., Accuracy of a commercial optical 3D surface imaging system for realignment of patients for radiotherapy of the thorax. *Phys Med Biol*, 2007. **52**: 3949–63.
13. Litzenberg, D.W. et al., Positional stability of electromagnetic transponders used for prostate localization and continuous, real-time tracking. *Int J Radiat Oncol Biol Phys*, 2007. **68**: 1199–206.
14. Herman, M.G. et al., Clinical use of electronic portal imaging: Report of AAPM Radiation Therapy Committee Task Group 58. *Med Phys*, 2001. **28**: 712–37.
15. Yin, F.F. et al., The role of in-room kv x-ray imaging for patient setup and target localization. Report of AAPM Task Group 104. 2009. American Association of Physicists in Medicine. Available from http://www.aapm.org/pubs/reports/detail.asp?docid=104 ISBN: 978-1-888340-89-1
16. Molloy, J.A. et al., Quality assurance of U.S.-guided external beam radiotherapy for prostate cancer: Report of AAPM Task Group 154. *Med Phys*, 2011. **38**: 857–71.
17. Bissonnette, J.P. et al., Quality assurance for image-guided radiation therapy utilizing CT-based technologies: A report of the AAPM TG-179. *Med Phys*, 2012. **39**: 1946–63.
18. Willoughby, T. et al., Quality assurance for nonradiographic radiotherapy localization and positioning systems: Report of Task Group 147. *Med Phys*, 2012. **39**: 1728–47.
19. Kutcher, G.J. et al., Comprehensive QA for radiation oncology: Report of AAPM Radiation Therapy Committee Task Group 40. *Med Phys*, 1994. **21**: 581–618.
20. Klein, E.E. et al., Task Group 142 Report: Quality assurance of medical accelerators. *Med Phys*, 2009. **36**: 4197–212.
21. Langen, K.M. et al., QA for helical tomotherapy: Report of the AAPM Task Group 148. *Med Phys*, 2010. **37**: 4817–53.
22. Dieterich, S. et al., Report of AAPM TG 135: Quality assurance for robotic radiosurgery. *Med Phys*, 2011. **38**: 2914–36.
23. Biggs, P.J., M. Goitein, and M.D. Russell, A diagnostic X ray field verification device for a 10 MV linear accelerator. *Int J Radiat Oncol Biol Phys*, 1985. **11**: 635–43.
24. Morrow, N.V. et al., Impact of computed tomography image quality on image-guided radiation therapy based on soft tissue registration. *Int J Radiat Oncol Biol Phys*, 2012. **82**: e733–8.

25. Handsfield, L.L. et al., Determination of optimal fiducial marker across image-guided radiation therapy (IGRT) modalities: Visibility and artifact analysis of gold, carbon, and polymer fiducial markers. *J Appl Clin Med Phys*, 2012. **13**: 3976.
26. Stock, M. et al., Image quality and stability of image-guided radiotherapy (IGRT) devices: A comparative study. *Radiother Oncol*, 2009. **93**: 1–7.
27. Bissonnette, J.P., D.J. Moseley, and D.A. Jaffray, A quality assurance program for image quality of cone-beam CT guidance in radiation therapy. *Med Phys*, 2008. **35**: 1807–15.
28. Staton, R.J. et al., Dosimetric effects of rotational output variation and x-ray target degradation on helical tomotherapy plans. *Med Phys*, 2009. **36**: 2881–8.
29. Yadav, P. et al., The effect and stability of MVCT images on adaptive TomoTherapy. *J Appl Clin Med Phys*, 2010. **11**: 3229.
30. Bel, A. et al., A computerized remote table control for fast on-line patient repositioning: Implementation and clinical feasibility. *Med Phys*, 2000. **27**: 354–8.
31. Meyer, J. et al., Positioning accuracy of cone-beam computed tomography in combination with a HexaPOD robot treatment table. *Int J Radiat Oncol Biol Phys*, 2007. **67**: 1220–8.
32. Guckenberger, M. et al., Precision of image-guided radiotherapy (IGRT) in six degrees of freedom and limitations in clinical practice. *Strahlenther Onkol*, 2007. **183**: 307–13.
33. Pepin, E.W. et al., Correlation and prediction uncertainties in the CyberKnife Synchrony respiratory tracking system. *Med Phys*, 2011. **38**: 4036–44.
34. Solberg, T.D. et al., Commissioning and initial stereotactic ablative radiotherapy experience with Vero. *J Appl Clin Med Phys*, 2014. **15**: 4685.
35. Kamino, Y. et al., Development of an ultrasmall C-band linear accelerator guide for a four-dimensional image-guided radiotherapy system with a gimbaled x-ray head. *Med Phys*, 2007. **34**: 1797–808.
36. Kamino, Y. et al., Development of a four-dimensional image-guided radiotherapy system with a gimbaled X-ray head. *Int J Radiat Oncol Biol Phys*, 2006. **66**: 271–8.
37. Boswell, S.A. et al., A novel method to correct for pitch and yaw patient setup errors in helical tomotherapy. *Med Phys*, 2005. **32**: 1630–9.
38. Mamalui-Hunter, M., H. Li, and D.A. Low, Linac mechanic QA using a cylindrical phantom. *Phys Med Biol*, 2008. **53**: 5139–49.
39. Li, W. et al., Accuracy of automatic couch corrections with on-line volumetric imaging. *J Appl Clin Med Phys*, 2009. **10**: 3056.
40. Fenwick, J.D. et al., Quality assurance of a helical tomotherapy machine. *Phys Med Biol*, 2004. **49**: 2933–53.
41. Cheng, C.W. et al., Commissioning and clinical implementation of a sliding gantry CT scanner installed in an existing treatment room and early clinical experience for precise tumor localization. *Am J Clin Oncol*, 2003. **26**: e28–36.
42. Lutz, W., K.R. Winston, N. Maleki, A system for stereotactic radiosurgery with a linear accelerator. *Int J Radiat Oncol Biol Phys*, 1988. **14**: 373–81.
43. Rahimian, J. et al., Geometrical accuracy of the Novalis stereotactic radiosurgery system for trigeminal neuralgia. *J Neurosurg*, 2004. **101**(Suppl. 3): 351–55.
44. Glide-Hurst, C. et al., Commissioning of the Varian TrueBeam linear accelerator: A multi-institutional study. *Med Phys*, 2013. **40**: 031719.
45. Mutic, S. et al., Quality assurance for computed-tomography simulators and the computed-tomography-simulation process: Report of the AAPM Radiation Therapy Committee Task Group No. 66. *Med Phys*, 2003. **30**: 2762–92.
46. Langen, K.M., S.L. Meeks, and J. Pouliot, Quality assurance of onboard megavoltage computed tomography imaging and target localization systems for on- and off-line image-guided radiotherapy. *Int J Radiat Oncol Biol Phys*, 2008. **71**: S62–65.
47. Huq, M.S. et al., The report of Task Group 100 of the AAPM: application of risk analysis methods to radiation therapy quality management. *Med Phys*. 2016;43:4209-62.
48. Bissonnette, J.P. et al., Quality assurance for the geometric accuracy of cone-beam CT guidance in radiation therapy. *Int J Radiat Oncol Biol Phys*, 2008. **71**: S57–61.

49. Keall, P.J. et al., The management of respiratory motion in radiation oncology report of AAPM Task Group 76. *Med Phys*, 2006. **33**: 3874–900.
50. Jiang, S.B., J. Wolfgang, and G.S. Mageras, Quality assurance challenges for motion-adaptive radiation therapy: Gating, breath holding, and four-dimensional computed tomography. *Int J Radiat Oncol Biol Phys*, 2008. **71**: S103–7.
51. Timmerman, R. et al., Accreditation and quality assurance for Radiation Therapy Oncology Group: Multicenter clinical trials using Stereotactic Body Radiation Therapy in lung cancer. *Acta Oncol*, 2006. **45**: 779–86.
52. Bayouth, J. et al., Evaluation of 4DRT: CT acquisition and gated delivery system. *Med Phys*, 2006. **33**: 2188–9.
53. Jiang, S.B., Technical aspects of image-guided respiration-gated radiation therapy. *Med Dosim*, 2006. **31**: 141–51.
54. Shirato, H. et al., Real-time tumour-tracking radiotherapy. *Lancet*, 1999. **353**: 1331–2.
55. Mageras, G.S. et al., Fluoroscopic evaluation of diaphragmatic motion reduction with a respiratory gated radiotherapy system. *J Appl Clin Med Phys*, 2001. **2**: 191–200.
56. Neicu, T. et al., Synchronized moving aperture radiation therapy (SMART): Improvement of breathing pattern reproducibility using respiratory coaching. *Phys Med Biol*, 2006. **51**: 617–36.
57. Berbeco, R.I. et al., A technique for respiratory-gated radiotherapy treatment verification with an EPID in cine mode. *Phys Med Biol*, 2005, **50**: 3669–79.
58. McIntosh, A. et al., Quantifying the reproducibility of heart position during treatment and corresponding delivered heart dose in voluntary deep inhalation breath hold for left breast cancer patients treated with external beam radiotherapy. *Int J Radiat Oncol Biol Phys*, 2011. **81**: e569–576.
59. Ng, J.A. et al., Quality assurance for the clinical implementation of kilovoltage intrafraction monitoring for prostate cancer VMAT. *Med Phys*, 2014. **41**: 111712.
60. Santanam, L. et al., Quality assurance for clinical implementation of an electromagnetic tracking system. *Med Phys*, 2009. **36**: 3477–86.
61. Jung, J. et al., Verification of accuracy of CyberKnife tumor-tracking radiation therapy using patient-specific lung phantoms. *Int J Radiat Oncol Biol Phys*, 2015. **92**: 745–53.
62. Depuydt, T. et al., Initial assessment of tumor tracking with a gimbaled linac system in clinical circumstances: A patient simulation study. *Radiother Oncol*, 2013. **106**: 236–40.
63. Krauss, A., S. Nill, and U. Oelfke, The comparative performance of four respiratory motion predictors for real-time tumour tracking. *Phys Med Biol*, 2011. **56**: 5303–17.
64. Depuydt, T. et al., Geometric accuracy of a novel gimbals based radiation therapy tumor tracking system. *Radiother Oncol*, 2011. **98**: 365–72.
65. Depuydt, T. et al., Treating patients with real-time tumor tracking using the Vero gimbaled linac system: Implementation and first review. *Radiother Oncol*, 2014. **112**: 343–51.
66. Sawant, A. et al., Management of three-dimensional intrafraction motion through real-time DMLC tracking. *Med Phys*, 2008. **35**: 2050–61.
67. Poulsen, P.R. et al., Image-based dynamic multileaf collimator tracking of moving targets during intensity-modulated arc therapy. *Int J Radiat Oncol Biol Phys*, 2012. **83**: e265–271.
68. Graves, Y.J. et al. A deformable head and neck phantom with in-vivo dosimetry for adaptive radiotherapy quality assurance. *Med Phys*, 2015. **42**: 1490–7.
69. Bissonnette, J.P. et al., Cone-beam computed tomographic image guidance for lung cancer radiation therapy. *Int J Radiat Oncol Biol Phys*, 2009. **73**: 927–34.
70. Sonke, J.J. et al., Frameless stereotactic body radiotherapy for lung cancer using four-dimensional cone beam CT guidance. *Int J Radiat Oncol Biol Phys*, 2009. **74**: 567–74.
71. Galerani, A.P. et al., Dosimetric impact of online correction via cone-beam CT-based image guidance for stereotactic lung radiotherapy. *Int J Radiat Oncol Biol Phys*, 2010. **78**: 1571–8.
72. Ikushima, H. et al., Daily alignment results of in-room computed tomography-guided stereotactic body radiation therapy for lung cancer. *Int J Radiat Oncol Biol Phys*, 2011. **79**: 473–80.
73. Masi, L. et al., On-line image guidance for frameless stereotactic radiotherapy of lung malignancies by cone beam CT: Comparison between target localization and alignment on bony anatomy. *Acta Oncol*, 2008. **47**: 1422–31.

74. Verellen, D. et al., Gating and tracking, 4D in thoracic tumours. *Cancer Radiother*, 2010. **14**: 446–54.
75. Purdy, J.A., Quality assurance issues in conducting multi-institutional advanced technology clinical trials. *Int J Radiat Oncol Biol Phys*, 2008. **71**: S66–70.
76. Middleton, M. et al., Successful implementation of image-guided radiation therapy quality assurance in the Trans Tasman Radiation Oncology Group 08.01 PROFIT Study. *Int J Radiat Oncol Biol Phys*, 2011. **81**: 1576–81.
77. Galvin, J., TH-A-M100E-05: Credentialing IGRT Verification Techniques for Clinical Trials. *Medical Physics*. 2007;34:2616 -16.
78. Potters, L. et al., American Society for Therapeutic Radiology and Oncology (ASTRO) and American College of Radiology (ACR) practice guidelines for image-guided radiation therapy (IGRT). *Int J Radiat Oncol Biol Phys*, 2010. **76**: 319–25.
79. Cui, Y. et al., Multi-system verification of registrations for image-guided radiotherapy in clinical trials. *Int J Radiat Oncol Biol Phys*, 2011. **81**: 305–12.
80. Cui, Y. et al., Implementation of remote 3-dimensional image guided radiation therapy quality assurance for radiation therapy oncology group clinical trials. *Int J Radiat Oncol Biol Phys*, 2013. **85**: 271–7.
81. Alvarez, P. et al., Results of irradiations performed on radiological physics center's anthropomorphic lung phantom and respiratory simulating motion table, 2013.
82. Dempsey, J. et al., A real-time MRI guided external beam radiotherapy delivery system. *Med Phys*, 2006. **33**: 2254.
83. Olsen, J. et al., Feasibility of single and multiplane cine MR for monitoring tumor volumes and organs-at-risk (OARs) position during radiation therapy. *Int J Radiat Oncol Biol Phys*, 2012. **84**: S742.
84. Green, O. et al., TH-AB-303-12: Commissioning of Magnetic Resonance Imaging-Based Tumor Tracking and Beam Control. *Med Phys*, 2015. **42**: 3713.
85. Sawant, A. et al., Failure mode and effect analysis-based quality assurance for dynamic MLC tracking systems. *Med Phys*, 2010. **37**: 6466–79.

PART 3

PRACTICE OF IGRT FOR LUNG CANCER

7

L-shaped linacs

DAVID HOFFMAN, JULIAN PERKS, STEVE GOETSCH,
AND STANLEY BENEDICT

7.1 INTRODUCTION

Linear accelerators (linacs) have been in use since 1953 when a device built by Metropolitan-Vickers was installed at Hammersmith Hospital in London, England with a photon energy of 8 megavoltage (MV). Subsequently, two 4 megaelectron volt (MeV) machines manufactured by Mullard Equipment Company (a division of Philips Medical, later acquired by Elekta) were installed at other hospitals in England [1]. A 6-MeV machine built by a research group at Stanford University was used to treat patients in 1956 [2]. These machines rapidly proved their value and made an important contribution to radiation therapy. The first machines were very long (up to 3 meters!) and ungainly. Some of the early machines could not rotate around the patient. Varian installed its first machine, a 6-MV fully isocentric unit, at the University of California at Los Angeles (UCLA)

Medical Center in Los Angeles in 1962. At that time, there were only 15 clinical linear accelerators in the world, plus a number of Van de Graaf units and about 50 betatrons [1].

Modern linear accelerators have become more compact, far more stable, and are capable of producing a number of photon and electron energies [2]. The rotational stability of these units has markedly improved; they can achieve a mechanical accuracy of 1 millimeter or less in three rotational directions. Beginning in the early 1980s, after the early success of the Leksell Gamma Knife, several centers experimented with add-on devices to direct a small, precise beam of photons through a circular collimator to an intracranial stereotactic target. Soon, several manufacturers were selling add-on accessories and planning systems for linac-based stereotactic treatments.

The latest generation of linacs offers a full panoply of radiation modalities, including multiple electron and photon energies, conventional or flattening filter-free (FFF) modes (up to 2400 MU/minute), and micro-multileaf collimators (MLC) and/or circular collimators for precise small field treatments. A wide range of on-board imaging capabilities are offered, including kilovoltage (kV) and MV digital flat-film detectors, kV and MV cone beam computed tomography (CBCT) capabilities, infrared and/or cross-firing x-ray position detection devices, and now also video positioning devices. Immobilization technology for patients has made possible a wide range of stereotactic radiosurgery and stereotactic radiotherapy applications. The most recent innovation in treatment delivery, known as intensity-modulated arc therapy (IMAT), is an advanced form of rotational therapy, taking advantage of modulation of output, gantry speed, and precise movements of MLCs. This advanced treatment capability has been incorporated into modern treatment planning systems and now permits very complex treatments to be delivered to a patient in one or two arcs in a period of 2–3 minutes [3].

7.2 OVERVIEW OF THE CURRENTLY COMMERCIALLY AVAILABLE L-SHAPED LINACS

This chapter compares three commercially available linacs: the Elekta Versa HD™ (Figure 7.1), the Varian TrueBeam™ (Figure 7.2), and the Brainlab Novalis® (Figure 7.3). The characteristics of these three linac accelerators and their treatment couches are summarized in Tables 7.1 and 7.2, respectively.

7.2.1 Elekta Versa HD

The Elekta Versa HD was introduced into clinical practice in April 2013. This accelerator draws its RF power from a magnetron, using a non-gridded heated tungsten filament electron gun. The available photon energies are 6, 10, 15, and 18 MV and the electron energies are 6, 9, 12, 15, 18, and 20 MeV; these energies are generated by the power applied to the waveguide. The waveguide itself is of the traveling design, and after acceleration, the electron beam passes through a set of bellows and is transported to the beam bending system. This bending system comprises an achromatic triple magnet array (slalom) to double focus the electron beam; the beam deflected an effective 112° (from 22° above horizontal to 90° below). A FFF mode is available for the Versa HD capable of 2200 MU/min for 6-MV x-rays. The MLC of the Versa HD consists of 80 pairs of 5-mm leaves for a maximum field size of 40 × 40 cm. The maximum leaf speed is 65 mm/s and the machine can deliver both intensity-modulated radiation therapy (IMRT) and volumetric modulated arc therapy (VMAT) in addition to traditional fields [4].

The imaging system of the Versa HD is a pair of amorphous silicon panels, one in the beam line and the other perpendicular to it. The in-line panel provides standard, mega-voltage portal imaging and the perpendicular system provides kV CBCT. The CBCT system provides a set of protocols of varying kV, mAs, frame-rate, and field size for the clinical range of anatomic sites. All the imaging parameters are customizable by the user for specific needs, e.g., the kV can be adjusted from 100 kV up to 150 kV and the volumetric images can be formed from arc lengths from 200° up to 360°. The customization allows the user to optimize the scans as a balance of imaging dose and image quality. A four-dimensional (4D) CBCT scan is also available to capture

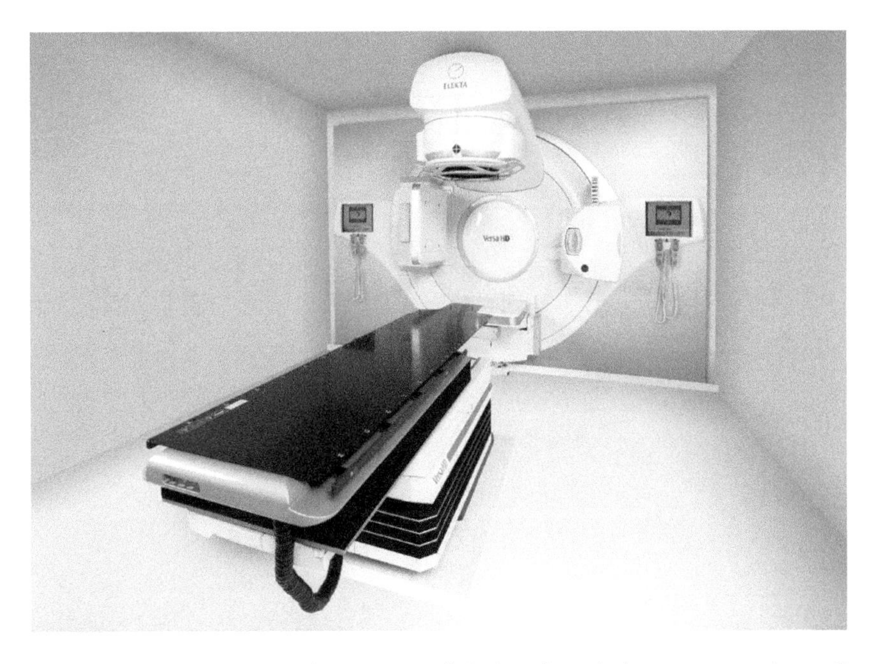

Figure 7.1 The Elekta Versa HD™ provides an array of IGRT tools, including two amorphous silicon panels for MV portal imaging, perpendicular kV imaging, and kV CBCT. 4D CBCT is possible to characterize patient motion, especially useful in the case of lung lesions.

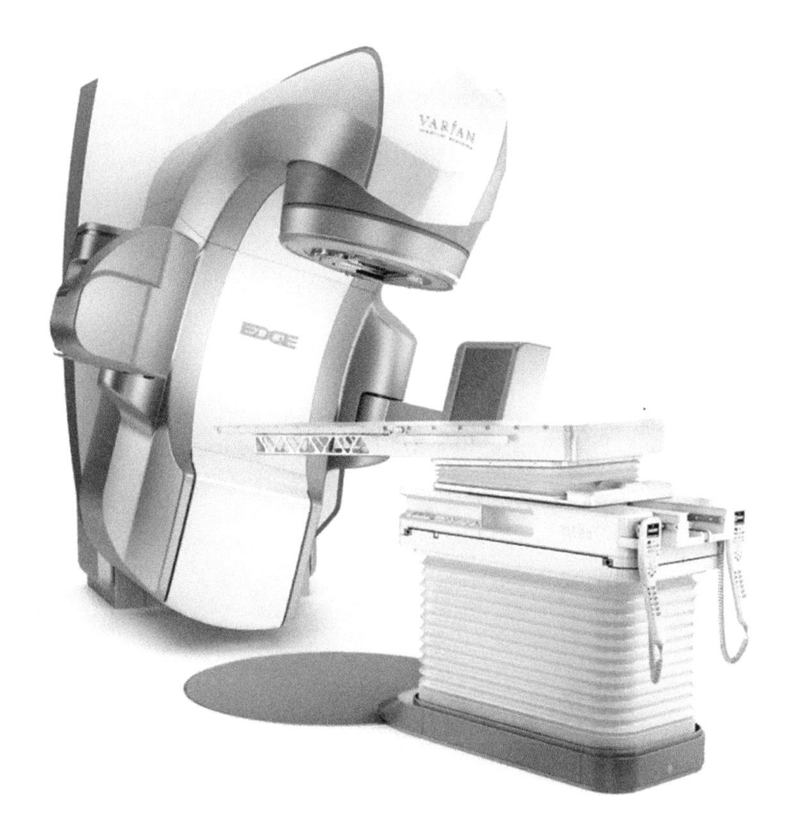

Figure 7.2 The Varian TrueBeam™ linac may be incorporated into the Edge radiosurgery system, which incorporates perpendicular gantry mounted MV electronic portal imaging and kV imaging for planar, fluoroscopic, and CBCT image guidance.

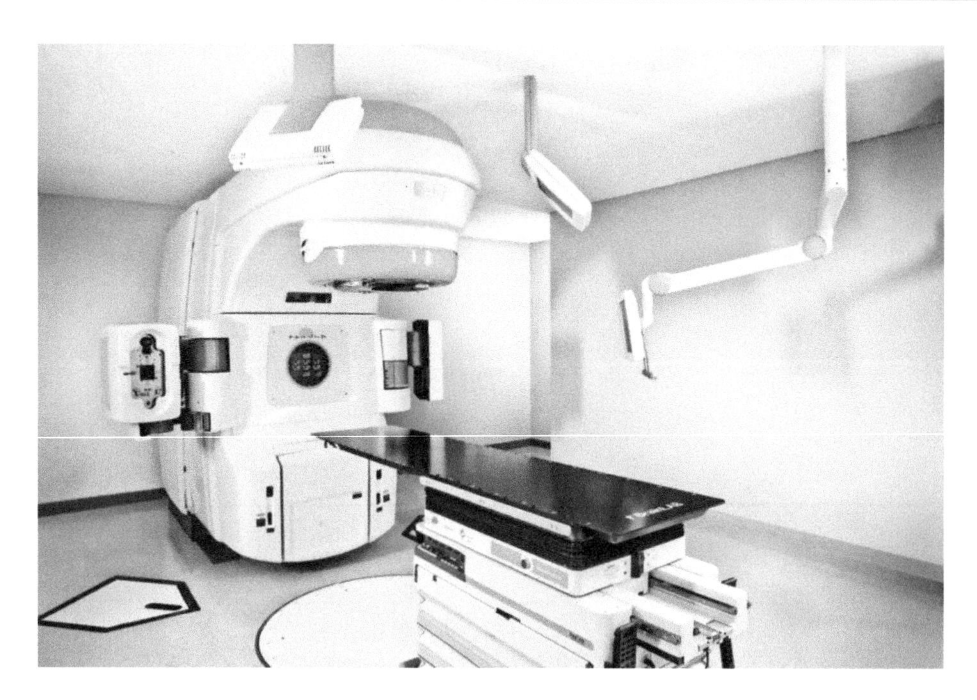

Figure 7.3 The Novalis® system has IGRT tools including MV electronic portal imaging and kV planar, fluoroscopic, and CBCT.

Table 7.1 Linac Characteristics

Manufacturer	Elekta	Varian	Brainlab
Linac	Versa HD™	TrueBeam™	Novalis®
RF source	Magnetron	Klystron	Klystron
Flattened Photon Configuration	6 MV, 10/15/18 MV	6 MV	6 MV, 10/15/18/20 MV
FFF Photon Configuration	6 MV	6 MV, 10 MV	None
Electron energies	Yes	No	Yes
MLC leaf size	5 mm	2.5 mm (central) 5 mm (peripheral)	2.5 mm (central) 4 mm (peripheral)
MLC leaf speed	65 mm/s	2.5 cm/s	25 mm/s
Maximum static field size	40 × 40 cm (35 cm with corners)	40 × 22 cm	40 × 22 cm
Maximum dose rate	2200 MU/minute	2400 MU/minute	1000 MU/minute
Gating capability	Yes	Yes	Yes
Gating input	Response™ interface	Real-time Position Management™/Open	Open
Treatment delivery capabilities	3D, IMRT, VMAT	3D, IMRT, VMAT	3D, IMRT, VMAT

Table 7.2 Treatment Couch Characteristics

Manufacturer	Elekta	Varian	Brainlab
Linac	Versa HD	TrueBeam	Novalis
Degrees of motion	3 degrees	6 degrees	6 degrees
Weight capacity	200 kg	150 kg	–
Setup indexing configuration	BodyFIX® 14	Vac-Q-Fix indexer	Indexed Immobilization®

breathing motion for lung cases, a 20-cm-long volumetric imaging of lungs, split into 10 binned phases, can be formed from a single arc CBCT where the gantry motion is slowed to capture the breathing motion; this scan take approximately 3 min.

7.2.2 Varian TrueBeam

The Varian TrueBeam was introduced in 2010. It is designed to be a linear accelerator with capabilities for every kind of radiation therapy procedure likely to be needed in a modern radiation oncology department. Six photon energies are available at 4, 6, 8, 10, 15, and 20 MV with an output of 600 MU/min at every energy except 4 MV (250 MU/min). FFF modes are available at 6X (1400 MU/min) and 10X (2400 MU/min). The linac also offers eight electron energies at 6, 9, 12, 15, 16, 18, 20, and 22 MeV. Two special high-dose total skin electron modes (HDTSE) are available at 6 and 9 MeV (1000 MU/min). The TrueBeam utilizes the Millennium™ 120-leaf MLC with 40 leaf pairs at 5 mm width and 20 pairs at 10 mm width, with a total field size of 40 by 40 cm [5].

The TrueBeam is equipped with the PerfectPitch™ couch with six degrees of freedom, making it a fully robotic couch. The gantry and collimator are specified to have rotational accuracy less than or equal to 0.5 mm and the gantry, collimator, and couch have a rotational accuracy of less than or equal to 0.75 mm. The gantry is warranted to have a rotational accuracy of less than or equal to 0.3°.

The imaging system for the TrueBeam includes kV planar imaging, kV Conebeam CT, and fluoroscopy. The pixel matrix is 2048 by 1536 or 1024 by 768. The Calypso® 4D Localization System™ is provided for alignment of any body site except lung. It utilizes markers surgically implanted in the target volume with RFID tracking devices. The system reports marker position 25 times/s and automatically shuts off the beam if the target moves out of position. The Calypso system also includes the Surface Beacon® transponder for external placement to track lung movement.

7.2.3 Novalis system

The Novalis system was the result of collaboration between Varian Medical Systems (Palo Alto, CA) and Brainlab (Munich, Germany). The original Novalis system was an upgraded Varian Clinac 600 SR linac, capable of one photon energy (6 MV) and no electron capability. It was installed at UCLA Medical Center, Department of Radiation Oncology in 1997 and included a miniature MLC permanently installed to the linac. It could also use cylindrical circular collimators on an accessory mount [6]. The dose rate was 800 MU/min and the useful field size was 9.8 by 9.8 cm^2. The original system featured the ExacTrac® x-ray (ETX) system of ceiling-mounted orthogonal x-ray generators with floor-mounted amorphous silicon solid state detectors to localize patient markers and/or patient anatomy. The original "Classic Novalis" unit was linked to the BrainScan treatment planning software. Later units were supplied with a detachable Brainlab MLC. The original UCLA unit included an interlock system which detected the presence and size of the cylindrical add-on collimator, while later versions of this unit lacked this important safety interlock.

The Novalis system evolved into the Novalis Tx in 2007, based on the Varian Tx linac supplied with the Varian High Definition Multileaf Collimator (HDMLC), featuring 6 MV, 15 MV, and 6 MV photon high-dose (1000 MU/min) dose rate modes [7, 8].

The Novalis system is currently offered by Varian Medical and Brainlab as the TrueBeam STx with Novalis Radiosurgery system as well as the Novalis Tx image-guided radiosurgery linear accelerator system. Both use the iPlan treatment planning software, ExacTrac x-ray system, infrared patient positioning system, and six-dimensional (6D) robotic couch. Each can treat up to 40 by 40 cm^2 field sizes, and have high-dose-rate FFF modes.

The Novalis Tx offers up to five photon energies (6–25 MV), with 1000 MU/min in stereotactic radiosurgery mode and six electron beams (4–22 MeV). The Novalis Tx is equipped with the HD 120 MLC with 120 leaves, including 64 2.5-mm inner leaves and 56 5-mm outer leaves with a maximum field size of 40 × 22 cm^2. The maximum leaf speed is 25 mm/s. The maximum dose rate is 600 MU/min for IMRT treatments and 1000 MU/min in the radiosurgery mode. The Novalis imaging capabilities include MV electronic portal imaging devices (EPID) imaging (PortalVision a S1000) with 1024 by 768 pixels (400 by 300 mm^2 field size) and the Paxscan 4030 CB CBCT with 2048 by 1536 pixels (400 by 300 mm^2 field size. The ExacTrac infrared patient position and tracking system and x-ray 6D system is an optional accessory. The optional PortalVision portal dosimetry records the intensity distribution of IMRT fields. The real-time position management (RPM) system permits respiratory gating for motion management of patient treatments. The 6D Adaptive Gating Module is also available for high-resolution scans of moving targets during treatment. RapidArc IMRT treatment is available with this system.

The TrueBeam STx linear accelerator is the stereotactic option of the TrueBeam linear accelerator [5]. The STx option includes four photon energies (6, 8, 10, and 15 MV, 600 MU/min) with FFF modes at 6 and 10 MV (1400 and 2400 MU/min, respectively). The High Definition Multileaf Collimator (HD-MLC) with 2.5-mm central leaves is standard with the TrueBeam STx, while the Millennium MLC is standard with the TrueBeam system (5-mm central leaf width). The gantry and collimator isocenter accuracy is specified as 05 mm or less, while the gantry, collimator, and couch isocenter accuracy is specified as 0.75 mm or less, with a rotational accuracy of 0.5° or less. Glidehurst et al. report gantry/collimator of 0.265–0.283 mm for five different linacs [5].

The amorphous silicon onboard 6-MV imager has a pixel matrix of 1024 by 768 pixels with an active imaging area of 30.1 by 40.1 cm^2. The kV imager operates at 75, 100, or 125 kVp and uses amorphous silicon detectors with 2048 by 1536 pixels (39.7 by 29.8 cm^2 area). The kV CBCT system operates at 100 kVp with a 512 by 512 matrix and 2-mm slice thickness.

7.3 IGRT ON L-SHAPED LINACS

Image-guided radiation therapy (IGRT) refers to the general principle where a patient set for radiation treatment is aligned to the beam by a captured image. Using an image to position the patient acknowledges that patient anatomy differs on a daily basis, and that accurate beam delivery requires knowledge of the internal anatomy to align to the beam. Numerous studies have confirmed the requirement for on-set imaging, and further reports exist on how frequent the imaging should be (daily or less than), the size of the shift discrepancy to be expected, and intervention protocols [9].

Many technologies have been developed to address on-board imaging (OBI) and they have progressed from two-dimensional projections to three-dimensional (3D) datasets and most recently four-dimensional (4D) scans that can capture a motion component as well as overall anatomy. Initially, on-board imaging was achieved with film in a cassette, placed perpendicular to the beam line at an extended source-to-surface distance (SSD), typically 140 cm. Without CT, aided planning, and virtual simulation, this port film was compared with an image formed by a conventional simulator, i.e., an isocentric kV x-ray set.

The development of flat-panel imaging systems, including ion chamber arrays and amorphous silicon, allowed for faster clinical implementation of 2D IGRT. Ion chamber panels are filled with isooctane and the 1-mm layer of this liquid is where the ionization takes place. The image is formed by a 256 × 256 matrix of switches and electrometers which pixelate the ionization space. Recently, amorphous silicon has replaced liquid ionization as the detector medium; this has allowed increased pixel counts.

With the limitations posed by 2D planar imaging, there is a clear advantage of volumetric imaging for image guidance in radiation therapy. The first solution to CT scanning a radiation therapy patient in the treatment was to introduce a diagnostic CT scanner into the treatment room. This so-called CT-on-rails was usually placed with the axis of the bore at 90° to the unrotated treatment couch. Then, through a series of couch rotations and translations, the patient was put through the CT scanner, imaged, set to (virtual) isocenter, and translated back to the treatment isocenter. This clearly relies on high-precision couch movements as the shifts needed to correct a patient position are of the order of millimeters, and so the mechanical accuracy of the CT scanner and couch mechanism needs to be about a magnitude better.

Due to the geometric convenience of mounting the CT imaging equipment on the x-ray beam gantry CT-on-rails has been superseded by cone beam CT. The concept of CBCT, where a volumetric dataset is created by one rotation around the patient, was well established for dental imaging before its use in radiation therapy.

The concept is that a square-based cone (pyramid) of image information can be collected during a rotation of the x-ray around the subject. The advantage of conventional sliced CT techniques is that only one rotation is needed; however, the increased photon scatter as the data are collected degrades the image, reducing resolution.

Tables 7.3 and 7.4 summarize the characteristics of the kV image guidance and the MV image guidance, respectively, for the three commonly available commercial linac accelerators. Figure 7.4 illustrates the typical lung cancer patient IGRT on L-shaped linac.

7.3.1 MV PORTS

Using the treatment beam to image a radiation oncology patient on set is possibly the most intuitive form of image formation. The advantages for using the treatment beam include the patient being ready for treatment immediately before the image is taken, the alignment of the beam to the treatment isocenter, and the imaging dose can sometimes be considered as "free." An MV radiation treatment beam should be aligned to the room isocenter to within 2 mm [10]. MV portal imaging can take advantage of this alignment by the treatment beam being the source of photons for the image formation. The image itself is formed on a panel which extends on an armature to catch the transmitted beam, it transmits the patient, and then forms an image from that flux. As the treatment beam is used with the patient on set any misalignments of the patient can be swiftly corrected and implemented with couch shifts, and a second confirmation image can then be taken if desired. In certain circumstances, the photons which form the image may even be the first part of the planned treated field, e.g., a four-field pelvis treatment with large orthogonal fields [11].

As with all imaging methodologies, there are drawbacks and compromises associated with MV portal imaging. First, the beam energy of 6 MV (peak and thus 2-MV average) is not ideal. Fully in the Compton scatter dominant range of the kV–MV spectrum, there is a predominance of scatter in the patient which leads to blur and contrast reduction in the image. The contrast reduction is quite marked at this imaging beam energy and it is typical to have only bony anatomy visible, and even the trained eye can only distinguish gross displacements with orthogonal imaging. The portal images obtained on set are compared to digitally reconstructed radiographs (DRR), which are formed from the CT data during treatment planning. Image resolution, of both the DRR and the MV port, limit the accuracy to which MV portal imaging can be applied. The MV port is formed on an amorphous silicon panel, which needs to be notably thick to stop sufficient photons

Table 7.3 kV Image Guidance

Manufacturer	Elekta	Varian	BrainLab
Linac	Versa HD™	TrueBeam™	Novalis®
2D radiograph	Yes	Yes	Yes
Fluoroscopy	Yes	Yes	Yes
CBCT	Yes	Yes	Yes
CBCT field of view	50 × 26 cm		39.7 × 29.8 cm
4D CBCT	Yes	No	No
Tube current range	40 mA	0.1–1000 mAs	
Tube voltage range	100–150 kV	40–140 kVp	40–150 kVp

Table 7.4 MV Image Guidance

Manufacturer	Elekta	Varian	BrainLab
Linac	Versa HD™	TrueBeam™	Novalis®
2D Portal Image	Yes	Yes	Yes
Fluoroscopy	Yes	Yes	Yes
CBCT	No	No	No

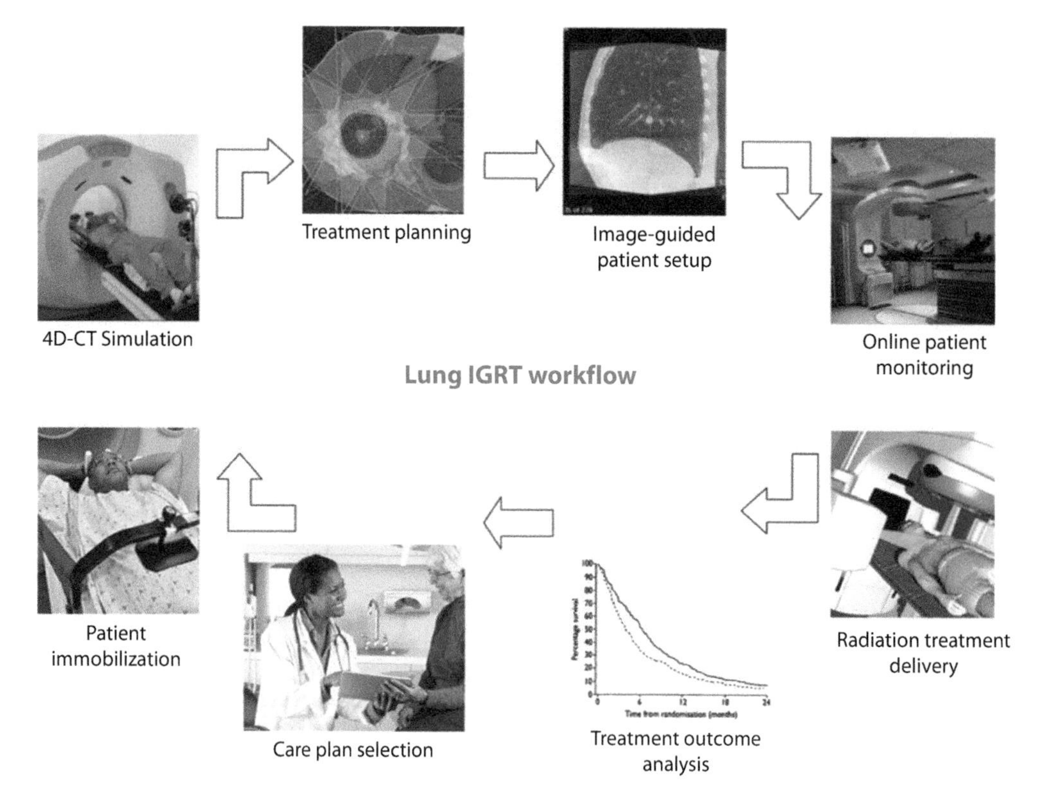

Figure 7.4 The clinical work flow for typical lung cancer patient treated with IGRT. The clinical work flow connects with the clinical outcomes analysis that informs care plan selection and improvement of the entire process

to form an image; this leads to a decrease in the portal image resolution. Overall, MV portal imaging can provide translational accuracy only (not enough information for rotational corrections) with a resolution of 3–5 mm minimal shift.

7.3.2 MV FLUOROSCOPY

As the MV portal image is formed by the treatment beam after it exits the patient, theoretically any number of images can be taken during the beam on time. The number of images would be limited somewhat by the refresh rate of the imaging panel; also, the usefulness of the imaging information would be limited by the nature of the MV port, namely that only bony anatomy would be seen and only the anatomy which is being irradiated. That said, there is no additional imaging dose to the patient. So, if gross, bony shifts are a concern, they can be resolved through a cine series of MV ports, and then an MV fluoroscopic mode could be used clinically.

7.3.3 kV RADIOGRAPH

While two-dimensional in nature, kV planar images offer a significant resolution improvement over MV ports due to lower x-ray energy yielding an increased probability of photoelectric interaction in the patient. This leads to reduced scatter in the image. Additionally, a thinner and more sensitive panel can be used with kV imaging. To this extent, kV portal imaging has the resolution to allow clinical use of non-orthogonal images for matching and patient registration. From a QA standpoint the additional consideration of a kV imaging system is that it requires alignment with the room isocenter; the increased image quality comes with the price of extra QA checks [12].

7.3.4 kV FLUOROSCOPY

One further advantage of kV imaging is the rapidity with which images can be taken linked to the relatively low dose of each exposure. As the treatment beam does not have to be interrupted to take a kV image, several images can be taken to confirm and reconfirm positional information, to the extent of facilitating beam gating-based breathing patterns.

Rapidly acquired kV images can also be easily linked and played as a cine loop. The main use of this technique is to acquire a fluoroscopic view of a patient's breathing pattern and diaphragm motion. Typically around 100–150 frames are captured, each being 120 kV and 50 ms long [13].

7.3.5 kV CBCT (4D CBCT)

For a linear accelerator fitted with a kV imaging set, mounted isocentrically off the MV beam line, the formation of a CT dataset can be facilitated by "snapping" numerous frames of image data as the gantry is rotated. If sufficient planar images are taken, then software back-projection techniques can be employed to generate the 3D dataset. The principle of back-projection for cone beam images differs somewhat from more traditional single- or multi-slice CT, but CBCT algorithms are well established and validated [14].

The advantages of kV CBCT are that a volumetric dataset is generated as opposed to planar, projection images. The additional patient dose from the multiple projections is balanced by the advantages of the full CT reconstruction and the patient dose per CBCT is typically 1–3 mGy [15]. The 6D correction aspects are present with kV CBCT, as it is with stereoscopic planar projections, but the advantage of the full 3D dataset is that the parameters of the matching algorithm can be selected to preferentially favor a soft tissue match or a bony match, whichever is preferred for the given anatomy being imaged.

Additionally, a set of CBCT images taken through the patient treatment course will show how the treatment area (both tumor and surrounding tissues) is changing over time. This is one of the first crucial steps toward adaptive radiation therapy. In one interpretation, the adaptive approach, the temporal changes in the target area are tracked until some dosimetric threshold is reached, at which point a new plan is implemented. This could be as simple as one replan being applied in response to a patient losing weight after two weeks of the four-week course. A more intensive interpretation of adaptive radiation therapy would rely heavily on on-board, daily CT imaging; here the daily plan is adapted based on the target and organ at risk positions as they exist with the patient on set.

7.3.6 FIXED FLOOR MOUNTED 2D-3D REGISTRATION: BRAINLAB

The Brainlab ExacTrac system is an in-room system that utilizes two, floor-mounted, kV x-ray units positioned for stereoscopic projection with two ceiling-mounted detector panels. Images from the kV system are compared to digitally reconstructed radiographs, which are generated from the planning CT scan. The treatment planning software is programmed with the camera orientations and focal lengths so comparisons can be made between the DRR from the planning system and the on-set image(s). By utilizing two stereoscopic projections six degrees of positioning are afforded, three rotations and three translations [16].

7.3.7 LINAC WITH IN-ROOM CT

In-room CT was a forerunner of the gantry-mounted imaging system preceding CBCT. The premise here is that an anatomical assessment in the form of a 3D scan of the patient at the time of treatment is so useful that the technical difficulties of a diagnostic CT scanner in the room are justified. The main technical difficulties of a full, diagnostic type scanner in the treatment room include the size of the scanner itself, which prevents the scanner being mounted isocentrically. To overcome this, there is generally a very precise table repositioning mechanism to move the patient from CT scanning, through repositioning (the daily image guidance), to the treatment isocenter; this may even mean swinging the patient on the treatment table through 90 degrees [17].

7.4 IN-ROOM PATIENT SETUP AND MOTION-MONITORING STRATEGIES

There are several technologies that have been developed to guide radiation delivery and account for patient setup vitiations and target motion during treatment.

7.4.1 Calypso (prostate)

The Calypso system is a set of implanted tracking markers for positioning any body site except the lung during radiation delivery. The majority of clinical experience with Calypso is for prostate alignment and tracking. The system consists of three marker beacons, which are implanted into the prostate prior to patient CT planning, and a tracking station, which monitors the beacon position when the patient in under treatment. The beacons are about the size of a grain of rice and consist of an iron core, wrapped in copper wire and sleeved in a sterile glass tube. To track the beacon, an electric coil array is placed over the patient; when an alternating, pulsing pattern of electric current passes in the array a resonant frequency is created in beacons, which is detected by the same panel. Each of the three implanted beacons has different resonant frequencies so spatial differentiation is possible. Then, spatial localization and tracking is achieved by signal triangulation. Three beacons are recommended for the most accurate function but the system can function (both localize and track) if only two beacons are present [18].

The beacons are placed in a triangular pattern in the prostate via transrectal ultrasound guidance, nominally in the left, right, and apex positions. The beacons are identified during treatment planning and the 3D DICOM coordinates are entered into the Calypso control console, along with the isocenter coordinates. At the time of treatment, the patient is sent to the isocenter as usual and then the Calypso system is brought in to localize and then track the prostate. An in-room Geiger counter is also included in the system; this records when the treatment beam is on. At the end of the treatment, a report is produced to show the treatment team the shifts that were required to bring the beacons to the isocenter and how the beacons tracked in position with bars added to show the beam-on times.

7.4.2 Non-ionizing techniques with video/IR: AlignRT

Patient positioning and repositioning daily is an important challenge in radiation therapy. Treatment techniques have evolved to become more precise, with smaller margins. This has led to the rise of patient immobilization devices and in-room imaging systems. Milliken et al. at the University of Chicago Medical Center reported on a video image subtraction system to help position a patient at the time of treatment as closely as possible to the position the patient occupied at the time of radiation therapy simulation [19]. This technique was based on photogrammetry, a field which dates to the dawn of photography. Stereo photogrammetry is a specialized field which utilizes two or more images to accurately localize an object in 3D space. Yan et al. at Stanford University Medical Center advanced the field by developing a system with three video cameras which compared real-time patient surface images to DRRs [20]. This technique is now referred to as Surface Guided Radiation Therapy, or SGRT [21].

Vision RT (London, England) was founded in 2001 and began marketing its AlignRT® product in 2006. Bert et al. at Massachusetts General Hospital reported on this system in 2006 [22], quoting mean displacements of 7.3 mm and 7.6 mm for laser and port films, respectively. More recently, Cervino et al. at the University of California San Diego Medical Center reported on the use of Align RT with 23 patients undergoing frameless mask-less stereotactic radiosurgery [23]. They used the video system to set up patients and then confirmed their positions with CBCT. They found average shifts of 1.85-mm AP and 1.0-mm lateral and superior/inferior directions. The AlignRT system utilizes two or three ceiling-mounted camera units which project a pattern onto the patient and measure the reflection at up to 7.5 frames/s. Proprietary image evaluation software can be interfaced with the linear accelerator to initiate a treatment stop if the patient moves out of the specified alignment parameters.

C-Rad (Uppsala, Sweden) introduced a similar product called Catalyst in 2011 [24]. The optical surface scanning system also projected deviation from the planned treatment position onto the patient's skin in real time. The system used three high-powered light-emitting diodes to project three different colors of light (blue, green, and red) always. The blue light (405 nm) is used for position detection while the red (624 nm) and green (528 nm) lights are used to project deviations. Stieler et al. reported reproducibility with human patients was reported as 0.25 ± 0.21 cm, while accuracy was 0.52 ± 0.42 cm [24].

7.4.3 Implanted markers

Implanted markers have been used to delineate tumor boundaries since the dawn of the radiological era. Surgical clips have been implanted for decades by surgeons to mark the boundaries of a surgical resection, with the anticipation of "consolidation" radiation therapy to follow. This was often the only way that a radiation oncologist (who was also typically a radiologist by training during the first 50–60 years of radiation therapy) could outline the radiation fields to treat on a patient.

The dawn of the CT era in 1971 led to the implantation of radiologically opaque markers designed to be easily visible on an imaging study [25]. The markers were usually made of a high atomic number metabolically inert metal, such as gold, and were typically a few millimeters in size, and spherical or cylindrical in shape. The first noted use of these markers was to help delineate the apex of the prostate, which is difficult to see on ordinary transmission x-rays. Another early reported use was implanted skull markers for frameless stereotactic radiosurgery [26].

One disadvantage of implanted markers is that they must be surgically implanted, usually by a surgeon or an interventional radiologist. The recent rapid growth of IMRT has created the demand for 3D localization of the entire target volume, often on a real-time basis. This usually requires implantation of at least three well-spaced fiducials, which may be difficult to achieve. Nevertheless, implanted fiducials have been successfully used for treatment of lung and liver tumors [27].

Another disadvantage of implanted markers is their tendency to migrate from their initial positions. Radiation oncologists have warned patients for years that prostate seed implants (often with 100 or more seeds) have a possibility of migrating to the lungs or brain [28]. One study followed 32 patients with 147 implanted lung markers and found a mean migration of 1.28 mm (range 0.78–2.63 mm) [29]. Blockage of fiducials by moving MLC during VMAT can be minimized by re-optimization [7].

7.5 ONGOING DEVELOPMENTS OF L-SHAPED LINACS

Technological research continues to address the various challenges lung IGRT poses to optimal radiation therapy treatment. These new technologies allow for increased treatment planning flexibility and shorter treatment delivery time, and they can account for target volume motion.

7.5.1 MLC tumor tracking with MLC

Conforming a radiotherapy dose distribution to an irregular shape allows for simultaneous tumor treatment and normal tissue sparing, and thus is one of the guiding tenets of treatment. Many techniques have been developed to match the radiation field to complex, 3D, even folded tumors but, during treatment planning, they all rely on the target being stationary. However, it is easy to understand that extra-cranial targets vary in position on both an intra- and an interfractional basis. Many techniques have been put forward to account for tumor motion. One of the most technologically innovative is MLC tracking. The concept here is that imaging technology is employed throughout the treatment fraction to accurately locate and then continuously track the target. While the target motion is tracked the motion data are fed to the MLC processors and the MLC leaf positions are adjusted to cover the target as it moves [30].

7.5.2 4 Pi DELIVERY

The use of IMRT has grown dramatically since its introduction in 2000 [31]. Yet, the use of non-coplanar beams with dynamic movement of the linear accelerator gantry, MLC, beam intensity, and couch angle has not yet reached its full potential [32]. A new technique called 4 Pi Non-coplanar IMRT has been proposed by Sheng et al. at UCLA Medical Center [33]. This technique, not yet used clinically, involves using the full capability of the linear accelerator and patient support assembly to create new combinations of non-coplanar beams and variable source surface distances.

The keys to this new proposed treatment technique are (1) a novel algorithm developed at Erasmus Medical Center, Rotterdam, The Netherlands, called iCycle [34], which uses Pareto optimization to search over a multi-dimensional surface of possible irradiation methods until an optimum is achieved and (2) an extremely reliable computer-assisted design (CAD) model of the linear accelerator gantry and couch had to be created which eliminates the possibility of any form of collision involving linac with the couch or the patient [35]. The authors of the second study from UCLA and the University of Michigan Medical Centers retrospectively replanned 10 liver stereotactic body radiation therapy (SBRT) cases and reduced 50% dose spillage volume by 2% and integral dose by 19%.

The technique involves sweeping arcs with full MLC motion (as in VMAT), but also including full rotational motion of the patient support assembly from left to right and raising or lowering the couch above and below the isocenter to change the source surface distance.

REFERENCES

1. Karzmark, C.J. and N.C. Pering, Electron linear accelerators for radiation therapy: History, principles and contemporary developments. *Phys Med Biol*, 1973. **18**(3): 321–54.
2. Thwaites, D.I. and J.B. Tuohy, Back to the future: The history and development of the clinical linear accelerator. *Phys Med Biol*, 2006. **51**(13): R343–62.
3. Bortfeld, T. and R. Jeraj, The physical basis and future of radiation therapy. *Br J Radiol*, 2011. **84**(1002): 485–98.
4. Narayanasamy, G. et al., Commissioning an Elekta Versa HD linear accelerator. *J Appl Clin Med Phys*, 2016. **17**(1): 5799.
5. Glide-Hurst, C. et al., Commissioning of the Varian TrueBeam linear accelerator: A multi-institutional study. *Med Phys*, 2013. **40**(3): 031719.
6. Solberg, T.D. et al., Dynamic arc radiosurgery field shaping: A comparison with static field conformal and noncoplanar circular arcs. *Int J Radiat Oncol Biol Phys*, 2001. **49**(5): 1481–91.
7. Chang, Z. et al., Dosimetric characteristics of Novalis Tx system with high definition multileaf collimator. *Med Phys*, 2008. **35**(10): 4460–3.
8. Wurm, R.E. et al., Novalis frameless image-guided noninvasive radiosurgery: Initial experience. *Neurosurgery*, 2008. **62**(5 Suppl): A11–7; discussion A17–8.
9. De Los Santos, J. et al., Image guided radiation therapy (IGRT) technologies for radiation therapy localization and delivery. *Int J Radiat Oncol Biol Phys*, 2013. **87**(1): 33–45.
10. Herman, M.G. et al., Clinical use of electronic portal imaging: Report of AAPM Radiation Therapy Committee Task Group 58. *Med Phys*, 2001. **28**(5): 712–37.
11. Mubata, C.D. et al., Portal imaging protocol for radical dose-escalated radiotherapy treatment of prostate cancer. *Int J Radiat Oncol Biol Phys*, 1998. **40**(1): 221–31.
12. Sorcini, B. and A. Tilikidis, Clinical application of image-guided radiotherapy, IGRT (on the Varian OBI platform). *Cancer Radiother*, 2006. **10**(5): 252–7.
13. Werle, F. et al., Evaluation and choice of imaging protocols on the Elekta XVI (R) kilovoltage cone-beam computed tomography imaging system. *Cancer Radiother*, 2014. **18**(1): 47–54.
14. Lehmann, J. et al., Commissioning experience with cone-beam computed tomography for image-guided radiation therapy. *J Appl Clin Med Phys*, 2007. **8**(3): 2354.

15. Perks, J.R. et al., Comparison of peripheral dose from image-guided radiation therapy (IGRT) using kV cone beam CT to intensity-modulated radiation therapy (IMRT). *Radiother Oncol*, 2008. **89**(3): 304–10.
16. Jin, J.Y. et al., Use of the BrainLAB ExacTrac X-Ray 6D system in image-guided radiotherapy. *Med Dosim*, 2008. **33**(2): 124–34.
17. Ma, C.M. and K. Paskalev, In-room CT techniques for image-guided radiation therapy. *Med Dosim*, 2006. **31**(1): 30–9.
18. Willoughby, T.R. et al., Target localization and real-time tracking using the Calypso 4D localization system in patients with localized prostate cancer. *Int J Radiat Oncol Biol Phys*, 2006. **65**(2): 528–34.
19. Milliken, B.D. et al., Performance of a video-image-subtraction-based patient positioning system. *Int J Radiat Oncol Biol Phys*, 1997. **38**(4): 855–66.
20. Yan, Y., Y. Song, and A.L. Boyer, An investigation of a video-based patient repositioning technique. *Int J Radiat Oncol Biol Phys*, 2002. **54**(2): 606–14.
21. Willoughby, T. et al., Quality assurance for nonradiographic radiotherapy localization and positioning systems: Report of Task Group 147. *Med Phys*, 2012. **39**(4): 1728–47.
22. Bert, C. et al., Clinical experience with a 3D surface patient setup system for alignment of partial-breast irradiation patients. *Int J Radiat Oncol Biol Phys*, 2006. **64**(4): 1265–74.
23. Cervino, L.I. et al., Initial clinical experience with a frameless and maskless stereotactic radiosurgery treatment. *Pract Radiat Oncol*, 2012. **2**(1): 54–62.
24. Stieler, F. et al., A novel surface imaging system for patient positioning and surveillance during radiotherapy. A phantom study and clinical evaluation. *Strahlenther Onkol*, 2013. **189**(11): 938–44.
25. Sandler, H.M. et al., Localization of the prostatic apex for radiation therapy using implanted markers. *Int J Radiat Oncol Biol Phys*, 1993. **27**(4): 915–9.
26. Gall, K.P., L.J. Verhey, and M. Wagner, Computer-assisted positioning of radiotherapy patients using implanted radiopaque fiducials. *Med Phys*, 1993. **20**(4): 1153–9.
27. Wunderink, W. et al., Potentials and limitations of guiding liver stereotactic body radiation therapy set-up on liver-implanted fiducial markers. *Int J Radiat Oncol Biol Phys*, 2010. **77**(5): 1573–83.
28. Sugawara, A. et al., Incidence of seed migration to the chest, abdomen, and pelvis after transperineal interstitial prostate brachytherapy with loose (125)I seeds. *Radiat Oncol*, 2011. **6**: 130.
29. Hong, J.C. et al., Migration of implanted markers for image-guided lung tumor stereotactic ablative radiotherapy. *J Appl Clin Med Phys*, 2013. **14**(2): 4046.
30. Poulsen, P.R. et al., Image-based dynamic multileaf collimator tracking of moving targets during intensity-modulated arc therapy. *Int J Radiat Oncol Biol Phys*, 2012. **83**(2): e265–71.
31. Intensity Modulated Radiation Therapy Collaborative Working Group, Intensity-modulated radiotherapy: Current status and issues of interest. *Int J Radiat Oncol Biol Phys*, 2001. **51**(4): 880–914.
32. Sheng, K., D.M. Shepard, and C.G. Orton, Point/Counterpoint. Noncoplanar beams improve dosimetry quality for extracranial intensity modulated radiotherapy and should be used more extensively. *Med Phys*, 2015. **42**(2): 531–3.
33. Nguyen, D. et al., Integral dose investigation of non-coplanar treatment beam geometries in radiotherapy. *Med Phys*, 2014. **41**(1): 011905.
34. Breedveld, S. et al., iCycle: Integrated, multicriterial beam angle, and profile optimization for generation of coplanar and noncoplanar IMRT plans. *Med Phys*, 2012. **39**(2): 951–63.
35. Dong, P. et al., 4pi non-coplanar liver SBRT: A novel delivery technique. *Int J Radiat Oncol Biol Phys*, 2013. **85**(5): 1360–6.

8

TomoTherapy

KE SHENG

8.1 INTRODUCTION

8.1.1 Rotational IMRT and pre-helical TomoTherapy systems

Helical TomoTherapy® is an integrated software and hardware platform for image-guided intensity modulated radiotherapy (IMRT). The platform emerged as a marriage between arc therapy and static beam IMRT. There is a long history of using arcs for radiotherapy to improve dose conformity, homogeneity, and skin sparing [1]. The use of intensity modulation was first alluded to by Brahme in a rotational radiation therapy system to treat a ring structure [2]. The concept of modulating the fluency of intensity to improve the target dose homogeneity was then described by the same author [3]. The same group also suggested a device, named the multileaf collimator (MLC), for IMRT delivery [4]. The design and dosimetric characteristics of the device were then investigated [5]. Although the MLC was initially created for step-and-shoot IMRT on a C-arm gantry system, the first commercialized MLC used for patient treatment, interestingly enough, was for rotational delivery known as serial TomoTherapy [6,7]. The system, trademarked as Peacock by NOMOS, is illustrated in Figure 8.1. The 6 megavoltage (MV) therapeutic x-rays were collimated down to a slit fan beam. There were two

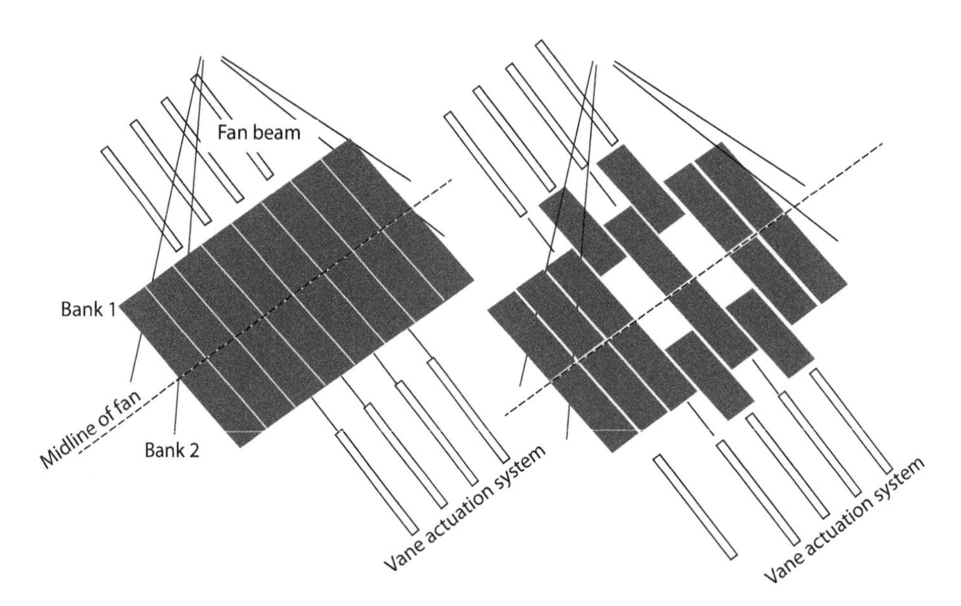

Figure 8.1 A schematic illustration of the slit beam of the MIMiC and its bixels. The left panel shows all leaves closed and the right panel shows two pairs of open leaves. (Modified from Mackie, T.R. et al., *Med Phys.*, 20, 1709–19, 1993.)

banks of opposing binary collimators that were trademarked as MIMiC. The mechanism allowed either fully opening or closing of a small beam aperture, which is also called a bixel in inverse optimization and treatment planning.

The serial TomoTherapy operated much like the CT scanners predating the helical CT scanner in that the couch was static during gantry rotation to allow treating one cranio-caudal segment of the patient before moving to the subsequent fan segments, until the entire treatment volume is covered. Different from the helical TomoTherapy system that is built on a dedicated rotational gantry platform, serial TomoTherapy was meant to be an add-on for the existing C-arm linacs. Serial TomoTherapy was one of the first systems that showed the feasibility of IMRT delivery by delivering concave isodose distributions that matched the calculated dose distribution. However, the serial TomoTherapy was limited in practicality. In addition to long delivery time, the static field junctions from stitching the slit fields together were prone to having dangerous hot and cold spots (over- and underdose volumes) for unavoidable slight filed mismatch.

8.1.2 Advent of helical TomoTherapy

A more practical design for rotational IMRT was first published in 1993 by T. Rock Mackie [8]. Based on a mechanism similar to the helical CT, the treatment couch moved continuously while the gantry rotated as radiation is being delivered. The helical trajectory largely mitigated the junction problem, and was significantly more efficient to deliver. This milestone paper conceptually described several key components of the helical TomoTherapy that later became widely available to treat patients. These components included binary MLCs, a CT detector array for the MV x-ray source, a slip ring, and adaptive radiotherapy based on the online CT images. The original design of the helical TomoTherapy system also included an orthogonal kV x-ray source and a separate detector array for kV fan beam CT, but the kV image system did not become part of the commercial system due to system complexity and cost concerns. The design decision was also due to the useable images obtained from the MV source and Xenon CT detectors [9].

The feasibility of TomoTherapy delivery as a valid concept was initially demonstrated using a Scanditronix Microtron MLC system and then single pencil beam produced from a conventional C-arm linac in 1997 [10]. After several more years of research, development, and commercialization, the first TomoTherapy prototype entered the clinic in 2000 and started to acquire MVCT images on animals and human patients. The system received FDA clearance in 2002 and was quickly adopted for treating cancer patients with a wide range of sites including brain, head and neck, prostate, and lung. To date, over 500 TomoTherapy systems have been installed worldwide.

8.2 TECHNICAL OVERVIEW OF HELICAL TOMOTHERAPY

8.2.1 Linac

A 6-MV S-band linac is used in TomoTherapy. The linac was initially supplied by Siemens Oncology Care Systems but later made in-house after TomoTherapy acquired a linac company. The Siemens linacs use a rotating target driven by cooling water. The design improved the cooling capacity, and allowed a smaller focal spot of approximately 1-mm, roughly half the size of a linac in a conventional C-arm system. The smaller focal spot is particularly important to the MVCT image quality. In the TomoTherapy system, the S-band linac was powered by a magnetron to produce 850 cGy/min at the isocenter, which is 850-mm away from the focal spot. The output was close to the higher end of the linac's capacity. The high demand on the linac compounded by the significantly higher monitor units in TomoTherapy treatment resulted in rapid deterioration of the linac and the target. In addition to overwhelming costs, the frequent service and replacement of linacs contributed to the downtime experienced by many early TomoTherapy adopters and created a significant burden on physicists for post-service calibration. After acquiring a linac manufacturer, TomoTherapy gradually replaced the Siemens linacs with the in-house linacs, which were characterized by slower deterioration, longer life span, and essentially the same focal spot, significant improvements in robustness over the Siemens linacs. The slightly lower energy (5.2 MV versus 5.7 MV) did not result in noticeable changes in the plan dosimetry [11].

Another important aspect of the TomoTherapy linac is that a flattening filter is not used, resulting in a tapered output toward the lateral edges of the field. This is acceptable for a system that exclusively uses IMRT. The x-rays are unattenuated without the flattening filter to improve delivery time and efficiency. The improvement is particularly significant for TomoTherapy, whose delivery efficiency using the fan beam geometry is considerably lower compared to platforms using the cone beam geometry. A typical TomoTherapy lateral profile is shown in Figure 8.2. The flattening-filter-free (FFF) field is also available in many C-arm linacs mainly for the purpose of high-dose treatment such as stereotactic radiosurgery (SRS) or stereotactic body radiation therapy (SBRT).

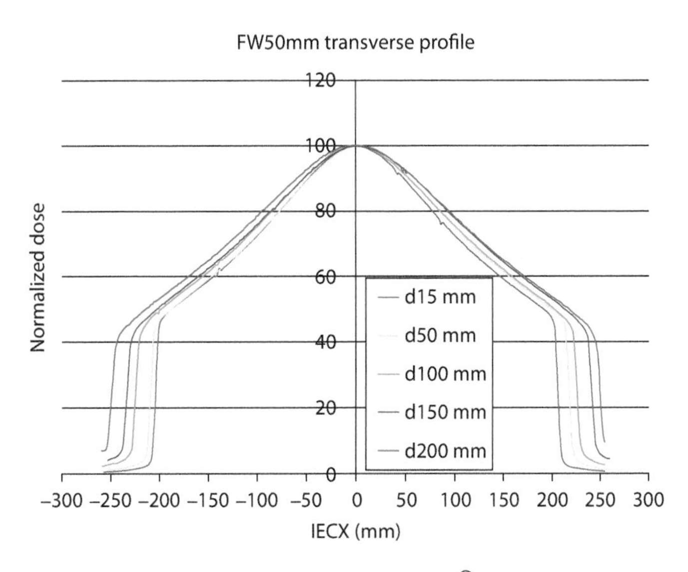

Figure 8.2 The lateral profile of a 5-cm jaw-open TomoTherapy® field at five different depths. The dose reduces to less than 50% of the its center value toward the edges of the field.

In contrast to C-arm linac systems, which are equipped with two pairs of orthogonal jaws to define square or rectangle fields, TomoTherapy uses one pair of jaws to define the narrow fan-fields in the superior/inferior direction. In the therapy mode, the jaws can be set to 1-cm, 2.5-cm, or 5-cm width measurements for treatment plans based on the size of the target and the varying needs for dose modulation resolution in the longitudinal direction. In the earlier TomoTherapy systems, a treatment plan was limited to using one fixed field width. The limitation resulted in compromised superior/inferior penumbra, poorer longitudinal modulation resolution, or prolonged delivery time for larger tumor targets. Dynamic jaws trademarked as TomoEdge™, which start and end a treatment with 1-cm jaw width and use wider field widths in between, have been implemented on later systems to overcome this limitation [12,13]. The lateral field size and modulation are determined by the TomoTherapy binary MLC, which will be introduced in the following section.

8.2.2 MVCT AND CT DETECTORS

As mentioned previously, due to the cost and complexity of integrating a kV system in TomoTherapy, kVCT is not included in the current generation of TomoTherapy systems. Instead of the kVCT, the same therapy MV x-ray source is matched with a Xenon linear CT detector array for MVCT imaging. Because of the significantly higher energy and lower cross intersection with Xenon gas, the pressurized chambers alone provide very low detector efficiency and signal-to-noise ratio. To mitigate this deficiency, the detector is offset from its originally intended location and moved closer to the MV source. As a consequence, the tungsten septa are not concentrically aligned to the source with increasing deviation toward the lateral channels. Because of the intentional misalignment, x-rays are intercepted by the septa that produce secondary charged particles for the Xenon chambers to absorb. The setup significantly increases the detector quantum efficiency but also results in a varying response that is low in the center and high toward the field edge. A typical lateral profile measured by the CT detector is shown in Figure 8.3. Compared to the profile measured using an ion chamber in the water, there is a sharp drop in the center channel signals; these channels are better aligned to the source and fewer photons are intercepted by the tungsten septa.

An additional function of the CT detector is to detect the exit x-ray from therapeutic beams. The CT detector is always active, recording the pulse-to-pulse signals after the x-rays penetrate the patient or phantom. The exit detector signal can be used to monitor the MLC leaf opening time [14], which in combination with the known patient geometry from the kVCT and MVCT has been shown to reconstruct the delivered dose with high accuracy [15].

To further improve the MVCT quality and reduce the imaging dose, the linac is detuned to produce lower energy x-rays (3.5 MV). The imaging system has proved to be able to produce images that are useful for patient alignment mainly based on bony anatomies and higher-contrast soft tissues, such as the contrast between fat and muscle. MVCT is also particularly useful to image patients with metal implants, where kVCT normally

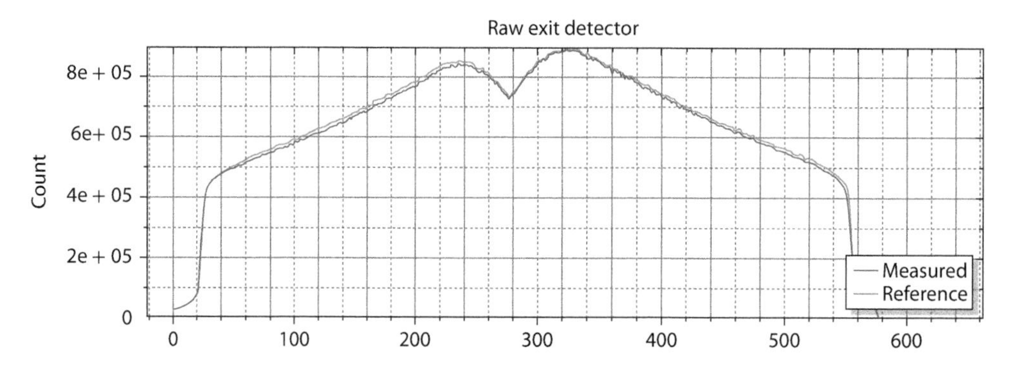

Figure 8.3 TomoTherapy® output measured using the on-board CT detector. Note the drop in signal at the center channels. The slight asymmetric shape is caused by the within-tolerance misalignment of the detector toward the target.

suffers from metal artifacts. Metal artifacts commonly affect the head and neck and prostate image quality from dental or prostheses implants. Metal implants for the spine can also affect the lung CT image quality.

MVCT imaging dose is comparable to that of the kV CBCT [16] but is considerably noisier. Although MVCT is less affected by the scatter artifacts that are prevalent in kV CBCT, the high noise level and low soft tissue contrast are commonly considered weaknesses when compared to kV images.

8.2.3 MLC

As mentioned, a distinct feature of TomoTherapy is its binary MLC. The MLC is divided into two opposing banks, each with 32 leaves (Figure 8.4). The width of the leaves is 6.25-mm projected to the isocenter. The opposing leaves are interleaved to cover a combined 40-cm field-of-view. The tungsten MLCs leaves are 10-cm deep with tongue-and-groove to reduce the overall leakage to less than 0.3% [17]. The MLC leaves are pneumatically driven by compressed air into one of only two positions, fully open or fully closed. The average leaf moving time is approximately 20 ms and neglected in the dose calculation.

8.2.4 Dose calculation and optimization algorithm

The dose calculation used in TomoTherapy planning systems was a collapsed cone convolution/superposition (CCC) initially developed by Mackie et al. and used in the Pinnacle planning system [18]. The algorithm is shown to be accurate in homogeneous and heterogeneous environments with noticeable error near tissue interfaces with large density differences. The error is typically small using TomoTherapy dose calculation for heterogeneous tissues with the exception of small lung tumors, where deviation above the 3% threshold for the dose received by 95% of the target volume was found [19,20] due to the lack of electron equilibrium

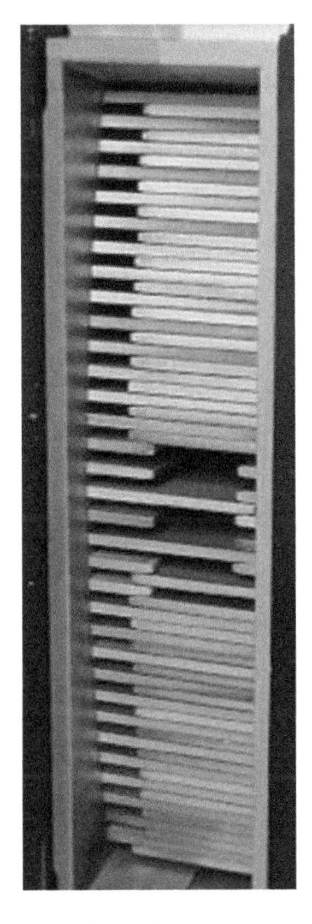

Figure 8.4 TomoTherapy® binary MLC are interleaved.

in these situations. The algorithm, initially developed in FORTRAN, was later written in more modern languages, C and C++, and improved in calculation speed. The single source algorithm was shown to be well suited for the TomoTherapy dose calculation due to its lack of flattening filter. Currently, two dose calculation approaches exist in parallel, depending on the computational platform. For the traditional CPU-based platform, the individual beamlets are precomputed for optimization using CCC. Each beamlet is a rectangle field projected by the opening of a single MLC leaf. For a typical TomoTherapy plan, tens of thousands of beamlets are needed, so this is a time-consuming step. However, once the beamlets are computed, the optimization iteration can be performed relatively quickly and the optimized dose is close to the final dose calculation. After beamlet calculation, the optimization problem is formulated as a quadratic cost function that is subsequently solved using the gradient descent method [21]. The second, more recent approach is based on a new computational graphic processing unit platform, which differs from the CPU platform by providing substantially more but simpler computational cores (a few thousand cores/GPU versus a few cores/CPU) for parallel computing. With this platform, the full dose for a given MLC pattern can be quickly computed during optimization iteration. Furthermore, by adopting a non-voxel-based broad-beam (NVBB) framework, the time-consuming dose calculation using CCC for the large number of beamlets is no longer necessary [22]. The approach allows an immediate start of optimization without waiting for the beamlets to be calculated. The error caused by using ray tracing and total attenuation as the dose surrogate is corrected by performing a full dose calculation using CCC periodically during iteration, which is made possible by the fast GPU dose calculation platform. The GPU-based dose calculation was compared to the CPU-based dose calculation and found essentially equivalent in accuracy with significant improvement in computational speed [23]. In another comparison study for total marrow irradiation, using GPU versus CPU translated into a 20-fold improvement in the overall planning time [24].

8.3 TREATMENT PLANNING FOR LUNG CANCER

8.3.1 Dosimetric characteristics

For TomoTherapy dose calculation and optimization, a full arc delivery is simulated by 51 equally spaced discrete beams at 7° apart. The weight of a beamlet is proportional to the leaf opening time. Because of the continuous gantry rotation, the actual beamlet location is blurred by the motion and spread in to a 7° arc. Although the blurring effect is not modeled in the planning system, its effect is negligible for targets closed to the isocenter and moderate-to-off-centered target [21,25]. It was later found that off-centered small targets can be underdosed due to the blurring effect. A software patch was installed to remedy this problem for all existing TomoTherapy TPS. As a result, TomoTherapy dose to the target natively tends to be highly homogenous [26]. This dosimetric characteristic is desired for many non-SBRT treatments but may be considered a limitation in SBRT treatments, which have been traditionally less homogeneous, allowing a more substantial hot spot in the target in exchange for superior dose gradient outside the target.

As mentioned previously, standard TomoTherapy provides three fixed jaw sizes that not only determine the longitudinal intensity modulation but also the craniocaudal penumbra when the two larger 2.5-cm or 5-cm jaw sizes are selected. Although a 1-cm jaw is significantly superior in the craniocaudal jaw penumbra, its low output factor and small field coverage are drawbacks in the SBRT treatment that requires a high dose in a single fraction. The limitation has been mitigated with the release of the dynamic jaw mode in TomoTherapy. The dynamic jaw mode, trademarked as TomoEdge, starts and ends a treatment with 1-cm jaw but increases the jaw opening to the user-selected maximal jaw size of either 2.5-cm or 5-cm in between. Consequently, the craniocaudal penumbra is reduced without the penalty of increasing treatment time [27]. Figure 8.5 shows the isodose comparison with or without TomoEdge. A sharper dose gradient in the superior and inferior edges was achieved using TomoEdge compared to the plan using a 2.5-cm fixed jaw size.

TomoTherapy uses constant rotational periods for the entire treatment and the gantry rotational period is determined by the longest leaf opening time. The ratio between the longest leaf opening time and the average leaf opening time is termed the modulation factor, which is a user-selected parameter. Clearly, a higher

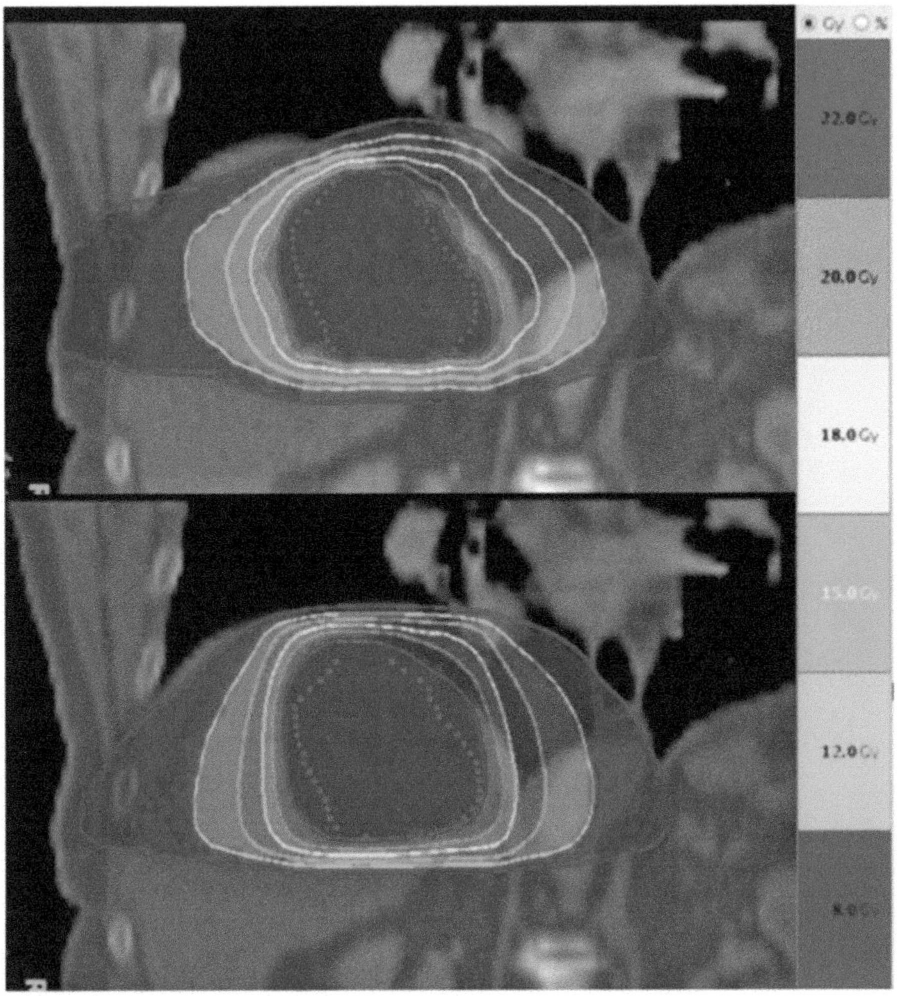

Figure 8.5 Dose comparison with (bottom) or without (top) TomoEdge™. A sharper dose gradient in the superior and inferior edges was achieved using TomoEdge compared to the plan using 2.5-cm fixed jaw.

modulation factor allows greater variation in the leaf opening time and slower gantry rotation time to deliver the small number of long leaf opening times. On the other hand, plans with large modulation factors are less efficient, requiring more monitor units and longer treatment time to deliver.

Unlike in-plane modulation, the longitudinal intensity modulation is achieved by partially overlapping helical bands, whose width is determined by the selected jaw size. The number of overlap is reciprocal of another user-selected parameter termed pitch. Smaller pitch allows more overlaps and more intensity modulation in the longitudinal direction. However, there are three other considerations when choosing pitch. First, tight pitch generally leads to slower delivery except for plans with high fractional doses, which will be explained later in this paragraph. The second is the gantry rotation time. For a conventionally fractionated plan delivering 2 Gy to the isocenter, using tight pitch (smaller value) could lead to fast gantry rotation (approaching 5 RPM) and fast MLC movement, which tend to increase delivery error. For SBRT treatment delivering a larger dose, using coarse pitch could lead to gantry rotation speed slower than the lowest limit (1 RPM) and then require the plan to be split into multiple passes. In this case, tighter pitch may allow single-pass delivery and actually save time compared to plans using a coarser pitch. The third consideration is dose fluctuation caused by the imperfect match of the helical beams, a phenomenon known as the thread effect, which was first characterized by Kissick [28]. Based on a simple geometric model, Kissick derived pitches that minimized the undesired thread effect. The recommended values were refined by Chen in 2011 [29] for both on- and off-isocenter targets. A typical lung SBRT dosimetry by TomoTherapy is shown in Figure 8.6.

The user interface of TomoTherapy optimization is shown in Figure 8.7. The interface allows the dosimetrist to interact with the optimization process on the fly. The dosimetrist first sets the prescription, which is a hard constraint typically in the form of dose to certain percentage of the PTV, and initial set of constraints on the PTV and OARs. The constraints can be maximal dose, minimal dose, or dose volume points.

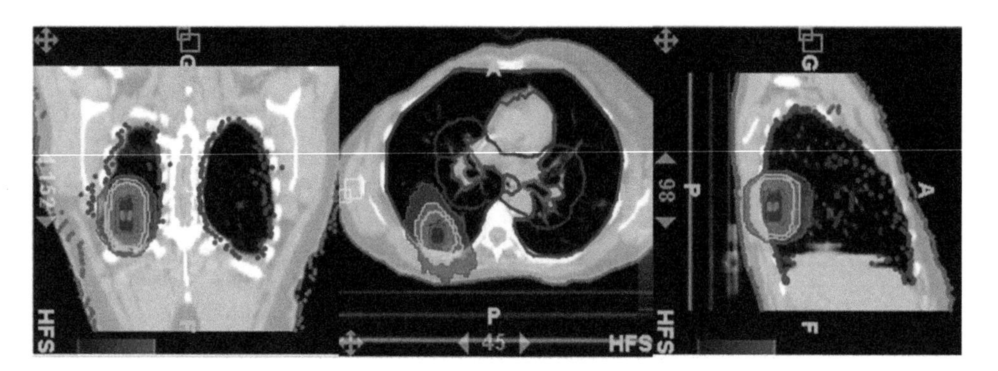

Figure 8.6 A typical TomoTherapy® SBRT plan for a small peripheral lung tumor.

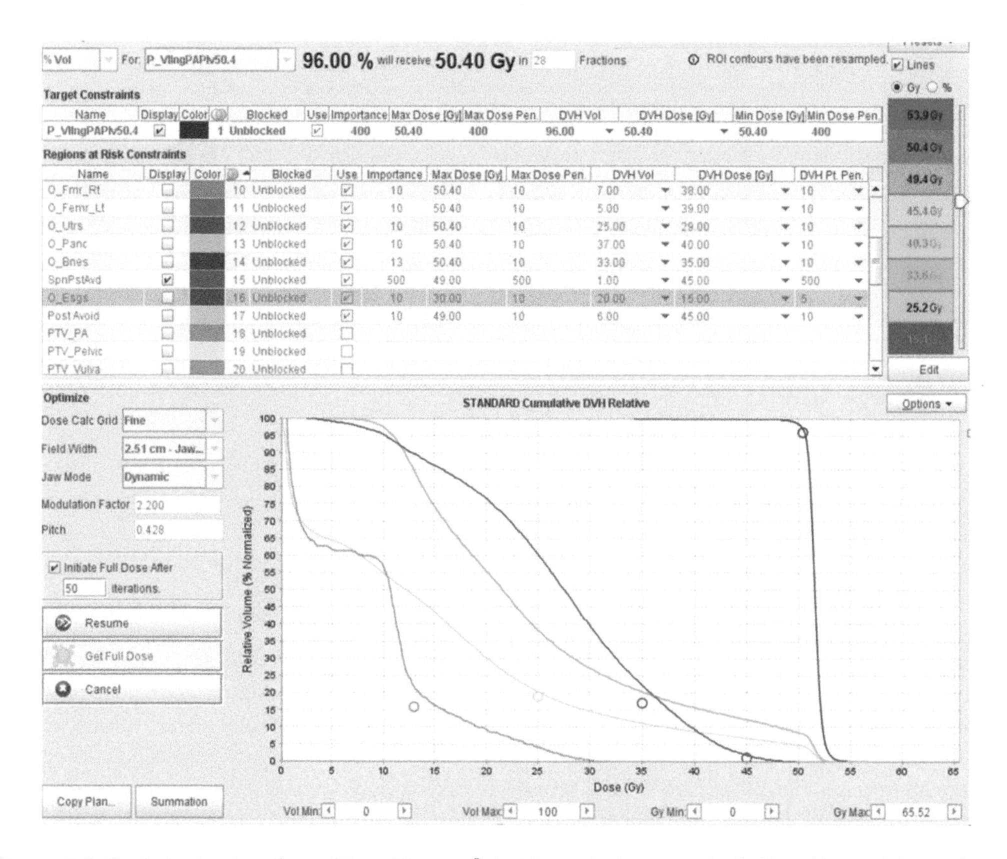

Figure 8.7 Optimization interface of TomoTherapy®. In this particular case, the field width, modulation factor, and pitch are set as 2.5-cm, 2.2-cm, and 0.428-cm, respectively. Dynamic jaws are used. The DVH points are shown as circles in the DVH plots.

Priorities and weights can be assigned to individual structures. Separate penalties can be assigned to the dose constraint points. The dose distribution and dose volume histogram are updated with each iteration. The dosimetrist can choose to pause the optimization process and then adjust the weights and penalties, and add or remove a dose constraint point. The typical numbers of iterations are 100 or more. Because of the dose volume constraints, the TomoTherapy objective function is not strictly convex and does not guarantee global optimality. The optimization results depend on the history of computer–dosimetrist interactive history. When satisfactory dosimetry is not obtained after many iterations, or there is a need to change the jaw size or pitch, the current iteration needs to be aborted, and then restarted after resetting these parameters. TomoTherapy delivery is strictly coplanar. Although small couch yaw in the gantry bore is theoretically feasible, dosimetric gains from the small non-coplanar angles are insignificant [30].

In addition to the helical mode, TomoTherapy has a fixed beam mode where the gantry remains at a fixed angle while the couch translates longitudinally during beam delivery [31]. This mode, trademarked as TomoDirect™ [32], was mainly developed to answer the need for breast radiotherapy by mimicking the tangential beams. Because of its insignificant role in lung cancer therapy, TomoDirect is not discussed further in this chapter.

8.3.2 Dosimetric comparison between IMRT and VMAT

Conformality index (CI), which is defined as the ratio between 100% isodose volume and PTV, R50, which is the 50% isodose volume divided by PTV, homogeneity index (HI), defined by the minimum dose delivered to 5% of the PTV receiving the highest dose divided by the minimum dose delivered to 95% of the PTV, is commonly used to describe the PTV coverage and high dose spillage. OAR doses are individually defined based on the organ radiobiological features. For serial and centrally located organs, the dose limit is determined by the highest dose received by a small volume of the organ. For parallel organs such as the lung, the mean dose and the volume of organ receiving a specific percentage of prescription doses are used as tolerance. In a study of TomoTherapy lung SBRT, using the RTOG 0236 lung SBRT protocol as a reference [33], it was found that the lung volume receiving 20 Gy or more (V20) can be met using TomoTherapy with adequate sparing of serial organs including heart, trachea, major blood vessels, and the bronchus for peripheral early stage lung cancer. R50 was not evaluated for several reasons, including that the R50 criterion was thought unrealistic for coplanar beams and dose calculation with tissue heterogeneity correction.

Dosimetric comparisons between TomoTherapy and other treatment modalities for lung cancer treatment planning hVW been performed. However, although quantitative criteria have been used, the treatment planning process is highly variable and subjective. The comparison results also depend on different software versions and hardware platforms, including the MLC resolution. Therefore, it is not surprising that the conclusions from various dosimetric studies may not always be consistent. For example, in a study comparing lung SBRT plans for TomoTherapy, VMAT, and fixed beam IMRT, Weyh et al. [34] showed that TomoTherapy is superior in CI, HI, and R50 to both VMAT and IMRT. The OAR doses were not significantly different except the maximal rib dose is lowest using TomoTherapy. VMAT delivered 60% faster than TomoTherapy and 40% faster than IMRT. In a study comparing TomoTherapy and VMAT, it was found that with essentially the same PTV coverage, TomoTherapy is superior to VMAT in OAR sparing and the dosimetric advantage is consistent even with more than two arcs being used in the VMAT plan [35]. However, in a study using radiobiological measures, fixed beam IMRT was shown to achieve greater tumor control probability than TomoTherapy with the same normal tissue toxicity [36]. In a recent study, the dosimetries of TomoTherapy, VMAT, and CyberKnife® for centrally located lung cancer were compared [37]. CyberKnife was shown to deliver greater dose gradient outside the PTV, largely owing to its non-coplanar beam capacities, although its dose is less homogeneous in the PTV. Using whole lung or ipsilateral lung volume, CyberKnife and VMAT were shown to result in lower probability of radiation pneumonitis compared to TomoTherapy. However, it is worth pointing out that CyberKnife is restricted from using many posterior beam angles that can lead to significantly greater lung dose when treating a posterior lung tumor [38].

8.3.3 Image quality of MVCT

TomoTherapy utilizes the same x-ray target for both imaging and therapy. In the imaging mode, the x-ray energy is detuned to achieve slightly better detecting efficiency and substantially lower output. MVCT image quality of TomoTherapy was compared to other major vendors by Chan et al. [39] using a Catphan CT phantom. The spatial resolution and low-contrast tests are shown in Figures 8.8 and 8.9. Compared to the kV KBCT from Varian and Elekta, TomoTherapy MVCT resulted in significantly poorer resolution (3–5 lp/cm versus 8–10 lp/mm) and sensitivity to low contrast (3% versus <1%). Its image noise level is 2–4 times greater than kV CBCT. Therefore, the TomoTherapy MVCT quality is considerably worse than the kV CBCT used by Varian and Elekta. However, MVCT is unaffected by scatter artifacts due to its fan beam geometry and more robust image artifacts caused by beam hardening effects. Specifically, for the lung region, kV CBCT typically shows more severe artifacts due to the large tissue density heterogeneity. In practice, the difference in image quality is not as great as what the phantom tests suggest. Furthermore, MVCT is advantageous in providing accurate electron density measurement for dose calculation compared to the kVCT.

There are a number of studies attempting to improve the MVCT image quality. The desired method would be to improve the detector quantum efficiency to MV x-rays without increasing the imaging dose. Several experimental solid-state CT detectors [40,41] have been tested to increase MV x-ray DQE but none of them was clinically or commercially adopted. Alternatively, a straightforward way is to increase the MVCT dose, thus increasing the number of photons detected [42]. By increasing the imaging dose from 2.2 cGy to 8.5 cGy, the image noise decreased from 5.2% to 2.6%.

For standard MVCT reconstruction, filtered back-projection was used. Different denoising methods have been attempted to improve the image quality. For example, iterative algebraic reconstruction has been used for kVCT to reconstruct suboptimal projection data, including low mAs, incomplete projections, and the presence of metal artifacts, and shows more robust results than the back-projection approach under these conditions [43]. This method also can be readily formulated as a least-square L1-type of regularization problem to exploit the piecewise continuity typically assumed for human anatomy [43,44]. Recently, Gao et al. used tight framelet regularization, a type of L1 norm, to reconstruct MVCT images showing cleaner

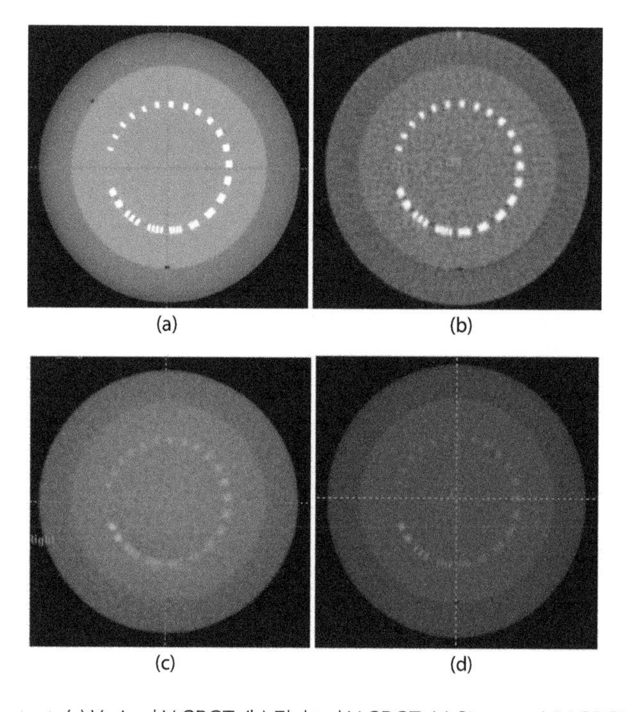

Figure 8.8 Resolution test. (a) Varian kV CBCT; (b) Elekta kV CBCT; (c) Siemens MV CBCT; (d) Tomo MV FBCT.

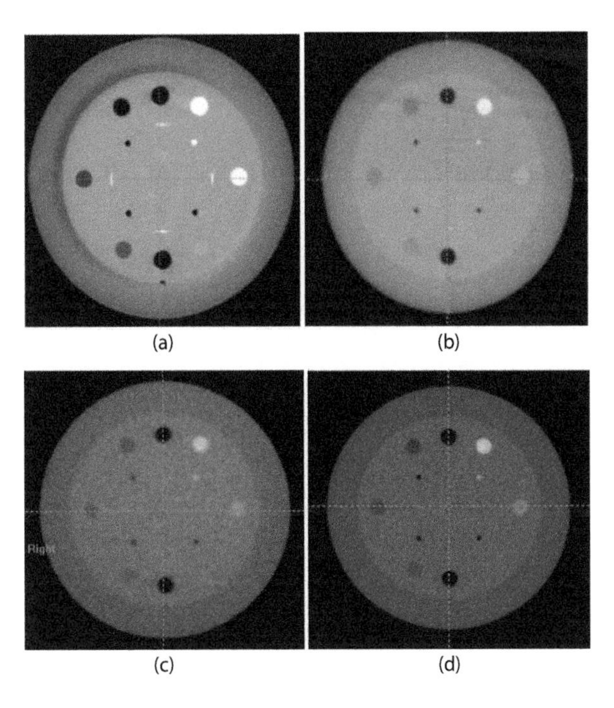

Figure 8.9 Low contrast test. (a) Varian kV CBCT; (b) Elekta kV CBCT; (c) Siemens MV CBCT; (d) Tomo MV FBCT.

images with reduced noise and well-preserved edges [45]. On the other hand, this method resulted in reduced resolution and did not improve low-contrast object conspicuity. Imaging post-processing methods take a different approach to denoising the filtered back-projection MVCT images. An anisotropic diffusion (AD) filter was used to prepare the MVCT image for deformable registration [46]. In a separate study, an adaptive Gaussian filter was applied to the MVCT image for noise reduction and MVCT-based contouring consistency improvement [47]. These methods showed varying levels of noise reduction while preserving "hard" edges between bones and soft tissue. However, they did not improve the conspicuity of low-contrast fine structures and often degraded the contrast of fine features and textures that are important for organ delineation. Sheng et al. applied a non-local means denoising filter, block matching 3D, on MVCT images and showed a 10-fold increase in the contrast-to-noise ratio and the ability to preserve fine structures in the resultant images [48]. These methods have yet to be integrated into clinical TomoTherapy.

8.3.4 Clinical implementations and trials using helical TomoTherapy for lung SBRT

The TomoTherapy system is one of the earliest clinical systems that provided volumetric images for image-guided radiation therapy (IGRT). Although the MVCT images show relatively poor soft tissue contrast, these are adequate for patient positioning based on bony anatomies [49]. For patients with lung cancer, the large contrast between the tumor and the lung parenchyma allows localization using the tumor directly, which is important for lung tumors that often move relative to the bones. Even for sub-centimeter small lung tumors, MVCT can provide useful visualization for precise patient positioning (Figure 8.10). Tumors of this size would be difficult to visualize in 2D radiography, the technology in use before CT was available for image-guided radiotherapy. The IGRT workflow of TomoTherapy was well integrated compared to early competing platforms offering IGRT, making it well suited for the lung SBRT treatment. In a study including eight patients treated with 3–5 SBRT fractions, sub-millimeter accuracy of MVCT registration was shown to be attainable [50].

Consequently, with adequate geometrical margins included in the planning target volume, high fractional doses to a highly mobile small lung tumor can be accurately delivered using TomoTherapy. The outcome

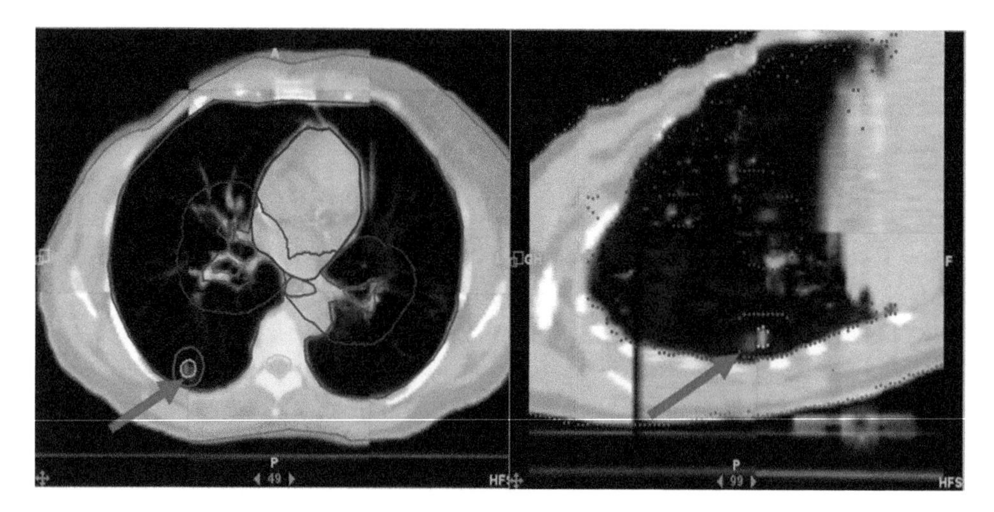

Figure 8.10 Lung SBRT patient setup based on MVCT kVCT registration. The lung tumor diameter was 9-mm.

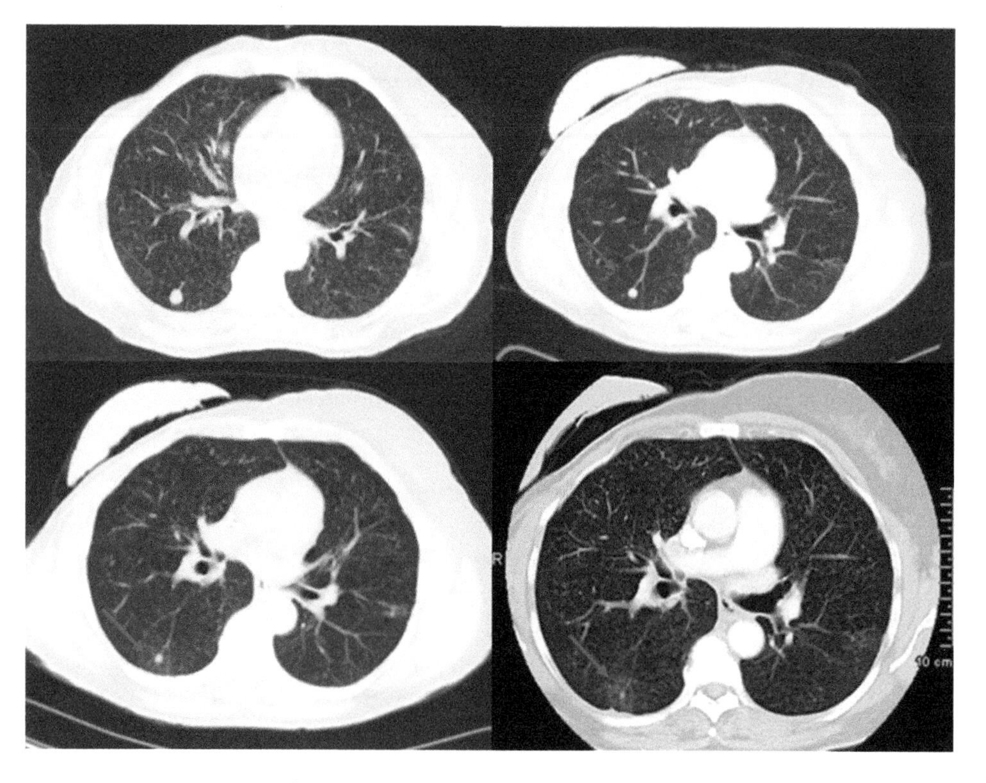

Figure 8.11 Treatment outcomes follow-up by CT showing reduction in tumor sizes and spherical ground-glass lung tissue change centered to the lung tumor after the treatment. The sequential images show pre-treatment CT, and 2 months post-, 3 months post-, and 6 months post- treatment CT.

of such a treatment is shown in Figure 8.11. The tumor shrank substantially 3 months after the treatment. 6 months after the treatment, a spherical ground-glass consolidation pattern centered to the original tumor formed, demonstrating the accuracy of treatment.

Because of the readiness of IGRT and its relatively advanced IMRT planning system compared to systems at the same period, TomoTherapy was widely popular and clinically adopted in the first few years when it became commercially available. At the same time, lung SBRT has emerged as a promising treatment modality for patients with inoperable early stage non-small-cell lung cancer (NSCLC) in contrast to disappointing conventionally fractionated dose escalation studies. The University of Wisconsin first showed the feasibility of lung SBRT on TomoTherapy without major technical limitations or acute toxicities [51]. Dunlap et al. reported excellent local control using TomoTherapy to treat early stage NSCLC [52]. Aibe reported excellent local control and survival for early stage lung cancer patients using TomoTherapy [53]. The GTV size-dependent severe toxicity rate was low (6.7%). More recently, Nagai et al. showed that TomoTherapy is safe and effective for lung treatment via SBRT [54]. For patients with multiple pulmonary metastases, Kim showed that TomoTherapy offers safe effective local control [55]. A major concern for lung SBRT was the central organ toxicity when the location of the tumor is near these organs [56–60]. TomoTherapy was used to create a steep dose gradient between the tumor and adjacent central organs [61] that may have reduced the risk of severe toxicity.

8.4 MOTION MANAGEMENT WITH HELICAL TOMOTHERAPY

8.4.1 Interfractional motion management

TomoTherapy manages interfractional motion based on the on-board MVCT images. For rigid interfractional motion, the translation motion can be corrected by couch shifts. The roll is corrected by gantry rotation. The yaw and pitch cannot be automatically corrected (incremental couch vertical and lateral translations with couch longitudinal motion were suggested to correct yaw and pitch [62] but the method has not been implemented in production of TomoTherapy systems). Large yaw and pitch shifts have to be corrected by manually shift and adjustment of patient immobilization. However, for most patients eligible for the lung SBRT treatment involving limited craniocaudal tumor extension, yaw and pitch are generally negligible [63].

The efficacy of setting up lung cancer patients based on MVCT was shown previously in Figure 8.7. Statistically, without such image guidance by MVCT and using the surface markers alone, significant setup errors could occur. Zhou et al. reported −1.1±2.8-mm, −2.5±8.7-mm, and 4.1±2.6-mm error for a total of 225 lung isocenters of patients immobilized using the state-of-the-art BodyLoc double vacuum system [50]. Schubert et al. [64] reported an average of 3.2-mm translational error without MVCT guidance for lung tumor treatment.

The correction of rigid shifts is straightforward but for tumors showing response to the treatment, new radiation therapy plans adapted were considered desirable [65–68]. The response of NSCLC during SBRT treatment was considered negligible [69] but a recent study of lung tumor response to the SBRT treatment showed that a more significant tumor shrinkage may happen for protracted SBRT treatment, such as once or twice a week, that took 2–5 weeks to complete [70], although the shrinkage could be tumor histopathology dependent. By adapting to the reduced tumor volume, the volume of normal tissue irradiated to high doses may be reduced to decrease toxicities. TomoTherapy with its MVCT image capacity would be conducive to such adaptation but to the best of the author's knowledge, a clinical study of adaptive lung SBRT has not been reported on this platform.

8.4.2 Intrafractional motion management and interplay effect

It has been increasingly recognized that internal organ motion during the treatment can have adverse dosimetric impacts by causing geometric misses and increasing normal tissue exposure to ionizing radiation. The intrafractional organ motions can have different temporal frequencies. For slower non-periodic motion, because of the slow CT acquisition speed, MVCT can be seen as an average CT image of the moving lung tumor. Two studies independently used repeating TomoTherapy MVCT to quantify the motion amplitude [50,71]. Both studies show that for well-immobilized patients using a double vacuum body lock system, the average location of the lung tumor drifted less than 1-mm.

The other, faster source of internal organ motion is respiratory motion that affects thoracic and upper abdominal organs. A significant portion of medical physics research in the past decade has been dedicated to characterizing its dosimetric implications and developing motion management of lung tumor motions. The extensive studies characterizing the lung tumor motion are beyond the scope of this chapter but a short summary will follow. First, the lung tumor motion is quasi-periodic. The inhalation and exhalation give basic periodicity but it is further modulated by irregularities including changes in breathing patterns, baseline drifts and lung hysteresis. Second, the motion amplitude varies substantially between patients and locations of the tumor. Third, although most tumors exhibit dominant craniocaudal motion, large anterior/posterior or mediolateral tumor motion is not uncommon.

The most straightforward way to manage lung tumor motion and avoid geometric misses, is by including the motion excursions in the internal target volume (ITV) [72], which is further expanded to PTV account for setup uncertainties. 4D-CT and dynamic MRI [73,74] have been used to estimate the patient- and tumor-specific motion excursion. A maximum intensity projection is typically adopted to simply determine the ITV. Once the PTV is defined, motion management using TomoTherapy in principle is not different from other treatment modalities but there are several caveats that are worth mentioning. First, 4D-CT is shown to underestimate the motion excursion of lung tumors of patients with highly variable breathing patterns [75], resulting in a potential underdosing of the tumor. On the other hand, to account for the entire motion excursion based on dynamic MRI, a large ITV expansion is needed, increasing the normal tissue exposure to radiation. It has been shown that instead of using the maximum intensity projection, a mid-position strategy may be adequate for most lung tumors, except those that are small and move more than 10-mm [76]. Another concern for TomoTherapy is that the treatment delivery is typically long, increasing the chance of additional patient shift and baseline drifts, although they were shown to be small in two separate studies [50,71].

Moreover, the interplay effects between dynamic IMRT delivery and the tumor motion has been a research topic of interest. Specifically for TomoTherapy, the additional constant gantry rotation in addition to the MLC motion warrants a close inspection of the problem.

The interplay effect between TomoTherapy sliding window and the moving tumor was first described by Yang, several years before the actual machine materialized [10]. It was concluded that if the tumor and the gantry move in synchrony, gross deviation from the intended dose could happen. However, since the gantry rotation is significantly slower (more so for TomoTherapy SBRT treatment that uses gantry period over 30 s) than normal breathing motion, the interplay effect was expected to be small. In a study investigating a one-dimensional model to evaluate on-axis intensity variations due to the interplay between sliding jaw motion and respiratory motion the possibility of substantial undesired dose heterogeneity greater than 50% of the prescription dose was reported [77]. Error of this magnitude would raise significant concern for lung radiotherapy. In 2005, the interplay effect was studied in a refined model for fractionated treatment [78]. It was concluded that indeed the interplay effect for a combination of fast-moving couch and high-motion amplitude tumors can result in an approximately 20% dose heterogeneity. The magnitude of dose heterogeneity was later experimentally reproduced for plans with short gantry period and long breathing cycle (10 s) [79]. On the other hand, due to the random breathing phase at each treatment fraction, the interplay-induced dose heterogeneity is expected to reduce to less than a few percent. The conclusion is consistent with Bortfeld's estimate of the interplay effect of MLC and tumor motion [80]. The interplay effect was experimentally studied by Kanagaki [81] using EDR2 film and a motion phantom. For various TomoTherapy planning parameters and longitudinal motion profiles, other than the cold spots at the edges of the PTV due to expected dose convolution with the motion, the interplay effect was not observed. In a 4D Monte Carlo treatment planning study, the interplay effect was found to contribute negligibly to the final dose distribution for simultaneous integrated boost (SIB) and hypo-fractionated lung cancer treatment [82]. It was then also concluded that accounting for intrafractional motion through the definition of an ITV was adequate. When anterior/posterior and lateral motion are included, however, the dose delivery is sensitive to the interplay between the tumor motion and the MLC motion, showing up to 29% cold spots in the PTV [79]. It is reasonable to believe that these extreme cases are unlikely to occur among patients whose breathing cycles are well separated from the gantry periods of typical TomoTherapy lung SBRT plans. Furthermore, the patient breathing patterns are not perfectly periodic within a treatment fraction. The interplay effect greatly diminishes without the perfect synchrony of the gantry cycle and the breathing cycle.

Although a properly implemented ITV approach provides adequate lung tumor coverage and OAR sparing in many cases, it unavoidably increases the normal tissue exposure to ionizing radiation. The increase is particularly significant for tumors that move more than 1-cm. In modern radiation therapy, probability density function (PDF)-based, gated, or motion adaptive radiation therapy have been considered for lung tumors with large motion amplitude.

Instead of treating the PTV to a uniform dose in PDF-based treatment planning, it was hypothesized that by optimizing a heterogeneous dose to the PTV based on the probability of a tumor's sub-volume at the location, the normal tissue dose may be reduced compared to the standard ITV approach. Trofimov reported dosimetric gain using this approach and efficiency advantage compared to the gated radiotherapy approach [83]. On a simplified TomoTherapy simulation platform, Sheng showed that by incorporating the lung tumor PDF into the optimization cost function, the lung V10 and V20 can be substantially reduced by up to 40–50% [84]. The drawback of this approach, however, is that the treatment is extremely sensitive to the reproducibility of PDF, which may differ from the time of simulation and the time of treatment. Since PDF is a result of cumulative lung tumor position, it cannot be measured based on instantaneous online images. The treatment would quickly become complicated to adapt for the PDF reproducibility issues although ongoing research in this direction is still being reported [85].

Gated and motion adaptive radiotherapy have been clinically adopted in various forms but this is an area more challenging to TomoTherapy than competing platforms. Gated radiotherapy [86–90] was developed to treat a moving tumor at specific phase of its motion trajectory so the ITV margin can be effectively reduced at a cost of reduced duty cycle and prolonged treatment time. For lung SBRT treatment, typically the gating position is established based on 4D-CT. At the time of treatment, an external or internal surrogate is used to indicate the tumor location, which may further be verified by intrafractional x-ray images. The radiation beam is then controlled by the gating signal to treat the lung tumor within the specific gating window. For fixed beam IMRT technique, the beam control component is relatively straightforward, requiring a simple beam switch. For dynamic arc delivery, it is considerably more difficult. Due to inertia, a rotating gantry cannot instantaneously stop and then start moving. The difficulty is even greater for TomoTherapy, which can only treat a slice of the tumor at a time and the slice is perpendicular to the primary tumor motion direction. In order to catch up with the motion, the tumor needs to be treated in multi-passes. The theoretical feasibility of such respiratory gated TomoTherapy was described by Kim et al. [91] but was not developed beyond simulation due to its conceivable complexity, further prolonged treatment duration, and questionable robustness.

Tumor motion adaptive radiotherapy was developed as an alternative to gated radiotherapy [92,93]. It has a smaller impact on the duty cycle and greater flexibility to manage tumor deformation. On conventional C-arm linac, theories and apparatus for these types of treatments have been extensively reported on, but due to the complexity, have not been performed on patients. On the other hand, motion adaptive treatment based on active tumor tracking has been conducted clinically using CyberKnife [94,95]. Under the trademark of Synchrony®, CyberKnife utilizes its highly nimble robotically mounted linac to track the tumor motion, which is predicted by a mathematical model. The prediction is updated or corrected in real-time based on stereotactic x-ray images of the implanted marker or external surrogates. Unfortunately, there is no current corresponding production solution for TomoTherapy despite conceptual and experimental studies to demonstrate the possibility. Based on deformable registration, Zhang et al. [96] showed that the respiratory motion can be incorporated in TomoTherapy treatment planning in the form of deformed beamlets. The 4D treatment can then be performed synchronized to the breathing trace acquired at the time of treatment [97]. Lu [98–100] described a multi-pass motion-adaptive-optimization (MAO) for TomoTherapy that delivers partial dose synchronized to the respiratory cycle. The method is shown to compensate largely for the motion-induced dose degradation as shown in Figure 8.12. However, this approach has not been further developed and commercialized. Other than the continuous rotating ring gantry, inflexible fan beam treatment geometry, the lack of real-time monitoring owing to the bore occlusion was the main reason that motion adaptive radiotherapy cannot be reliably delivered on current TomoTherapy. Major changes to its hardware platform appear to be needed to enable this advanced motion management method.

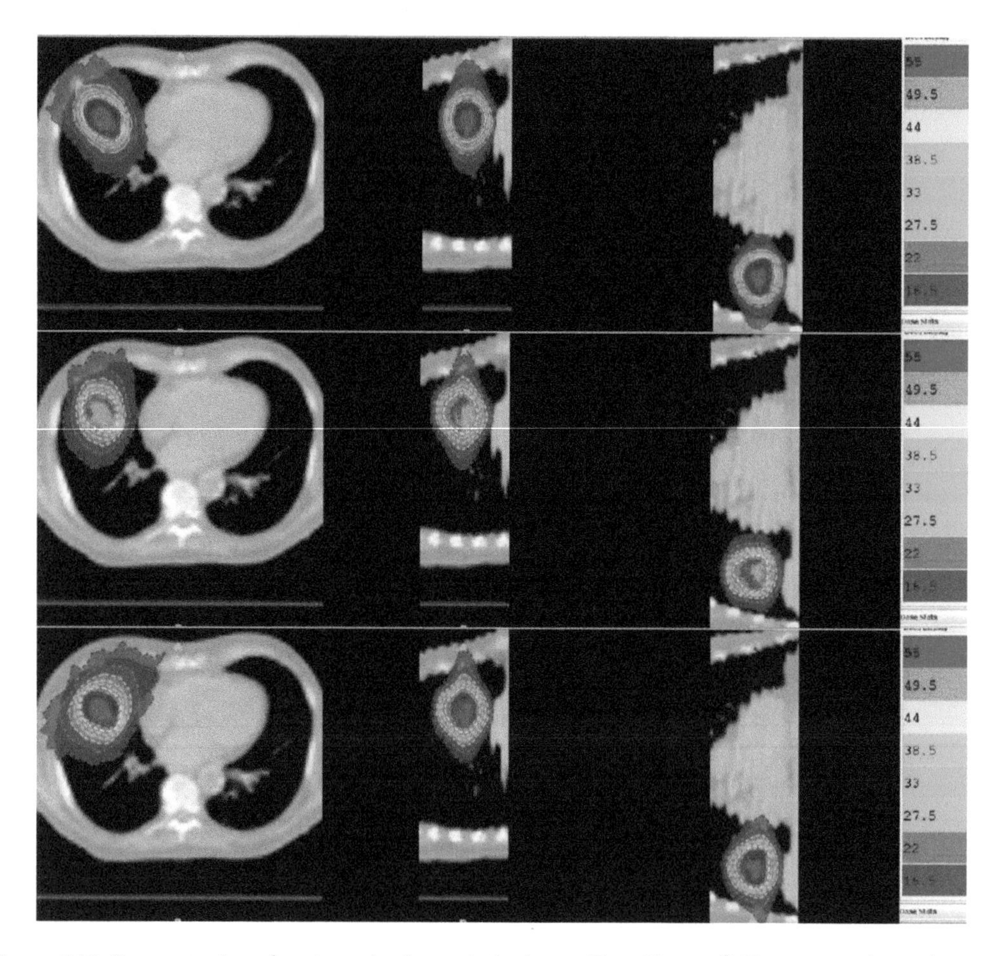

Figure 8.12 Demonstration of motion adaptive optimization on TomoTherapy®. The top row shows the transversal (T), sagittal (S), and coronal (C) views of the static delivery dose distribution, the middle row shows, TSC views of the motion without-compensation delivery dose distribution, and the bottom row shows, TSC views of the MAO dose distribution. The unit of isodose lines is the Gy. (From Lu, W. et al., *Phys Med Biol*, 54(14): 4373–98, 2009. With permission.)

8.5 FUTURE DEVELOPMENT OF HELICAL TOMOTHERAPY

TomoTherapy was introduced to the clinic nearly 15 years ago had a major impact on radiation therapy practice. It has motivated the development of rotational IMRT on other platforms, including the widely popular VMAT on the C-arm platform [101,102]. The history of TomoTherapy coincided with the development and adoption of lung SBRT, which has been shown to be vastly more effective than conventionally fractionated radiotherapy for early stage lung cancers. TomoTherapy provides a well-integrated, easy-to-use treatment planning, imaging, and delivery platform that has been instrumental to the success of lung SBRT.

However, TomoTherapy in its current form suffers from a number of limitations. As mentioned previously, the constant gantry rotation speed used in TomoTherapy forces the user to choose between reduced dose modulation and increased treatment time. The constant gantry rotation tends to deliver a more homogeneous target dose that is less steep in the dose gradient. It also struggles to deliver intended heterogeneous target dose for simultaneous integrated boost [103]. The lack of non-coplanar beams is a deficiency that cannot be ignored. The non-coplanar IMRT beams have been shown to markedly improve the compactness of dose distribution and OAR sparing, compared to coplanar arc beams [104]. The ring gantry platform is not easily worked to provide motion management that is particularly important in the lung SBRT treatment.

To perform gated or 4D treatment on lung tumors, their positions need to be visualized during treatment, which is hampered by the lack of real-time imaging in the current generation of TomoTherapy.

During the same period of TomoTherapy development, IGRT, optimization, and delivery on conventional C-arm gantry have improved and matured. The advent of VMAT has provided similar workflow for treatment plan creation and delivery, making TomoTherapy less unique in this regard. The robotic tracking system from CyberKnife has provided a compelling tool for lung cancer treatment. In many senses, the landscape has changed for lung cancer treatment and the change has been less favorable of utilizing TomoTherapy for such indication.

To stay relevant, TomoTherapy must evolve its technology and align with the future development of lung SBRT, which aims at increasing its patient eligibility to locally advanced tumors [105], retreatment [106], and tumors at more challenging locations, such as centrally located lung tumors [107–109]. To treat these tumors using the aggressive lung SBRT doses, the dose conformity as well as the dose gradients between the tumor and nearby critical organs needs to be significantly improved. Moreover, with the available molecular images, it is appealing to selectively boost the volumes showing greater metabolic activities [110], hypoxia, or proliferation.

Some of the possible improvements to TomoTherapy are listed here to conclude the chapter. Variable gantry speed may help achieve a better balance between the delivery efficiency and dosimetry quality. Variable gantry speed is also valuable for delivering a simultaneous integrated boost where a large amount of dose needs to be delivered from selective angles. To provide non-coplanar beams, either the bore diameter needs to be significantly increased to accommodate couch kick or the x-ray beam needs to be tilted. However, these concepts were already unsuccessfully tested in Vero and rejected for various reasons, including the cost and inability to cover the entire 4π Steradian angles [111]. Reinvigorating the original idea of having an on-board kVCT may be critical. The kV imager would not only provide superior image quality but also facilitate the real-time monitoring of the tumor location for 4D radiotherapy. Robust and easy-to-use 4D treatment methods would have to be implemented to offset the adverse impact of lung tumor motion. Exit dosimetry using the MVCT detector [14,15] is a currently underutilized asset that may provide real-time dose reconstruction for lung SBRT in combination with real-time imaging.

REFERENCES

1. Nuttall, A.K., Dose distribution in arc therapy. *Br J Radiol*, 1956. **29**(338): 110–20.
2. Brahme, A., J.E. Roos, and I. Lax. Solution of an integral equation encountered i+n rotation therapy. *Phys Med Biol*, 1982. **27**(10): 1221–9.
3. Brahme, A. Optimization of stationary and moving beam radiation therapy techniques. *Radiother Oncol*, 1988. **12**(2): 129–40.
4. Kallman, P. et al. Shaping of arbitrary dose distributions by dynamic multileaf collimation. *Phys Med Biol*, 1988. **33**(11): 1291–300.
5. Galvin, J.M. et al., Evaluation of multileaf collimator design for a photon beam. *Int J Radiat Oncol Biol Phys*, 1992. **23**(4): 789–801.
6. Oldham, M. and S. Webb, Intensity-modulated radiotherapy by means of static tomotherapy: A planning and verification study. *Med Phys*, 1997. **24**(6): 827–36.
7. Carol, M.P., Peacock™: A system for planning and rotational delivery of intensity-modulated fields. *Int J Imag Syst Tech*, 1995. **6**(1): 56–61. doi:10.1002/ima.1850060108.
8. Mackie, T.R. et al., TomoTheraphy: A new concept for the delivery of dynamic conformal radiotherapy. *Med Phys*, 1993. **20**(6): 1709–19.
9. Ruchala, K.J. et al., Megavoltage CT on a tomotherapy system. *Phys Med Biol*, 1999. **44**(10): 2597–621.
10. Yang, J.N. et al., Thomadsen BR. An investigation of tomotherapy beam delivery. *Med Phys*, 1997. **24**(3): 425–36.
11. Movahed, A. and B. Rabbani, Experience with helical tomotherapy commissioning and quality assurance of twin peaks linac vs. earlier models. *Med Phys*, 2010. **38**(6).

12. Rong, Y. et al., Helical tomotherapy with dynamic running-start-stop delivery compared to conventional tomotherapy delivery. *Med Phys*, 2014. **41**(5): 051709.
13. Sterzing, F. et al., Dynamic jaws and dynamic couch in helical tomotherapy. *Int J Radiat Oncol Biol Phys*, 2010. **76**(4): 1266–73.
14. Chen, Q. et al., TomoTherapy MLC verification using exit detector data. *Med Phys*, 2012. **39**(1): 143–51.
15. Sheng, K. et al., 3D dose verification using tomotherapy CT detector array. *Int J Radiat Oncol Biol Phys*, 2012. **82**(2): 1013–20.
16. Shah, A., E. Aird, J. Shekhdar, Contribution to normal tissue dose from concomitant radiation for two common kV-CBCT systems and one MVCT system used in radiotherapy. *Radiother Oncol*, 2012. **105**(1): 139–44. doi:10.1016/j.radonc.2012.04.017.
17. Balog, J.P. et al., Multileaf collimator interleaf transmission. *Med Phys*, 1999. **26**(2): 176–86.
18. Mackie, T.R., J.W. Scrimger, J.J. Battista, A convolution method of calculating dose for 15-MV x rays. *Med Phys*, 1985. **12**(2): 188–96.
19. Sterpin, E. et al., Monte Carlo evaluation of the convolution/superposition algorithm of Hi-Art tomotherapy in heterogeneous phantoms and clinical cases. *Med Phys*, 2009. **36**(5): 1566–75.
20. Zhao, Y.L. et al., Monte Carlo evaluation of a treatment planning system for helical tomotherapy in an anthropomorphic heterogeneous phantom and for clinical treatment plans. *Med Phys*, 2008. **35**(12): 5366–74.
21. Shepard, D.M. et al., Iterative approaches to dose optimization in tomotherapy. *Phys Med Biol*, 2000. **45**(1): 69–90.
22. Lu, W., A non-voxel-based broad-beam (NVBB) framework for IMRT treatment planning. *Phys Med Biol*, 2010. **55**(23): 7175–210.
23. Chen, Q. et al., Validation of GPU based TomoTherapy dose calculation engine. *Med Phys*, 2012. **39**(4): 1877–86.
24. Nalichowski, A. and J. Burmeister, Dosimetric comparison of helical tomotherapy treatment plans for total marrow irradiation created using GPU and CPU dose calculation engines. *Med Phys*, 2013. **40**(7): 071716.
25. Shepard, D.M. et al., A simple model for examining issues in radiotherapy optimization. *Med Phys*, 1999. **26**(7): 1212–21.
26. Sheng, K., J.A. Molloy, P.W. Read, Intensity-modulated radiation therapy (IMRT) dosimetry of the head and neck: A comparison of treatment plans using linear accelerator-based IMRT and helical tomotherapy. *Int J Radiat Oncol Biol Phys*, 2006. **65**(3): 917–23.
27. Rudofsky, L. et al., Lung and liver SBRT using helical tomotherapy—A dosimetric comparison of fixed jaw and dynamic jaw delivery. *J Appl Clin Med Phys*, 2014. **15**(3): 114–21.
28. Kissick, M.W. et al., The helical tomotherapy thread effect. *Med Phys*, 2005. **32**(5): 1414–23.
29. Chen, M. et al., Theoretical analysis of the thread effect in helical TomoTherapy. *Med Phys*, 2011. **38**(11): 5945–60.
30. Yang, W. et al., Feasibility of non-coplanar tomotherapy for lung cancer stereotactic body radiation therapy. *Technol Cancer Res Treat*, 2011. **10**(4): 307–15.
31. McIntosh, A. et al., Evaluation of coplanar partial left breast irradiation using tomotherapy-based topotherapy. *Int J Radiat Oncol*, 2008. **71**(2): 603–10. doi:10.1016/j.ijrobp.2008.01.047.
32. Catuzzo P, et al., Technical note: Patient-specific quality assurance methods for TomoDirect™ whole breast treatment delivery. *Med Phys*, 2012. **39**(7): 4073–8.
33. Baisden JM, et al. Dose as a function of lung volume and planned treatment volume in helical tomotherapy intensity-modulated radiation therapy-based stereotactic body radiation therapy for small lung tumors. *Int J Radiat Oncol*, 2007. **68**(4): 1229–37. doi:10.1016/j.ijrobp.2007.03.024.
34. Weyh A, Konski A, Nalichowski A, Maier J, Lack D. Lung SBRT: Dosimetric and delivery comparison of RapidArc, TomoTherapy, and IMR. *J Appl Clin Med Phys*, 2013. **14**(4): 4065.
35. Chi A, et al. Critical structure sparing in stereotactic ablative radiotherapy for central lung lesions: Helical tomotherapy vs. volumetric modulated arc therapy. *PLOS ONE*, 2013. **8**(4):e59729.

36. Mavroidis, P. et al., Treatment plan comparison between helical tomotherapy and MLC-based IMRT using radiobiological measures. *Phys Med Biol*, 2007. **52**(13): 3817–36.
37. Kannarunimit, D. et al., Analysis of dose distribution and risk of pneumonitis in stereotactic body radiation therapy for centrally located lung tumors: A comparison of robotic radiosurgery, helical tomotherapy and volumetric modulated arc therapy. *Technol Cancer Res Treat*, 2015. **14**(1): 49–60.
38. Ding, C. et al., A dosimetric comparison of stereotactic body radiation therapy techniques for lung cancer: Robotic versus conventional linac-based systems. *J Appl Clin Med Phys*, 2010. **11**(3): 3223.
39. Chan, M. et al., Evaluation of imaging performance of major image guidance systems. *Biomed Imaging Interv J*, 2011. **7**(2):e11. Epub 2012/01/31. doi:10.2349/biij.7.2.e11.
40. Monajemi, T.T. et al., A bench-top megavoltage fan-beam CT using CdWO4-photodiode detectors. II. Image performance evaluation. *Med Phys*, 2006. **33**(4): 1090–100.
41. Monajemi, T.T. et al., Modeling scintillator-photodiodes as detectors for megavoltage CT. *Med Phys*, 2004. **31**(5): 1225–34.
42. Westerly, D.C. et al., High-dose MVCT image guidance for stereotactic body radiation therapy. *Med Phys*, 2012. **39**(8): 4812–9.
43. Jia, X. et al., GPU-based iterative cone-beam CT reconstruction using tight frame regularization. *Phys Med Biol*, 2011. **56**(13): 3787–807.
44. Tian, Z. et al., Low-dose CT reconstruction via edge-preserving total variation regularization. *Phys Med Biol*, 2011. **56**(18): 5949–67.
45. Gao, H. et al., Megavoltage CT imaging quality improvement on TomoTherapy via tensor framelet. *Med Phys*, 2013. **40**(8): 081919.
46. Lu, W. et al., Deformable registration of the planning image (kVCT) and the daily images (MVCT) for adaptive radiation therapy. *Phys Med Biol*, 2006. **51**(17): 4357–74.
47. Martin, S. et al., Evaluation of tomotherapy MVCT image enhancement program for tumor volume delineation. *J Appl Clin Med Phys*, 2011. **12**(3): 3505.
48. Sheng, K. et al., Denoised and texture enhanced MVCT to improve soft tissue conspicuity. *Med Phys*, 2014. **41**(10): 101916.
49. Boswell, S. et al., Automatic registration of megavoltage to kilovoltage CT images in helical tomotherapy: An evaluation of the setup verification process for the special case of a rigid head phantom. *Med Phys*, 2006. **33**(11): 4395–404.
50. Zhou, J.N. et al., Image-guided stereotactic body radiotherapy for lung tumors using Bodyloc with tomotherapy: Clinical implementation and set-up accuracy. *Med Dosim*, 2010. **35**(1): 12–8.
51. Hodge, W. et al., Feasibility report of image guided stereotactic body radiotherapy (IG-SBRT) with tomotherapy for early stage medically inoperable lung cancer using extreme hypofractionation. *Acta Oncol*, 2006. **45**(7): 890–6.
52. Dunlap, N.E. et al., Size matters: A comparison of T1 and T2 peripheral non-small-cell lung cancers treated with stereotactic body radiation therapy (SBRT). *J Thorac Cardiovasc Surg*, 2010. **140**(3): 583–9.
53. Aibe, N. et al., Outcome and toxicity of stereotactic body radiotherapy with helical tomotherapy for inoperable lung tumor: Analysis of Grade 5 radiation pneumonitis. *J Radiat Res*, 2014. **55**(3): 575–82. Epub 2014/01/25.
54. Nagai, A. et al., Safety and efficacy of intensity-modulated stereotactic body radiotherapy using helical tomotherapy for lung cancer and lung metastasis. *Biomed Res Int*, 2014. **2014**: 473173.
55. Kim, J.Y. et al., Helical tomotherapy for simultaneous multitarget radiotherapy for pulmonary metastasis. *Int J Radiat Oncol Biol Phys*, 2009. **75**(3): 703–10. Epub 2009/05/08. doi:10.1016/j.ijrobp.2008.11.065; S0360-3016(09)00196-5 [pii]. PubMed PMID: 19419818.
56. Rowe, B.P. et al., Stereotactic body radiotherapy for central lung tumors. *J Thorac Oncol*, 2012. **7**(9): 1394–9.
57. Haasbeek, C.J. et al., Outcomes of stereotactic ablative radiotherapy for centrally located early-stage lung cancer. *J Thorac Oncol*, 2011. **6**(12): 2036–43. Epub 2011/09/06.
58. Song, S.Y. et al., Fractionated stereotactic body radiation therapy for medically inoperable stage I lung cancer adjacent to central large bronchus. *Lung Cancer*, 2009. **66**(1): 89–93.

59. Joyner, M. et al., Stereotactic body radiation therapy for centrally located lung lesions. *Acta Oncologica*, 2006. **45**(7): 802–7.
60. Timmerman, R. et al., Excessive toxicity when treating central tumors in a phase II study of stereotactic body radiation therapy for medically inoperable early-stage lung cancer. *J Clin Oncol*, 2006. **24**(30): 4833–9.
61. Chi, A. et al., Feasibility of helical tomotherapy in stereotactic body radiation therapy for centrally located early stage nonsmall-cell lung cancer or lung metastases. *Int J Radiat Oncol Biol Phys*, 2011. **81**(3): 856–62.
62. Boswell, S.A., et al., A novel method to correct for pitch and yaw patient setup errors in helical tomotherapy. *Med Phys*, 2005. **32**(6): 1630–9.
63. Kaiser, A. et al., Pitch, roll, and yaw variations in patient positioning. *Int J Radiat Oncol Biol Phys*, 2006. **66**(3): 949–55.
64. Schubert, L.K. et al., A comprehensive assessment by tumor site of patient setup using daily Mvct imaging from more than 3,800 helical tomotherapy treatments. *Int J Radiat Oncol*, 2009. **73**(4): 1260–9.
65. Ramsey, C.R. et al., A technique for adaptive image-guided helical tomotherapy for lung cancer. *Int J Radiat Oncol Biol Phys*, 2006. **64**(4): 1237–44.
66. Sonke, J.J. and J. Belderbos, Adaptive radiotherapy for lung cancer. *Semin Radiat Oncol*, 2010. **20**(2): 94–106.
67. Guckenberger, M. et al., Adaptive radiotherapy for locally advanced non-small-cell lung cancer does not underdose the microscopic disease and has the potential to increase tumor control. *Int J Radiat Oncol Biol Phys*, 2011. **81**(4):e275–82.
68. Guckenberger, M. et al., Potential of adaptive radiotherapy to escalate the radiation dose in combined radiochemotherapy for locally advanced non-small cell lung cancer. *Int J Radiat Oncol Biol Phys*, 2011. **79**(3): 901–8.
69. Haasbeek, C.J. et al., Is adaptive treatment planning required for stereotactic radiotherapy of stage I non-small-cell lung cancer? *Int J Radiat Oncol Biol Phys*, 2007. **67**(5): 1370–4.
70. Tvilum, M. et al., Clinical outcome of image-guided adaptive radiotherapy in the treatment of lung cancer patients. *Acta Oncol*, 2015: 1–8.
71. Boggs, D.H. et al., Stereotactic radiotherapy using tomotherapy for early-stage non-small cell lung carcinoma: Analysis of intrafraction tumour motion. *J Med Imag Radiat Oncol*, 2014. **58**(6): 706–13.
72. Gregoire, V. and T.R. Mackie, ICRU committee on volume and dose specification for prescribing, recording and reporting special techniques in external photon beam therapy: Conformal and IMRT. *Radiother Oncol*, 2005. **76**: S71.
73. Chi, T.W. and S.H. Chen, Dynamic magnetic resonance imaging used in evaluation of female pelvic prolapse: Experience from nine cases. *Kaohsiung J Med Sci*, 2007. **23**(6): 302–8.
74. Cai, J. et al., Evaluation of the reproducibility of lung motion probability distribution function (PDF) using dynamic MRI. *Phys Med Biol*, 2007. **52**(2): 365–73.
75. Cai, J. et al., Estimation of error in maximal intensity projection-based internal target volume of lung tumors: A simulation and comparison study using dynamic magnetic resonance imaging. *Int J Radiat Oncol Biol Phys*, 2007. **69**(3): 895–902.
76. Wanet, M. et al., Validation of the mid-position strategy for lung tumors in helical TomoTherapy. *Radiother Oncol*, 2014. **110**(3): 529–37.
77. Yu, C.X., D.A. Jaffray, J.W. Wong, The effects of intra-fraction organ motion on the delivery of dynamic intensity modulation. *Phys Med Biol*, 1998. **43**(1): 91–104.
78. Kissick, M.W. et al., Confirmation, refinement, and extension of a study in intrafraction motion interplay with sliding jaw motion. *Med Phys*, 2005. **32**(7): 2346–50.
79. Kim, B. et al., Motion-induced dose artifacts in helical tomotherapy. *Phys Med Biol*, 2009. **54**(19): 5707–34.
80. Bortfeld, T. et al., Effects of intra-fraction motion on IMRT dose delivery: Statistical analysis and simulation. *Phys Med Biol*, 2002. **47**(13): 2203–20.
81. Kanagaki, B. et al., A motion phantom study on helical tomotherapy: The dosimetric impacts of delivery technique and motion. *Phys Med Biol*, 2007. **52**(1): 243–55.

82. Sterpin, E. et al., Helical tomotherapy for SIB and hypo-fractionated treatments in lung carcinomas: A 4D Monte Carlo treatment planning study. *Radiother Oncol*, 2012. **104**(2): 173–80.
83. Trofimov, A. et al., Temporo-spatial IMRT optimization: Concepts, implementation and initial results. *Phys Med Biol*, 2005. **50**(12): 2779–98.
84. Zhao, W.H., et al., Apoptosis induced by preoperative oral 5'-DFUR administration in gastric adenocarcinoma and its mechanism of action. *World J Gastroenterol*, 2006. **12**(9): 1356–61.
85. Watkins, W.T. et al., Multiple anatomy optimization of accumulated dose. *Med Phys*, 2014. **41**(11): 111705. Epub 2014/11/06. doi:10.1118/1.4896104.
86. Berbeco, R.I. et al., Residual motion of lung tumors in end-of-inhale respiratory gated radiotherapy based on external surrogates. *Med Phys*, 2006. **33**(11): 4149–56.
87. Korreman, S. et al., Comparison of respiratory surrogates for gated lung radiotherapy without internal fiducials. *Acta Oncol*, 2006. **45**(7): 935–42.
88. Underberg, R.W. et al., A dosimetric analysis of respiration-gated radiotherapy in patients with stage III lung cancer. *Radiat Oncol*, 2006. **1**: 8.
89. Jin, J.Y. et al., A technique of using gated-CT images to determine internal target volume (ITV) for fractionated stereotactic lung radiotherapy. *Radiother Oncol*, 2006. **78**(2): 177–84.
90. Underberg, R.W. et al., Benefit of respiration-gated stereotactic radiotherapy for stage I lung cancer: An analysis of 4DCT datasets. *Int J Radiat Oncol Biol Phys*, 2005. **62**(2): 554–60.
91. Kim, B. et al., Feasibility study of multi-pass respiratory-gated helical tomotherapy of a moving target via binary MLC closure. *Phys Med Biol*, 2010. **55**(22): 6673–94.
92. Keall. P.J. et al., On the use of EPID-based implanted marker tracking for 4D radiotherapy. *Med Phys*, 2004. **31**(12): 3492–9.
93. Neicu, T. et al., Synchronized moving aperture radiation therapy (SMART): Average tumour trajectory for lung patients. *Phys Med Biol*, 2003. **48**(5): 587–98.
94. Ozhasoglu, C. et al., Synchrony—CyberKnife respiratory compensation technology. *Med Dosim*, 2008. **33**(2): 117–23.
95. Casamassima, F. et al., Use of motion tracking in stereotactic body radiotherapy: Evaluation of uncertainty in off-target dose distribution and optimization strategies. *Acta Oncologica*, 2006. **45**(7): 943–7.
96. Zhang, T. et al., Treatment plan optimization incorporating respiratory motion. *Med Phys*, 2004. **31**(6): 1576–86.
97. Zhang, T. et al., Breathing-synchronized delivery: A potential four-dimensional tomotherapy treatment technique. *Int J Radiat Oncol Biol Phys*, 2007. **68**(5): 1572–8.
98. Lu, W. et al., Real-time motion-adaptive-optimization (MAO) in TomoTherapy. *Phys Med Biol*, 2009. **54**(14): 4373–98.
99. Lu, W., Real-time motion-adaptive delivery (MAD) using binary MLC: I. Static beam (topotherapy) delivery. *Phys Med Biol*, 2008. **53**(22): 6491–511.
100. Lu, W., Real-time motion-adaptive delivery (MAD) using binary MLC: II. Rotational beam (tomotherapy) delivery. *Phys Med Biol*, 2008. **53**(22): 6491–511.
101. Yu, C.X., Intensity-modulated arc therapy with dynamic multileaf collimation: An alternative to tomotherapy. *Phys Med Biol*, 1995. **40**(9): 1435–49.
102. Otto, K., Volumetric modulated arc therapy: IMRT in a single gantry arc. *Med Phys*, 2008. **35**(1): 310–7.
103. Yang, W. et al., Standardized evaluation of simultaneous integrated boost plans on volumetric modulated arc therapy. *Phys Med Biol*, 2011. **56**(2): 327–39.
104. Dong, P. et al., 4pi noncoplanar stereotactic body radiation therapy for centrally located or larger lung tumors. *Int J Radiat Oncol Biol Phys*, 2013. **86**(3): 407–13.
105. Karam, S.D. et al., Dose escalation with stereotactic body radiation therapy boost for locally advanced non small cell lung cancer. *Radiat Oncol*, 2013. **8**: 179.
106. Parks, J. et al., Stereotactic body radiation therapy as salvage for intrathoracic recurrence in patients with previously irradiated locally advanced non-small cell lung cancer. *Am J Clin Oncol*, 2014.

107. Chang, J.Y., A. Bezjak, and F. Mornex. Stereotactic ablative radiotherapy for centrally located early stage non-small-cell lung cancer: What we have learned. *J Thorac Oncol*, 2015. **10**(4): 577–85.
108. Schanne, D.H. et al., Stereotactic body radiotherapy for centrally located stage I NSCLC: A multicenter analysis. Strahlentherapie und Onkologie: Organ der Deutschen Rontgengesellschaft [et al.], 2015. **191**(2): 125–32.
109. Shen, G. et al., Stereotactic body radiation therapy for centrally-located lung tumors. *Oncol Lett*, 2014. **7**(4): 1292–6.
110. Henriques, B. et al., Use of FDG-PET to guide dose prescription heterogeneity in stereotactic body radiation therapy for lung cancers with volumetric modulated arc therapy: A study of feasibility. *Int J Radiat Oncol*, 2014. **90**: S902–S3.
111. Solberg, TD et al., Commissioning and initial stereotactic ablative radiotherapy experience with Vero. *J Appl Clin Med Phys*, 2014. **15**(2): 4685.

9

Robotic arm linac

JUN YANG, ANDREW CARDIN, JING FENG, XING LIANG, AND ENMING WANG

9.1 INTRODUCTION

Lung tumors can present a challenge to those who wish to deliver an exceptionally precise radiation treatment such as stereotactic body radiation therapy (SBRT). Complicating factors include proximity to critical structures, significant tissue density heterogeneities, and relatively large and irregular motion caused by patient respiration. The robotic radiosurgery system, CyberKnife®, provides several technologies to achieve an accurate and precise treatment for lung cancer patients.

The CyberKnife system is a frameless robotic stereotactic radiosurgery system. As shown in Figure 9.1, the system is composed of several main components; (1) a small X-band linear accelerator that produces 6 MV photon beams which are collimated by either fixed conical collimators, a 12-sided IRIS dynamic collimator, or a newly designed multi-leaf collimator; (2) a six-jointed industrial robotic arm (the manipulator) to which the linear accelerator is attached; (3) a standard or robotic treatment couch; and (4) a pair of orthogonal kV

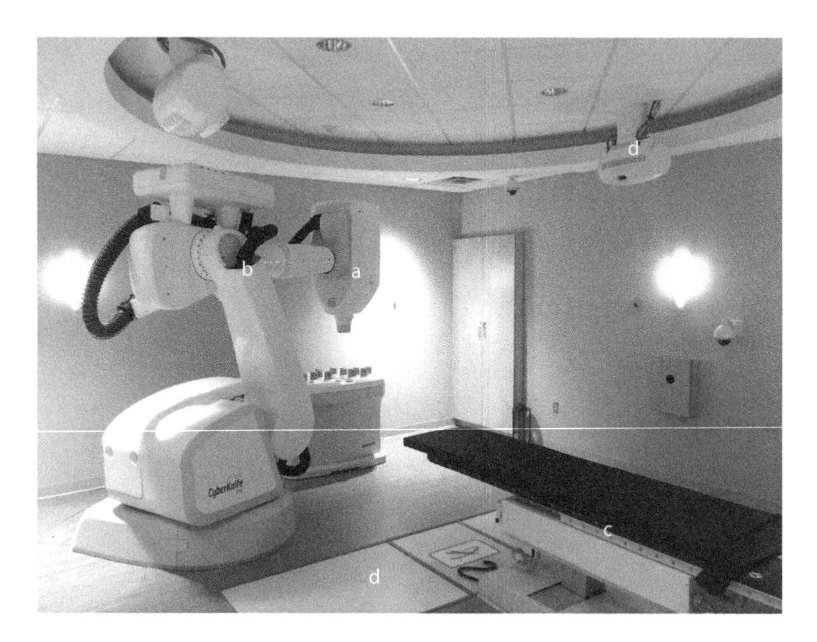

Figure 9.1 A typical CyberKnife® treatment room (Model G4). Components are labeled: (a) X-band linear accelerator, (b) six-jointed industrial robotic arm, (c) a standard treatment couch, and (d) x-ray tubes and detectors.

x-ray tubes and detectors. Unlike a conventional "C-arm" -based medical accelerator, the treatment radiation beams delivered by the CyberKnife system are always delivered in a non-coplanar fashion, which can reduce the dose delivered to healthy tissue surrounding the targeted area. Additionally, the CyberKnife system is equipped with an advanced tracking system, which is especially useful for managing tumor motions while maintaining a high degree of accuracy and precision. This tracking system provides four main modes of anatomical tracking: (1) six-dimensional (6D) Skull, which is exclusively used for intracranial treatments; (2) Xsight®, which is further divided into Xsight-Spine for the tracking of spine anatomy and Xsight-Lung for the tracking of lung anatomy; (3) fiducial tracking which accurately tracks the locations of implanted fiducials; and (4) Synchrony®, which uses external light-emitting diode (LED) markers as a surrogate in order to track the motion of a tumor in real time. These imaging modalities ascertain the true location of the tumor with sub millimeter accuracy during treatment. The difference between this true location and the planned location is compensated for by the robotic manipulator during treatment, even while the radiation is being delivered and the tumor is in motion. This ensures that the radiation beam is always incident upon the intended area.

In this chapter, the motion management technologies of the CyberKnife system will be described, as well as considerations specific to lung treatment. We then provide an overview of how the CyberKnife system is applied clinically and explain workflow of its use in treating a lung tumor. Finally, some techniques are suggested for performing quality assessment (QA) and quality control of lung tumor treatments.

9.2 MOTION MANAGEMENT

Motion management is always a concern in radiotherapy for lung tumors. Depending on the location of the tumor within the lung and the patient's depth of breath, the range of motion of a lung tumor can be anything from no motion at all to several centimeters of motion. Additionally, respiratory motions can be irregular and display hysteresis, so it is important to individualize the motion management of each patient. Common methods of motion management, fully described in the AAPM Task Group 76 Report [1], include encompassing the motion of the tumor within the full radiation beam, respiratory gating of the radiation beam, breath-holding, forced shallow breathing, and real-time tumor tracking. The CyberKnife system employs this latter method, as well as motion encompassing methods when necessary. Real-time tumor tracking is accomplished using the Synchrony system, both with or without fiducials, and when this is not feasible, an internal target volume (ITV) is generated to encompass the tumor's motion within the radiation field.

9.2.1 Fiducial tracking and Synchrony tracking with fiducials

The CyberKnife system has two tracking options that involve fiducial recognition: fiducial tracking alone or fiducial tracking with Synchrony. In general, fiducial tracking is used to track markers located in or near a radiotherapy target and to automatically correct for their displacement. This tracking method requires the implantation of radiopaque fiducial markers in or near the target volume prior to the radiation planning computed tomography (CT) scan. If a target does not move with the patient's breathing, then fiducial tracking by itself is sufficient. However, for targets that do move with respiration, fiducial tracking is used cooperatively with the Synchrony system. In either case, fiducial markers represent the treatment target's position and, if three or more are implanted, the treatment geometry.

Synchrony is capable of tracking tumors whose motion can be correlated to the motion of some external surrogate on the surface of the patient, which makes it ideal to treat those that move with respiratory motion. Its real-time tracking capabilities allow radiation beams to continuously follow and treat the target while it moves. Both prior to and during a Synchrony treatment session, the location of the tumor is determined radiographically by the orthogonal x-ray imaging system and, at the same time, the motion due to respiration is determined by an optical tracking system that is fixed to the patient's abdomen. A mathematical motion predictive model is then generated based on the correlation between the synchronized tumor location data and respiratory motion data. With this model, the live respiratory motion data are used to proactively determine the tumor's position in three dimensions and thus synchronize the motion of the robot with the motion of the tumor. The system is also designed to adapt to changes in the patient breathing pattern, such that the motion model periodically updates itself by taking new radiographs throughout the treatment session. This allows the patient to breathe in a relaxed and unrestricted manner without compromising the accuracy of the treatment delivery. Still, breath coaching is crucial to minimize drastic changes in breathing pattern. Details about the Synchrony tracking algorithms are published and available [2]. Considerable research has affirmed the Synchrony system's accuracy and demonstrated its sub millimeter capabilities [3–6].

The use of fiducials is the standard of practice for CyberKnife treatment of lung tumors. Delivering a treatment using fiducial tracking is easy due to software-assisted fiducial lock-on, and visual confirmation of the lock-on is usually obvious. Fiducial placement, however, requires an invasive procedure and therefore has an associated risk. Indeed, fiducial implantation comes with the risk of complications such as pneumothorax, which has been shown to occur in a large percentage of patients who undergo percutaneous fiducial implantation [7,8.] In addition to the risk of an invasive implantation procedure, there are two other potential disadvantages of using fiducials: fiducial migration and fiducial positioning. Specifically, it is not uncommon for implanted fiducials to migrate at any time after implantation, both before or after CT simulation. If this is the case, new fiducials must be implanted before treatment can proceed. If the fiducials migrate after CT simulation, and no new fiducials are implanted, then it is very probable that the treatment will be inaccurate. Indeed, tracking may not even be possible. To avoid this potential complication, it is recommended that lung patient simulation be performed at least 1 week after fiducial placement. This gives time for a fiducial to settle into the tissue and thus minimizes the risk of fiducial migration between CT simulation and treatment delivery. As mentioned, the position of the fiducials is also a concern. If fiducials are placed outside the target, or they are not evenly distributed around the target, the tissue between the fiducials and target may deform during respiration. This could lead to higher uncertainty in treatment targeting and thus an inaccurate treatment.

9.2.2 Lung treatment without fiducials

Lung Optimized Treatment (LOT) is a set of tracking solutions designed as an available option to avoid using fiducials. LOT is divided into three tracking options: 0-View Tracking, 1-View Tracking, and 2-View Tracking (also known as Xsight Lung Tracking, or XLT). Which tracking option a clinical user decides to use is dependent on the tumor's visibility in the x-ray images; tumors visible on both orthogonal x-ray images can be treated with

2-View Tracking, those visible in only one x-ray image are treated with 1-View Tracking, and those not visible at all are treated with 0-View Tracking. However, the choice of option may clinically depend on other factors such as respiratory motion of the tumor, proximity to critical structures, and the overall health condition of the patient. In the 1-View Tracking option, the manipulator compensates for the tumor motion in the plane in which the tumor is visible, and in the axis orthogonal to this plane a partial internal target volume (ITV) is created. This is the motion encompassing method, mentioned in the previous section, which is used to compensate for the loss of motion information that would otherwise be captured in 2-View Tracking. To correctly position the treatment target at the imaging center, the patient is initially set up by aligning the bones of the spine to match the digitally reconstructed radiographs (DRRs) from treatment planning, and then a pre-calculated couch shift is applied to bring the partial ITV into the treatment area. Synchrony Respiratory Tracking is then used in combination with either 2- or 1-View Tracking to follow the tumor motion during treatment. 0-View Tracking is essentially the same as the traditional motion-encompassing method; the patient is initially aligned to nearby vertebral bodies, and then a planning target volume (PTV), generated from a full ITV and clinical target volume (CTV), is treated without any real-time tracking or motion compensation by the manipulator. The imaging, alignment, and target locating algorithm, in this case, is identical to Xsight-Spine Tracking.

9.2.2.1 LOT SIMULATION PLAN

LOT also allows for the generation of a simulation treatment plan to be used for the determination of the optimal tracking mode. This simulation plan is based on a pair of normal expiration-hold and inspiration-hold CT scans, and the expiration-hold CT scan is used for treatment planning dosimetry and DRR generation. For the treatment plans to be valid, the two CT scans must be registered together, either by acquiring the scans during the same study or by performing an image registration in the treatment planning system. If the two CT scans are registered in the treatment planning system, then the region of registration should be the spine. After completion, the simulation plan becomes available in a dedicated application of the treatment delivery console and allows the user to discover any limitations of the LOT tracking. This is accomplished by taking several x-ray images of the patient in the treatment position while lying on the treatment couch. Images are taken at each phase of the patient's respiratory cycle and the images from each x-ray source are evaluated separately based on the visibility of the target volume. By performing this procedure, the user can more reliably determine the optimal tracking method for the patient. Once the optimal tracking mode has been determined, the CTVs are contoured in each of the CT scans and are then used to automatically generate the full, or partial, ITV using an automated procedure in the treatment planning system.

Since these CT scans will eventually be used as the basis for the treatment planning process, it is critically important that they represent the extent of breathing motions of the patient during treatment. Exaggerated breath-holding during CT acquisition will result in the formation of an inaccurate ITV and therefore, unnecessary radiation exposure to healthy lung tissue. This can be avoided in several ways and the method of quality control is dependent on the available technology and clinical preference. Some quality control methods include: (1) acquiring a free-breath, slow CT, and fusing this to the expiration-hold CT; (2) acquiring a four-dimensional (4D) CT scan, extracting the expiration and inspiration phases, and either using these directly to generate the simulation plan or using them to confirm the validity of the breath-hold scans; and (3) using external markers (light-emitting or IR-reflective) to observe and/or quantify the motion/position of the patient's chest both during free-breathing (as if during treatment) and during a breath-hold. Additionally, the use of two breath-hold CT scans for ITV generation assumes a linear translation of the target volume, which may not be the case. Therefore, it may be necessary to discern the true trajectory of the target volume, typically by 4D CT acquisition, to ensure accurate ITV generation.

9.2.2.2 0-VIEW TRACKING

0-View Tracking does not actually track the tumor, but instead tracks the nearby vertebral bodies of the spine. This tracking only corrects for gross patient motion during the treatment and does not track the motion of the tumor caused by respiration. As mentioned before, a tumor-motion encompassing ITV is irradiated, and it is very important that the treatment planner contours the ITV based on the tumor's true trajectory and does not assume that it can be contoured by a linear translation of the CTV between inspiration and expiration phases.

9.2.2.2.1 Patient selection and considerations for 0-View Tracking

0-View Tracking is most appropriate for tumors that are not visible in either orthogonal x-ray image. This can occur in several situations and depends on several different factors. Tumors that are small or diffuse can lack sufficient contrast to be distinguishable from surrounding tissue, or conversely, the thick tissue of a heavy patient may obscure the image of a lung tumor that would otherwise be noticeable. To simplify, the tumor may be blocked from view by nearby dense anatomy such as the heart, great vessels, or spine.

Since 0-View Tracking requires a full ITV, this tracking mode will necessarily irradiate surrounding lung tissue within the PTV and may increase tissue toxicity. Therefore, it is important that clinicians evaluate the risk of this tissue toxicity relative to the risks associated with fiducial implantation. It may, in fact, be a prudent clinical policy to only use 0-View Tracking with lung tumors that exhibit minimal respiratory motion, such as those that appear in the upper lobe of the lung.

As a final patient selection criterion, it is preferable to limit 0-View Tracking patients to those whose tumors are near the spinal column. This is because the positional uncertainty is greater when using bony anatomy as a surrogate landmark for aligning an ITV [9].

9.2.2.3 1-VIEW TRACKING

As stated previously, 1-View Tracking is used to locate and track tumors that are visible in only one of the two x-ray images. The need for 1-View Tracking usually arises when a tumor is large enough to be visible, but is blocked from view on one of the x-ray images by major structures such as the heart or spine.

1-View Tracking takes advantage of the fact that the CyberKnife's x-ray imaging system shares an inferior/superior axis. Because the two imagers share this axis, the inferior/superior component of the tumor's motion can be determined using only one of the two imagers. A depiction of the different tracking modes, including 1-View Tracking, is shown in Figure 9.2. For lung tumors that move significantly with respiration, the inferior/superior direction is the major component of the motion, so 1-View Tracking accommodates most of the tumor's motion. As in 2-View Tracking, this two-dimensional position and motion information is sent to the Synchrony system and allows the robotic manipulator to follow the tumor's motion while irradiating. However, the one-dimensional information parallel to the x-ray source-detector axis cannot be determined, and, as mentioned earlier, this is compensated for with a partial ITV. This partial ITV is not a simple combination of inhale CTV and exhale CTV, but rather a volume expansion in the untracked direction. It is automatically generated correctly in the treatment planning system application given correctly delineated CTVs.

9.2.2.4 2-VIEW TRACKING

2-View Tracking, also known as Xsight Lung Tracking (XLT), can recognize the tumor area on the orthogonal x-ray images because of the difference in density between the tumor and the surrounding lung tissue. This density difference causes contrast in the image which allows it to be identified by back-projection algorithms programmed into the tracking software. The position of the tumor in the images is used to calculate the position of the tumor in three dimensions. To continuously track the location of the tumor, XLT is used in combination with, which detects the real-time positions of LEDs placed on the patient's chest and correlates this information with the tumor position information. Using this information, the linac head can both irradiate, and synchronously move with, the tumor. With this real-time tracking of the moving target, a CTV is used instead of an ITV and greater sparing of healthy tissue is achieved.

Two-View Tracking is performed by a two-step procedure. First, the patient is positioned on the treatment couch in the same position as during the CT scan. As is done for 0-View Tracking, the Xsight-Spine Tracking algorithm is then used to compute the translational and rotational couch corrections based on the vertebrae nearest to the lung tumor. In transition to the second step, a couch shift is performed such that the imaging center becomes coincident with the tumor region. Then, before irradiating, several pairs of orthogonal x-ray images are taken while the Synchrony cameras track the position of LEDs that rest on the patient's chest or abdomen. While not of great significance, it is best to position the LEDs and Synchrony camera such that the LEDs move perpendicular to the central axis of the camera, and to place the LEDs on an area of the patient that moves the most with respiration. Once an adequate correlation model is built, the treatment begins,

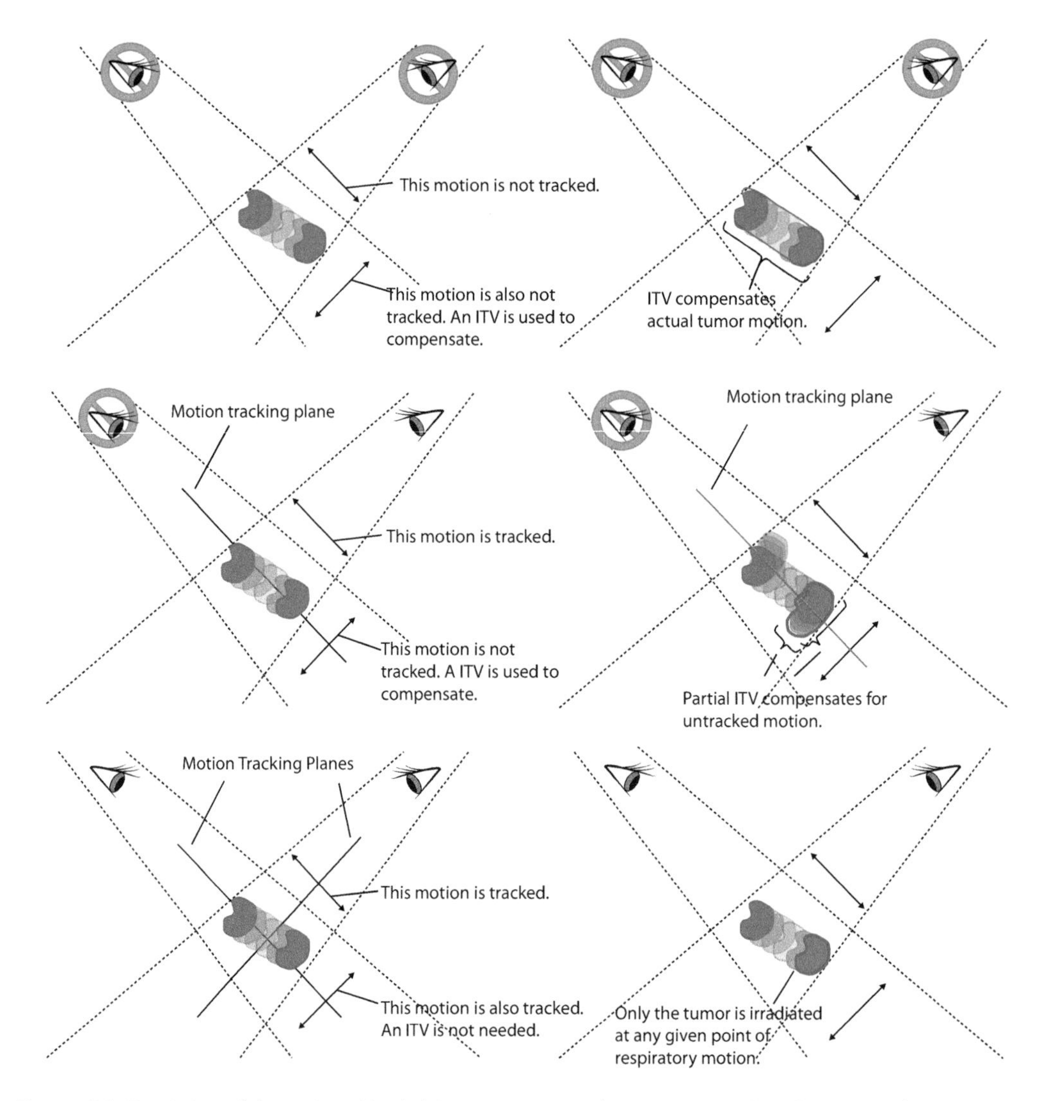

Figure 9.2 Depiction of the various Xsight® Lung motion-tracking concepts. Top: 0-View Tracking: No component of the tumor's motion is visible; therefore the ITV encompasses the entire volume of tumor motion. (middle) 1-View Tracking: A component of the tumor's motion is visible to one of the x-ray imagers and not visible to the other. The component of the tumor's motion that is visible is that component which is perpendicular to the central axis of the x-ray imager. The partial ITV used to encompass the tumor's non-tracked motion is delineated by brackets. Bottom: 2-View Tracking: The tumor's motion is visible in all three directions; therefore no ITV is necessary. The PTV is generated directly from the CTV.

and additional orthogonal x-ray images are periodically taken to track the tumor and update the correlation model. In a recent version of software, the volume that is tracked by XLT is based on the Tumor Region DRR. The Tumor Region DRR is generated only from the volume of the CT scan in and close to the tumor. This Tumor Region DRR serves as a model which allows the tracking algorithm to identify the tumor's density pattern in the live x-ray images. While the tumor is being tracked, real-time translational corrections are applied but rotational corrections are not applied because the Synchrony system builds a correlation model that specifically correlates the LED position to the centroid of the tumor region, and rotations cannot be calculated based on one point.

As previously stated, 2-View is only used to treat patients in whom a lung tumor is visible in both x-ray images. It is not enough, though, that the tumor is visible to human users; it must also be identifiable in both images by the tracking algorithm. Therefore, 2-View is usually reserved for treatment of solid tumors

1.5 cm or larger. The patient selection considerations for 2-View are the same as those factors mentioned in the 0-View subsection that work to obscure the visibility of a lung tumor, that is, factors such as patient chest wall thickness, tumor location, and obstruction of view by other anatomical structures. Given these considerations, a challenge of 2-View Tracking is human visual verification of the tracking accuracy on both x-ray images. Thus, appropriate patient selection as outlined above is central to successful and confident treatment delivery. Based on practical experience so far, the usage of 2-View is typically limited to about 30% of the lung patients.

9.3 CLINICAL PROCESS

9.3.1 FIDUCIAL AND FIDUCIAL PLACEMENT

If it is decided that fiducials are necessary to properly track and treat a tumor, treatment management starts with the implantation of fiducial markers. For lung patients, it is important that fiducials be implanted either inside or very close to the targeted tumor. Several different methods of implantation and types of fiducials are available to the physician to perform this task. Typically, an interventional radiologist implants one or more standard cylindrical gold markers percutaneously under image or video guidance. The gold markers are 0.8–1.2 mm in diameter and 3–6 mm in length, and are pre-loaded in 17- or 18-gauge needles. Due to the risk of pneumothorax in lung patients, there are more advanced placement procedures. Bronchoscopic implantation is accurate and has a smaller chance of causing pneumothorax [10,11]. A recent technological advancement in bronchoscopy, called electromagnetic navigation bronchoscopy (ENB), is minimally invasive and used for hard-to-reach locations in the lung. An example is the superDimension™ lung navigation system (Medtronic, Inc., Minneapolis, MN). This technology allows physicians to perform fiducial placements using an electromagnetic guidance system, like a GPS for the small spaces of lung bronchioles. Other types of fiducials such as the VISICOIL™ (Core Oncology, Santa Barbara, CA) and Gold Anchor fiducial are also available for clinical use implanted percutaneously using a thinner needle. Gold Anchor fiducials have a lower chance of migrating after implantation because the fiducial folds and scrunches into a ball shape within the tissue, immobilizing it immediately after placement. This reduced chance of migration has been substantiated by research [12]. The three different types of fiducials discussed here are shown in Figure 9.3.

While the optimal number of fiducial markers is still debated [13], the CyberKnife manufacturer recommends 3–6 fiducials be implanted to allow for translational and rotational information to be determined by the tracking system. Having multiple fiducials also allows for a comparison of fiducial position to detect any migration. If multiple fiducials are implanted, they should be spaced at least 2 cm apart. This spacing increases the certainty of the rotational corrections computed by the tracking system during treatment, and reduces the chance that the fiducials will appear to overlap each other in the obliquely acquired x-ray images. Alternatively, one can place a single, central fiducial in the tumor and, as proposed by Wu et al., estimate the margin to compensate for the tumor's deformation during respiration [14]. This is a generally accepted

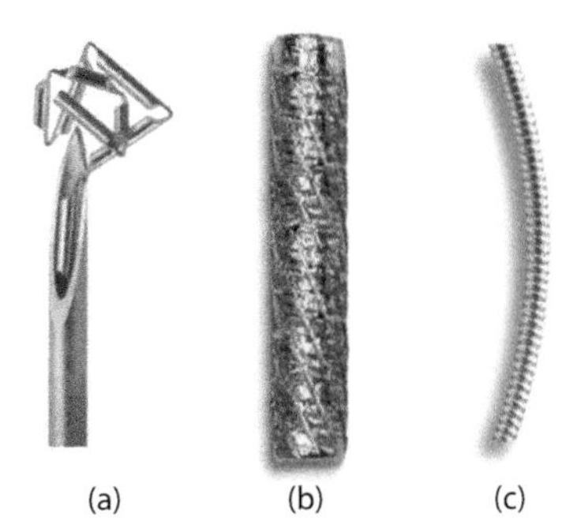

Figure 9.3 Fiducial marker examples used for CyberKnife® lung SBRT: (a) Gold Anchor™ fiducial marker, (b) Civco Cyber Mark™ cylindrical fiducial marker, and (c) VISICOIL™ fiducial marker.

method and further reduces the risk of pneumothorax; however, it requires the operators to carefully exclude the possibility of fiducial migration during the treatment.

9.3.2 Pre-treatment imaging

Many image series can be acquired prior to treatment, but one scan that is usually included is a noncontrast breath-hold planning CT to be used for dosimetry calculations and for generating the DRR images that are required for target tracking. Additional imaging modalities may be indicated, such as PET/CT and contrast-enhanced CT. It is a common practice to acquire a CT scan with IV contrast on patients who have a central lung lesion because the contrast more clearly defines the target and nearby organs at risk. All the scans that are necessary for planning are eventually co-registered with the planning CT to effectively delineate the tumor and critical structures during the contouring phase of treatment planning.

Like a conventional C-arm linac, lung patients are scanned head first in the supine position. Patients receiving treatment of the lung can be immobilized in a device such as a Vac-Lok cushion (Civco Medical Solutions, Kalona, IA). It is important to consider the potential advantages of immobilization while considering the chance that the immobilization device may make the patient less comfortable during a long treatment, and thus motivate the patient to move due to discomfort. It may be preferable to use a Vac-Lok cushion so that the patient's shoulder position is reproducible. Patients who experience discomfort in a Vac-Lok device can alternatively be placed on a soft pad. In this case, it can be advantageous to use a pad with a large thickness, such as the pad developed by Jim Hevezi, to allow the patient's arms to fall below their body and thus provide access to more posterior lateral radiation beams [15].

Lung patients being treated with CyberKnife should be imaged using a fast spiral multiple slice CT scanner. Since patients must hold their breath during a scan, the scanner should have at least 64 rows of detectors (64-slice) to keep the scanning time to a minimum. Contiguous thin-slice (1–2 mm) scans are ideal, and should cover the patient's full circumference. To acquire a sufficient volume for treatment planning, the CT scan should start about 20 cm superior to the target and end 20 cm inferior to the target. As mentioned previously, expiration-hold and inspiration-hold CT scans should be performed on lung patients [16]. It is common practice to use the expiration CT as the radiation planning CT, and then estimate the total motion of the target and nearby critical structures due to respiratory motion by performing a spine-based rigid-body registration between the inspiration and expiration CT scans. This allows the practitioner to better determine the appropriate tracking method, as well as the treatment margins. In addition to the breath-hold CT scans, it is ideal to also acquire a 4D CT scan and then generate a maximum intensity projection (MIP) CT series based on the individual series associated with each respiratory phase. This MIP series highlights the tumor position at all phases of the patient's respiratory cycle. This is advantageous because the respiratory motion of many patients' tumors is not linear, but rather elliptical in three dimensions. Thus, a more accurate ITV can be delineated based on the additional information provided by the MIP series. In addition, this pattern of the target's respiratory motion can help therapists during treatment delivery by indicating to them some expectation of how the tumor should move. This can facilitate the Synchrony model-building process as the therapists are required to visually verify the automatic image recognition performed by the delivery software. Therefore, this target motion pattern can serve as a reference in treatment quality control [16], as explained later in the quality control section.

9.3.3 Treatment planning

The CyberKnife system includes its own dedicated treatment planning system (TPS) called MultiPlan. This TPS provides the user with a step-by-step, task-oriented process and is quite user friendly. The planning process effectively selects an optimal subset of groups of beams to be used for treatment from a set of predefined "nodes," where each node is a potential group of treatment beams. These nodes are distributed on the surface of a virtual sphere, the center of which is coincident with the image tracking center. This imaging center can be visually approximated in Figure 9.1, directly above the blue logo located between the two imaging panels on the floor, approximately at the height of the treatment couch. The radius of this approximate sphere varies from 800 to 850 mm for intracranial treatment, and for extracranial treatments this node-space more closely resembles an ellipsoid, with a radius ranging from 800 to 1000 mm. Each of these two sets of predefined nodes is called a "path." The intracranial path has about 130 nodes and the extracranial path has about 110 nodes, about 20 nodes less in the apex direction compared to the intracranial path. Depending on the parameters of the treatment and the customized optimization, the TPS generates several candidate beams per node. The total number of possible beams deliverable by the CyberKnife ranges from 1200 to 6000 beams. Most clinical plans range from 50 to 250 beams.

9.3.4 Dose calculation

The CyberKnife is a single-energy machine, producing photons nominally rated at 6 MV. Therefore, the output of the CyberKnife is calibrated in a fashion similar to conventional C-arm linear accelerators. One monitor unit (MU) is calibrated to deliver 1 cGy at a distance of 800-mm source-axis distance (SAD) and a depth of 15 mm in water (d_{max} of a 6-MV photon beam) on the central axis of the 60-mm cone collimator. By default, the MultiPlan TPS uses a ray-tracing dose calculation algorithm. This ray-tracing function calculates the dose contribution from each beam in the treatment plan to each voxel in the user-defined calculation area. The sum of the contributions creates the complete dose distribution of the treatment plan. This algorithm is based on look-up procedures of tabulated beam data (measured and recorded during commissioning of the system), and its simplicity allows for rapid dose calculation. Heterogeneity corrections are performed using effective path length, and contour corrections are applied by casting multiple rays within each beam. The dose is calculated per the equation,

$$\frac{\text{Dose}}{\text{MU}} = \text{OCR} \times \text{IVS} \times \text{TPR} \times \text{OF}$$

where OCR is the off-central ratio, IVS is the inverse square $(800/\text{SAD})^2$, TPR is the tissue-phantom ratio, and OF is the output factor.

MultiPlan can also perform Monte Carlo calculations for more accurate dosimetry, which is particularly desirable in lung patient treatments. Monte Carlo is generally regarded as the most accurate algorithm for dosimetric calculations, and it is especially advantageous when calculating dose to area of tissue with various densities [17]. Research has reported that the ray-tracing algorithm overestimates the dose to lung lesions by 5–25% due to its simple heterogeneity correction calculations. While these corrections are sufficient for simple cases such as brain metastases, they do not compensate for the build-up that occurs from low-density lung tissue to higher-density tumors [6,18]. An example is shown in Figure 9.4, where the dose distribution of a treatment plan is shown calculated using the ray-tracing algorithm and the Monte Carlo algorithm. Because of this, Monte Carlo should be used for dosimetry of all lung cancer patients. To be consistent with traditional

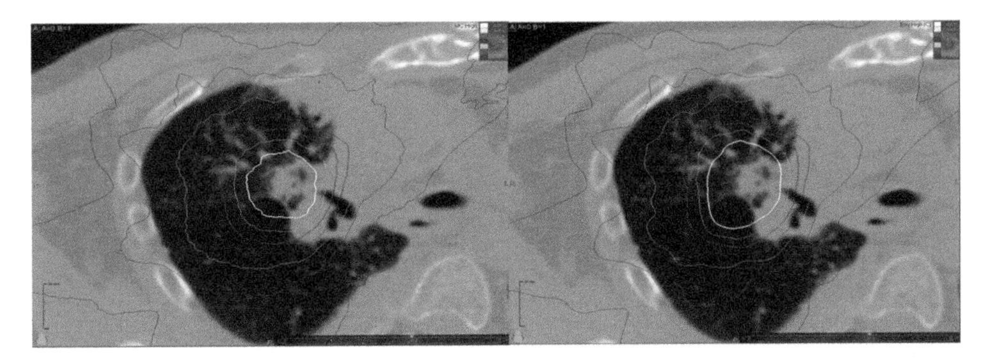

Figure 9.4 Comparison of Monte Carlo calculation (left) and ray-tracing calculation (right) on the same patient using the same treatment plan and normalization. One can clearly see the white Rx isodose line (4000 cGy) encompasses a larger volume using the ray-tracing algorithm, indicating an overestimate of the dose in that region compared to the dose calculated by the Monte Carlo algorithm.

dosage using the ray-tracing algorithm, Van der Voort van Zyp et al. have suggested lowering the prescription dose for lung tumors by 10% when the Monte Carlo algorithm is used and prescribing a lower isodose line to maintain sufficient coverage [19].

9.3.4.1 DOSIMETRIC CONSIDERATIONS RELATED TO TUMOR TRACKING

Generally, the accuracy of the CyberKnife system and its non-coplanar approach to treatment delivery provide a dosimetric outcome that is very sparing to normal tissue. Specifically, the dose gradient outside a planning treatment volume is much greater than most intensity-modulated radiation therapy cases. This can be seen in Figure 9.5, where the dosimetry of three different treatment modalities is visually compared. However, within the context of the advantages offered by the CyberKnife system, there are still subtle dosimetric complications that are peculiar to moving lung lesions and should be regarded during the treatment planning process. There are four adverse dosimetric effects that arise when treating an ITV instead of a GTV using live tracking. First, and most obviously, there is additional lung tissue included in the ITV that is not included in the GTV, and this lung tissue will therefore receive the prescription dose or possibly even more than the prescription dose due to tissue heterogeneities. This is significant because the typical SBRT prescription dose is usually higher than lung tissue dose tolerance. Second, the dose gradient around a large treatment volume is generally less than the gradient around a smaller PTV. Therefore, for larger treatment volumes, it is possible for the surrounding tissue to receive a dose that is less than the prescription dose but higher than the tissue's tolerance. Third, if the direction of the tumor's motion during respiration is toward a nearby organ at risk, planning on an ITV will generate a higher dose to the organ at risk than what would be generated when planning on only a GTV. Lastly, because the treatment is planned on a static 3D volume, the dose to the tumor that is displayed on the treatment planning system is likely to be somewhat different than the dose that is cumulatively received by the tumor as it moves within the ITV during treatment. This also means that the dose to nearby critical structures could be higher than planned if they move into or very close to the ITV during respiration. This increases the likelihood of exceeding the tissue tolerance of these critical structures, especially if the patient had previous radiation therapy in the same or nearby region. Thus, for larger tumor respiratory motion there is greater uncertainty between the calculated dose during treatment planning and the actual dose delivered to the tumor.

While the dose difference between what was planned and what is received might be negligible for homogenous dose distributions and conventionally fractionated treatment, this dose difference should not be considered negligible when the dose to the target volume is heterogeneous and when the treatment is hypo-fractionated, as is the case for SBRT treatments. While the first three dosimetric effects can be quantified in the treatment planning system, the fourth is difficult if the software does not have 4D capabilities. Therefore, it is important to understand how these dose differences can arise as well as how they can be mitigated during treatment planning. Based on the above considerations, a good rule of thumb is to use 0-View Tracking only if the tumor's total respiratory motion is less than 5~10 mm and the center of the tumor is no more than about 10 cm away from the center of the spine.

One technique that can be applied to 0-View and 1-View Tracking is to use a CT density override on the ITV. This would prevent the planning system from overestimating the number of monitor units needed to deliver the prescription dose to the low-density lung tissue inside the ITV. This is particularly important when using the Monte Carlo algorithm, which does correctly account for tissue heterogeneities and would therefore correctly (but undesirably) calculate the high monitor units necessary to deliver a large dose to such

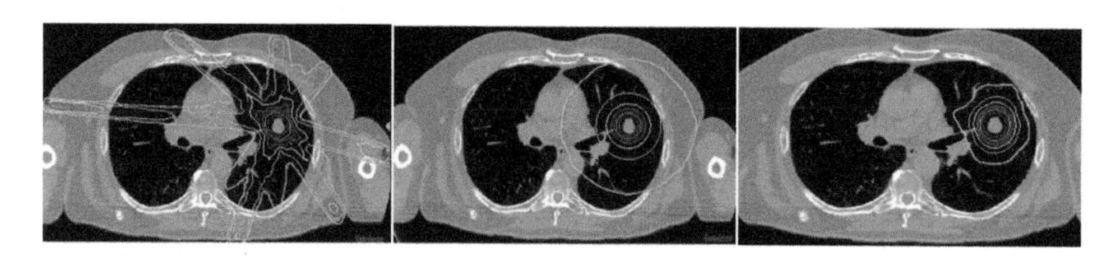

Figure 9.5 Comparison of treatment plans: Left: 7-beam intensity-modulated radiotherapy (IMRT). Middle: VMAT SBRT. RIght: Non-coplanar CyberKnife® plan. All three techniques give similar dose to the tumor, but the surrounding tissue dose is reduced using the non-coplanar technique.

low-density tissue. Lung lesions are approximately the same density as other soft tissues, so overriding the density to be equivalent to water is sufficient for this technique. One last subtlety that can be detected and corrected in the treatment planning system is the minimum beam MU; this should be adjusted so that the minimum beam on duration is equal to or greater than the respiratory period.

9.3.5 Treatment delivery

As with conventional radiation therapy, treatment begins with laying the patient on the treatment table and, using the same immobilization and support devices, reproducing the position of the patient during the CT simulation. Therapists should be especially attendant to the patient's comfort to minimize the chance that the patient will move during the long treatment. Once the patient's body is in the same general position as it was during the CT simulation, therapists manually move the treatment table until the target is close to the imaging center. In-room lasers that focus on the imaging center are often used to guide the therapists. Next, a pair of x-ray images is taken to more accurately determine how the patient should be moved to accurately reproduce their position. Alignment is performed either automatically by the image-guidance system, or manually by matching the anatomy in the x-ray images to the DRR overlay images. In either case, the treatment table automatically translates and rotates per the therapists' adjustments. Additional x-ray images are then acquired as needed, and adjustments are made to the patient's position, until the image guidance system and the therapists both confirm an accurate lock-on. The image guidance system always displays its calculated estimates of how the patient should be moved. The manufacturer's treatment limits on these estimates are 10 mm and 1 degree, but clinically it is both easy and prudent to maintain smaller estimates of 1–2 mm and 1 degree. Even if the guidance system determines that the patient is laterally displaced from their CT simulation position by several millimeters, this deviation is corrected automatically during treatment by the robotic arm. For tumors that are tracked by Synchrony, an additional step must be completed before treatment. In this step, the Synchrony model is built by acquiring x-ray images at different respiratory phases. Therapists correct any computer errors in tumor/fiducial recognition and treatment then begins. Some images pertaining to a typical lung treatment are shown in Figure 9.6.

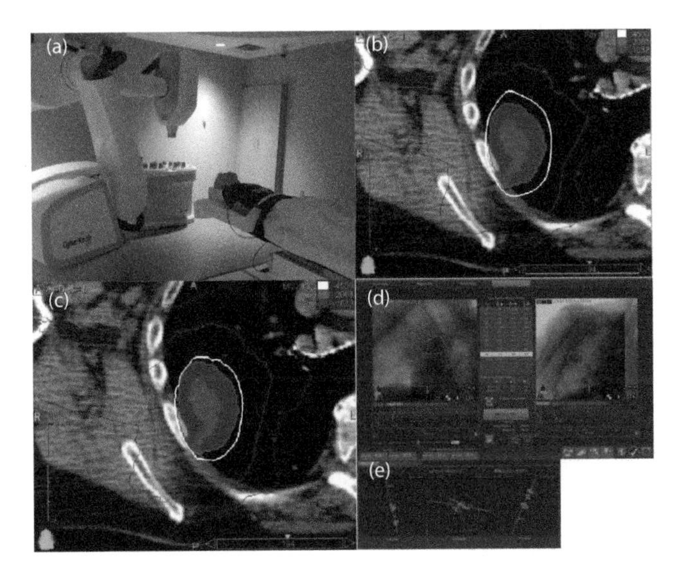

Figure 9.6 Example of 2-view Xsight® Lung treatment. (a) Patient setup for Xsight Lung treatment. The patient wears the Synchrony® vest upon which three optical markers are secured by Velcro. (b) Isocentric treatment plan for a 2-cm lung lesion with a 5-mm margin, and dose calculated using the ray-tracing algorithm. (c) The same plan as shown in (b), recalculated using the Monte Carlo algorithm. The 45-Gy isodose line (white) is tighter around the PTV after Monte Carlo calculation than it is after ray-tracing calculation. (d) Screenshot of treatment console during Xsight Lung treatment with the tumor as the tracking objective. The tumor (outlined) was identified in the live x-ray images based on the DRR. (e) Screenshot of the same treatment console showing the Synchrony correlation model. Each data plot corresponds to one dimension of motion (inf/sup, left/right, ant/post).

A clinically developed approach to setting up a patient for fiducial tracking involves a two-stage procedure. In this approach, a set of coordinates is used to define the imaging centers of each stage. In the treatment plan, the tracking center (X1, Y1, Z1) is defined on the expiration-hold CT coordinates as either the geometric center of the fiducials or the centroid of the targeted tumor. Additionally, a setup plan is created in which a spine-tracking imaging center (X2, Y2, Z2) is defined on the spine nearest to the treatment target. In this way, a pre-calculated couch shift (X1–X2, Y1–Y2, Z1–Z2) can be calculated and used during patient setup. The therapists use the setup plan until they have adequately positioned the patient's spine, and then apply the couch shift to move the patient into treatment position. In this way, the patient's body is aligned and the fiducials appear in the middle of the image after the couch shift. Naturally, this also acts as a quality assurance measure to ensure that the fiducials have not migrated since the treatment planning CT scan; if the patient is imaged during the expiration phase and the fiducials do not closely match those in the DRR, it is likely that the fiducials have migrated.

During CyberKnife treatment, the robotic arm moves through pre-defined positions, or nodes, to deliver beams from the treatment plan. The movement is optimized by a path traversal algorithm such that the robot skips those nodes for which there are no treatment beams. At the active nodes, the robotic arm corrects its translational and rotational positions based on the latest image guidance to compensate for target movement. The frequency of x-ray image guidance can be adjusted by the users on a clinical basis. At some nodes, patient images may be blocked by the robotic arm or the linac, in which case the last valid image will be adopted for motion tracking. If the target movement or patient motion exceeds the clinical tolerance, the treatment is paused automatically so that the user can adjust patient positioning. The treatment can also be stopped automatically if the robotic arm moves within 5 cm of a "safe zone." The safe zone can be defined by the user based on the size of the patient and the couch position. Another safety feature of the system includes touch sensors on the linac head, which will induce an emergency stop once it is triggered. The system generates a make-up plan if the interrupted plan needs to be continued at a different time.

Treatment time is composed of imaging time, robotic arm movement time, and beam-on time. When using Synchrony, the Synchrony model buildup time, which normally ranges from 5 to 10 minutes, also needs to be included in the total treatment time. The average treatment time for lung SBRT using V8.5 CyberKnife is approximately 40 minutes.

9.4 QUALITY ASSESSMENT AND QUALITY CONTROL

The most generally relevant guidelines for the quality assurance and quality control of the CyberKnife system is the Task Group 135 by the American Association of Medical Physicists [20], entitled "Quality Assurance for Robotic Radiosurgery." This report, as well as Task Groups 51 and 101 on clinical reference dosimetry of high-energy photons and on stereotactic body radiation therapy (SBRT), respectively [21,22], provides sufficient guidance for general quality assurance of both the CyberKnife system and of the stereotactic treatments that it delivers. While physicists are the primary audience of Task Group 101, this report provides a broad overview of the technical aspects pertaining to SBRT and gives many specific recommendations that are applicable to lung treatments. Physicists should follow the guidelines in these documents on a regular basis to assure and control a non-patient-specific quality of radiation treatment. The next two sections discuss some recommendations specific to CyberKnife lung treatment.

9.4.1 Quality assessment

An anthropomorphic lung phantom called the XLT Phantom is available for end-to-end (E2E) QA testing. This phantom is designed to model a human upper body, with a radiographically equivalent lung, chest wall, spine and ribs. A rod inserted into the "lung" is pulled and pushed in the superior/inferior direction by an electric motor to simulate respiratory motion. Inside the rod is a small cube with a plastic sphere inside, which represents a lung tumor. The cube is designed to hold an axial and a sagittal radio chromic film. This phantom, as well as sample films and E2E analysis, is shown in Figure 9.7.

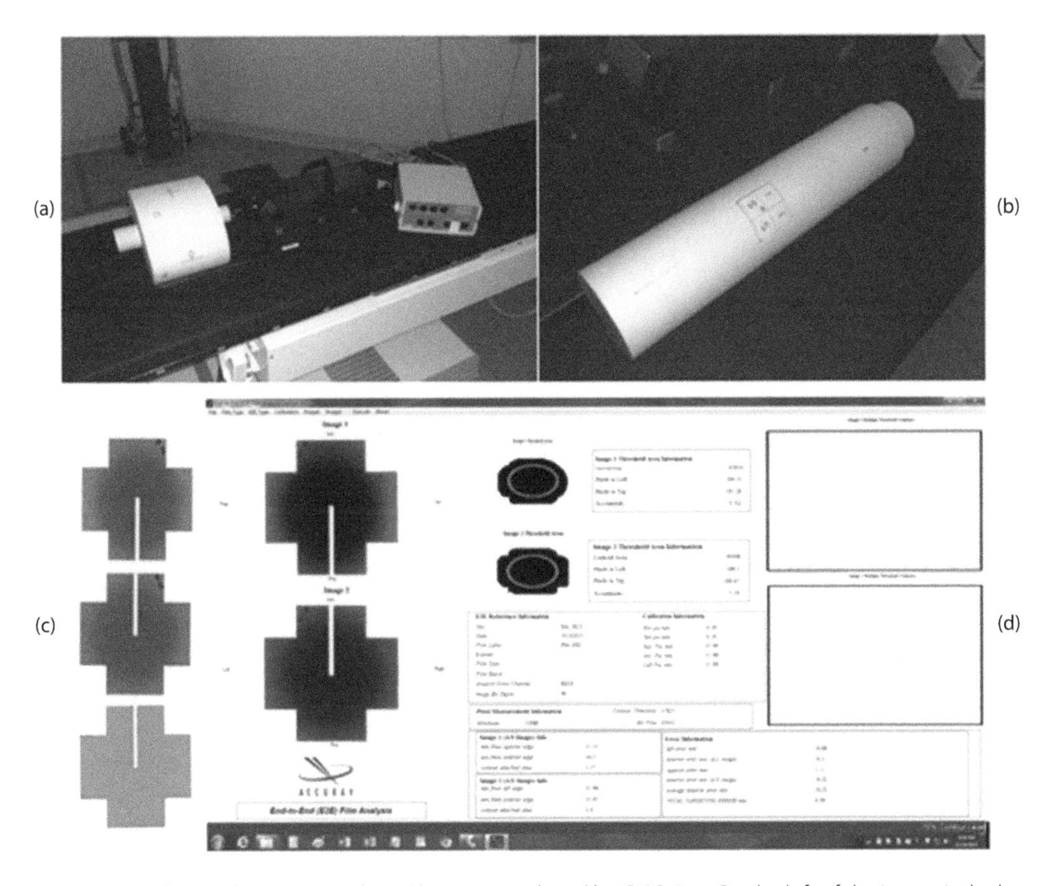

Figure 9.7 (a) The Xsight® Lung Tracking Phantom produced by CIRS, Inc. On the left of the image is the lung phantom with inserted rod. (b) The rod containing the cube in which films are inserted. (c) An example of films irradiated during a QA plan delivery. The circular cross section of the planned spherical dose cloud is clearly visible on the top two films, whereas the bottom film serves as a background. (d) A screenshot of the E2E software analysis.

A QA plan is created on a CT scan of the XLT phantom. It is designed such that a spherical shaped dose cloud is centered within the film cube, concentric with the plastic sphere (tumor) inside the cube. After delivery of the QA plan, E2E software analyzes the film to quantify delivery accuracy.

The plastic sphere in the phantom can be visualized in both x-ray images which means it can be tracked using 2-View Tracking. While a LOT specific QA device designed for 1-View or 0-View is not currently available, site physicists can still use the XLT phantom for 1-View and 0-View Tracking QA by creating new QA treatment plans and delivering them on the XLT phantom using one of these tracking methods.

It is generally recommended that a patient-specific delivery QA be performed in order to analyze the actual dose distribution delivered to a phantom by the patient's treatment plan. For IMRT with a C-arm linac, this is usually accomplished using a diode detector array. However, since the dose distribution delivered to most lung patients is small, a diode detector array does not have sufficient resolution to adequately assess the accuracy of the distribution. Therefore, any patient-specific delivery QA should be performed using film. When the CyberKnife cones or Iris collimators are planned to deliver the patient's treatment, patient-specific delivery QA is encouraged but not required. This is because the dose information used for dosimetric calculations in the TPS comes directly from the commissioning measurements, much like the dose information used in other modern TPSs to calculate the dose from a square 10-×-10-cm field from a C-arm linac. A 10-×-10-cm treatment field delivered by a C-arm linac under routine physicist quality control does not require any delivery quality assurance as it would be quite unnecessary and redundant. However, also similar to the C-arm linac situation, if the patient's CyberKnife treatment is collimated by a multi-leaf collimator (MLC), then patient-specific delivery QA is required.

9.4.2 Quality control

Due to the factors that affect patient selection for lung optimized treatments, like tumor size and location, it can be challenging to visually verify the lock-on of the target locating system. Consequently, a quality control (QC) procedure is outlined below that can assist the operator in verifying the software's image recognition results. This QC procedure compares the tumor position during the expiration phase of the patient's respiration and the total respiratory motion of the tumor during treatment with what was estimated during treatment planning:

1. Estimate tumor respiratory excursion during simulation and treatment planning: Acquire one expiration-hold CT scan and one inspiration-hold CT, and use the expiration-hold CT as the planning CT. Fuse the inspiration-hold CT with expiration-hold CT based on a spine match, and have the same clinician contour the tumor volumes on both CT scans. Record the magnitude of the tumor respiratory motion as the relative distance between the centroids of the two tumor volumes.
2. Validation based on expiration of tumor position during treatment setup: After spine alignment, the couch shifts to the tumor region and x-ray images are acquired during patient's expiration phase to lock onto the tumor. If minimal couch corrections are reported from lock-on, this verifies that the lock-on is consistent with what was planned.
3. Validation based on tumor excursion during Synchrony setup: Additional x-ray images are obtained at different respiratory phases. The reported location of the tumor at inspiration is then compared to the location of the tumor at expiration. The difference in location is the magnitude of the tumor respiratory excursion as determined by the target locating system. Alternatively, one can build the Synchrony respiratory model first, and the total respiratory motion can be estimated from the Synchrony model graphs. In either case, if the excursion measured during setup is in the same range and trends the same as the estimated excursion during treatment planning, this is a second validation that the lock-on is consistent with the treatment plan.

Due to the complicated concepts associated with multiple tracking options and their subtle technical details, a physicist should be actively involved in all steps of the LOT procedure: patient evaluation, simulation, planning, and treatment supervision. The physics department should educate the clinical team to understand the concepts involved with LOT treatments and to implement the QC procedure.

References

1. Keall, P.J. et al., The management of respiratory motion in radiation oncology report of AAPM Task Group 76. *Med Phys*, 2006. **33**(10): 3874–900.
2. Sayeh, S. et al., Respiratory motion tracking for robotic radiosurgery, in *Treating Tumors That Move with Respiration*, H.C. Urschel et al., Editors. 2007, Berlin: Springer. pp. 15–29.
3. Muacevic, A. et al., Technical description, phantom accuracy, and clinical feasibility for single-session lung radiosurgery using robotic image-guided real-time respiratory tumor tracking. *Technol Cancer Res Treat*, 2007. **6**(4): 321–8.
4. Wong, K.H. et al., Quantitative measurement of CyberKnife robotic arm steering. *Technol Cancer Res Treat*, 2007. **6**(6): 589–94.
5. Nioutsikou, E. et al., Dosimetric investigation of lung tumor motion compensation with a robotic respiratory tracking system: An experimental study. *Med Phys*, 2008. **35**(4): 1232–40.
6. Hoogeman, M. et al., Clinical accuracy of the respiratory tumor tracking system of the CyberKnife: Assessment by analysis of log files. *Int J Radiat Oncol Biol Phys*, 2009. **74**(1): 297–303.
7. Bhagat, N. et al., Complications associated with the percutaneous insertion of fiducial markers in the thorax. *Cardiovasc Intervent Radiol*, 2010. **33**(6): 1186–91.
8. Kothary, N. et al., Safety and efficacy of percutaneous fiducial marker implantation for image-guided radiation therapy. *J Vasc Interv Radiol*, 2009. **20**(2): 235–9.

9. Guckenberger, M. et al., Cone-beam CT based image-guidance for extracranial stereotactic radiotherapy of intrapulmonary tumors. *Acta Oncol*, 2006. **45**(7): 897–906.
10. Reichner, C.A. et al., The placement of gold fiducials for CyberKnife stereotactic radiosurgery using a modified transbronchial needle aspiration technique. *J Bronchol*, 2005. **12**(4): 193–5.
11. Anantham, D. et al., Electromagnetic navigation bronchoscopy-guided fiducial placement for robotic stereotactic radiosurgery of lung tumors: A feasibility study. *Chest*, 2007. **132**(3): 930–5.
12. Hong, J.C. et al., High retention and safety of percutaneously implanted endovascular embolization coils as fiducial markers for image-guided stereotactic ablative radiotherapy of pulmonary tumors. *Int J Radiat Oncol Biol Phys*, 2011. **81**(1): 85–90.
13. Wu, X., S. Dieterich, and C.G. Orton, Point/counterpoint. Only a single implanted marker is needed for tracking lung cancers for IGRT. *Med Phys*, 2009. **36**(11): 4845–7.
14. Wu, X. et al., Patient alignment and target tracking in radiosurgery of soft-tissue tumors using combined fiducial and skeletal structures tracking techniques, in *Treating Tumors That Move with Respiration*, H.C. Urschel et al., Editors. 2007, Berlin: Springer. pp. 31–6.
15. Hevezi, J.M., A new patient support pad for CyberKnife planning & delivery—A technical note. *Cureus*, 2010. **2**(10): e16.
16. Yang, J. et al. A quality control procedure for using Xsight® lung. CyberKnife® Users' Meeting. 2009, Munich, Germany.
17. Papanikolaou, N. et al., Tissue inhomogeneity corrections for megavoltage photon beams, in *Report of Task Group No. 65 of the Radiation Therapy Committee*. 2004, American Association of Physicists in Medicine, One Physics Ellipse, College Park, MD.
18. Mardirossian, G. et al., Validation of accuray MultiPlan® Monte Carlo treatment plans. CyberKnife® Users' Meeting. 2009, Munich, Germany.
19. van der Voort van Zyp, N.C. et al., Clinical introduction of Monte Carlo treatment planning: A different prescription dose for non-small cell lung cancer according to tumor location and size. *Radiother Oncol*, 2010. **96**(1): 55–60.
20. Dieterich, S. et al., Report of AAPM TG 135: Quality assurance for robotic radiosurgery. *Med Phys*, 2011. **38**(6): 2914–36.
21. Almond, P.R. et al., AAPM's TG-51 protocol for clinical reference dosimetry of high-energy photon and electron beams. *Med Phys*, 1999. **26**(9): 1847–70.
22. Benedict, S.H. et al., Stereotactic body radiation therapy: The report of AAPM Task Group 101. *Med Phys*, 2010. **37**(8): 4078–101.

10

Proton therapy

CLEMENS GRASSBERGER, GREGORY C. SHARP, AND HARALD PAGANETTI

10.1 INTRODUCTION

10.1.1 Rationale for proton therapy

10.1.1.1 INTRODUCTION TO PROTON THERAPY PHYSICS

The interest in proton therapy originates from the physical properties of proton beams resulting in dose distributions that are generally advantageous to the ones achievable in photon therapy. The expectation is that this leads to potentially fewer side effects and/or the potential for tumor dose escalation.

After a short build-up, photon depth-dose curves show an exponentially decreasing energy deposition with increasing depth in tissue and exit radiation after penetrating the patient. In contrast, protons slowing down in tissue eventually stop. The combination of more and more protons stopping and the fact that the energy transferred to tissue increases with decreasing proton energy leads to the Bragg peak at a well-defined depth in tissue. This maximum dose peak can be positioned within the target for each beam direction by adjusting the beam energy. Another advantage is that, due to the lack of exit dose, one can point a dose towards a critical structure. These advantages are correlated with the depth-dose curve. In contrast, protons offer little advantage in lateral beam penumbra, particularly at large depths.

The idea for using proton beams to treat cancer dates to the 1940s [1]. Initially, proton therapy was restricted to physics research laboratories, but since the 1990s it became more and more established in hospital environments. Proton therapy is still offered only at a few centers due to high cost and challenging technology, but this is gradually changing. The technology is now becoming widely available with currently 17 centers in operation in the United States alone.

Proton therapy reduces the "integral dose" (total energy deposited in the patient) by about a factor of 2–3 compared to photon techniques [2]. This is independent of the photon or proton delivery technique (Figure 10.1 [3]). There is a true reduction in integral dose, other than in intensity-modulated photon therapy (IMRT) versus 3D conformal photon therapy, where the integral dose stays largely the same but the dose distribution can be shaped more favorably when using IMRT as it allows to redistribute dose within the irradiated area. Thus, from a purely dosimetric standpoint, proton therapy offers an advantage for all radiation therapy patients. There is clearly more sparing of normal structures with protons (Figure 10.2 [4]). Dosimetric advantages may, however, not necessarily translate into significant clinical gain.

Proton therapy, when using intensity-modulated proton therapy (IMPT), not only has an advantage in integral dose but also in shaping the dose distribution. This is because the energy of the proton beam entering the treatment room or the rotational gantry can be adjusted to place the Bragg peak at a prescribed depth in the patient, adding an additional degree of freedom in treatment planning compared to photon techniques. As this will be discussed below, range uncertainties require proton therapy specific margins but even with current range uncertainty margins, the high dose volume with protons is always smaller compared to photon treatments.

A consequence of the reduced integral dose and end of range when using protons is that proton therapy typically administers fewer beams compared to photon-based treatment plans. Photon treatments require

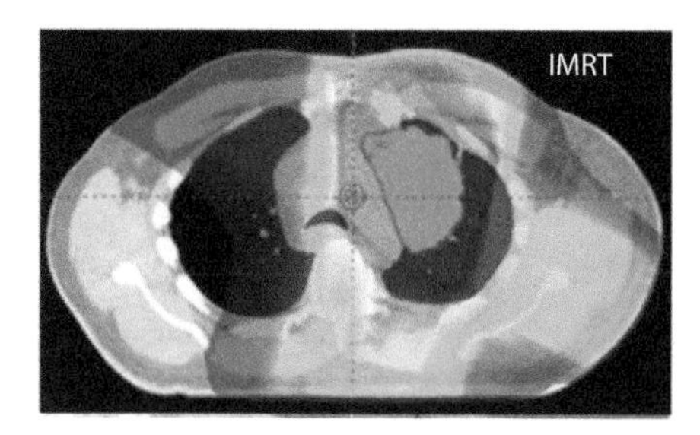

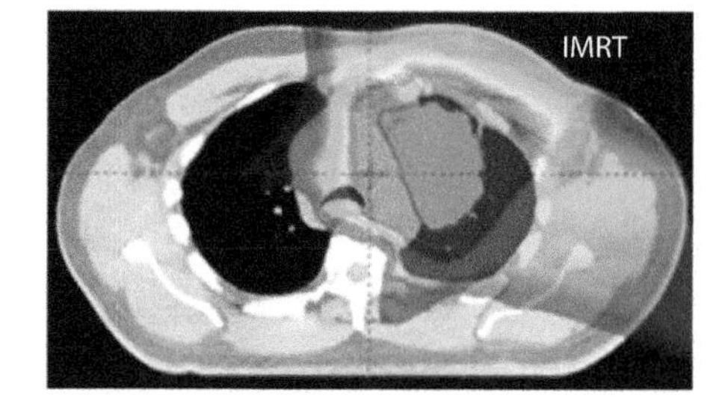

Figure 10.1 Illustration of the reduced integral dose when using proton (right) compared to photon (left) treatments. Note the slightly higher dose conformity with photons due to range uncertainty margins in proton therapy. (From Chang, J.Y. et al., *Int J Radiat Oncol Biol Phys.*, 90, 809–818, 2014. With permission.)

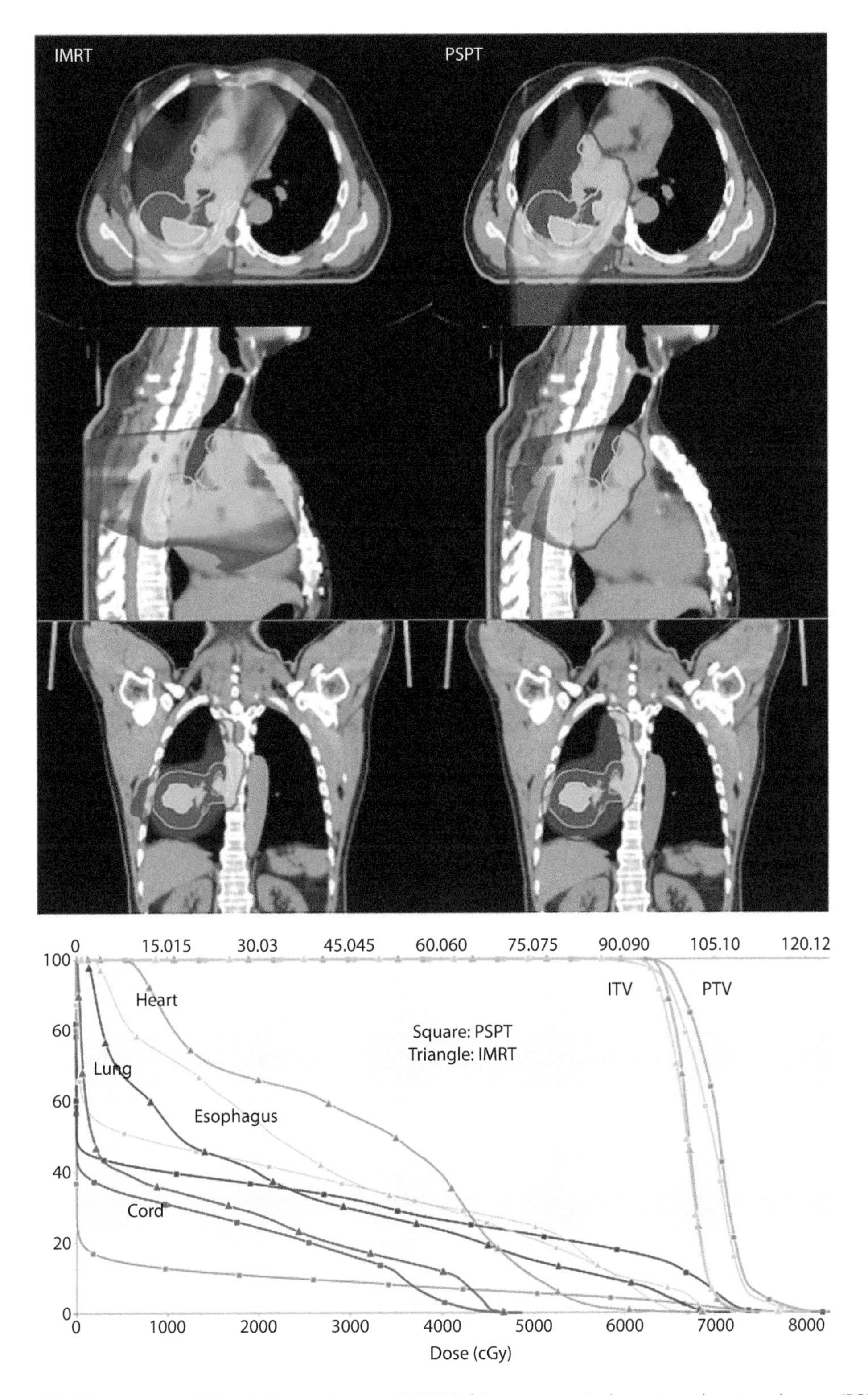

Figure 10.2 Intensity-modulated photon therapy (IMRT, left) versus passively scattered proton therapy (PSPT, right) for an NSCLC patient illustrating the dosimetric advantage of a proton therapy plan. (From Wink, K.C. et al., *Front Oncol.*, 4, 1–15, 2014. With permission.)

many beam angles to achieve a homogeneous dose plateau in the target. Using protons, a single field can achieve a homogeneous target dose by modulating individual Bragg-peaks into a spread-out Bragg peak (SOBP). An SOBP is a combination of various pristine, mono-energetic, peaks. Nevertheless, multiple beam angles are also used in proton therapy to further optimize the dose distribution and lower the dose to the skin, as protons offer generally less skin sparing than high-energy photons.

An accelerated proton beam is relatively small with a width of typically a few mm (sigma of a Gaussian distribution). Scattering systems have been used since the beginning of proton therapy to broaden this beam so that it can cover the shape of the target in the beam's eye view [5]. This delivery technology has several shortcomings. First, the materials in the beam path used for scattering and thus broadening the beam produce secondary radiation such as neutrons. Furthermore, the energy and thus range of the beam is constant across the field so that a patient specific compensator is needed to modulate the range across the field, and the nominal circular shaped beam is larger in area than the target so that a patient specific aperture is needed. Lastly, depth modulation is only feasible to conform the dose distribution to the distal end of the target, not the proximal end.

A different method is currently introduced at most proton centers, i.e. beam scanning [6]. The idea to use scanned beam delivery has been around for decades but only now are we confident to be able to deliver scanned beams with the required accuracy and safety. In scanned beam delivery, individual beam spots of small size (a few mm in sigma width) can be steered magnetically to place the Bragg peak at a designated position in the patient. When using scanned beams, the dose can be conformed to both proximal and distal edges without the use of patient-specific hardware such as apertures and compensators. Furthermore, scatterers can typically be avoided (although pre-absorbers may be needed for shallow tumors or because of limitations in minimum energy for some delivery systems). Most importantly, when using scanned beams IMPT can be delivered which allows more flexibility in avoiding critical structures [7,8]. In IMPT the pencil spot map is optimized in treatment planning leading to inhomogeneous dose distributions per field comparable to IMRT. Note that in IMRT only the fluence is modulated whereas in IMPT fluence as well as beam energy can be varied, offering more flexibility. Thus, proton therapy shows distinct advantages particularly for geometrically challenging geometries due to superior ability to shape the dose distribution. Figure 10.3 [9] illustrates the difference between passive scattering beam delivery, scanned beam delivery, and scanned beam delivery using IMPT.

The discussion about the pros and cons of proton therapy are not about the physics of protons, which clearly show an advantage to photon therapy, but whether this advantage in physics matters in terms of clinical outcome.

10.1.1.2 INTRODUCTION TO THE RESULTING CLINICAL BENEFITS

Roughly 45%–50% of all cancer patients receive radiation therapy at some point during their treatment. From a local control perspective, radiation therapy is very effective but normal tissues are inevitably irradiated resulting in toxicity and a reduction of the quality of life [10,11]. The appearance and severity of side effects are influenced by many factors, of which many are patient specific, such as radiosensitivity, and potentially determined by genetic markers.

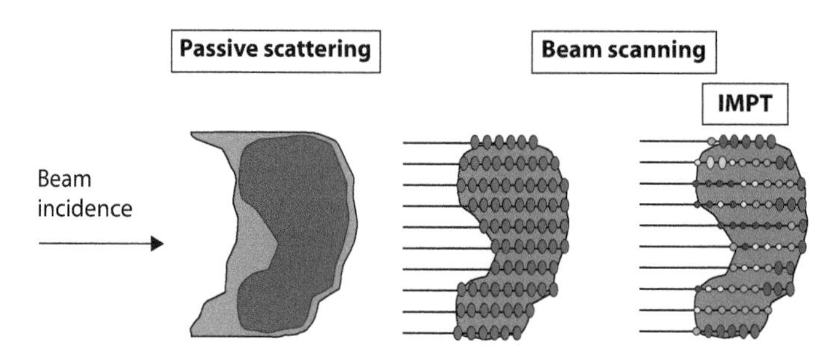

Figure 10.3 Illustration of the advantage of beam scanning and intensity-modulated proton therapy (IMPT) compared with passive delivery (Adapted from Paganetti, H. and H. Kooy, *Expert Rev Med Devices*, 7, 275–85, 2010. With permission.)

The likelihood of toxicities does depend on dose and on the irradiated volume [12–14]. Dose distributions are typically analyzed using dose-volume histograms (DVH) and parameters extracted from them. Biophysical models based on parameters deduced from clinical studies can be used to predict clinical outcome in lung [15]. Typically, single parameters are extracted from DVHs such as V20 and mean lung dose, which are related to radiation pneumonitis for thoracic tumors [14]. In photon therapy, strong correlations have also been found between V20 and the mean lung dose ($r > 0.94$) [16].

While many outcome predictions are being made based on mean doses to critical structures, not only in lung cancer, caution should be used. Regional differences of lung tissue response to radiation were reported in experiments with rodents [17–21]. It has also been demonstrated that radiation-induced effects in the lung are not limited to the irradiated lung area [19,20,22]. Regional differences are seen in patients as well. For instance, dose to the lower parts of the lung is more predictive of radiation pneumonitis than dose to the upper parts [23–25]. It is also known that lung function is affected by dose to the heart from experiments in rodents [19,21,26]. Clinically, this has been confirmed in patients as well [27].

These and other factors make it difficult to assess the potential clinical benefit due to a reduction in lung dose when using protons. In other words, the clear advantage in integral dose may not result in an advantage in outcome, depending on the distribution of dose. This is the main motivation for clinical trials comparing proton with photon treatments. In 2012, the Emerging Technology Committee of the American Society for Radiation Oncology (ASTRO) concluded, "Current data do not provide sufficient evidence to recommend proton beam therapy outside of clinical trials in lung cancer" [28]).

10.1.1.3 RATIONALE FOR PROTON THERAPY FOR LUNGS

For non-small cell lung cancer (NSCLC), treatment dose and efficacy are limited by the risk of severe toxicities [29–31]. Proton therapy, with its reduced integral doses and advanced dose shaping capabilities, offers the potential for escalating doses to the target without increasing doses to the lung or heart [32,33]. Typically, fewer fields are needed to deliver a conformal dose distribution when using protons as compared to photons. In fact, typically only two to three fields are being used in proton therapy for lung cancer treatments (Figures 10.1 and 10.2). The reduced irradiated volume has a large effect on expected toxicities, i.e. proton therapy patients are expected to show a lower risk for radiation-induced lung injuries [34,35].

Various studies have compared proton and photon therapy for early-stage lung cancer and have demonstrated a clear dosimetric advantage of protons [36–42]. Advantages were shown particularly for larger and/or centrally located tumors. Chang et al. [32] have published results from a comparative treatment planning study with 25 patients comparing 3D-conformal photon therapy, IMRT, and proton therapy. The radiation dose to the lungs, the spinal cord, the heart, and the esophagus was reduced when using protons because of the overall lower integral dose. This should offer the potential for dose escalation. Interestingly, the RTOG lung trial 0617 using dose escalation did surprisingly not show an advantage as 74 Gy given in 2-Gy fractions was not better than 60 Gy, when both were administered with concurrent chemotherapy for patients with stage III NSCLC [43].

Photon techniques such as stereotactic ablative body radiation (SABR) have been successfully used but large or centrally located lung tumors are often difficult to treat due to risk of toxicities [44]. While there is the potential for hypofractionation also when using photons, the reduced dose bath with proton therapy offers even greater potential in this regard because of the reduced normal tissue dose [45]. Dose escalation potential when using protons has been shown to be on the order of 30%–40% [46]. When evaluating fractionation regimens, we must be aware of the difference in dose distribution between photon and proton treatments [47].

Proton therapy for lung has been used extensively in many centers and various reviews have been published [48–51]. Clinical results on proton therapy for lung cancer are summarized in the next section.

10.2 CLINICAL RESULTS

There are a growing number of published clinical results available for proton therapy in the treatment of lung cancer of various stages. We have divided the available literature in the early-stage and locally advanced diseases, and grouped the studies by location to exhibit the evolution of therapy with clinical experience in specific centers. This also eases identification of possibly overlapping study populations in some reports from the same institution. The few publications that contained a wide array of clinical stages were reported in the section (early stage vs locally advanced) in which most patients fell.

Only standard abbreviations were used below, overall survival (OS), disease-free survival (DFS), local control (LC), disease-specific survival (DSS), radiation pneumonitis (RP), and fractionation schemes are denoted as XXGy(RBE)/YYfx, i.e. XXGy(RBE) total dose given in YY daily fractions five times per week, if not denoted otherwise. Unless otherwise indicated, all patients in the studies reported below were treated with passively scattered proton therapy.

10.2.1 Early-Stage NSCLC

Bush and colleagues published a series of outcome and toxicity results for a cohort of patients treated at Loma Linda University Medical Center starting in the 1990s [36,41,52–54]. In their earliest studies [52–54] they compared photon-proton combination treatments (45Gy(RBE) photons to mediastinum + 28.8Gy (RBE) proton boost to the gross tumor volume (GTV)) for patients with good cardiopulmonary function to proton-only treatments to 51Gy(RBE) in 10 fractions. The 2-year disease-free survival for early-stage patients was 86% and compared favorably with other reports at the time [53]. Furthermore, the reported pulmonary toxicities in the proton-only group were lower than in the combined treatment group [52,54].

Based on this experience, a phase II trial was designed in which the dose was first escalated from 51 to 60, and subsequently to 70Gy(RBE) delivered in 10 fractions [36,41]. In the final analysis of 111 patients, 64 of them T2 and 22 with gross disease > 5 cm, they observed increased OS with dose level, i.e. 18%, 32%, and 51% at 4 years with 51, 60 and 70Gy(RBE), respectively. The tumor location, i.e. central versus peripheral, did not correlate with outcome. No case of significant radiation pneumonitis necessitating steroid therapy was observed in that series and pulmonary function was well maintained 1 year after treatment.

Chang et al. at the M.D. Anderson Cancer Center conducted a phase I/II study containing 18 patients with larger peripheral (T2–T3) or central (T1) tumors to a total dose of 87.5Gy(RBE) in fractions of 2.5Gy(RBE) [55]. Follow-up was short (16.3 months median) which impacts the interpretation of the results. The LC was reported to be 89%, DFS and OS 53% and 93% at 1 year, and 46% and 55% at 2 years. No grade 4/5 toxicity was reported. The most common toxicities included dermatitis (67% grade 2; 17% grade 3), followed by grade 2 fatigue (44%), grade 2 pneumonitis (11%), and grade 2 esophagitis (6%). Due to the long treatment time of 7 weeks, all patients had an additional four-dimensional computer tomography (4D-CT) during week 3 or 4 and the treatment plans were adapted if necessary (which was the case in 45% of patients).

Westover et al. analyzed a series of 15 stage I NSCLC patients treated at Massachusetts General Hospital with 42–50Gy(RBE) in 3–5 fractions [42]. Patients were selected based on comorbidities, e.g. severe chronic obstructive pulmonary disease (COPD) or interstitial lung disease (n = 8), multiple primaries and/or prior RT (n = 7). After a median follow-up of over 2 years, LC and OS were 100% and 64%, respectively. Toxicities included grade 2 fatigue and dermatitis (n = 1 each), rib fracture (n = 3) and one case of grade 3 RP in one of the patients with severe COPD.

The experience at the proton center at the University of Tsukuba is outlined in a series of papers describing proton treatments of lung patients going back to 1983 [37,56–58]. The earliest study [57] reports on the outcome of 51 NSCLC patients (37 stage I–II, 9 stage III–IV, 5 recurrent) treated with a median fraction size of 3Gy(RBE) (range 2–6) to a median total dose of 76Gy(RBE) (range 49–93). The 5y-OS was 29% for all patients, 70% for stage Ia and 16% for stage Ib. Note that most of these patients were treated in the pre-PET era, i.e. the true stage distribution was most probably skewed towards higher stages. Treatment was well tolerated, though, with no grade 4+, one grade 3, and three grade 2 acute lung toxicities and no significant late toxicities.

Based on this initial experience they started studying hypo fractionation, first with 50Gy(RBE)/10fx, then 60Gy(RBE)/10fx [37], and finally with a protocol prescribing 72.6Gy(RBE)/22fx to centrally located tumors and 66Gy(RBE)/10–12fx to peripherally located ones [56,58]. The latest published study from Tsukuba reports outcomes for 74 stage I NSCLC patients with a 3-year OS of 77% for all patients, and 3-year LC of 86% for stage Ia and 67% for stage Ib. The dose level turned out to be a significant predictor for recurrence, 3y-LC was 64%/88% for centrally versus peripherally located tumors, respectively. Toxicities included three grade 2 (dermatitis/esophagitis), two grade 3 (RP, skin ulcer), and 11 rib fractures (14%).

Nihei et al. [59] published a study analyzing 37 patients treated in Chiba to four different dose levels, 70/80/88/94Gy(RBE) in 3.5–4.5Gy(RBE)/fx, with most patients treated to 80 or 88Gy(RBE). The 2-year local progression-free survival (PFS) and OS were 80% and 84%, respectively, with a 2y-DFS of 58%. Acute toxicity was minor, with only three grade 1 cases. Late pulmonary toxicities however were common, three grade 2 and three grade 3 cases, i.e. 16% of patients experienced late-toxicity grade ≥2. This could be related to the high total dose delivered, but also to tumor shrinkage during the 4–5 weeks of treatment (longer than most other schedules) and the resulting higher normal tissue dose.

The experience at the proton therapy center in Tohoku (Japan) is published in two recent reports, one describing only their protocol for peripheral tumors treated to 66Gy(RBE) in 10 fractions [60], while the other also includes central tumors treated to 80Gy(RBE) in 25 fractions [61]. They report excellent outcomes for the 50 patients treated on the peripheral protocol, with 3-year OS, LC, and PFS standing at 88%, 96%, and 76%, respectively, though median follow-up was only 23 months. Only one patient experienced grade 2 RP on this protocol. The protocol treating central tumors to 80Gy(RBE) in 25 fractions led to similarly good outcomes, albeit with elevated toxicity. Of the 32 patients treated with 66Gy(RBE) and 24 patients treated with 80Gy(RBE), 9% and 33% experienced grade 2+ dermatitis, 9% and 29% grade 2+ rib fractures, and 16% and 21% grade 2+ RP, respectively. No grade 4/5 toxicity was reported in either of the studies [60,61].

Iwata, Fujii and co-workers published three articles describing the outcomes of patients treated at the Hyogo Ion Beam Facility with protons and carbon ions from 2003 to 2009. The results discussed here refer to the proton population only [62–64]. Initially, the treatment schedule was 80Gy(RBE) in 20 fractions for the first 20 patients, with further shortening of the treatment regimen to 60Gy(RBE)/10fx after evaluation of acute and medium-term toxicity [64]. After 57 patients and a median follow-up of 3 years, their 3-y OS/LC was 90/61% and 83/81% for the 80/60Gy(RBE) arms, respectively, with no significant difference between the groups.

In a subsequent report, Iwata et al. focus on T2a-bN0M0 tumors, i.e. a challenging patient cohort for SBRT [63]. They added two additional fractionations regimens, one longer (70.2/26fx) and one more hypofractionated (52.8/4fx). The results highlight the minimal toxicity that conformal techniques such as proton therapy can achieve, even for patients with large (T2b, >5 cm) and centrally located tumors. Though limited by a relatively small number of patients (n = 43), they note no significant difference between outcome for T2a and T2b patients.

In the report by Fujii et al. [62] covering a similar treatment period, only the smaller T2a tumors (<5 cm) are included together with T1 patients. They showed excellent outcomes for the 70 patients analyzed, i.e. a 3y-OS of 72% and LC of 81%. It should be noted that the outcome is very similar to the T2 tumor study described above, which reports a 3-year OS and LC of 74% and 78%, respectively. Note that this is the case even though the former consists mostly of T1 patients, while the other contains only T2 tumors, suggesting that outcomes for these 2 groups are similar.

The studies listed above represent a wide spectrum of patient characteristics in terms of geographical locations as well as in time. Certain aspects should be considered in their interpretation. The oldest studies reach back to the 1980s, before PET was used routinely for staging of lung cancer, and their results are hard to compare to modern studies, as a significant number of those patients might have been restaged if PET were available. Similarly, the stage distributions listed in Table 10.1 reflect the staging system in use at that time. For example, pre-2010 studies classified large tumors (>7 cm) as T2, which would be T3 in the current TNM-classification [65]. Reflecting a difference in the practice of treating lung cancer, Japanese studies can contain a significant amount of medically operable patients that refused surgery, while their American counterparts often include only medically inoperable patients [36,55,62,64].

Generally, it seems that over the last three decades a similar evolution has occurred in several centers. First, doses have been intensified keeping the fractions size at 2–3Gy(RBE), then with the advent of hypo fractionation more centers have started shortening the treatment to <10 fractions. Experience from different centers now show that protons can treat central tumors up to doses of 70Gy(RBE) in 10 fractions, and produce outcomes like those for peripheral lesions if normal tissue constraints are respected.

Toxicities are generally manageable. Although grade 4/5 toxicities are very rare, they tend to increase with increasing fraction size. Several of the studies above reported clinically significant dermatitis and frequent rib fractures. The risk for both can be minimized by using multiple beam ports, which some authors recommend

Table 10.1 Published studies reporting results for early-stage patients

Treatment center	Authors	Timeframe	# of patients	Stage distribution	Fractionation scheme
Loma Linda Cancer Center	Bush et al. [53,54] Bonnet et al. [52]	1994–1998	37	27 I, 2 II, 8 IIIA	Proton boost or 51Gy(RBE)/10fx
	Bush et al. [36]	1995–2002	68	29 T1, 39 T2	51Gy(RBE)/10fx; 60Gy(RBE)/10fx
	Bush et al. [41]	1999–2010	111	47 T1, 64 T2	51Gy(RBE)/10fx; 60Gy(RBE)/10fx; 70Gy(RBE)/10fx
M.D. Anderson	Chang et al. [55,66]	2006–2009	18	4 T1, 13 T2, 1 T3	87.5Gy(RBE)/35fx
Massachusetts General Hospital	Westover et al. [42]	2008–2010	15 (20 tumors)	16 IA, 2 IB, 2 IIA	42–50Gy(RBE)/3–5fx
University of Tsukuba	Shioyama et al. [57]	1983–2000	51	28 I, 9 II, 8 III, 1 IV	49–93Gy(RBE)/8–46fx
	Hata et al. [37]	2002–2005	21	11 IAa, 10 IB	50–60Gy(RBE)/10fx
	Kanemoto et al. [56]	1997–2011	74 (80 tumors)	59 IA, 21 IB	66Gy(RBE)/10–12fx peripheral; 72.6/22fx central
Chiba	Nihei et al. [59]	1999–2003	37	17 IA, 20 IB	70–94Gy(RBE)/20fx
Southern Tohoku Proton Beam Therapy Center	Makita et al. [61]	2009–2012	56	24 IA, 19 IB, 13 IIA	66Gy(RBE)/10fx peripheral; 80Gy(RBE)/25fx central
	Hatayama et al. [60]	2009–2014	50 (52 tumors)	44 IA, 8 IB, peripheral only	66Gy(RBE)/10fx
Hyogo Ion Beam Medical Center	Iwata et al. [64]	2003–2007	57	27 IA, 30 IB	80Gy(RBE)/20fx, 60Gy(RBE)/10fx
	Iwata et al. [63]	2003–2009	43	30 T2a, 13 T2b	52.8Gy(RBE)/4x 60–66/10fx 70.2Gy(RBE)/26fx 80Gy(RBE)/20fx
	Fujii et al. [62]	2003–2009	70	8 T1a, 28 T1b, 34 T2a	52.8Gy(RBE)/4x 60–66/10fx 70.2Gy(RBE)/26fx 80Gy(RBE)/20fx

Note: Outcome and toxicity are not included because of variable stage distribution, inclusion/exclusion criteria. Care should be taken in the interpretation of the stage distribution of older studies, which were partly staged without PET, and many of them classified per older AJCC TNM classification (pre-2010).

especially for large fraction sizes and tumors located close to the chest wall. IMPT, which allows shaping of the proximal edge, enables better sparing of the chest wall and could lead to lower rate of rib fractures.

10.2.2 Locally advanced lung cancer

The group from the M.D. Anderson Cancer Center has published their extensive experience treating locally advanced NSCLC with protons in a series of publications [66–70]. In their earliest article [67] they report the toxicity in a cohort of 66 patients treated to a median total dose of 74Gy(RBE) in 2Gy(RBE) fractions. Grade 3+ pneumonitis and esophagitis was lower (2% and 5%, respectively) than in a retrospective comparison with photon patients (30% and 18% in 3D-conformal photons, 9% and 44% in IMRT). This has led to design of a phase III trial (NCT00495040), whose results will be discussed below.

Chang et al. [66] report the results of a prospective phase II study involving 44 stage III NSCLC patients treated to 74Gy(RBE) in 37 fractions. An interesting detail about the study is that patients underwent additional 4DCT imaging after 3 weeks of treatment to assess the need for treatment adaptation, which was performed in 9 (20%) of the patients [71]. Median OS was 29.4 months while 1y-OS and 1y-PFS were 86% and 63%, respectively. None of the patients experienced grade 4 or 5 proton-related adverse events.

The latest report [68] describes excellent long-term (median follow-up 4.7y) outcomes for 134 stage II–III patients (population not overlapping with the previous study). Most patients were treated to 75Gy(RBE) in 37 fractions. Five-year DFS rates were 17.3% and 18% for stages II and III, respectively. The toxicity was reported to be tolerable with one grade 4 esophagitis and 16 grade 3 events (8 dermatitis, 6 esophagitis, 2 pneumonitis). In all three series from the M.D. Anderson group reporting on concurrent chemo-radiation, the concurrent chemotherapy regimen is very homogeneous for all patients, i.e. consisting of weekly paclitaxel 50 mg/m2 and carboplatin AUC 2 (see Table 10.2). Induction and adjuvant regimen were allowed in addition, though timing, dosage and type were at the discretion of the treating physician.

Gomez et al. reported the result of a phase I intermediate hypofractionation study in 25 patients treated to 45–60 Gy (RBE) in 15 fractions without concurrent chemotherapy [69]. Their findings are preliminary (13 months median follow-up) and focus on toxicity: only 2 patients experienced severe grade 3+ dose-limiting events possibly related to radiation therapy.

McAvoy et al. has published the results from a cohort of 102 patients re-irradiated to a median dose of 60.5Gy(RBE) in 2Gy(RBE) fractions [70]. The median time from initial radiation therapy to re-irradiation was 17 months and concurrent chemotherapy as well as higher dose was associated with improved OS. However, the achieved 1-year loco-regional control and median OS were poor, 49.2% and 14.7 months, respectively, and severe esophageal and pulmonary toxicity related to concurrent chemotherapy and dose were evident. However, it was noted that re-irradiation with definitive intent is feasible with proton therapy as 97% of the patients completed the planned course of irradiation. The local control did impact survival as patients experiencing local failure frequently died of the resulting complications.

A technical study published by the M.D. Anderson group reported on the implementation of IMPT for 34 thoracic cancer patients treated to 45–78Gy(RBE) (median 66Gy(RBE)), focusing on the dosimetric results and robustness towards uncertainties [3]. They concluded that their approach was safe for the treatment of thoracic malignancies with motion amplitudes up to 5 mm.

The latest study from M.D. Anderson is a Bayesian randomized trial [72] comparing passively scattered proton therapy to IMRT, which was presented at the 2016 American Society of Clinical Oncology (ASCO) Meeting. The trial, which enrolled 255 patients, 149 randomized, was not able to show a statistically significant difference in incidence of local recurrence or grade 3+ radiation pneumonitis. This could have several reasons, among them the fact that patients were only randomized if both plans satisfied constraints, that proton therapy patients had larger tumors, or that high dose regions were generally larger in the proton therapy group.

Hoppe et al. published a series reporting the early results (median follow-up 16 months) for 19 locally advanced NSCLC patients treated in Florida to a dose range of 62–80Gy(RBE) in 2Gy(RBE)/fraction [73]. Acute grade 3+ toxicity occurred in 5 patients, late toxicity grade 3+ in 3 patients, where one patient exhibiting poor performance status developed grade 4 esophagitis and fatigue during treatment.

Colaco et al. report the only published series on SCLC treated with protons [74]. Even though follow-up in this study was also limited (median 12 months) and patient numbers are low (n = 6), they report robust 1y-OS of 83% and 1y-PFS of 63% using 60–66Gy(RBE) in 30–34 fractions. No cases of 3+ esophagitis, 2+ pneumonitis and no other 3+ hematological toxicities arose in these patients.

Two cohorts of patients have been treated at the University of Tsukuba, i.e. one cohort of 57 patients without concurrent chemotherapy and fraction sizes from 2–6.6Gy(RBE) to total doses of 50–84.5Gy(RBE) [79] and one cohort of 15 patients with concurrent chemotherapy and conventional fractionation [80]. In the first study, 3 patients were unable to complete treatment due to comorbidities. Furthermore, the target volume had

Table 10.2 Overview of clinical studies on locally advanced lung disease

Treatment center	Authors	Timeframe	# of patients	Stage distribution	Fractionation scheme	Chemotherapy
M.D. Anderson Cancer Center	Sejpal et al. [67]	2006–2008	62	2 IB, 5 IIB, 25 IIIA, 17 IIIB, 5 IV, 8 recurrent	Median total dose 74Gy(RBE), 2 Gy(RBE)/fraction	All patients had concurrent weekly paclitaxel 50 mg/m2, carboplatin AUC 2 mg/ml/min; induction/ adjuvant also allowed; type, dosing, timing at discretion of treating physician
	Chang et al. [55,66]	2006–2009	44	21 IIIA, 23 IIIB	74Gy (RBE)/37fx	
	Nguyen et al. [68]	2006–2010	134	6 IIA 15 IIB 70 IIIA 43 IIIB	74Gy (RBE)/37fx 57% of patients received 74Gy(RBE)	
	Gomez et al. [69]	2010–2012	25	-	45Gy(RBE)/15fx 52.5Gy(RBE)/15fx 60Gy(RBE)/15fx	Not allowed
	McAvoy et al. [70]	2006–2013	102 (99 completed)	20 IA, 9 IB, 11 IIA, 5 IIB, 31 IIIA, 14 IIIB, 9 IV	Median dose 60.5 EQD2 Gy(RBE) [25.2–155], median 30 fractions [10–58]	~30% of patients had concurrent chemotherapy
	Chang et al. [3]	2011–2013	34	1 I, 1 II, 17 III, 1 IV, rest not primary lung cancer	Median total dose 66Gy(RBE) [45–78]	–
	Liao et al. [72]	–	57 protons 92 IMRT	–	74Gy (RBE)/37fx	Concurrent weekly paclitaxel 50 mg/m2, carboplatin AUC 2 mg/ml/min
University of Florida Proton Therapy Institute	Hoppe et al. [73]	2008–2010	19	1 IIB 15 IIIA 3 IIIB	Median total dose 74Gy(RBE) (range 62–80), 2Gy(RBE)/ fraction	Concurrent for all patients, induction in 7, variety of regimen

(Continued)

Table 10.2 (Continued) Overview of clinical studies on locally advanced lung disease

Treatment center	Authors	Timeframe	# of patients	Stage distribution	Fractionation scheme	Chemotherapy
University of Florida Proton Therapy Institute	Colaco et al. [74]	2009–2012	6	LS-SCLC	60–66Gy(RBE)/30–34fx 45Gy (RBE)/30fx twice daily (n = 1)	Concurrent (n = 5) and induction (n = 1) cisplatin and etoposide
University of Pennsylvania	Remick et al. [75]	2011–2014	17	4 IA-IIB, 13 IIIA or higher	Median total dose 54Gy (RBE) [50–67Gy(RBE)]	2 neoadjuvant, 11 adjuvants, 4 concurrent
	Remick et al. [76]	2011–2014	27 protons 34 IMRT	–	50.4/54.0Gy(RBE) median dose for protons/IMRT	–
Proton Collaborative Group	Badiyan et al. [77]	2010–2015	96	22% II 54% IIIA 24% IIIB	Median total dose 70Gy(RBE) [48–75], in 35fx	80% received chemotherapy, 70% concurrently
University of Tsukuba	Nakayama et al. [78]	2001–2008	35	5 II, 12 IIIA, 18 IIIB	Median total dose 78Gy(RBE) [67–91], most commonly 77Gy(RBE)/35fx	No concurrent chemotherapy
	Oshiro et al. [79]	2001–2010	57 (51 completed)	24 IIIA, 33 IIIB	Median total dose 74Gy(RBE) [50–84.5], fraction size 2.0–6.6Gy (RBE)	
	Oshiro et al. [80]	2010–2013	15	4 IIIA, 11 IIIB	66Gy (RBE)/33fx to CTV 74Gy(RBE)/37fx to primary tumor	Monthly concurrent cisplatin (80 mg/m2 day1) and vinolrebine (20 mg/m2 day1+8), two courses administered during RT
Southern Tohoku Proton Beam Therapy Center	Hatayama et al. [60]	2009–2013	27	14 IIIA 13 IIIB	Median dose 77Gy(RBE), 60.6–86.4Gy(RBE)/25–37fx 2–3.2 Gy(RBE)/fx	11 patients received chemotherapy, various agents

Note: Outcome and toxicity are not included because of variable stage distribution, inclusion/exclusion criteria.

to be adapted in 44 (78%) of the patients due to tumor shrinkage (in one case even three times). Even though most patients in this study were not suitable for chemotherapy or failed chemotherapy already, treatment was relatively well tolerated, with grade 3 lung toxicity in 6 patients and no grade 3+ esophagitis or cardiac toxicity. Outcome compares well given this challenging patient cohort, i.e. a median OS of 21 months and 2-year OS, PFS, and LC of 39%, 25%, and 64%, respectively. The second study [80] reports the outcome of 15 patients treated to 74Gy(RBE) in 37 fractions with concurrent monthly cisplatin and vinolrebine. The reported mean survival of 26.7 months is comparable to other reports, but a high rate of myelosuppression was observed and nearly half the patients were not able to complete chemotherapy.

Remick et al. recently presented their preliminary findings from proton beam therapy used in 17 patients as post-operative radiotherapy (PORT) [75], and also published a larger cohort with proton and IMRT patients [76]. PORT is routinely applied in NSCLC in the setting of mediastinal N2 disease and positive margins after surgical resection. There is an intense discussion about the risk/benefit ratio of the procedure. Proton therapy may be able to offer a benefit in this challenging scenario, where the therapeutic window is particularly narrow. The results of proton-based PORT to a median dose of 50.4 Gy(RBE) indicate similar short-term outcome and toxicity compared to IMRT to 54Gy(RBE), though longer follow-up might be able to reveal differences in outcome [76].

Badiyan et al. [77] reported preliminary results from the Proton Collaborative Group, including 96 patients from four centers. The patient population mainly consisted of high-risk cases with poor pulmonary function and other comorbidities that were not eligible for RTOG1308 (see clinical trial section below). With estimated median, 1- and 2-year OS of 13.2 months, 53.4%, and 39.4%, and 6% acute grade 3/4 toxicities, the results show that proton therapy can offer an effective therapy option with limited toxicity in this challenging patient population.

Lately, the results of RTOG0617 have shown lower survival in a high dose (74Gy(RBE)) group relative to a low dose (60Gy(RBE)) group, revealing the limits of dose escalation with photons [43]. However, there is evidence that higher radiation doses could still improve local control and survival, although this is still subject to debate [81]. The outcomes described above indicated that proton therapy may be one way to safely escalate dose and produce excellent results, with 3-year OS >40%, and manageable side effects with grade 3 toxicities around 10% and a very low incidence of grade 4 toxicities.

10.2.3 Comparison to photons

There are numerous publications showing planning comparisons between photon and proton therapy [32,82]. However, clinical comparisons are rare and few clinical trials have been conducted. On one hand, this is because up until recently, only few centers have had the experience and capabilities to treat lung cancer with protons. On the other hand, some insurance providers are reluctant to cover proton therapy for lung malignancies.

Grutters et al. have performed a meta-analysis of observational studies from different centers [83]. Furthermore, the studies by Bush et al. [52–54] compared proton-only to proton-photon treatments, although including only very few patients.

An extensive clinical comparison is an effort by Sejpal et al. [67], who analyzed a total of 202 patients receiving concurrent chemo-radiation with proton therapy, conventional RT or IMRT. They concluded that even though the median total dose delivered with proton therapy was more than 10Gy (RBE) higher, grade 3+ RP and esophagitis were significantly lower in the proton group (2% and 5%, respectively). This has driven the design of a randomized trial comparing IMRT to proton therapy (NCT00915005), which was presented at the ASCO 2016 meeting [72], though could not determine a statistically significant difference between passively scatted protons and IMRT for induction of RP and local recurrence.

The largest retrospective study to date has been conducted by Higgins et al. [84], who queried the National Cancer Database for all NSCLC patients treated from 2004–2012. A total of 243,474 photon patients and 348 proton patients were included into the outcome analysis, demonstrating significantly better survival for proton therapy patients. A propensity-matched analysis indicated 22% OS at 5 years for protons compared to 16% for the photon cohort.

These studies highlight the difficulties in investigating eventual outcome differences between protons and photons owing to trial design, patient selection, and the rapidly developing treatment technology.

10.2.4 Ongoing clinical trials

There are a plethora of clinical trials underway to define the emerging role of proton therapy in thoracic malignancies. In the United States alone, there are 17 studies active. This section does not give a comprehensive overview over all currently active studies, but rather highlights the significant trials grouped by thematic area:

1. *The role of protons versus photons:* RTOG 1308 (NCT01993810) is a multi-center randomized phase III study for stage II–IIIB NSCLC, delivering 70Gy(RBE)/35fx with photons or protons. NCT01629498 is a non-randomized phase I/II trial of image-guided, IMRT or IMPT at M.D Anderson Cancer Center. Both arms use a simultaneous integrated boost to escalate the dose to the GTV.
2. NCT00915005 is a randomized protocol treating to 74Gy(RBE)/37fx with both photons and protons with the primary objective to compare the incidence of grade 3+ RP or local failure. First results have recently been reported in an ASCO abstract [72], though long-term follow-up and survival for the cohorts will reveal additional insight. The OncoRay center in Dresden (Germany) is running a similar study (PRONTOX), a proton-photon comparison treating to 66Gy(RBE)/33fx.
3. *Optimal fraction size:* NCT01770418 is a multi-center, hypofractionated protocol for stage II–III NSCLC, treating to 60Gy(RBE) in 4 fraction sizes from 2.5 to 4Gy(RBE)/fx. Washington University has a similar phase I study (NCT02172846), also shortening the treatment time to 3 weeks. Loma Linda University Medical Center had a similar protocol (now terminated, no results published, NCT00614484), treating concurrently with Taxol and carboplatin to 76Gy(RBE) in 5 weeks.
4. *The role of protons in resectable disease:* The role of protons in tri-modality treatments, i.e. including surgery, is currently investigated in the pre- and post-operative setting. The Massachusetts General Hospital has conducted a phase I trial (NCT01565772) exploring hypo-fractionated proton therapy with cisplatin and etoposide in 3 weeks to 45–55Gy(RBE), followed by surgery. The University of Pennsylvania is currently also investigating pre-operative proton therapy with concurrent chemotherapy in a phase I/II study, though over 5.5–7.5 weeks (NCT01076231). The OncoRay center (Dresden, Germany) is planning a study to investigate the value of accelerated schedules (7 fractions per week at 2 Gy (RBE)/fx, PORTAF, NCT02189967).
5. *Technical aspects:* To date the M.D. Anderson Cancer Center is the only institution to have published results of lung cancer patients treated with IMPT [3]. They continue to investigate the clinical promise of IMPT in a protocol explicitly using only IMPT to deliver proton therapy (NCT01629498). Other technical aspects being worked on by multiple groups include better image guidance and motion mitigation techniques.

Other trials and current updates can be found at clincaltrials.gov and on the website of the particle cooperative group (ptcog.ch).

10.3 TREATMENT PLANNING

10.3.1 Target volume definition with respect to motion

Intra-fractional motion due to respiration, is an important consideration for radiotherapy of lung cancer, because the tumor motion affects the tumor dose. Treatment volume definitions have been strongly influenced by International Commission on Radiation Units and Measurements (ICRU) 62, which specifies that a tumor clinical target volume (CTV) may be expanded per an internal margin to create an internal target volume (ITV). However, the use of an ITV for proton therapy is problematic, because tumor motion changes not only the geometric location of the tumor, but also changes its radiological depth. For this reason, several alternative target definition strategies have been proposed, and there is not yet a complete consensus as to which strategy is best.

An early strategy developed for proton therapy of lung cancer involved modifying aperture and range compensator shapes for ensuring coverage with passively scattered plans. Moyers et al. used a PTV to encompass both the setup and internal margin, but then modified the aperture margin, bolus smearing, and proximal margin to cover setup and motion margins [85]. Engelsman and Kooy quantified the effect of different aperture margins and bolus smearing on EUD (equivalent uniform dose) in a phantom [86]. Engelsman et al. then compared treatment plan quality with target volumes defined on free-breathing, mid-inspiration, and 4D-CT [87]. For the 4D-CT case, they defined an aperture and bolus based on the maximum lateral displacements and maximum water-equivalent depth needed for coverage on all breathing phases. Their conclusion was that an aperture and bolus expansion created on mid-inspiration CT is adequate, and one created on 4D-CT provided the best coverage.

While bolus and aperture expansion remain a popular strategy, it is possible to achieve a similar effect by creating modified target volumes in a 3D scan. This idea was introduced by Koto et al. for carbon ion therapy [88]. In their approach, planning was based on an exhale CT for gated therapy. Recognizing that gated delivery may differ from gated simulation, they constructed an ITV volume, and the Hounsfield unit (HU) values for voxels within the ITV volume were replaced with HU values of the maximum intensity projection (MIP). HU numbers may be modified in the target volume and entrance path to ensure coverage at any breathing phase. The aperture and bolus are then created from the modified ITV directly. Subsequently, Kang et al. introduced an alternative approach, where an average intensity projection (AIP) CT is used, but voxels within the internal gross tumor volume (iGTV) replaced with a constant density of 100 HU [89]. They produced comparison treatment plans with free-breathing, AIP, and MIP CT scans, and concluded that the density assignment strategy was superior. Another strategy, introduced by Bert and Rietzel [90], optimizes the density values for each voxel in the ITV in a beam-dependent manner. For a given beam direction, the maximum water-equivalent path length (WEPL) to each location is computed. Then, densities are assigned to voxels in the ITV to ensure that the WEPL to voxels in the optimized ITV are equal to the maximum WEPL. This approach was improved by Rietzel and Bert to better account for moving structures in the entrance region [91], and by Park et al. to account for setup error [92]. Adequate coverage in the case of setup error is assured by considering the maximum WEPL within a neighborhood of each voxel rather than at a single voxel. A similar approach, called raITV, is introduced by Knopf et al. [93], which achieves coverage by optimizing the target contour on a reference image without modifying target voxels. The different concepts are illustrated in Figure 10.4.

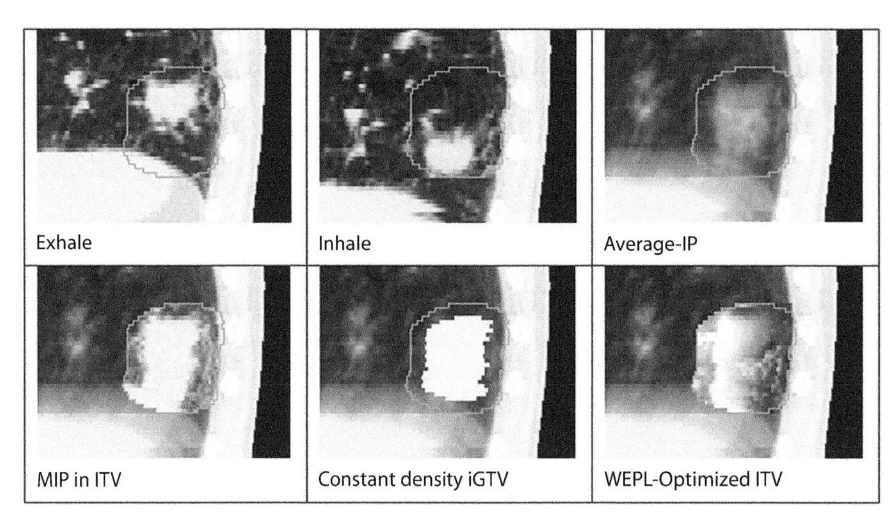

Figure 10.4 Proton treatment planning structures for lung treatments. Upper row: Tumor in exhale (left), inhale (middle), and average intensity projection (right). Lower row: maximum intensity projection (MIP) as ITV ([88], left), constant density iGTV ([89], middle), and WEPL-optimized ITV ([91], right).

10.3.2 TREATMENT PLANNING CONSIDERATIONS

10.3.2.1 SINGLE FIELD UNIFORM DOSE VERSUS IMPT

IMPT plans can deliver highly conformal dose distributions to target volumes of complex geometrical shape by accumulating the contributions from individually inhomogeneous treatment fields. A recurrent confusion is the definition of Single Field Uniform Dose (SFUD), and its discrimination from IMPT. The fundamental challenge is the following: on one hand, no SFUD field is fully uniform, as even advanced scanning system struggle to deliver completely uniform target coverage with a single field, especially in geometrically challenging lung cases. On the other hand, an IMPT plan does not necessarily have to include the very sharp dose gradients that make treatment plans susceptible to uncertainties. Dowdell et al. [94] have addressed this problem in a systematic fashion by defining all active scanning treatment plans as $IMPT_{H\%}$, where H defines the maximum inhomogeneity allowed based on the common inhomogeneity definition:

$$H = \frac{D_{max} - D_{min}}{D_{mean}}, \ \forall \text{ fields in the plan.}$$

This removed the inherent ambiguity in the SFUD definition, i.e. an SFUD-like plan in which only 2% inhomogeneity is allowed is termed $IMPT_{2\%}$, a plan in which no constraint is applied is denoted as $IMPT_{full}$. Examples for lung treatment plans using different degrees of in-field homogeneity are displayed in Figure 10.5.

The dependence on matching sharp inhomogeneities within the treatment fields leads to an increased sensitivity of IMPT towards a range of uncertainties. Lomax has studied this problem for calculation [95] and setup uncertainties [96]. Albertini et al. have shown that the degree of intensity modulation influences the

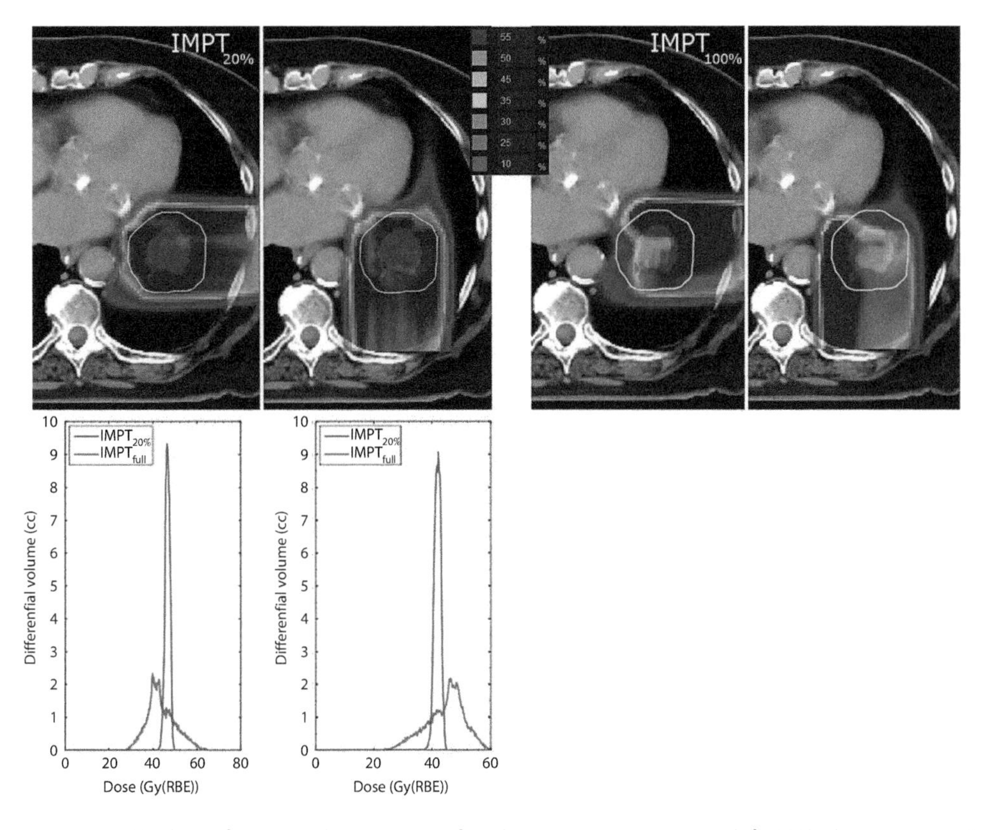

Figure 10.5 IMPT plans of varying inhomogeneity for a lung cancer patient. Top left: 20% inhomogeneity. Top Right: no constraint posed on inhomogeneity, i.e. $IMPT_{full}$. Bottom Left: DVHs for both plans. (Data courtesy of Dr. Stephen Dowdell.)

robustness of a treatment plan [97], Dowdell et al. investigated this subject in detail for lung cancer treatments under the influence of systemic versus random setup uncertainties [94]. The main conclusions from these studies can be summarized as follows:

- The higher the modulation within a field, i.e. the steeper the dose gradients, the less applicable are "PTV"-based margin concepts taken over from photon therapy.
- For conventionally fractionated treatments, systematic setup errors constitute a greater challenge than random ones.
- Fractionation is a powerful tool to mitigate effects of random setup errors, and conclusions from studies using >30 fractions are not necessarily transferrable to more hypofractionated regimens.

This underscores the importance of using comprehensive, robust multi-criteria optimization approaches [98], which encompass a host of parameters including setup uncertainties, beams angles [99], number of fields, and possible changes in patient and tumor geometry [100,101]. All these areas are active fields of research, though they have not yet been implemented clinically.

10.3.2.2 RANGE UNCERTAINTIES

Proton dose distributions are more sensitive to inter- and intra-fractional anatomical changes compared to photon dose distributions because geometrical changes can affect the beam range. Range uncertainties are present for all proton treatments. Consequently, in proton therapy the homogeneous PTV expansion used in photon therapy planning is applicable only when considering lateral uncertainties. Range uncertainties require a separate margin along the beam direction. The concept of raITV has been discussed in Section 10.3.1. Range uncertainties do depend on the patient geometry and beam angle. Clinically, most centers apply a distal uncertainty margin on the order of 2.5%–3.5% of the prescribed range plus an additional 1–3 mm water-equivalent depth, resulting in significant overshoot and irradiation of healthy tissues to ensure tumor coverage [102]. These effects need to be understood by treatment planners. They are magnified in lung cancer because the tumor is often surrounded by low-density lung tissue, i.e. every water-equivalent millimeter added to the range due to these uncertainties translates to 3–4 mm dose to the normal lung [103]. Range uncertainties are an additional effect to a blurring of the dose distribution in the presence of motion which compromises lateral conformity to the target volume both in photon and in proton therapy [104,105].

Because of the low density of lung tissue, ranges are often reported as WEPL instead of absolute distance. Water-equivalent path length translates to a substantial overshoot in the lung due to the low lung density. Thus, these fluctuations can result in an excessive dose to distal critical structures. In addition to lung tissue being replaced by higher density tumor tissue (or vice versa), rib cage motion can result in significant changes in WEPL as well. Figure 10.6 [106] illustrates the effect in an idealized geometry assuming a circular shaped tumor in two dimensions. Visualization of the water-equivalent path length variations can be helpful during treatment planning [107]. Water-equivalent path length fluctuations in proton therapy treatment plans for lung tumors have been studied by Mori et al. [108]. They showed variations up to 2.2 cm for ITV-based planning and 1 cm for gated ITV-based delivery.

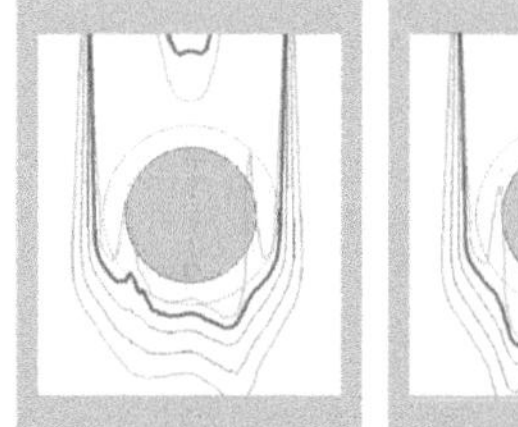
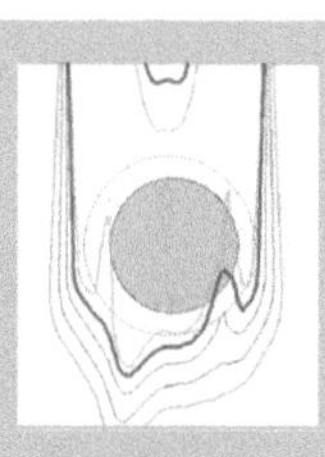
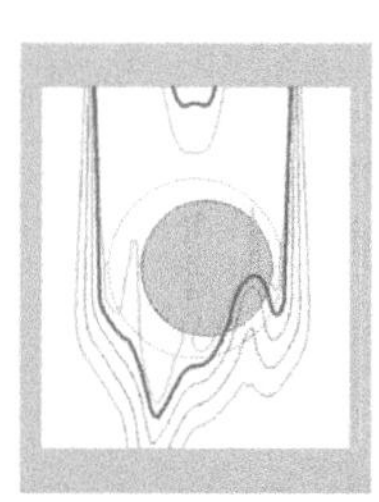
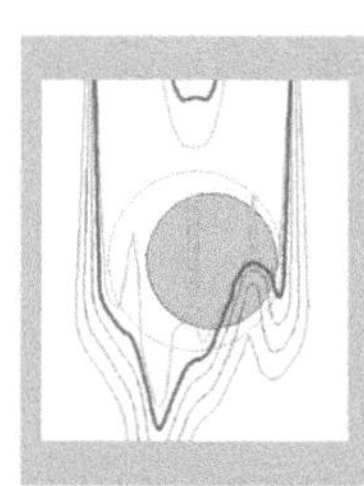
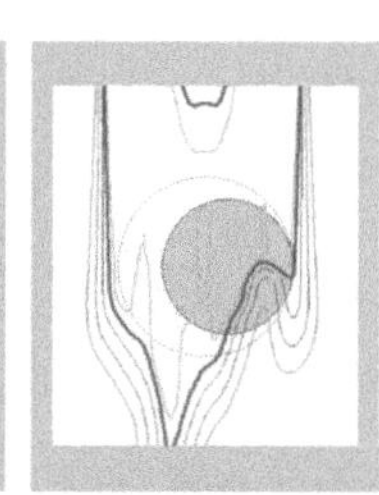

Figure 10.6 Distortion of a proton dose distribution (beam entering from the top) assuming a circular-shaped target under motion (From Knopf, A. and S. Mori, In I.J. Das and H. Paganetti [ed.], *Principles and Practice of Proton Beam Therapy*, Madison, Medical Physics Publishing, 2015. With permission.)

In addition to applying a range margin, passive scattered proton therapy also uses compensator smearing to account for range uncertainties due to setup errors and inter-fractional geometry changes or motion changes in lung tumors [85,87,109]. Compensator smearing cannot be used in pencil beam scanning. Thus, in this case such uncertainties must be covered by range uncertainty margins [92,93].

In general, the effect of range uncertainties can be more complex in beam scanning (due to, for example, interplay effects discussed below). Dowdell et al [94] studied dosimetric effects in intensity-modulated proton therapy assuming setup uncertainties of ± 5 mm. The dosimetric effect of setup uncertainties was larger in full IMPT for both systematic and random setup uncertainties compared to IMPT limiting the variation in dose within a field to 20%. The impact of motion (dose blurring as well as interplay effect) combined with random setup uncertainties for a conventionally fractionated treatment was quite small for large beam spot sizes but substantial for smaller spot sizes.

In addition to uncertainties due to motion or setup, there are also discrepancies between dose calculated in the planning system, which is typically based on analytical dose calculation algorithms, and the truly delivered dose. Monte Carlo based dose calculation has been shown to calculate dose more accurately (Figure 10.7 [110]) [111,112]. It has been shown that analytical dose calculation algorithms in treatment planning systems may overestimate tumor control probabilities by up to 11% for lung [111]. Furthermore, range differences of several mm have been reported [103]. Range uncertainty margins of ~6% of the prescribed range would be needed to ensure tumor coverage for 95% of the patients and for every single field [103]. However, this holds if a generic margin is being used. Treatment planners use smaller margins and add additional range for certain scenarios based on their experience and beam orientation. The accuracy of dose calculation and range prediction in the lung may also depend on the CT resolution [113].

There is also range uncertainty associated with the relative biological effectiveness (RBE) of proton beams. Although a generic RBE of 1.1 is being applied clinically, the RBE is likely increasing with depth and thus can cause a shift of the distal dose-fall-off if RBE-weighted doses based on a variable RBE would be considered [114–116].

10.3.2.3 4D TREATMENT PLANNING AND PLAN ROBUSTNESS

As discussed above, in contrast to photon therapy, the proton dose distribution is significantly affected by the change in patient geometry. Furthermore, the susceptibility of treatment plans to dose distribution perturbations due to motion depends on the delivery method. In passive scattering, the field is essentially delivered simultaneously. When applying beam scanning, treatment fields are delivered as a series of iso-energy layers and beam spots covering each layer to the prescribed dose. The consequence is a motion effect that is specific to scanning, the interplay effect between beam motion (within a layer or when going from one layer to the next) and organ motion (see also 10.4).

Methods have been developed to design treatment plans that are less sensitive to uncertainties in general or geometrical changes i.e. treatment plan optimization that can be done in a robust way. There are

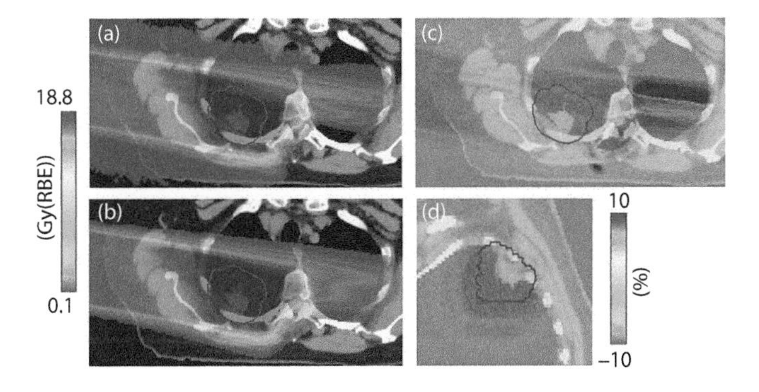

Figure 10.7 Differences in the dose distributions between (a) Monte Carlo simulation and (b) analytical calculation (c) shows the dose difference between a and b in axial view and (d) the dose difference in coronal view (From Paganetti, H. et al., In I.J. Das and H. Paganetti [ed.], *Principles and Practice of Proton Beam Therapy*, Madison, Medical Physics Publishing, 2015. With permission.)

several methods of robust optimization and evaluation of plan robustness such as the "worst-case" method [98,117,118], the "mini-max" approach [119] and the probabilistic approach [120]. In the worst-case approach, several dose distributions are considered, each based on a particularly scenario. The worst-case dose distribution may be very conservative and thus overestimate the true impact of uncertainties. The mini-max approach is very similar but less conservative as it considers rankings of objectives. A different strategy is the basis for probabilistic robust optimization. It may be the best strategy, but is computationally more demanding. Here, uncertainties are introduced in the optimization as random variables based on probability distributions. The dose distribution is then optimized based on the expected value of the objective function. These approaches were designed for general robust optimization but can be used similarly also for robust 4D optimization. Robustness comes at a price, i.e. a potential reduction in target dose conformity or an increased volume of critical normal tissue being irradiated. Probabilistic approaches are more promising for 4D optimization because they add less treatment volume. Parameters to generate probability density functions for the optimization routine must be deduced from the 4D-CT dataset or multiple 4D-CT datasets.

Robust optimization methods have been introduced first to consider motion in IMRT [121]. While the principle is the same for proton therapy one must consider the additional effect of range uncertainties which makes proton therapy less forgiving towards uncertainties. On the other hand, a treatment modality offering more degrees of freedom in planning, such as proton therapy, has more options regarding techniques for plan robustness. Plan robustness has been introduced particularly for mitigating range uncertainties in IMPT [120]. Intensity-modulated proton therapy, due to its additional degrees of freedom, allows the design of treatment plans that are potentially less affected by motion. This can be achieved, for instance, by manipulating the spot map distribution. For example, less steep dose gradients per field reduces the interplay effect and the sensitivity to random and systematic setup uncertainties [122].

10.3.2.4 INTERFRACTIONAL MOTION VARIATIONS

The patient's breathing pattern might change from fraction to fraction [123]. The 4D-CT dataset typically taken for treatment planning reflects only one breathing pattern. This breathing pattern may look different during treatment and may also change during a fractionated treatment resulting in a baseline drift. Furthermore, a 4D-CT does not provide continuous motion information because only 10 idealized waveforms are generated from the raw data.

Consequently, treatment margins must be chosen conservatively to ensure tumor coverage not only considering the beams-eye view as in photon therapy but also considering potential range changes when treating with protons. Even small deviations from the motion captured in the 4D planning CT can have significant impact on tumor coverage. It is thus important to estimate the tolerance level of planning margins with respect to expected or known breathing variations even if the motion exceeds the motion amplitude shown in the 4D-CT dataset. A method to estimate the dose delivered to a tumor for any input breathing function without limits on the range of tumor positions has been described by Philips et al. [124]. It is based on 1D or 3D waveforms that can be captured at the treatment day. The dose distributions are transformed from a Cartesian space into a beam-specific radiological depth space where they are invariant towards density changes and can be weighted and summed per the deduced trajectory. The resulting dose distribution can then be transformed back into Cartesian space to estimate the motion effect and the resulting tumor coverage at the day of treatment.

10.3.2.5 IMPORTANCE OF PLAN ADAPTATION/TARGET SHRINKAGE

Inter-fractional changes generally include anatomical changes due to tumor shrinkage [125] or weight loss or due to daily positioning uncertainties [109]. It has been shown that up to 25% of the CTV could be missed during 7 weeks of radiation therapy for lung cancer if setup relies on skin markers, only emphasizing the need for daily bone registration [109]. Tumor shrinkage is less significant in hypo-fractionated regimens.

Hui et al. have studied the effects of inter-fractional motion and anatomic changes on proton therapy dose distribution in lung cancer based on weekly 4D-CT scans [109]. They found that for 7 out of 8 patients' tumor coverage was maintained during treatment with no need for adaptive therapy. This conclusion depends on the patient characteristics and assigned treatment planning margins. Adaptive re-planning may be required if normal tissue toxicity is a concern clinically or if the CTV coverage is compromised by more than 2% [109]. Clinical studies treating lung cancer with proton therapy on conventionally fractionated treatment schedules sometimes report a substantial fraction of patients being re-planned due to target volume shrinkage, up to 78% [3,55,79].

10.4 TREATMENT DELIVERY

Proton therapy treatment delivery for lung cancer is largely like delivery for other sites, with the additional consideration of motion management. Like photon delivery, a lateral excursion of the treatment target outside of the beam port will cause an under dose. However, proton therapy is also subject to tumor underdose or organs-at-risk (OAR) overdose for target lateral excursions within the planned beam port. Furthermore, treatments with scanned beams are subject to hot and cold spots within the target caused by organ motion that happens between the delivery of individual spots. For these reasons, motion management at the time of delivery is a key element of lung cancer treatment, and is a complementary requirement to planning margins. Motion management can be considered part of robust treatment delivery as compared to robust treatment planning discussed earlier [120,126,127].

How much lung tumors typically move is shown in Figure 10.8 based on 20 studies reporting the motion amplitude of lung tumors and lymph nodes in patients undergoing radiotherapy [128]. Inferred from these publications, the average motion is 7.7 mm based on 509 patients, 28% of the tumors move more than 10 mm (based on 356 patients) and 9% > 20 mm (based on 288 patients). However, tumor motion is correlated to other factors as well, such as clinical stage (larger tumors tend to move less) and performance status of the patient, as patients with better performance status and pulmonary reserve tend to exhibit larger tumor motion amplitudes. This distribution is an estimate and dependent on geographical location and clinical practice, as it also depends on the amount of medically operable patients coming to radiotherapy.

Motion mitigation can be done applying gating or tracking. Gating describes the restriction of treatment delivery to certain phases of the breathing cycle, and needs knowledge of the current breathing phase. Tracking implies continuous delivery of the treatment while "tracking" the tumor's path, and necessitates online imaging capability [129].

10.4.1 Motion management

10.4.1.1 BREATH HOLD AND GATING

A simple and effective method for reducing respiratory motion during therapy is the breath-hold technique, in which organ motion is reduced or nearly eliminated by stopping respiration. Breath hold may be voluntary

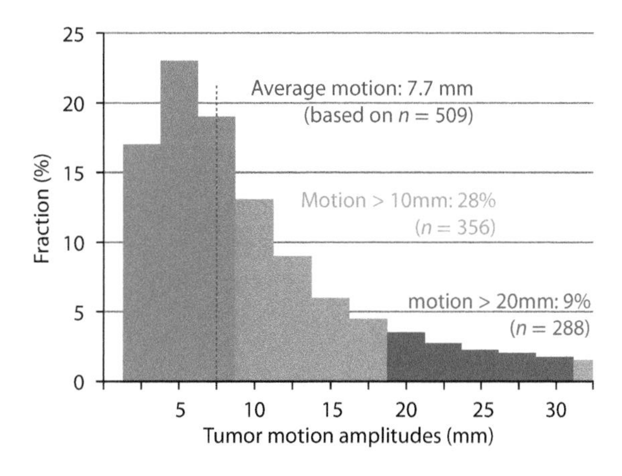

Figure 10.8 Spectrum of lung tumor motion amplitudes in radiotherapy patients based on 20 studies [128]. We included only publications that report unbiased estimations of patient populations, i.e. studies investigating gating were excluded, as they tend to select for patients with significant motion amplitude.

or involuntary, it may be held at exhale, inhale, or any other pulmonary volume, and it may be performed with and without either coaching or monitoring. The use of breath hold can benefit from a patient selection process that assesses both patient tolerance and compliance with instructions. It is expected that on average, a patient will tolerate breath-hold maneuvers of about 15 seconds, with intra-session reproducibility of about 2.5 mm [130,131]. A comprehensive survey on the use of the breath hold technique in photon radiotherapy is found in the report of Keall et al. [132].

Respiratory gating reduces organ motion by limiting beam delivery based on respiratory state [133,134]. In its most common form, a patient breathes freely, and an automated monitoring system tracks the respiration. The treatment beam is enabled at exhale, which is the most stable respiratory state, and disabled at inhale. Respiratory gating is well tolerated, but treatment time is increased due to beam-on and beam-off cycles.

Both breath-hold and respiratory-gated treatments have been implemented in proton and ion therapy centers since at least the early 2000s [135]. When the target is in position for treatment, the respiratory monitoring device signals the accelerator to enable beam. In the case of a synchrotron, beam extraction can occur only during the flat-top part of the synchrotron's magnet excitation cycle. If a variable cycle time is used, a proton spill can be held in the synchrotron ring until the patient respiration is ready, increasing treatment delivery [136]; see Figure 10.9.

For passively scattered protons, there is an additional consideration that the delivery of partial or incomplete SOBPs be avoided. A simple method to achieve this is to deliver a discrete number of complete SOBPs during each extraction [137], if the range modulation device operates with a sufficiently short period. For active scanning systems, the raster scan or spot scan pattern is stopped and then restarted at the appropriate location in the scanning pattern [138,139]. If available, a higher beam current can be used improve delivery efficiency.

A very sophisticated, combined implementation of the techniques described above has been performed at Chiba using scanned carbon ions, as described by Mori and colleagues [140]. They use amplitude-gated phase-controlled rescanning for moving lung and liver tumors preserving target coverage also under irregular respiratory conditions.

10.4.1.2 TRACKING

In contrast to gating systems, which halt the beam delivery when the target is out of position, beam tracking systems attempt to provide continuous directional control of the beam to aim it at a moving target. In photon therapy, tracking systems have been clinically implemented with robotic linac positioning, gimballed linac positioning, and for prostate, with dynamic multileaf collimator (MLC) motions [141–143]. Geometric accuracy of the tumor position is verified in real-time, usually using x-ray imaging, implanted transponders, or optical markers.

A tracking system for proton therapy must continuously control both the lateral position and the range of the beam. Tracking systems have not been proposed for passively scattered proton therapy, because real-time

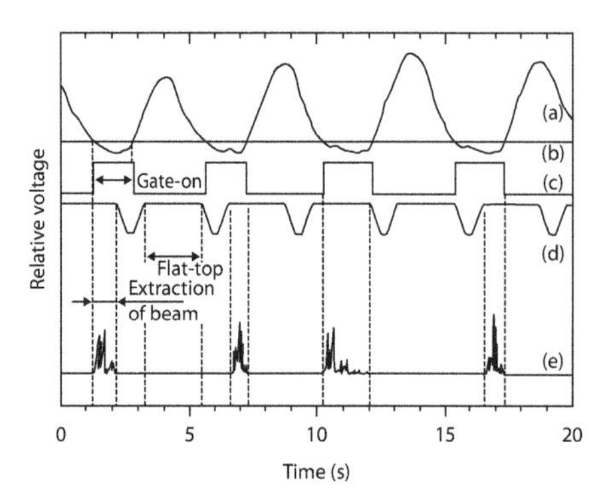

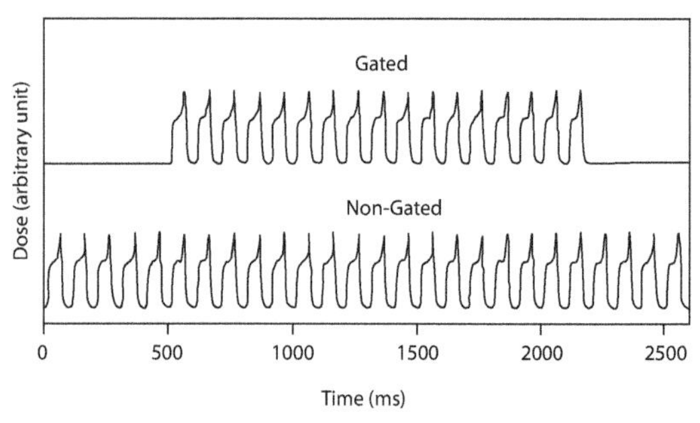

Figure 10.9 Left: Respiratory gating in a synchrotron. (a) respiratory waveform; (b) gating threshold; (c) gate-on signal; (d) synchrotron bending magnets; (e) extracted beam. (From Minohara, S. et al., *Int J Radiat Oncol Biol Phys*, 47, 1097–1103, 2000. With permission). Right: Respiratory gating in a passively scattered cyclotron (From Lu, H.M. et al., *Med Phys*, 34, 3273–3278, 2007. With permission.)

control of position and energy presents a serious engineering challenge. Instead, beam tracking is considered feasible only for active scanning systems, where steering magnets can accurately adapt pre-programmed beam spot locations to account for lateral tumor motion [144]. Real-time control of the beam energy can be achieved through a motorized paired wedge system [145]. At GSI, adaptation of lateral positions was demonstrated with a latency of about 1 ms and energy was adapted with a latency of about 25 ms [146]. Alternatively, energy can be adapted using a fast energy switching beamline. The beamline developed at PSI was demonstrated to be capable of energy changes at speeds of up to 80 ms [147]. Zhang et al. have investigated tracking comprehensively, using an approach termed 're-tracking', where rescanning is used in addition to mitigate the residual uncertainties and motion effects from tracking [129]. Tracking with particle beams has not yet been attempted in patients, though multiple groups are working on the clinical implementation of this challenging technique [148].

10.4.2 Interplay effect in beam scanning

Besides blurring of the dose distribution due to motion at the edges of the tumor, active scanning proton therapy can cause degradation of the dose distribution within the target. This interference between the dynamic pencil beam delivery and the motion of the tumor is called interplay effect. In intensity-modulated photon therapy the changing field is caused by movement of the multi-leaf collimator, while in intensity-modulated proton therapy the pencil beam spot is magnetically steered across the target. The interplay effect has been extensively studied for photon therapy [89,149–153]. These investigators concluded that the interplay effect is insignificant for fractionated photon techniques, where small effects are likely to wash out over the course of treatment. Subsequently, there have been many studies on interplay in proton therapy [122,154–162).

The interplay effect can potentially be more significant in proton therapy for three reasons. First, the motion of the beam spots is typically more regular in proton therapy where spots of equal size are moved along straight lines. Second, the time to change the energy to move to the next iso-energy layer might be on the same order as the breathing phase for some hardware settings. Third, the beam range varies with the water-equivalent thickness of the material in the beam path, which can change due to motion.

The interplay effect has typically very little impact on the mean dose to the target but will degrade dose homogeneity and can thus lead to underdosage (or overdosage) of parts of the target volume, which could negatively impact tumor control [8,163]; see Figure 10.10 for an example. The interplay effect is patient specific, depending on the motion amplitude, tumor location and the delivery parameters.

The necessary condition for the occurrence of the interplay effect is the discrete time structure of the dose delivery to the different voxels, i.e. it is an *intra* fraction effect that occurs for all active scanning proton

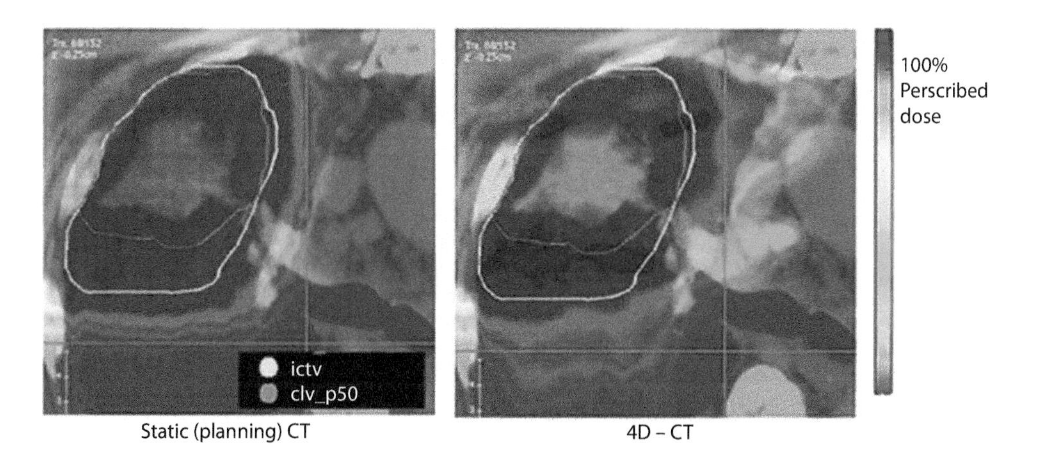

Figure 10.10 Two dose distributions in the patient. Left: simulated on the static CT. Right: simulated on the 4D-CT including respiratory motion. The orange contour shows the position of the target at the end of exhalation and the yellow contour the envelope of tumor motion over all breathing phases. The color bar is in percent of prescribed dose to the target. (C. Grassberger, unpublished data.)

therapy treatments, no matter the extent of intensity-modulation within the field. Dowdell et al. [122] investigated how the extent of intensity-modulation impacts the dose degradation due to interplay and concluded that the differences are clinically significant only for patients with very large motion amplitudes, in which case mitigating procedures would be undertaken in any case.

The key messages concerning interplay in lung tumors are as follows:

- The effect is very patient specific; tumor motion amplitude is not a good predictor.
- Fractionation effectively mitigates the effect to a large extent; therefore, care has to be exercised especially for hypofractionated protocols.
- Spot size is the most important delivery parameter. Very small spot sizes may not be well suited for moving targets. But the spot size can easily be increased if needed.
- Steep in-field gradients in IMPT do not impact the effect significantly. Therefore, plan quality does not have to be sacrificed for fear of increased interplay. However, inter-fraction and inter-field setup uncertainty affect highly modulated IMPT plans.

In the following sections, we will first discuss the patient specificity of the interplay effect, including the impact of fractionation, further how it is influenced by the technical machine parameters, and how it can be actively mitigated.

10.4.2.1 PATIENT SPECIFICITY

Lambert et al. [160] concluded that proton beam scanning should be applied only for targets with motion smaller than 10 mm. This seems too restrictive. In fact, the interplay effect depends on many delivery parameters such as the time to change the energy between layers, the scan time within an iso-energy layer, the scanning direction, the beam spot size, the beam spot spacing, the fractionation, and the initial treatment breathing phase. Furthermore, it depends on patient specific parameters such as the target size, tumor motion amplitude and frequency. General conclusions are difficult to draw.

Even though the interplay effect is caused by motion, it is hard to predict its exact magnitude based on the tumor motion amplitude. Grassberger et al. [161] used four-dimensional Monte Carlo dose calculation to study the interplay effect in 10 patients of varying motion amplitude and concluded that motion amplitude is not a reliable predictor of the TCP loss due to interplay, similar conclusions can be drawn from studies by Bert et al. [155].

All investigations into the interplay effect demonstrate the influence of the starting phase, i.e. in which breathing phase dose delivery starts [154–156,161]. This is of great importance, because it determines the effect of fractionation on the interplay effect. As dose delivery is usually started at a random moment in the breathing cycle for every fraction, fractionation leads to a statistical averaging of the different dose distributions, and results in a significant mitigation of the interplay effect [94,161]. This is demonstrated in Figure 10.11, which shows the dose distributions for different starting phases, together with the average after a conventionally fractionated treatment for a patient with unusually large motion amplitude (> 30 mm).

10.4.2.2 TECHNICAL DELIVERY PARAMETERS

Grassberger et al. and Dowdell et al. have shown that even for patients with lung tumor motion up to 20 mm, scanning is a feasible treatment option depending on the beam spot size [161,162]. Smaller spot sizes ($\sigma \approx 3$ mm) were more sensitive to motion, decreasing target dose homogeneity on average by a factor of ~3 compared to larger spot sizes ($\sigma \approx 12$ mm). For an extreme case, assuming treatment of a tumor with 30-mm motion amplitude with very small spots the 2-year local control was reduced from 87.0% to 71.6% with conventional fractionation. Many modern proton therapy facilities aim for very small spot sizes because it allows superior dose shaping. Caution should be taken if these small spots are used to treat lung tumors. Fortunately, a beam spot can always be artificially increased if there is a concern with respect to interplay effects.

The time to deliver the field has a considerable impact as well. Especially for shorter delivery times, the initial breathing phase can have a significant impact [162]. Daily variation in starting phase will decrease the dosimetric degradation that interplay causes. In general, longer delivery times led to lower interplay effects, due to averaging out of interplay effects. Obviously, a very short delivery time, far shorter than one breathing

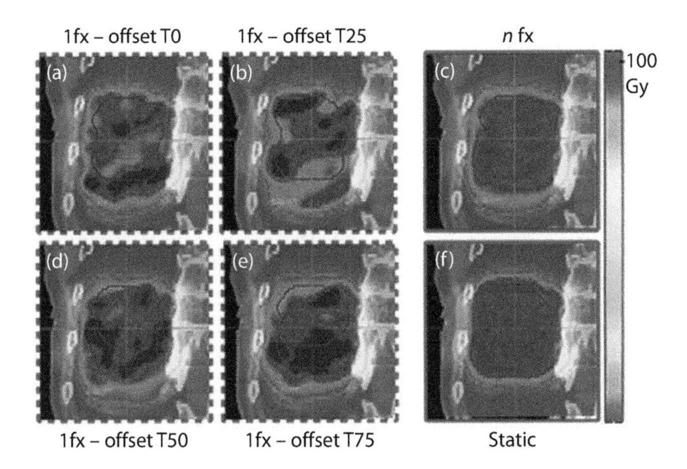

Figure 10.11 Sagittal view of the dose distributions for a patient with 30 mm tumor motion amplitude. Clinical target volume (red, small contour) and internal clinical target volume (pink, large contour) contoured in end-exhale phase. Panels (a) through (d) denote the 1-fraction cases for the 4 initial starting phases (T50: end-exhale, T0: peak-inhale), panel (e) the n-fraction (conventional fractionation), and panel (f) of the static case (simulated on static CT). (From Grassberger, C. et al., *Int J Radiat Oncol Biol Phys*, 86, 380–386, 2013. With permission.)

period (<0.5s), would mitigate interplay almost entirely. Thus, the times in between these two extremes are most susceptible to interplay. Particularly, the time it takes to switch the energy from one layer to the next is critical because the time it takes to scan within one layer is typically very small compared to breathing motion.

While studies in rigid phantoms have shown that the interplay effect depends on the direction of spot scanning [104,144,155,160], it has been demonstrated that for patient scenarios, there is no significant difference in interplay when scanning either parallel or perpendicular to the predominant axis of motion [162]. Reducing the spacing between adjacent spots makes the plan less susceptible to interplay [155,162].

Dowdell et al. have investigated how the amount of intensity modulation within an IMPT treatment plan impacts the interplay effect [122]. They concluded that the differences in interplay due to differences in intensity modulation between plans are small, outweighed by other factors such as starting phase, and only clinically significant in patients with very large tumor motion (>20 mm), which would be actively mitigated in any case.

In general, it has been shown that the interplay effect typically has little dosimetric consequences for a 30-fraction treatment and becomes significant only for small spot sizes, small number of fractions, and large tumor motion amplitude if no gating is being used, the latter being unlikely for such a scenario.

10.4.2.3 MITIGATION TECHNIQUES

Three main techniques exist to mitigate the interplay effect: rescanning (of different flavors), gating and tracking. In rescanning, the dose is delivered in n scans with $1/n$ of the original spot weight to mitigate the interplay effect through statistical averaging [104], in this sense it is identical to mitigation through fractionation, as explained above. The main flavors of rescanning are volumetric, layered and breath-sampled. In volumetric rescanning, the whole volume is scanned at once and the rescans are applied continuously; i.e. the system starts the next scan as soon as the last scan has finished. In layered rescanning, each energy layer is rescanned continuously to the prescribed dose before moving to the next energy. In breath-sampled rescanning, also termed phase-controlled rescanning, the volumetric rescans are not executed continuously, but evenly spaced in time over the breathing cycle [91,159,164].

It has been shown that all three techniques can mitigate the interplay effect appropriately. For rescanning, it has been shown that around six repetitions are adequate and that layered rescanning is more robust and faster than volumetric rescanning, similar to what has been demonstrated in liver tumors [154,159,165]. The main differences between rescanning and gating is the dose to the surrounding normal tissue: gating significantly reduces the dose to normal lung compared to rescanning, at the expense of longer treatment time, while rescanning is better able to mitigate hotspots in normal tissue distal to the target [159].

10.5 OUTLOOK

From the clinical perspective, the current role of proton therapy depends on the lung cancer stage. For early-stage lung cancer, proton therapy is in the process of establishing itself as an effective treatment option for tumors with clinically challenging location, larger size, and patients with limited pulmonary reserve or other severe comorbidities, combining good outcomes with minimal toxicity.

In locally advanced disease, the place of proton therapy in the spectrum of therapeutic options is still being actively defined. Outcomes in locally advanced lung cancer have improved from around 20% 2-year-and-9-months' median survival in the 1980s to over 50% 2-year and >24 months' median survival today [43,166], reflecting more accurate staging, increased conformity of radiation fields and better systemic therapy. The main question being answered in this and the next generation of clinical trials is the following: "Will proton therapy allow us to continue this trend and further increase local control and overall survival with reduced toxicity, or have we reached a plateau in the localized treatment of this aggressive disease, and completely new approaches (targeted agents, immunotherapy) are necessary?"

Currently, the dosimetric advantages of protons are opening new avenues in the practice of thoracic radiation oncology. In the phase I study by Gomez et al. [69], the treatment time was shortened and the dose/fraction was escalated, thus demonstrating how the physical advantages of protons widen the possible treatment options and enable us to ask new questions. Especially the optimal fraction size and treatment duration with and without concurrent chemotherapy is going to be investigated in exploratory proton therapy trials that simply could not be undertaken with photons due to inherent limits regarding normal tissue dose.

Other clinical questions in which proton therapy will be further investigated include its role in postoperative RT [75] and non-NSCLC thoracic malignancies [74]. Proton therapy is also used for other malignancies located in the thoracic region, such as oligo metastases to the lung [167], mediastinal lymphoma [168], and other rare cases [169].

Technically, the treatment of moving targets with proton beams can be more challenging compared to photon treatments. Range uncertainties caused by motion as well as potential interplay effects need to be considered. An up-to-date resource on the current state-of-the-art in the treatment of moving tumors with protons is the report of the annual international 4D particle treatment planning workshop [148].

REFERENCES

1. Wilson, R.R., Radiological use of fast protons. *Radiology*, 1946. **47**: 487–91.
2. Lomax, A.J. et al., A treatment planning inter-comparison of proton and intensity modulated photon radiotherapy. *Radiother Oncol*, 1999. **51**: 257–71.
3. Chang, J.Y. et al., Clinical implementation of intensity modulated proton therapy for thoracic malignancies. *Int J Radiat Oncol Biol Phys*, 2014. **90**(4): 809–18.
4. Wink, K.C. et al., Particle therapy for non-small cell lung tumors: Where do we stand? A systematic review of the literature. *Front Oncol*, 2014. **4**(Article 292): 1–15.
5. Koehler, A.M., R.J. Schneider, and J.M. Sisterson. Flattening of proton dose distributions for large-field radiotherapy. Med Phys, 1977. **4**: 297–301.
6. Pedroni, E. et al., The 200-MeV proton therapy project at the Paul Scherrer Institute: Conceptual design and practical realization. *Med Phys*, 1995. **22**: 37–53.
7. Lomax, A., Intensity modulation methods for proton radiotherapy. *Phys Med Biol*, 1999. **44**: 185–205.
8. Lomax, A.J. et al., Intensity modulated proton therapy: A clinical example. *Med Phys*, 2001. **28**: 317–24.
9. Paganetti, H. and H. Kooy, Proton radiation in the management of localized cancer. *Expert Rev Med Devices*, 2010. 7(2): 275–85.

10. Bentzen, S.M., Preventing or reducing late side effects of radiation therapy: Radiobiology meets molecular pathology. *Nat Rev Cancer*, 2006. **6**(9): 702–13.
11. Langendijk, J.A. et al., Impact of late treatment-related toxicity on quality of life among patients with head and neck cancer treated with radiotherapy. *J Clin Oncol*, 2008. **26**(22): 3770–6.
12. Deasy, J.O. et al., Radiotherapy dose-volume effects on salivary gland function. *Int J Radiat Oncol Biol Phys*, 2010. **76**(3 Suppl):S58–63.
13. Michalski, J.M. et al., Radiation dose-volume effects in radiation-induced rectal injury. *Int J Radiat Oncol Biol Phys*, 2010. **76**(3 Suppl):S123–9.
14. Marks, L.B. et al., Radiation dose-volume effects in the lung. *Int J Radiat Oncol Biol Phys*, 2010. **76**(3 Suppl): S70–6.
15. Semenenko, V.A. and X.A. Li, Lyman-Kutcher-Burman NTCP model parameters for radiation pneumonitis and xerostomia based on combined analysis of published clinical data. *Phys Med Biol*, 2008. **53**(3): 737–55.
16. Fay, M. et al., Dose-volume histogram analysis as predictor of radiation pneumonitis in primary lung cancer patients treated with radiotherapy. *Int J Radiat Oncol Biol Phys*, 2005. **61**(5): 1355–63.
17. Khan, M.A., R.P. Hill, and J. Van Dyk, Partial volume rat lung irradiation: An evaluation of early DNA damage. *Int J Radiat Oncol Biol Phys*, 1998. **40**(2): 467–76.
18. Khan, M.A. et al., Partial volume rat lung irradiation; assessment of early DNA damage in different lung regions and effect of radical scavengers. *Radiother Oncol*, 2003. **66**(1): 95–102.
19. Novakova-Jiresova, A. et al., Changes in expression of injury after irradiation of increasing volumes in rat lung. *Int J Radiat Oncol Biol Phys*, 2007. **67**(5): 1510–8.
20. Travis, E.L., Z.X. Liao, and S.L. Tucker, Spatial heterogeneity of the volume effect for radiation pneumonitis in mouse lung. *Int J Radiat Oncol Biol Phys*, 1997. **38**(5): 1045–54.
21. van Luijk, P. et al., Radiation damage to the heart enhances early radiation-induced lung function loss. *Cancer Res*, 2005. **65**(15): 6509–11.
22. Coppes, R.P. et al., Volume-dependent expression of in-field and out-of-field effects in the proton-irradiated rat lung. *Int J Radiat Oncol Biol Phys*, 2011. **81**(1): 262–9.
23. Hope, A.J. et al., Modeling radiation pneumonitis risk with clinical, dosimetric, and spatial parameters. *Int J Radiat Oncol Biol Phys*, 2006. **65**(1): 112–24.
24. Seppenwoolde, Y. et al., Regional differences in lung radiosensitivity after radiotherapy for non-small-cell lung cancer. *Int J Radiat Oncol Biol Phys*, 2004. **60**(3): 748–58.
25. Yorke, E.D. et al., Correlation of dosimetric factors and radiation pneumonitis for non-small-cell lung cancer patients in a recently completed dose escalation study. *Int J Radiat Oncol Biol Phys*, 2005. **63**(3): 672–82.
26. van Luijk, P. et al., The impact of heart irradiation on dose-volume effects in the rat lung. *Int J Radiat Oncol Biol Phys*, 2007. **69**(2): 552–9.
27. Huang, E.X. et al., Heart irradiation as a risk factor for radiation pneumonitis. *Acta Oncol*, 2011. **50**(1): 51–60.
28. Allen, A.M. et al., An evidence based review of proton beam therapy: The report of ASTRO's emerging technology committee. *Radiother Oncol*, 2012. **103**(1): 8–11.
29. Choi, N. et al., Predictive factors in radiotherapy for non-small cell lung cancer: Present status. *Lung Cancer*, 2001. **31**(1): 43–56.
30. Maguire, P.D. et al., 73.6 Gy and beyond: Hyperfractionated, accelerated radiotherapy for non-small-cell lung cancer. *J Clin Oncol*, 2001. **19**(3): 705–11.
31. Willner, J. et al., Dose, volume, and tumor control prediction in primary radiotherapy of non-small-cell lung cancer. *Int J Radiat Oncol Biol Phys*, 2002. **52**(2): 382–9.
32. Chang, J.Y. et al., Significant reduction of normal tissue dose by proton radiotherapy compared with three-dimensional conformal or intensity-modulated radiation therapy in Stage I or Stage III non-small-cell lung cancer. *Int J Radiat Oncol Biol Phys*, 2006. **65**(4): 1087–96.
33. van Baardwijk, A. et al., Mature results of an individualized radiation dose prescription study based on normal tissue constraints in stages I to III non-small-cell lung cancer. *J Clin Oncol*, 2010. **28**(8): 1380–6.

34. Rancati, T. et al., Factors predicting radiation pneumonitis in lung cancer patients: A retrospective study. *Radiother Oncol*, 2003. **67**(3): 275–83.
35. Hernando, M.L. et al., Radiation-induced pulmonary toxicity: A dose-volume histogram analysis in 201 patients with lung cancer. *Int J Radiat Oncol Biol Phys*, 2001. **51**(3): 650–9.
36. Bush, D.A. et al., Hypofractionated proton beam radiotherapy for stage I lung cancer. *Chest*, 2004. **126**: 1198–203.
37. Hata, M. et al., Hypofractionated high-dose proton beam therapy for stage I non-small-cell lung cancer: Preliminary results of a phase I/II clinical study. *Int J Radiat Oncol Biol Phys*, 2007. **68**(3): 786–93.
38. Hoppe, B.S. et al., Double-scattered proton-based stereotactic body radiotherapy for stage I lung cancer: A dosimetric comparison with photon-based stereotactic body radiotherapy. *Radiother Oncol*, 2010. **97**(3): 425–30.
39. Kadoya, N. et al., Dose-volume comparison of proton radiotherapy and stereotactic body radiotherapy for non-small-cell lung cancer. *Int J Radiat Oncol Biol Phys*, 2011. **79**(4): 1225–31.
40. Register, S.P. et al., Proton stereotactic body radiation therapy for clinically challenging cases of centrally and superiorly located stage I non-small-cell lung cancer. *Int J Radiat Oncol Biol Phys*, 2011. **80**(4): 1015–22.
41. Bush, D.A. et al., High-dose hypofractionated proton beam radiation therapy is safe and effective for central and peripheral early-stage non-small cell lung cancer: Results of a 12-year experience at Loma Linda University Medical Center. *Int J Radiat Oncol Biol Phys*, 2013. **86**(5): 964–8.
42. Westover, K.D. et al., Proton SBRT for medically inoperable stage I NSCLC. *J Thorac Oncol*, 2012. **7**(6): 1021–5.
43. Bradley, J.D. et al., Standard-dose versus high-dose conformal radiotherapy with concurrent and consolidation carboplatin plus paclitaxel with or without cetuximab for patients with stage IIIA or IIIB non-small-cell lung cancer (RTOG 0617): A randomised, two-by-two factorial phase 3 study. *Lancet Oncol*, 2015. **16**(2): 187–99.
44. Timmerman, R. et al., Excessive toxicity when treating central tumors in a phase II study of stereotactic body radiation therapy for medically inoperable early-stage lung cancer. *J Clin Oncol*, 2006. **24**(30): 4833–9.
45. Gomez, D.R. and J.Y. Chang, Accelerated dose escalation with proton beam therapy for non-small cell lung cancer. *J Thorac Dis*, 2014. **6**(4): 348–55.
46. Zhang, X. et al., Intensity-modulated proton therapy reduces the dose to normal tissue compared with intensity-modulated radiation therapy or passive scattering proton therapy and enables individualized radical radiotherapy for extensive stage IIIB non-small-cell lung cancer: A virtual clinical study. *Int J Radiat Oncol Biol Phys*, 2010. **77**: 357–66.
47. Unkelbach, J. et al., The dependence of optimal fractionation schemes on the spatial dose distribution. *Phys Med Biol*, 2013. **58**(1): 159–67.
48. Giap, H., D. Roda, and F. Giap, Can proton beam therapy be clinically relevant for the management of lung cancer? *Transl Cancer Res*, 2015. **4**(4): E3–15.
49. Berman, A.T., S.S. James, and R. Rengan, Proton beam therapy for non-small cell lung cancer: Current clinical evidence and future directions. *Cancers*, 2015. **7**(3): 1178–90.
50. Schild, S.E. et al., Proton beam therapy for locally advanced lung cancer: A review. *World J Clin Oncol*, 2014. **5**(4): 568–75.
51. Oshiro, Y. and H. Sakurai, The use of proton-beam therapy in the treatment of non-small-cell lung cancer. *Expert Rev Med Devices*, 2013. **10**(2): 239–45.
52. Bonnet, R.B. et al., Effects of proton and combined proton/photon beam radiation on pulmonary function in patients with resectable but medically inoperable non-small cell lung cancer. *Chest*, 2001. **120**(6): 1803–10.
53. Bush, D.A. et al., Proton-beam radiotherapy for early-stage lung cancer. *Chest*, 1999. **116**(5): 1313–9.
54. Bush, D.A. et al., Pulmonary injury from proton and conventional radiotherapy as revealed by CT. *AJR Am J Roentgenol*, 1999. **172**(3): 735–9.
55. Chang, J.Y. et al., Toxicity and patterns of failure of adaptive/ablative proton therapy for early-stage, medically inoperable non-small cell lung cancer. Int J Radiat Oncol Biol Phys, 2011. **80**(5): 1350–7.
56. Kanemoto, A. et al., Outcomes and prognostic factors for recurrence after high-dose proton beam therapy for centrally and peripherally located stage I non-small-cell lung cancer. *Clin Lung Cancer*, 2014. **15**(2):e7–12.

57. Shioyama, Y. et al., Clinical evaluation of proton radiotherapy for non-small-cell lung cancer. *Int J Radiat Oncol Biol Phys*, 2003. **56**: 7–13.
58. Nakayama, H. et al., Proton beam therapy for patients with medically inoperable stage I non-small-cell lung cancer at the university of tsukuba. *Int J Radiat Oncol Biol Phys*, 2010. **78**(2): 467–71.
59. Nihei, K. et al., High-dose proton beam therapy for Stage I non-small-cell lung cancer. *Int J Radiat Oncol Biol Phys*, 2006. **65**(1): 107–11.
60. Hatayama, Y. et al., Clinical Outcomes and Prognostic Factors of High-Dose Proton Beam Therapy for Peripheral Stage I Non-Small-Cell Lung Cancer. *Clin Lung Cancer*, 2015. **17**(5): 427–32.
61. Makita, C. et al., High-dose proton beam therapy for stage I non-small cell lung cancer: Clinical outcomes and prognostic factors. *Acta Oncol*, 2015. **54**(3): 307–14.
62. Fujii, O. et al., A retrospective comparison of proton therapy and carbon ion therapy for stage I non-small cell lung cancer. *Radiother Oncol*, 2013. **109**(1): 32–7.
63. Iwata, H. et al., Long-term outcome of proton therapy and carbon-ion therapy for large (T2a-T2bN0M0) non-small-cell lung cancer. *J Thorac Oncol*, 2013. **8**(6): 726–35.
64. Iwata, H. et al., High-dose proton therapy and carbon-ion therapy for stage I nonsmall cell lung cancer. *Cancer*, 2010. **116**(10): 2476–85.
65. Goldstraw, P. et al., The IASLC Lung Cancer Staging Project: Proposals for the revision of the TNM stage groupings in the forthcoming (seventh) edition of the TNM Classification of malignant tumours. *J Thorac Oncol*, 2007. **2**(8): 706–14.
66. Chang, J.Y. et al., Phase 2 study of high-dose proton therapy with concurrent chemotherapy for unresectable stage III nonsmall cell lung cancer. *Cancer*, 2011. **117**(20): 4707–13.
67. Sejpal. S. et al., Early findings on toxicity of proton beam therapy with concurrent chemotherapy for non-small cell lung cancer. *Cancer*, 2011. **117**(13): 3004–13.
68. Nguyen, Q.N. et al., Long-term outcomes after proton therapy, with concurrent chemotherapy, for stage II-III inoperable non-small cell lung cancer. *Radiother Oncol*, 2015. **115**(3): 367–72.
69. Gomez, D.R. et al., Phase 1 study of dose escalation in hypofractionated proton beam therapy for non-small cell lung cancer. *Int J Radiat Oncol Biol Phys*, 2013. **86**(4): 665–70.
70. McAvoy, S. et al., Definitive reirradiation for locoregionally recurrent non-small cell lung cancer with proton beam therapy or intensity modulated radiation therapy: Predictors of high-grade toxicity and survival outcomes. *Int J Radiat Oncol Biol Phys*, 2014. **90**(4): 819–27.
71. Koay, E.J. et al., Adaptive/nonadaptive proton radiation planning and outcomes in a phase II trial for locally advanced non-small cell lung cancer. *Int J Radiat Oncol Biol Phys*, 2012. **84**(5): 1093–100.
72. Liao, Z.X. et al., Bayesian randomized trial comparing intensity modulated radiation therapy versus passively scattered proton therapy for locally advanced non-small cell lung cancer. *J Clin Oncol*, 2016. **34**: 8500.
73. Hoppe, B.S. et al., Proton therapy with concurrent chemotherapy for non-small-cell lung cancer: Technique and early results. *Clin Lung Cancer*, 2012. **13**(5): 352–8.
74. Colaco, R.J. et al., Dosimetric rationale and early experience at UFPTI of thoracic proton therapy and chemotherapy in limited-stage small cell lung cancer. *Acta Oncol*, 2013. **52**(3): 506–13.
75. Remick, J., Schonewolf C, Gabriel P, Kralik JC. First clinical report of proton beam therapy versus intensity modulated radiation therapy for postoperative radiation therapy for non-small cell lung cancer. *Int J Radiat Oncol Biol Phys*, 2015. **93**(3): E422–3.
76. Remick, J.S. et al., First clinical report of proton beam therapy for post-operative radiotherapy for non-small cell lung cancer. *Clin Lung Cancer*, 2017. **18**(4): 364–71.
77. Badiyan, S.N. et al., Clinical outcomes of patients with stage II-III non-small cell lung cancer (NSCLC) treated with proton beam therapy (PBT) on the proton collaborative Group (PCG) prospective registry trial. *Int J Radiat Oncol Biol Phys*, 2016. **96**(2): E434–E5.
78. Nakayama, H. et al., Proton beam therapy of Stage II and III non-small-cell lung cancer. *Int J Radiat Oncol Biol Phys*, 2011. **81**(4): 979–84.
79. Oshiro, Y. et al., Results of proton beam therapy without concurrent chemotherapy for patients with unresectable stage III non-small cell lung cancer. *J Thorac Oncol*, 2012. **7**(2): 370–5.

80. Oshiro, Y. et al., High-dose concurrent chemo-proton therapy for Stage III NSCLC: Preliminary results of a Phase II study. *J Radiat Res*, 2014. **55**(5): 959–65.
81. Cox, J.D., Are the results of RTOG 0617 mysterious? *Int J Radiat Oncol Biol Phys*, 2012. **82**(3): 1042–4.
82. Nichols, R.C. et al., Proton radiation therapy offers reduced normal lung and bone marrow exposure for patients receiving dose-escalated radiation therapy for unresectable stage iii non-small-cell lung cancer: A dosimetric study. *Clin Lung Cancer*, 2011. **12**(4): 252–7.
83. Grutters, J.P. et al., Comparison of the effectiveness of radiotherapy with photons, protons and carbon-ions for non-small cell lung cancer: A meta-analysis. *Radiother Oncol*, 2010. **95**: 32–40.
84. Higgins, K.A. et al., National cancer database analysis of proton versus photon radiation therapy in non-small cell lung cancer. *Int J Radiat Oncol Biol Phys*, 2017. **97**(1): 128–37.
85. Moyers, M.F. et al., Methodologies and tools for proton beam design for lung tumors. *Int J Radiat Oncol Biol Phys*, 2001. **49**: 1429–38.
86. Engelsman, M. and H.M. Kooy, Target volume dose considerations in proton beam treatment planning for lung tumors. *Med Phys*, 2005. **32**(12): 3549–57.
87. Engelsman, M., E. Rietzel, and H.M. Kooy, Four-dimensional proton treatment planning for lung tumors. *Int J Radiat Oncol Biol Phys*, 2006. **64**: 1589–95.
88. Koto, M. et al., Local control and recurrence of stage I non-small cell lung cancer after carbon ion radiotherapy. *Radiother Oncol*, 2004. **71**(2): 147–56.
89. Kang, Y. et al., 4D Proton treatment planning strategy for mobile lung tumors. *Int J Radiat Oncol Biol Phys*, 2007. **67**(3): 906–14.
90. Bert, C. and E. Rietzel, 4D treatment planning for scanned ion beams. *Radiat Oncol*, 2007. **2**: 24.
91. Rietzel, E. and C. Bert, Respiratory motion management in particle therapy. *Med Phys*, 2010. **37**: 449–60.
92. Park, P.C. et al., A beam-specific planning target volume (PTV) design for proton therapy to account for setup and range uncertainties. *Int J Radiat Oncol Biol Phys*, 2012. **82**(2): e329–36.
93. Knopf, A.C. et al., Adequate margin definition for scanned particle therapy in the incidence of intrafractional motion. *Phys Med Biol*, 2013. **58**(17): 6079–94.
94. Dowdell, S. et al., Fractionated lung IMPT treatments: Sensitivity to setup uncertainties and motion effects based on single-field homogeneity. *Technol Cancer Res Treat*, 2015. **15**(5): 689–96.
95. Lomax, A.J., Intensity modulated proton therapy and its sensitivity to treatment uncertainties 1: The potential effects of calculational uncertainties. *Phys Med Biol*, 2008. **53**(4): 1027–42.
96. Lomax, A.J., Intensity modulated proton therapy and its sensitivity to treatment uncertainties 2: The potential effects of inter-fraction and inter-field motions. *Phys Med Biol*, 2008. **53**(4): 1043–56.
97. Albertini, F., E.B. Hug, and A.J. Lomax, Is it necessary to plan with safety margins for actively scanned proton therapy? *Phys Med Biol*, 2012. **56**(14): 4399–413.
98. Chen, W. et al., Including robustness in multi-criteria optimization for intensity-modulated proton therapy. *Phys Med Biol*, 2012. **57**(3): 591–608.
99. Cao, W. et al., Uncertainty incorporated beam angle optimization for IMPT treatment planning. *Med Phys*, 2012. **39**(8): 5248–56.
100. Albertini, F. et al., Sensitivity of intensity modulated proton therapy plans to changes in patient weight. *Radiother Oncol*, 2008. **86**(2): 187–94.
101. Li, H. et al., Robust optimization in intensity-modulated proton therapy to account for anatomy changes in lung cancer patients. *Radiother Oncol*, 2015. **114**(3): 367–72.
102. Paganetti, H., Range uncertainties in proton therapy and the role of Monte Carlo simulations. *Phys Med Biol*, 2012. **57**: R99–117.
103. Grassberger, C. et al., Quantification of proton dose calculation accuracy in the lung. *Int J Radiat Oncol Biol Phys*, 2014. **89**(2): 424–30.
104. Phillips, M.H. et al., Effects of respiratory motion on dose uniformity with a charged particle scanning method. *Phys Med Biol*, 1992. **37**: 223–34.
105. Seco, J. et al., Breathing interplay effects during proton beam scanning: Simulation and statistical analysis. *Phys Med Biol*, 2009. **54**(14): N283–94.

106. Knopf, A. and S. Mori, Motion management, in *Principles and Practice of Proton Beam Therapy*, I.J. Das and H. Paganetti, Editors. 2015; *Medical Physics Monograph No* 37, Madison, WI: Medical Physics Publishing, ISBN: 978-1-936366-43-9 2015. pp. 709–38.
107. Mori, S. and G.T. Chen, Quantification and visualization of charged particle range variations. *Int J Radiat Oncol Biol Phys*, 2008. **72**(1): 268–77.
108. Mori, S. et al., Quantitative assessment of range fluctuations in charged particle lung irradiation. *Int J Radiat Oncol Biol Phys*, 2008. **70**(1): 253–61.
109. Hui, Z. et al., Effects of interfractional motion and anatomic changes on proton therapy dose distribution in lung cancer. *Int J Radiat Oncol Biol Phys*, 2008. **72**(5): 1385–95.
110. Paganetti, H., J. Schuemann, and R. Mohan, Dose calculations for proton beam therapy: Monte Carlo, in *Principles and Practice of Proton Beam Therapy*, I.J. Das and H. Paganetti, Editors. 2015; Medical Physics Monograph No 37, Madison, WI: Medical Physics Publishing, ISBN: 978-1-936366-43-9 2015. pp. 571–94.
111. Schuemann, J. et al., Assessing the clinical impact of approximations in analytical dose calculations for proton therapy. *Int J Radiat Oncol Biol Phys*, 2015. **92**(5): 1157–64.
112. Schuemann, J. et al., Site-specific range uncertainties caused by dose calculation algorithms for proton therapy. *Phys Med Biol*, 2014. **59**(15): 4007–31.
113. Espana, S., and H. Paganetti, Uncertainties in planned dose due to the limited voxel size of the planning CT when treating lung tumors with proton therapy. *Phys Med Biol*, 2011. **56**(13): 3843–56.
114. Paganetti, H., Relative Biological Effectiveness (RBE) values for proton beam therapy. Variations as a function of biological endpoint, dose, and linear energy transfer. *Phys Med Biol*, 2014. **59**: R419–72.
115. Paganetti, H., Relating proton treatments to photon treatments via the relative biological effectiveness (RBE) – Should we revise the current clinical practice? *Int J Radiat Oncol Biol Phys*, 2015. **91**(5): 892–4.
116. Paganetti, H. et al., Relative biological effectiveness (RBE) values for proton beam therapy. *Int J Radiat Oncol Biol Phys*, 2002. **53**(2): 407–21.
117. Liu, W. et al., Robust optimization of intensity modulated proton therapy. *Med Phys*, 2012. **39**(2): 1079–91.
118. Pflugfelder, D. et al., A comparison of three optimization algorithms for intensity modulated radiation therapy. *Z Med Phys*, 2008. **18**(2): 111–9.
119. Fredriksson, A., A characterization of robust radiation therapy treatment planning methods-from expected value to worst case optimization. *Med Phys*, 2012. **39**(8): 5169–81.
120. Unkelbach, J. et al., Reducing the sensitivity of IMPT treatment plans to setup errors and range uncertainties via probabilistic treatment planning. *Med Phys*, 2009. **36**(1): 149–63.
121. Heath, E., J. Unkelbach, and U. Oelfke, Incorporating uncertainties in respiratory motion into 4D treatment plan optimization. *Med Phys*, 2009. **36**(7): 3059–71.
122. Dowdell, S., C. Grassberger, and H. Paganetti, Four-dimensional Monte Carlo simulations demonstrating how the extent of intensity-modulation impacts motion effects in proton therapy lung treatments. *Med Phys*, 2013. **40**(12): 121713.
123. Hugo, G. et al., Changes in the respiratory pattern during radiotherapy for cancer in the lung. *Radiother Oncol*, 2006. **78**(3): 326–31.
124. Phillips, J. et al., Computing proton dose to irregularly moving targets. *Phys Med Biol*, 2014. **59**(15): 4261–73.
125. Britton, K.R. et al., Assessment of gross tumor volume regression and motion changes during radiotherapy for non-small-cell lung cancer as measured by four-dimensional computed tomography. *Int J Radiat Oncol Biol Phys*, 2007. **68**(4): 1036–46.
126. Liu, W. et al., Effectiveness of robust optimization in intensity-modulated proton therapy planning for head and neck cancers. *Med Phys*, 2013. **40**(5):051711.
127. Stuschke, M. et al., Potentials of robust intensity modulated scanning proton plans for locally advanced lung cancer in comparison to intensity modulated photon plans. *Radiother Oncol*, 2012. **104**(1): 45–51.
128. Grassberger, C., Four-dimensional Monte Carlo simulation of lung cancer treatments with scanned proton beams. PhD thesis, 2014, ETH Zürich.

129. Zhang, Y. et al., Online image guided tumour tracking with scanned proton beams: A comprehensive simulation study. *Phys Med Biol*, 2014. **59**(24): 7793–817.
130. Wong, J.W. et al., The use of active breathing control (ABC) to reduce margin for breathing motion. *Int J Radiat Oncol Biol Phys*, 1999. **44**: 911–9.
131. Hanley, J. et al., Deep inspiration breath-hold technique for lung tumors: The potential value of target immobilization and reduced lung density in dose escalation. *Int J Radiat Oncol Biol Phys*, 1999. **45**: 603–11.
132. Keall, P.J. et al., The management of respiratory motion in radiation oncology report of AAPM Task Group 76. *Med Phys*, 2006. **33**(10): 3874–900.
133. Kubo, H.D. and B.C. Hill, Respiration gated radiotherapy treatment: A technical study. *Phys Med Biol*, 1996. **41**: 83–91.
134. Ohara, K. et al., Irradiation synchronized with respiration gate. *Int J Radiat Oncol Biol Phys*, 1989. **17**: 853–7.
135. Minohara, S. et al., Respiratory gated irradiation system for heavy-ion radiotherapy. *Int J Radiat Oncol Biol Phys*, 2000. **47**: 1097–103.
136. Tsunashima, Y. et al., Efficiency of respiratory-gated delivery of synchrotron-based pulsed proton irradiation. *Phys Med Biol*, 2008. **53**(7): 1947–59.
137. Lu, H.M. et al., A respiratory-gated treatment system for proton therapy. *Med Phys*, 2007. 34(8): 3273–8.
138. Furukawa, T. et al., Design study of a raster scanning system for moving target irradiation in heavy-ion radiotherapy. *Med Phys*, 2007. **34**(3): 1085–97.
139. Bert, C. et al., Gated irradiation with scanned particle beams. *Int J Radiat Oncol Biol Phys*, 2009. **73**(4): 1270–5.
140. Mori, S. et al., Amplitude-based gated phase-controlled rescanning in carbon-ion scanning beam treatment planning under irregular breathing conditions using lung and liver 4DCTs. *J Radiat Res*, 2014. **55**(5): 948–58.
141. Schweikard, A., H. Shiomi, and J. Adler, Respiration tracking in radiosurgery. *Med Phys*, 2004. **31**(10): 2738–41.
142. Matsuo, Y. et al., Evaluation of dynamic tumour tracking radiotherapy with real-time monitoring for lung tumours using a gimbal mounted linac. *Radiother Oncol*, 2014. **112**(3): 360–4.
143. Keall, P.J. et al., The first clinical implementation of electromagnetic transponder-guided MLC tracking. *Med Phys*, 2014. **41**(2): 020702.
144. Grozinger, S.O. et al., Simulations to design an online motion compensation system for scanned particle beams. *Phys Med Biol*, 2006. **51**(14): 3517–31.
145. Bert, C. et al., Target motion tracking with a scanned particle beam. *Med Phys*, 2007. **34**(12): 4768–71.
146. Saito, N. et al., Speed and accuracy of a beam tracking system for treatment of moving targets with scanned ion beams. *Phys Med Biol*, 2009. **54**(16): 4849–62.
147. Pedroni, E. et al., Pencil beam characteristics of the next-generation proton scanning gantry of PSI: Design issues and initial commissioning results. *Eur Phys J Plus*, 2011. **126**: 66.
148. Knopf, A. et al., Challenges of radiotherapy: Report on the 4D treatment planning workshop 2013. *Phys Med*, 2014. **30**(7): 809–15.
149. Bortfeld, T. et al., Effects of intra-fraction motion on IMRT dose delivery: Statistical analysis and simulation. *Phys Med Biol*, 2002. **47**: 2303–20.
150. Berbeco, R.I., C.J. Pope, and S.B. Jiang. Measurement of the interplay effect in lung IMRT treatment using EDR2 films. *J Appl Clin Med Phys*, 2006. **7**(4): 33–42.
151. Seco, J. et al., Effects of intra-fraction motion on IMRT treatments with segments of few monitor units. *IFMBE Proc*, 2007. **14**: 1763–5.
152. Ong, C. et al., Dosimetric impact of interplay effect on RapidArc lung stereotactic treatment delivery. *Int J Radiat Oncol Biol Phys*, 2011. **79**(1): 305–11.
153. Rao, M. et al., Dosimetric impact of breathing motion in lung stereotactic body radiotherapy treatment using intensity modulated radiotherapy and volumetric modulated arc therapy [corrected]. *Int J Radiat Oncol Biol Phys*, 2012. **83**(2): e251–6.
154. Knopf, A.C., T.S. Hong, and A. Lomax, Scanned proton radiotherapy for mobile targets-the effectiveness of re-scanning in the context of different treatment planning approaches and for different motion characteristics. , 2011. **56**(22): 7257–71.

155. Bert, C., S.O. Grozinger, and E. Rietzel, Quantification of interplay effects of scanned particle beams and moving targets. *Phys Med Biol*, 2008. **53**(9): 2253–65.
156. Kraus, K.M., E. Heath, and U. Oelfke, Dosimetric consequences of tumour motion due to respiration for a scanned proton beam. *Phys Med Biol*, 2011. **56**(20): 6563–81.
157. Kardar, L. et al., Evaluation and mitigation of the interplay effects of intensity modulated proton therapy for lung cancer in a clinical setting. *Pract Radiat Oncol*, 2014. **4**(6): e259–68.
158. Li, Y. et al., On the interplay effects with proton scanning beams in stage III lung cancer. *Med Phys*, 2014. **41**(2): 021721.
159. Grassberger, C. et al., Motion mitigation for lung cancer patients treated with active scanning proton therapy. *Med Phys*, 2015. **42**(5): 2462–9.
160. Lambert, J. et al., Intrafractional motion during proton beam scanning. *Phys Med Biol*, 2005. **50**: 4853–62.
161. Grassberger, C. et al., Motion interplay as a function of patient parameters and spot size in spot scanning proton therapy for lung cancer. *Int J Radiat Oncol Biol Phys*, 2013. **86**(2): 380–6.
162. Dowdell, S. et al., Interplay effects in proton scanning for lung: A 4D Monte Carlo study assessing the impact of tumor and beam delivery parameters. *Phys Med Biol*, 2013. **58**(12): 4137–56.
163. Tome, W.A. and J.F. Fowler, On cold spots in tumor subvolumes. *Med Phys*, 2002. **29**(7): 1590–8.
164. Takahashi, W. et al., Carbon-ion scanning lung treatment planning with respiratory-gated phase-controlled rescanning: Simulation study using 4-dimensional CT data. *Radiat Oncol*, 2014. **9**: 238.
165. Bernatowicz, K., A.J. Lomax, and A. Knopf, Comparative study of layered and volumetric rescanning for different scanning speeds of proton beam in liver patients. *Phys Med Biol*, 2013. **58**(22): 7905–20.
166. Slawson, R.G. et al., Once-a-week vs conventional daily radiation treatment for lung cancer: Final report. *Int J Radiat Oncol Biol Phys*, 1988. **15**(1): 61–8.
167. Sulaiman, N.S. et al., Particle beam radiation therapy using carbon ions and protons for oligometastatic lung tumors. *Radiat Oncol*, 2014. **9**: 183.
168. Li, J. et al., Rationale for and preliminary results of proton beam therapy for mediastinal lymphoma. *Int J Radiat Oncol Biol Phys*, 2011. **81**(1): 167–74.
169. Sugawara, K. et al., Proton beam therapy for a patient with a giant thymic carcinoid tumor and severe superior vena cava syndrome. *Rare Tumors*, 2014. **6**(2): 5177.

11

Application of IGRT for lung stereotactic body radiotherapy

JULIANNE M. POLLARD-LARKIN, PETER BALTER, AND JOE Y. CHANG

11.1 INTRODUCTION

Lung cancer is the leading cause of cancer death worldwide, with an estimated 1.8 million new cases and 1.6 million deaths annually [1,2]. Several treatment options have emerged to treat it. One of the latest treatment techniques is stereotactic body radiotherapy (SBRT), Also called stereotactic ablative radiotherapy (SABR), which can offer either improved outcomes or outcomes comparable to surgery [3]. The 5-year survival rate for medically inoperable stage I non-small-cell lung cancer (NSCLC) patients used to be 20%–30%, but with the use of SBRT, the 1–3-year overall survival rate ranges from 43% to 72% [4]. For operable stage I NSCLC, the 3 years' overall survival is up to 95% [3].

Lung cancer presents unique technical challenges to radiotherapy, because the tumor and normal tissue may move significantly (>1 cm)[5–8] during the time it takes to image or treat. In addition, the organ itself is generally more radiosensitive than the tumor. There also tends to be large differences in density between the various regions within the lung, making the development of a high-quality radiation therapy treatment plan difficult [9–13]. To overcome these challenges, modern radiation therapy for lung cancer, especially for SBRT, uses the combination of four-dimensional computer tomography (4D-CT) [8,14–16], IGRT [17–21] and intensity modulated radiotherapy (IMRT) [22,23], each of which is an important advancement in isolation but the best results come from the combination of all three [5,24]. The improvements in pre-and on-treatment imaging as well as improvements in planning algorithms have enabled a new use for SBRT or SABR.

11.2 IMAGE-GUIDED RADIOTHERAPY (IGRT) FOR SBRT

SBRT was possible prior to modern IGRT, but generally relied on an external frame or other coordinate systems [25–28], making this procedure time consuming and difficult. A critical component to the wide-scale implementation of SBRT was integration of high quality imaging with the treatment machine which offers direct setup to the tumor or a near-by fiducial based on kVp projection imaging or in-room volumetric imaging often referred to as image-guided radiation therapy (IGRT) [29]. IGRT provides the following:

1. Reduction of treatment field margins
2. Practical implementation of sharp dose gradients associated with SBRT
3. Practical implementation of reduced setup margins associated with SBRT [21]

The most common system for IGRT is a kVP imaging system, mounted on the gantry of a megavoltage linear accelerator (Figure 11.1) at a 90 degree offset from the treatment beam. These systems can be used to take individual kVp x-rays for setup based on bony anatomy or radio-opaque fiducials [30]. They can operate in fluoro-mode to watch physiological motion in real time. They also can acquire fluoro images while the gantry is rotating and use these to construct a CT scan [31]. In addition to the gantry mounted systems, at least two vendors have room-mounted systems [32,33], these systems use oblique orthogonal projection x-ray-based systems and cannot provide volumetric data but can monitor the patient in-real time during treatment. The choice of IGRT modality for SBRT depends on several factors including the radio-opacity of the lesion or its setup surrogate, the need to avoid nearby critical structures, the need to image with respect to time and respiration and, perhaps most importantly, the availability of equipment in the department.

In general, volumetric imaging, will give the most information about the target and the surrounding near-by structures and this is available as cone beam CT (CBCT) in most modern radiotherapy departments. CBCTs are acquired with a cone-shaped beam compared to the fan shaped beam in a traditional CT. CBCT have several limitations over traditional CT [17–18,34–36]. The biggest limitation comes from the gantry rotational speed, 1 min, which represents 10–20 respiratory cycles. This does give a time averaged image which is useful for setting up on the mean tumor position. However, the blurring associated with this process can make low contrast lesions or small lesions with large motions difficult or impossible to visualize. Another weakness of CBCT is that, unlike traditional CT, there is a significant amount of scatter in the field, this combined with the cone beam geometry, results in a lower overall image quality than traditional CT [37,38]. The last issue with CBCT is that the tube and detectors used in this system are not as well regulated as those in traditional CT so that the uncertainty in Hounsfield unit (HU) values is an order of magnitude greater. Even with these limitations, CBCT quality is sufficient to directly setup the patient using a soft tissue target of sufficient contrast. CBCT can also be combined with respiratory management, such as breath-hold and thus can be used for setup during these procedures and lower motion artifacts. One manufacturer has an option for reconstructing the CBCT as a 4DCT series allowing setup to moving targets [39].

IGRT paved the way for more aggressive radiation treatment regimens while reducing the complication rate. Examples of improved outcomes with the use of IGRT include prostate, head and neck, rectal, lung, vaginal and liver cancer [17,40–47]. IGRT in prostate cancer treatment has been used to reduce rectal and bladder complications, yet has improved biochemical control [41]. In head and neck cancer treatment, IGRT has been used to spare the parotid glands, decrease the incidence of xerostomia and thereby improves the quality of life for patients [21]. Another method of sparing normal tissue structures involves using patient daily imaging to

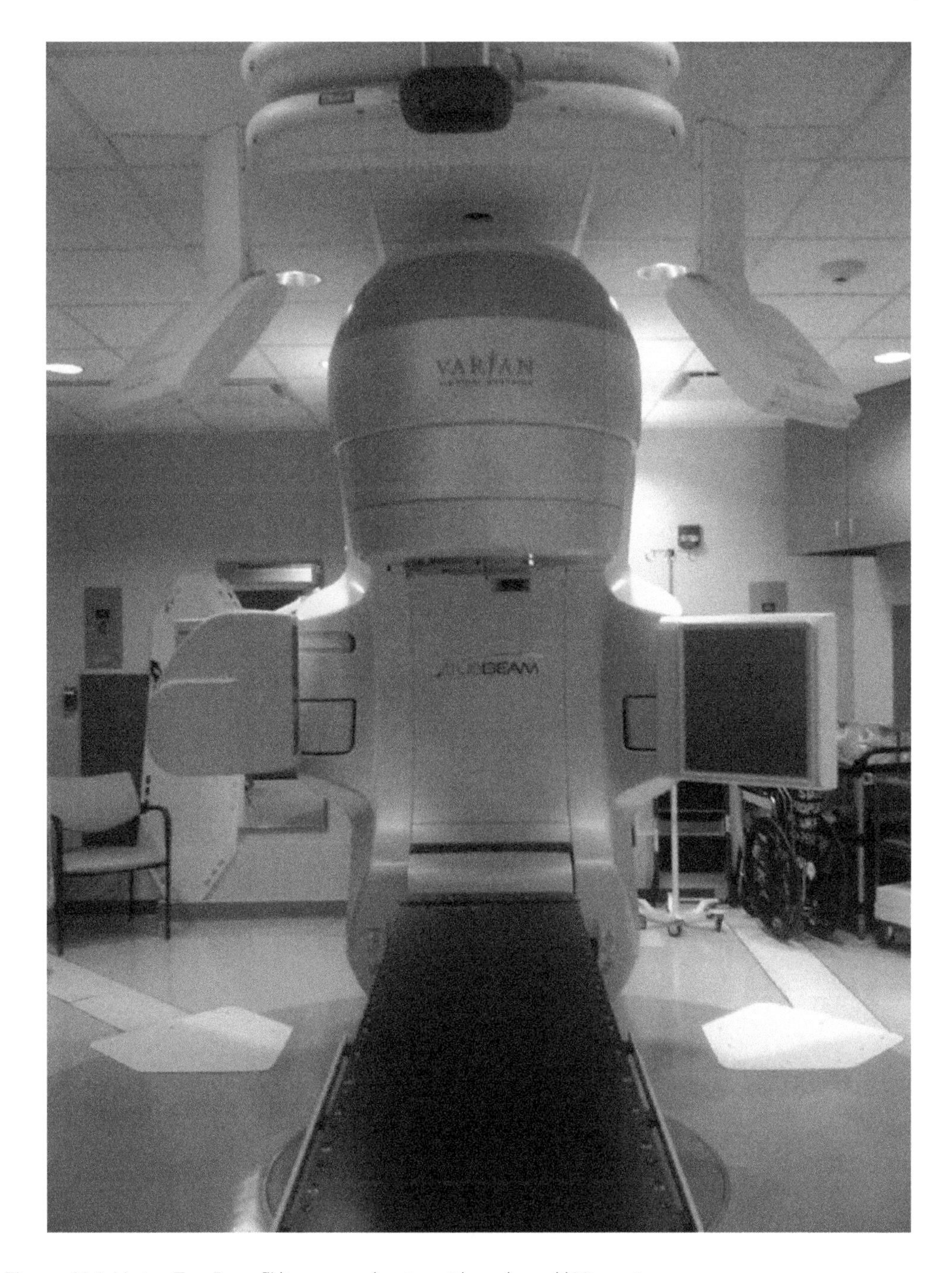

Figure 11.1 Varian TrueBeam™ linear accelerator with on-board kV imaging.

monitor tumor or anatomy changes and using this information to re-optimize the plan through a technique known as adaptive radiotherapy [15,40,48,49]

IGRT has helped to improve the precision of treatments, and simultaneously initiated a new interest in previously controversial fractionation schemes. Standard classical dose fractionation schemes involve 1.8–2 Gy per fraction for 30 or more total fractions over 5 or more weeks. Long treatment times for the patients and machines caused researchers in the 1960s to consider hypofractionation for breast cancer treatment, however, the results of these studies showed pronounced unfavorable outcomes due to normal tissue complications in the 3-day-a-week treatment compared to the standard 5-day-a-week regimen [50].

The higher dose per fraction, shorter treatment regimens were more problematic due to reduced time allowed for normal tissue sub-lethal repair to occur between fractions. Modern radiotherapy techniques allow us to create highly conformal dose distributions minimizing normal tissue doses and toxicity while IGRT allows us to still have confidence of our ability to cover the target with these tight dose distributions.

11.3 IMRT FOR SBRT

IMRT provides:

1. Improved normal tissue sparing compared to 3D conformal techniques
2. Heterogeneous dose distributions with rapid dose fall-off
3. The ability to dose escalate

Until the 1980s, radiation treatment planning was rudimentary and involved gross fields being drawn on planar x-ray films [51,52]. When computed tomography (CT) and multi-leaf collimators were introduced to radiotherapy, finally, radiation oncologists could fine tune field shapes with more detail that matched the target volume of interest, which was referred to as three-dimensional conformal radiotherapy (3D-CRT) [22,53]. While 3D-CRT methods were still being developed, the concepts of IMRT were being proposed [54]. IMRT is an improved version of 3DCRT that allows the planner to modify the intensity of each radiation beam in complex ways that provide the highest dose to the target of interest while sparing normal tissues [22]. The dose conformality provided by IMRT, paved the way for the next paradigm shift in radiation treatment regimens. With better dose fall-off available, radiation therapy was prepared to, once again, attempt to measure the feasibility of hypofractionation.

The appeal of hypofractionation is the reduced time for tumor cells to repopulate which increases the likelihood of tumor control probability [50,55,56]. Also, shortened overall treatment times facilitate less time on the machine, and a shortened stay at the treatment facility for patients.

11.4 SBRT

There are six essential characteristics of an SBRT:

1. Secure immobilization of patient (Figure 11.2)
2. Accurate repositioning of patient throughout process from simulation through treatment delivery
3. Minimized dose to normal critical structures by using multiple, non-opposing fields or arcs
4. Rigorously account for tumor motion at the time of simulation, planning and treatment
5. Stereotactically register the tumor targets and normal tissue avoidance structures to treatment machine
6. Deliver an ablative dose fractionation to the patient with sub-centimeter accuracy [57]

SBRT, or synonymously, SABR, utilizes all the principles of hypo-fractionation. SBRT delivers a high radiation dose capable of ablating the tumor in fewer than 5 fractions [58]. This fractionation scheme is also known as oligofractionation, using very few fractions, but delivering much higher doses per fraction [59]. Due to the previous history of late effects post hypo-fractionated treatments, early SBRT researchers used "dose-finding" studies to evaluate total dose, number of fractions, tumor target size, histology, and dose per fraction would limit toxicity while ensuring tumor control [59]. Several international phase I studies have shown SBRT's effectiveness in tumor control with limited toxicity in stage 1 patients and helped to identify dose and fractionation schemes to follow [60–62]. The tumor control rates in these early studies with SBRT were 80%–90%, almost two fold the control seen with conventional radiotherapy [63]. Recent studies indicate that SBRT might be comparable to surgery in specific settings [3,64,65]

Conventionally, fractionated radiotherapy gave 60–66 Gy in 1.8–2 Gy fractions with relatively poor 5-year local control, ranging from 30% to 50% and overall survival rates of 10%–30% in early stage inoperable patients [66]. These conventional radiotherapy regimens were based upon the "Four Rs" of radiation biology: normal

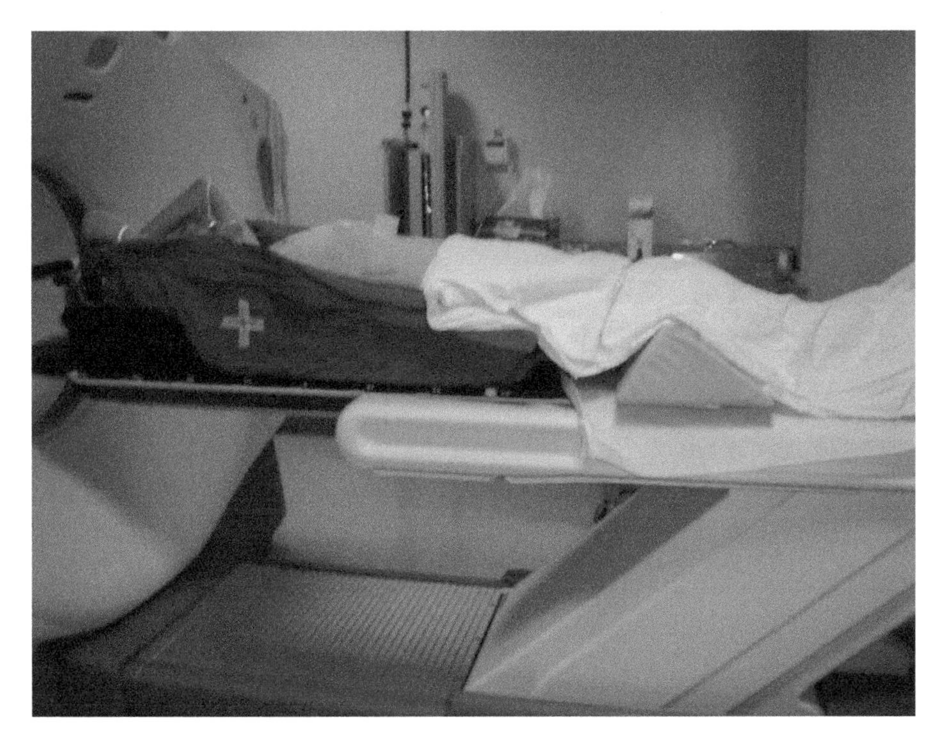

Figure 11.2 Example of SBRT immobilization at MD Anderson Cancer Center for a lung SBRT patient.

tissue repair of sub-lethal damage, repopulation, re-oxygenation and reassortment of cells in the cell cycle. This helps to give normal tissues a chance to rebound between radiotherapy fractions; however, this unfortunately also gives rebound times for the tumor. Protracted radiotherapy can offer surviving tumor cells time to repopulate and spread. SBRT reduces the overall treatment time and minimizes the chance for tumors to regrow during treatment. In addition, high radiation could damage cancer cells and release tumor associated antigen and danger signals that could function as a tumor specific vaccine in situ. In addition, high dose radiation can cause the damage of epithelial cell of small blood vessel in tumor bed and make it more accessible to immune cytotoxic T cells. However, the high doses delivered in SBRT's must be carefully chosen to spare normal tissues from harm.

In radiation biology, the biologically effective dose (BED) is a means to compare different fractionation regimens to assess their effect on tumor and normal tissues. The BED is calculated using the formula

$$\mathrm{BED} = n \times d[1 + d/(\alpha/\beta)]$$

where n is the number of fractions, d is the dose per fraction, the α/β ratio is the dose where cell killing from linear and quadratic components of the linear quadratic cell survival curve equation are equal. Typically, the α/β ratio is 10 Gy for acute effects and 3 Gy for late effects. [66]. After researchers have used varying high dose regimens with a wide array of BEDs, early stage patients who had been treated by SBRT with BEDs> 100 Gy performed better in a large Japanese multi-institutional study [66–68]. The overall survival rate of patients in the study who received BEDs ≥ 100 Gy had 5-year overall survival rate of 88.4% compared to 69.4% for patients with BEDs < 100 Gy [66].

11.4.1 SBRT PATIENT SELECTION CRITERIA

Early-stage NSCLC is typically treated with surgical resection and mediastinal lymph node dissection if the patient is medically operable, while inoperable patients and patients who refuse surgery are considered for stereotactic body radiation therapy. There is a growing body of retrospective evidence and population-based studies that suggest that local control, regional control, distant metastases, and overall survival can be comparable in matched cohort analyses for SBRT and surgery. A recently published pooled analysis from two independent randomized Phase III trials, StereoTActic Radiotherapy vs Surgery (STARS) and Radiosurgery or Surgery for Operable Early Stage non-small cell Lung cancer (ROSEL) of SBRT vs surgery in patients with operable Stage I NSCLC showed at least comparable outcomes between the two modalities [3]. However, only 58 patients were enrolled and evaluated in this pooled analysis, and additional randomized studies comparing these two modalities in operable patients will be warranted.

Although the selection criteria for SBRT patients are expanding to potentially include surgical candidates, there are instances that contra-indicate the use of SBRT. A lung lesion is considered centrally located if it is within 2 cm in each direction of the proximal bronchial tree (carina, right and left bronchi, bronchial tree to the second bifurcation, may include the esophagus, heart, brachial plexus, major vessels, spinal cord, phrenic nerve, recurrent laryngeal nerve and or adjacent to mediastinal or pericardial pleura [69]. Centrally located lesions have shown higher toxicity rates from SBRT than peripheral lesions [64] when using a 3-fraction dose regime. However, other studies have shown these lesions can be treated safely and effectively with alternative dose regimes. Two-year freedom from severe toxicity rates were only 54% for patients with centrally located tumors compared to 84% in peripheral tumors for a phase II study of 60–66 Gy in 3 fractions [64]. The main toxicities for patients with centrally located lesions treated were pleural effusion, pneumonia and worsening shortness of breath, fatal hemoptysis and fistula. The most common toxicities for SBRT treatments tended to be radiation pneumonitis, while rib fractures and chest wall pain can occur in patients with lesions close to their chest wall [64].

11.4.2 Dose-volume constraints

To avoid acute and chronic toxicity, it is very important to keep the dose volume of normal critical structures to a minimum. Most dose volume constraints have been developed based on experience with conventional fractionation regimens and RBE calculation. As we have developed experience with SBRT we could refine these, based on clinical experience with 4 fraction treatment regiments [70–73] for both 50 Gy in 10 fractions and 70 Gy in 10 fractions (Table 11.1)

If the potential SBRT patient has had previous radiation therapy treatment, then the attending radiation oncologist needs to evaluate the previous treatment plan, especially the dose delivered to critical structures, and make a clinical judgment based on BED, previous radiation therapy, and current SBRT doses using the above dose-volume constraints as a guide. A composite plan with the previous and current doses of radiation therapy is helpful when assessing the safety and quality of the current treatment plan.

Table 11.1 M. D. Anderson Cancer Center early-stage NSCLC with 50 Gy in 4 fractions prescribed to the PTV dose constraints

Total lung	**Mean lung dose ≤ 6 Gy; V5 ≤ 30%; V10 ≤ 17%; V20 ≤ 12%; V30 ≤ 7%**
Ipsilateral lung	Mean lung dose ≤ 10 Gy; V10 ≤ 35%; V20 ≤ 25%; V30 ≤ 15%
Esophagus	Dmax ≤ 35 Gy; V30 ≤ 1 cm^3
Trachea	V35 ≤ 1 cm^3
Bronchial tree	Dmax ≤ 38 Gy; V35 ≤ 1 cm^3
Heart	Dmax ≤ 45 Gy; V40 ≤ 1 cm^3; V20 ≤ 5 cm^3
Brachial plexus	Dmax ≤ 35 Gy; V30 ≤ 0.2 cm^3
Hilar major vessels	V40 ≤ 1 cm^3
Spinal cord	Dmax < 25 Gy; V20 < 1 cm^3
Chest wall	V30 < 30 cm^3
Skin	V30 < 50 cm^3

Source: Li, Q. et al., *Radiother Oncol.*, **112**, 2, 256–61, 2014; Welsh, J. et al., *Int J Radiat Oncol Biol Phys.*, **81**, 1, 91–6, 2011; Evans, J.D. et al., *Radiother Oncol.*, **109**, 1, 82–8, 2013; Chang, J. et al., *J Thorac Oncol.*, **10**, 4, 577–585, 2015.

11.4.3 SBRT PROGRAM REQUIREMENTS

11.4.3.1 PERSONNEL

11.4.3.1.1 Radiation oncologist

The radiation oncologist for SBRT should be certified in Radiation Oncology or Therapeutic Radiology by the American Board of Radiology or similar certifying body with proof of adequate physician training with specialty training in the delivery of SBRT. Also, it is recommended that the radiation oncologist have successfully completed an Accreditation Council for Graduate Medical Education (ACGME) approved residency program or similar approved residency program [74] (Table 11.2).

11.4.3.1.2 Qualified medical physicist

The qualified medical physicist for an SBRT program should be certified by the American Board of Radiology or a similar certifying body in a related subfield such as Therapeutic Radiological Physics or Radiological Physics and satisfy all state licensing criteria. The qualified medical physicist should also meet the ACR guidelines for Continuing Medical Education (CME). The qualified medical physicist is responsible each technical aspect of SBRT from imaging, treatment planning, dose delivery and quality assurance testing for the equipment and process.

Table 11.2 Roles of Personnel in SBRT Program Per American Society for Therapeutic Radiology and Oncology (ASTRO) and American College of Radiology (ACR) Practice Guideline for the Performance of Stereotactic Body Radiation Therapy

Personnel	Responsibility
Radiation Oncologist	Manage the overall-disease specific treatment regimen including post-treatment follow-up and receiving informed consent from patient regarding treatment.
	Determine and recommend proper patient positioning for simulation and treatment.
	Determine and recommend procedures to account for tumor volume motion.
	Supervise the patient's simulation to ensure proper imaging modalities are being used.
	Contour all necessary anatomy for radiation treatment plan.
	Prescribe the case-specific radiation dose, set limits for normal structures, participate in the treatment planning optimization process and approve the final treatment plan in collaboration with a medical physicist.
	Directly supervise and attend the actual treatment process.
Medical Physicist	Performing acceptance testing and commissioning of the SBRT system to ensure geometric and dosimetric accuracy.
	Implement and manage a quality control program to monitor the precision and accuracy of the entire SBRT system from the image guidance system to beam delivery.
	Directly supervise and check the treatment planning process.
	Establish a procedure or quality control checklist for the entire treatment process
	Communicate with the radiation oncologist to optimize treatment plan.
	Check the treatment plan approved by the radiation oncologist. Identify and correct any errors. Evaluate the appropriateness of the plan with respect to beam parameters and normal tissue constraints.
	Ensure that the treatment accurately fulfils the prescription approved by the radiation oncologist.
Radiation Therapist	Prepare the treatment room for the SBRT procedure.
	Assist the SBRT treatment team with patient positioning and immobilization.
	Operate the treatment unit after both the radiation oncologist and qualified medical physicist have given their approval for the clinical and technical aspects for beam delivery.

11.4.3.1.3 Radiation therapist

The radiation therapist for an SBRT program should fulfill all state licensing criteria as well as being certified by the American Registry of Radiologic Technologists (ARRT) in radiation therapy.

11.4.3.2 EQUIPMENT

Per the American Association of Physicists in Medicine (AAPM) Task Group 101 on SBRT, the current linear accelerators with image guidance capabilities should be adequate to perform SBRT [75] (Tables 11.2 and 11.3). The only difference in tolerance for SBRT linac requirements are covered in AAPM's Task Group 142 which specifies the following tolerances for SRS/SBRT linacs daily [76] (Table 11.4).

11.4.3.3 QUALITY ASSURANCE

As mentioned earlier, the qualified medical physicist is responsible for performing all quality assurance testing for the entire SBRT system. The acceptance testing, commissioning and routine quality assurance testing of all equipment, the record and verify system, the treatment planning software, the treatment plan, the training of the SBRT staff, and all other components of the SBRT program are the responsibility of the qualified medical physicist.

AAPM's Task Group 101 on SBRT suggests in full detail what needs to be covered by the qualified medical physicist's quality assurance program (Table 11.3). Namely, the physicist should ensure that their quality assurance program for their SBRT practice includes exhaustive testing of all components of the SBRT system, both individually and in conjunction with the other components. The tests should cover everything from the robustness of the simulation imaging dataset acquisition and subsequent transfer to the treatment planning software, to the dose calculation algorithms, MU calculation algorithms, secondary calculations, delivery precision and accuracy of small fields/MUs, patient immobilization devices, motion tracking, gating, and so forth. The AAPM and other organizations have published several task groups and reports that outline suggestions for commissioning and quality assurance for devices used in SBRT programs that should be consulted by the qualified medical physicist [35,74,76–83].

One of the most crucial aspects of SBRT treatment delivery that needs to be verified is the coincidence of the radiation, mechanical and imaging iso-centers [35,84]. This includes couch rotation and laser alignment which all should agree with the radiation iso-center. Several tests exist to help confirm this, such

Table 11.3 From AAPM Task Group 101, Comparison of 3D/IMRT and SBRT

Characteristic	3D/IMRT	SBRT
Dose/fraction	1.8–3 Gy	6–30 Gy
# of fractions	10–30	1–5
Target Definition	CTV/PTV (gross disease)	GTV/CTV/ITV/PTV (well-defined tumors, GTV=CTV)
Margin	cm	mm
Physics/Dosimetry monitoring	indirect	direct
Required Setup Accuracy	AAPM TG40	AAPM TG142
Primary Imaging modalities For treatment planning	CT	CT/MR/PET-CT
Maintenance of spatial accuracy Moderately enforced for entire treatment		Strictly enforced (rigid immobilization of patient)
Need for Respiratory management	Moderate	Highest
Staff training	Highest	Highest+special SBRT training
Technology implementation	Highest	Highest
Radiobiological Understanding	Moderately understood	Poorly understood
Interaction with systemic therapies	Yes	Yes

Table 11.4 AAPM's Task Group 142 which specifies the following tolerances for SRS/SBRT Linacs daily

Tolerance	Procedure
3%	Dosimetry, x-ray, and electron output constancy
1 mm	Laser localization and collimator size indicator
Functional	Machine safety features (door interlock, audiovisual monitors, etc)
AAPM's Task Group 142 specifies the following tolerances monthly for SBRT linacs:	
Tolerance	Procedure
2%	Dosimetry, x-ray, and electron output constancy (@stereo dose rate,MU)
1 mm/0.5°	Mechanicals (Laser localization, light/radiation coincidence, etc.)
Functional	Machine safety features (door interlock, audiovisual monitors, etc.)

as the Winston-Lutz test [85]. Other tests which may also help with end-to-end testing for localization accuracy, intrafraction targeting variability and positioning accuracy include stereo x-ray/DRR fusion, hidden target test with implanted fiducials in a phantom and portal image compared to cone beam CT image iso-center coincidence test [84–92]. It is highly recommended that an end-to-end test be performed before treating the first patient in a new SBRT program including any motion management used by the institution.

11.4.4 Simulation for SBRT

The radiation therapy treatment delivery process first begins with the patient simulation. The simulation is required to visualize the patient anatomy, and provide the treatment planning software with the necessary information for dose calculation and localization. The patient's simulation dataset is usually derived from a computed tomography scan performed in the treatment position with all necessary immobilization equipment in place. A well-conducted simulation will include the radiation oncologist, the qualified medical physicist and the therapist staff to ensure all information regarding the patient's specific medical history, SBRT target, normal structures and optimal treatment delivery technique is communicated effectively to all parties involved in the SBRT treatment. After the simulation, it is recommended to document all notes regarding the imaging and patient setup information in the patient's chart.

Target delineation for lung tumors is complicated due to the respiration-induced motion or interfractional tumor motion as this can lead to increased geometric uncertainty during radiation treatment. To safely and effectively treat tumors that move with respiration, a method must be developed to create treatment plans that are robust with respect to these motions. The most important step in doing so, is to build a target volume that that considers the changes in target position over the course of radiotherapy [93]. ICRU 62 established a framework for working with the uncertainness associated with target and normal tissue motion and deformation, the internal margin (IM), and with daily setup uncertainties, the setup margin (SM) [94,95]. This document, however, did not establish how to determine these margins or how best to design a treatment plan taking these margins into account. The most common method of incorporating these margins is to cover the entire envelope of motion of the clinical target volume (CTV) with the full prescription dose. Since this publication, several groups have investigated more complicated ways of ensuring good target coverage without expanding the margins to cover the entire range of respiratory motion [96–99], but this work is beyond the scope of this chapter.

11.4.5 4D-CT and free-breathing gated simulation

The simulation approach most widely used for SBRT lung tumors is 4D-CT where the 4th dimension is respiratory phase. In 4D-CT a series of three-dimensional (3D) CT datasets are created each of which represents the patient's anatomy during a different breathing phase [8,24,100–104]. There are two methods currently commercially available to create a 4D-CT dataset, one is based on a slow helical acquisition and the other is based on continuous axial sampling, cine mode. In either mode, the respiratory phase is determined by some type of respiratory monitor that uses the patient's external anatomy to estimate the respiratory phase. The two most common devices include, a reflective marker block that is placed on the patient's abdomen and is tracked by a computer [105–107], and the other measures the expansion of the abdomen using a belt [108–113]. Newer systems that determine breathing phase based on internal anatomy are becoming commercially available now (General Electric's "Smart Deviceless 4D") [114]. 4D-CT is commercially available for all major CT vendors. The choice of which system should be used is dependent on the individual institution's needs and resources as all system have benefits and drawbacks

The 4D-CT scan can be used for treatment planning of patients who will be treated with phase-based gating or with no gating using an internal target volume (ITV) approach. In phase-based gating the respiratory phase of the patient is monitored during treatment, and the treatment beam is only enabled during a restricted number of phases, generally those around end-exhale. If the patient will be treated with phase-based gating, the plan can be generated on a restricted set of the images from the 4D-CT that correspond to the phases that will be enabled for beam-on at the time of treatment. Several gating devices are available such as Varian's Real-time Position Management (RPM) system that was introduced in the early 2000s and Siemens' AZ-733C Anzai belt that measures respiratory signal with a strain gauge [2]. For an ITV approach all phases of the 4D-CT are used to create the target volume and no respiratory monitor is used during treatment.

If 4D-CT is not available, another approach to estimate the tumor position through the respiratory cycle is to use breath-hold scans at normal inhalation and exhalation [115–118]. To use these datasets, we assume that the union of the target volumes at full inhale and full exhale would give the complete trajectory of the tumor motion. For the patient to hold their breath at normal inhalation or exhalation, some form of feedback was required to help them get to the correct level and to hold their breath at that level throughout the scan. Even with this feedback, these techniques tended to overestimate tumor motion as the anatomy moves differently during normal breathing during breath-hold. If the patient was not given feedback, the breath-hold levels, as measured by tumor position, lung volume, or external fiducials, were often far more than the same parameters as measured during normal breathing [119]. However, these breath-hold methods are useful when 4D-CT is not available and can be quickly implemented on nearly any CT scanner with low cost equipment [120].

11.4.6 BH SIMULATION AND TREATMENT

An alternative approach to the management of respiratory motion is to image and treat under breath-hold. Breath-holds can be performed at inhale or exhale and can be voluntary as in the case of Varian's RPM device or forced as in the case of Elekta's "active-breathing control" (ABC) device [2,121]. Forced shallow breathing by way of abdominal compression, has also been investigated to minimize uncertainty in tumor position [122]. All systems for breath-hold require some type of feedback to the operator and/or patient on the level of the breath-hold maintained based on a surrogate. Furthermore, the reliability of the surrogate to predict the position of the tumor must also be determined on a patient-by-patient basis. When treating with breath-hold, it is also important to note that the patient's anatomy during breath-hold is not entirely representative of any of the phases of the 4D-CT.

The choice to treat with inhale or exhale should be made based on the changes in the tumor position and the normal anatomy. Typically, deep-inspiration breath-hold (DIBH) is chosen for breath-hold simulation and treatments in lung cases since it increases the distance between target and critical structures [2].

11.4.7 IMMOBILIZATION AND PATIENT POSITIONING

Patient positioning during the SBRT simulation and treatment delivery is critical to maintaining the tight margins associated with SBRT. It is important to reproduce the patient's positioning at the time of simulation during treatment. It is more important to maintain the relationship between the couch and the GTV throughout each fraction. This relationship is maintained by good immobilization that is indexed to the couch. This immobilization must be snug to the patient and rigid. The device should help to maintain body and arm position and be long enough to keep the abdomen aligned with the chest. The patient should have skin marks applied or have other anatomical landmarks that enable them to be reproducibility placed in the immobilization device each day.

At our institution, it is routine to utilize patient skin marks for aligning the patient in the craniocaudal axis to the immobilization device as well as use separate marks for determining the patient's rotation within the device. This should get the patient's position close enough to the final position as determined by in-room CT such that the magnitude of these shifts can be used as an effective QA on the position and should generally be less than 5 mm. In addition, if all the rules of good immobilization are followed on each day, the consistency of the couch coordinates can be used as a good QA metric.

The final treatment position decided upon for the patient should be comfortable enough for the patient to stay in place properly for the expected length of the treatment and simulation. Several SBRT immobilization products are available for use such as body aquaplast molds, vacuum molds, thermoplastic masks, immobilization cushions, compression devices, and others (Figure 11.2) [66,74,80,123–127].

11.4.8 Treatment planning for SBRT

In SBRT planning, the goal is to give a very high dose per fraction to the GTV with the maximum possible falloff to spare nearby critical structures [75]. This is generally accomplished by prescribing to a low iso-dose line to the planning target volume (PTV) (i.e. 80%) which simultaneously increases the dose to the GTV while better sparing nearby critical structures (Figure 11.3). This was intrinsic to 3D conformal radiotherapy, but with IMRT, this may not be necessary. However, some studies have indicated that hotspots within the central region of the target may be desirable, since radio resistant hypoxic tumor cells are thought to be in the interior of the tumor where the hot spots are generally located [75,128]. Recently, we analyzed our 1040 patients with stage I NSCLC treated with SBRT using 50 Gy in 4 fractions and 70 Gy in 10 fractions. We found that both PTVD95BED10 >85 Gy and PTVmeanBED10>130 Gy should be considered for optimal local control (Zhao et al., RED J 2016, in press). We recommend the minimum biologically effective dose (BED10) to 95% of planning target volume (PTVD95BED10) > 86 Gy (corresponding to PTV D95 physical dose of 42 Gy in 4 fractions or 55 Gy in 10 fractions) and PTVmean BED10 >130 Gy for PTVmean BED10 (corresponding to PTVmean physical dose of 55 Gy in 4 fractions or 75 Gy in 10 fractions). For our current practice, we intentionally create boosts to the GTV to increase mean GTV dose, while still sparing nearby critical structures as shown in Figures 11.3 and 11.4.

Treatment planning for lung tumors is made more difficult due to the presence of low-density lung tissue surrounding the lung tumors. In the case of lung SBRT fields, there is a loss of charged particle equilibrium that occurs when the lateral range of the incident electrons is on the order of size of the smaller field sizes and/or when there is not enough tissue around the target to establish electronic equilibrium [15]. This effect is worsened with higher energy beams due to the increased secondary electron ranges. Due to these issues, RTOG 0236 limits the use of field sizes less the 3.5 cm and energies above 10 MV [15,82,129,130]. Many groups have shown inaccuracies of dose calculations with pencil beam algorithms and AAPM Task Group 101 and others recommend that they not be used for Lung SBRT. Convolution superposition, Monte Carlo, and more recently, analytic algorithms have been validated for lung SBRT [11,131–135].

Treatment planning should be done with many beams (IMRT or 3D-CRT) or with sufficient arc angles (Conformal-Arc or Volumetric Arc Therapy (VMAT)) to ensure there is a sharp fall of outside of the target area and that skin dose is kept below constraints (Figures 11.3 and 11.4). RTOG 0813 recommends seven or more non-coplanar, non-opposing static beams should be used for static gantry delivery or 340 degrees for all arcs when using moving gantry delivery [136]. We have found that good plans can be developed using only co-planar beams which reduces the total volume of the lung in the treated volume as well as simplifies delivery. We have found that when using VMAT techniques, good plans can be achieved with arcs covering 200° of arc angle. In both IMRT and VMAT, we try to avoid beams that enter through the contralateral lung. This is consistent with our planning practice for non-SBRT cases and helps to avoid collisions at the time of treatment for lateral tumors.

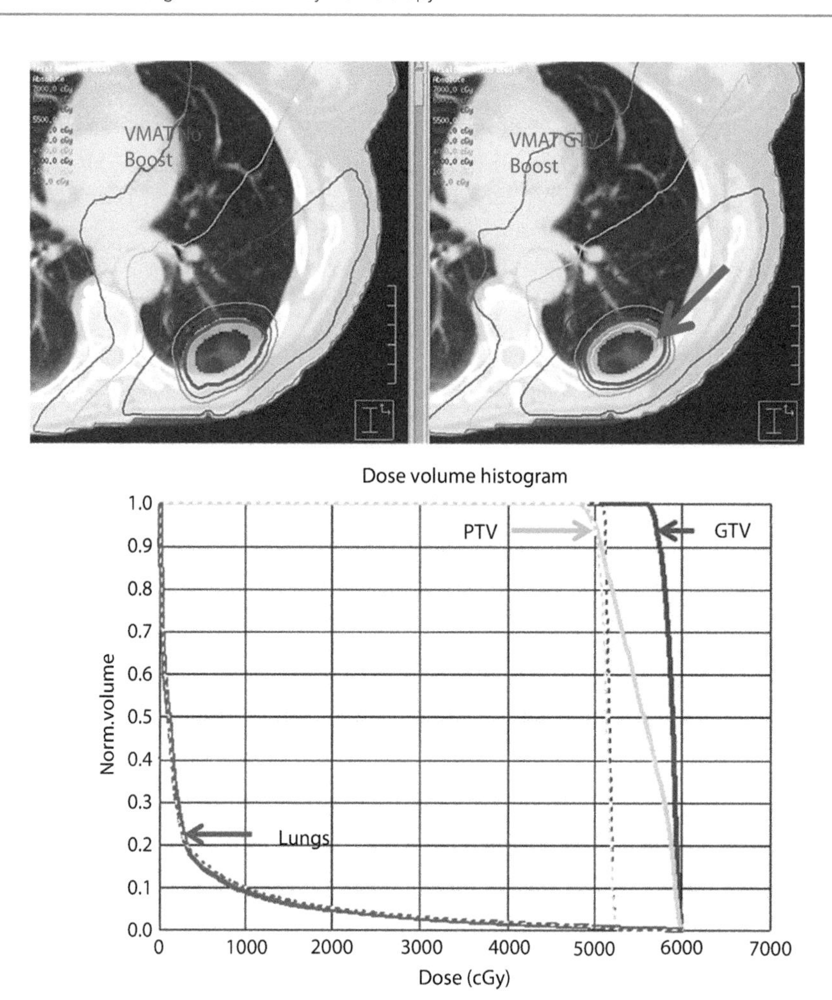

Figure 11.3 Transverse views of two SBRT VMAT plans are shown. Both plans were prescribed to 50 Gy in 4 fractions, but the plan without a boost was prescribed to 92% of maximum dose, while the boost plan was prescribed to 83% maximum dose. The yellow contour shown in the transverse views indicates the 55 Gy boost to the GTV in the boost plan. The DVH shows the coverage for the boost plan in solid lines and the coverage for the no boost plan is shown in dashed lines. Please note the increase in GTV mean dose from 51.7 Gy in the no boost plan to 58.7 Gy in the boost plan. Also, the PTV95BED10 > 85 Gy for both plans. The PTV mean physical dose > 55 Gy and the PTVmeanBED10 > 130 Gy in the boost plan.

When forward planning is used, the field aperture size and shape should be like the PTV's projection along the beam's-eye view. The 60%–90% prescription iso-dose lines should cover the PTV and hotspots should only be allowed in the target or GTV. We have found that placing the block edges at the edge of the PTV in the lateral and AP projections and a few mm greater than the PTV in the cranial-caudal directions gives good fall-off outside the PTV. When using inverse planning, constraints and false-structures should be used to achieve sharp falloff outside the PTV. Dose homogeneity constraints should not be used inside of the PTV.

11.4.9 Delivery systems and techniques for SBRT

Several treatment systems are available to perform SBRT including traditional linear accelerators (Linacs), proton accelerators and dedicated SBRT machines such as CyberKnife® and ViewRay®. In addition, on the Linacs, SBRT can be delivered with 3D-conformal, IMRT, or VMAT techniques. Protons may be

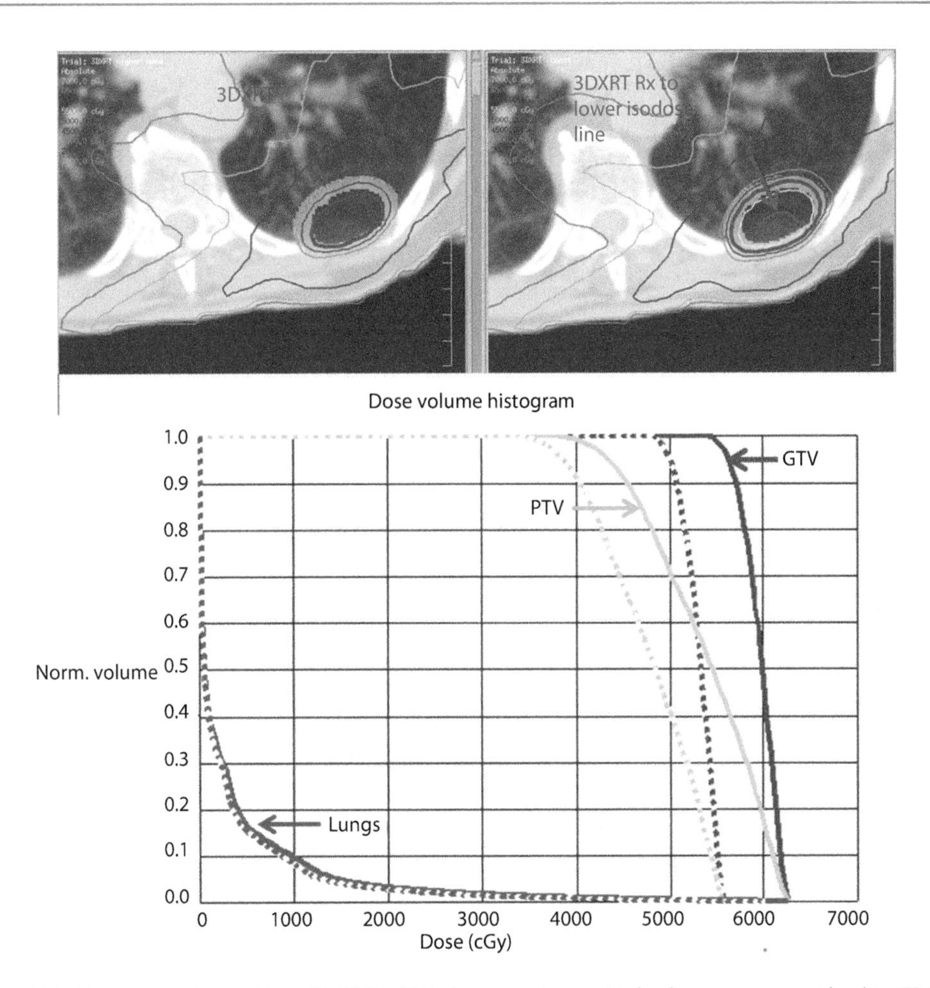

Figure 11.4 Transverse views of two SBRT 3DXRT plans are shown. Both plans were prescribed to 50 Gy in 4 fractions, but the first plan was prescribed to 90% of maximum dose, while the other plan was prescribed to a lower iso-dose line, 80% maximum dose. The red contour shown in the transverse views shows how the GTV is covered by the 60 Gy iso-dose line when the plan is prescribed to 80% maximum dose vs 90%. The DVH shows the difference in coverage for the lower iso-dose line prescribed plan in solid lines and the coverage for the higher iso-dose line prescribed plan is shown in dashed lines. Please note the PTV95BED10 > 85 Gy for both plans. The PTV mean physical dose was 55 Gy and the PTVmeanBED10 was 126 Gy for the 3DXRT lower prescribed iso-dose line plan.

produced as scattered or scanned beams. Each delivery system and technique has their advantages and disadvantages.

When using conventional Linacs to deliver SBRT treatments, there are several treatment options available for the SBRT treatment planner to use, such as standard 3D-conformal technique, IMRT, and volumetric arc therapy (VMAT).

Traditionally, 3D-CRT for SBRT would use 7–10 beams with couch kicks (i.e. non-coplanar beams) when needed to provide better tumor coverage, and dose fall-off with tight margins to spare nearby normal structures. 3D-CRT requires forward planning expertise since beam angles must be selected to produce the desired conformal target coverage while minimizing dose to critical structures. This forward planning process is manual and labor-intensive as beam weights, angles and MLC positions must be adjusted directly by the treatment planner.

In the case of IMRT or VMAT, inverse planning is employed. IMRT uses several beams collimated to the target with varying intensities all designed to target the tumor volume while sparing normal structures

[23]. The treatment planner creates optimization objectives, increase the weight on the objectives for target coverage and avoidance structures, avoid uniform dose objectives for target and use false treatment planning structures to create the desired steep dose fall-off. In addition to the benefits of IMRT, over 3D-conformal radiotherapy includes that IMRT plans may be easier to create than 3DCRT plans especially with modern automated optimization tools [137,138]. IMRT can also provide lower doses to nearby critical organs given its ability to modulate dose. However, IMRT may require more MUs or longer treatment times and there is the potential for interplay effect to occur if motion management is not used and the motion between the target and the MLCs is not synchronized [139] but this is small if the plan is generated with reasonable modulation [140].

VMAT is comparable to the delivery of several IMRT fields, but the treatment is delivered in arcs. VMAT can deliver treatment in a reduced amount of time, with increased high-dose conformality, when compared with IMRT. However, VMAT can create a larger volume of low dose in the surrounding tissues given the larger number of incident beam angles [136,139,141–143].

Proton therapy is another option for treating lung SBRT. The primary advantage of proton therapy is its characteristic Bragg Peak, which causes the proton beam to deliver most of its energy at the end of its finite range [144]. There are two main ways to deliver proton therapy: passive scattering or intensity modulated proton therapy (IMPT). Passive scattering proton therapy uses 3D-conformal proton treatment planning with compensators to form conformal dose distributions and an aperture to define the field shape [144]. Like IMRT for photons, IMPT uses scanning beam therapy to simultaneously optimize and adjust the intensities and energies of the pencil beams using similar objective functions to what is used in IMRT to target the tumor while sparing nearby critical structures. A treatment planning study by Register et al. showed IMPT capable of providing ablative doses to tumor targets and significantly sparing normal tissues compared to conventional 3D-conformal photon radiotherapy in stage 1 NSCLC centrally or superiorly located lesions [144]. However, the main concerns with proton treatments include range uncertainties, and the sensitivity of protons to any anatomic changes or target motion. Protons are greatly affected by the electron density they pass through, so in the case of lung SBRT, the effects of travelling through chest to lung must be considered. For optimal tumor coverage, one typically creates a less conformal high dose region to account for these uncertainties [145]. Also, any anatomic changes over the course of treatment can affect the proton dose distribution, therefore, adaptive planning is usually recommended for proton treatments. Finally, since lung lesions are mobile, caution should be used to validate tumor position when using proton techniques [144,146]. Most proton centers are limited to only having static on-board kilo-voltage x-ray imaging capabilities when volumetric imaging would be better-suited to assist with daily alignment.

CyberKnife is the alternative to typical rigid linac-based radiotherapy. This image-guided stereotactic imaging radiosurgery system utilizes a 6 MV linac mounted to a robotic arm capable of delivering 50–100 non-isocentric beams to targets within the patient [147–153]. CyberKnife uses an integrated stereoscopic kV imaging system to monitor patient position during the treatment. CyberKnife generally patients lie directly on the treatment couch with only fiducial markers placed on their anatomy which can be compared to their bony anatomy and digitally reconstructed radiographs (DRRs) derived from the CT simulation dataset to assess motion during treatment. CyberKnife uses the Synchrony® Respiratory Tracking system to dynamically compensate for respiratory motion. Synchrony optically tracks the external fiducial markers on the patient and predicts the tumor motion which then guides the robotic arm as it tracks the tumor. Studies have shown that although CyberKnife may give higher doses to normal lung for posterior tumors than other linac-based methods and require more MUs for treatment, it is comparable to standard rigid linac-based SBRT treatment methods [154]. CyberKnife SBRT treatment plans use more beams than regular linac-based treatments, on the order of >100 beams for CyberKnife in some cases compared to 7–10 beams for typical 3D-conformal treatments.

The most recent innovation in SBRT delivery is the use of magnetic resonance imaging (MRI) for real-time image guidance during treatment. A commercially available system (MRIdian®, ViewRay, Oakwood Village, OH) was released in 2014. The system provides simultaneous MR imaging and external beam radiotherapy from 3 ^{60}Co sources [155,156]. During treatment, targets or normal structures can be monitored in the sagittal plane at 4 frames/sec or in 3 parallel sagittal planes at 2 frames/sec. The system has an integrated adaptive radiotherapy treatment planning system with auto-contouring, Monte Carlo dose calculation and IMRT or 3D conformal planning capabilities which allows for adaptive planning each day since the dose calculations can be done in 30 seconds or less [156]. The drawbacks for this system include the low field strength of the magnet and the beam characteristics of ^{60}Co which include lower output, shallower penetration, larger penumbra and higher surface dose than a conventional linac [156,157].

11.4.10 SBRT TREATMENT DELIVERY

The treatment delivery process for thoracic SBRT cases depends upon the equipment chosen to deliver the treatment. For illustration of the process, we present the most common workflow in SBRT which is the delivery with a CBCT equipped traditional linear accelerator.

1. Perform necessary machine-specific QA to ensure imaging and treatment iso-centers are coincident. This may be covered by the normal daily QA of the treatment machine.
2. Prepare treatment couch with the patient-specific immobilization devices and other accessories present at simulation.
3. Setup patient into treatment position based upon the patient setup during simulation using a combination of setup notes, photographs and skin marks.
4. Image patient in treatment position to identify final iso-center as identified by volumetric or static kVp imaging. Note any day to day shifts in iso-center coordinates. Final review of the alignment to the GTV should be approved by the treating physician.
    a. For lung or liver SBRT, it is recommended that the tumor is referenced to some nearby bony anatomy and that if the alignment to the tumor and to the bony anatomy changes by greater than 5 mm from the simulation, repeat imaging is acquired to ensure the new position is stable.
5. Move couch to treatment position as identified by imaging and verify that all beams can be delivered without a collision.
6. Perform a final check of patient treatment position with an imaging system that is independent of the imaging modality chosen for initial imaging such as an MV portal.
7. Deliver treatment beams while monitoring the patient for movement. Repeat step 4 if any movement is suspected.

11.5 SUMMARY

Stereotactic body radiotherapy is a technologically advanced treatment option that utilizes precisely focused, high dose beams to treat tumors. It confers high rates of local control and survival with minimal toxicity in inoperable patients. Strict guidelines and quality assurance programs need to be adhered to for the safe practice of SBRT. The entire SBRT treatment team including attending physician, physicist, therapist and dosimetrist must be full participants in the SBRT quality assurance program. Several recommendations are published which offer guidance on each aspect of the SBRT process [19,23,75–77,81,83,115,158]. The physicist's role is instrumental in designing the SBRT quality assurance program for their center and this should include checklists for each treatment (Table 11.5). Recent studies have indicated that SBRT's role in lung cancer management may expand to include operable patients and, new developments of immunotherapy drugs combined with SBRT may show promising results for metastatic patients [65,159–161]. SBRT is a burgeoning field with growing pools of data and quality assurance protocols to ensure its safe delivery.

Table 11.5 MD Anderson's thoracic SBRT QA daily checklist

Date: ______	Initials: ______
☐ Ceiling Laser agree with crosshair within 1 mm at 0° Gantry	☐ Lasers agree with wall marks
☐ Couch set to 0°	☐ Couch locking pedal up
☐ Camera locked in position	☐ QA done for previous patient
☐ D&I/Dose Tracking checked-No Plan Change	☐ Images/Screen Shots Approved
☐ If Δ >5 mm, do 2nd CT or ensure consistent with previous fx	☐ CAT alignment scanned/sent
☐ Couch coord. ≤ 1 cm from previous fx	☐ All fields delivered

Alignment	Vrt 1:	Lng 1:	Lat 1:	Vrt 2:	Lng 2:	Lat 2:
Initial Couch						
Bone						
GTV						
Δ(bone-GTV)						
Alignment	Vrt 1:	Lng 1:	Lat 1:	Vrt 2:	Lng 2:	Lat 2:
Bone						
GTV						
Δ(bone-GTV)						
AVG GTV						

REFERENCES

1. Tanoue, L.T. et al., Lung cancer screening. *Am J Respir Crit Care Med*, 2015. **191**(1): 19–33.
2. Giraud, P. and R. Garcia, Respiratory gating for radiotherapy: Main technical aspects and clinical benefits. *Bull Cancer*, 2010. **97**(7): 847–56.
3. Chang, J.Y. et al., Stereotactic ablative radiotherapy versus lobectomy for operable stage I non-small-cell lung cancer: A pooled analysis of two randomised trials. *Lancet Oncol*, 2015. **16**(6): 630–7.
4. Kang, K.H. et al., Complications from stereotactic body radiotherapy for lung cancer. *Cancers (Basel)*, 2015. **7**(2): 981–1004.
5. Chang, J.Y. et al., Image-guided radiation therapy for non-small cell lung cancer. *J Thorac Oncol*, 2008. **3**(2): 177–86.
6. Koch, N. et al., Evaluation of internal lung motion for respiratory-gated radiotherapy using MRI: Part I-correlating internal lung motion with skin fiducial motion. *Int J Radiat Oncol Biol Phys*, 2004. **60**(5): 1459–72.
7. Liu, H.H. et al., Evaluation of internal lung motion for respiratory-gated radiotherapy using MRI: Part II-margin reduction of internal target volume. *Int J Radiat Oncol Biol Phys*, 2004. **60**(5): 1473–83.
8. Liu, H.H. et al., Assessing respiration-induced tumor motion and internal target volume using four-dimensional computed tomography for radiotherapy of lung cancer. *Int J Radiat Oncol Biol Phys*, 2007. **68**(2): 531–40.
9. Miyakawa, A. et al., Early response and local control of stage I non-small-cell lung cancer after stereotactic radiotherapy: Difference by histology. *Cancer Sci*, 2013. **104**(1): 130–4.
10. De La Fuente Herman, T. et al., Stereotactic body radiation therapy (SBRT) and respiratory gating in lung cancer: Dosimetric and radiobiological considerations. *J Appl Clin Med Phys*, 2010. **11**(1): 3133.
11. Liu, H.W. et al., Clinical impact of using the deterministic patient dose calculation algorithm Acuros XB for lung stereotactic body radiation therapy. *Acta Oncol*, 2014. **53**(3): 324–9.
12. Senthi, S. et al., Outcomes of stereotactic ablative radiotherapy for central lung tumours: A systematic review. *Radiother Oncol*, 2013. **106**(3): 276–82.

13. Zhuang, T. et al., Dose calculation differences between Monte Carlo and pencil beam depend on the tumor locations and volumes for lung stereotactic body radiation therapy. *J Appl Clin Med Phys*, 2013. **14**(2): 4011.
14. Ge, H. et al., Quantification and minimization of uncertainties of internal target volume for stereotactic body radiation therapy of lung cancer. *Int J Radiat Oncol Biol Phys*, 2013. **85**(2): 438–43.
15. Glide-Hurst, C.K. and I.J. Chetty, Improving radiotherapy planning, delivery accuracy, and normal tissue sparing using cutting edge technologies. *J Thorac Dis*, 2014. **6**(4): 303–18.
16. Liao, Z.X. et al., Influence of technologic advances on outcomes in patients with unresectable, locally advanced non-small-cell lung cancer receiving concomitant chemoradiotherapy. *Int J Radiat Oncol Biol Phys*, 2010. **76**(3): 775–81.
17. Bissonnette, J.P. et al., Cone-beam computed tomographic image guidance for lung cancer radiation therapy. *Int J Radiat Oncol Biol Phys*, 2009. **73**(3): 927–34.
18. De Los Santos, J. et al., Image guided radiation therapy (IGRT) technologies for radiation therapy localization and delivery. *Int J Radiat Oncol Biol Phys*, 2013. **87**(1): 33–45.
19. Murphy, M.J. et al., The management of imaging dose during image-guided radiotherapy: Report of the AAPM Task Group 75. *Med Phys*, 2007. **34**(10): 4041–63.
20. Potters, L. et al., American Society for Therapeutic Radiology and Oncology (ASTRO) and American College of Radiology (ACR) practice guidelines for image-guided radiation therapy (IGRT). *Int J Radiat Oncol Biol Phys*, 2010. **76**(2): 319–25.
21. Verellen, D., M. De Ridder, and G. Storme, A (short) history of image-guided radiotherapy. *Radiother Oncol*, 2008. **86**(1): 4–13.
22. Chan, C. et al., Intensity-modulated radiotherapy for lung cancer: Current status and future developments. *J Thorac Oncol*, 2014. **9**(11): 1598–608.
23. Ezzell, G.A. et al., Guidance document on delivery, treatment planning, and clinical implementation of IMRT: Report of the IMRT Subcommittee of the AAPM Radiation Therapy Committee. *Med Phys*, 2003. **30**(8): 2089–115.
24. Li, H. et al., Patient-specific quantification of respiratory motion-induced dose uncertainty for step-and-shoot IMRT of lung cancer. *Med Phys*, 2013. **40**(12): 121712.
25. Baumann, P. et al., Factors important for efficacy of stereotactic body radiotherapy of medically inoperable stage I lung cancer. A retrospective analysis of patients treated in the Nordic countries. *Acta Oncol*, 2006. **45**(7): 787–95.
26. Hansen, A.T., J.B. Petersen, and M. Høyer, Internal movement, set-up accuracy and margins for stereotactic body radiotherapy using a stereotactic body frame. *Acta Oncol*, 2006. **45**(7): 948–52.
27. Murray, B., K. Forster, and R. Timmerman, Frame-based immobilization and targeting for stereotactic body radiation therapy. *Med Dosim*, 2007. **32**(2): 86–91.
28. Wachter, T. et al., Extracranial stereotaxic body irradiation: Preliminary results and the Orleans hospital experience. *Bull Cancer*, 2008. **95**(1): 153–60.
29. Belderbos, J. and J.J. Sonke, State-of-the-art lung cancer radiation therapy. *Expert Rev Anticancer Ther*, 2009. **9**(10): 1353–63.
30. Nill, S. et al., Online correction for respiratory motion: Evaluation of two different imaging geometries. *Phys Med Biol*, 2005. **50**(17): 4087–96.
31. Kunos, C.A. et al., Dynamic lung tumor tracking for stereotactic ablative body radiation therapy. *J Vis Exp*, 2015. (100): e52875.
32. Adler, J.R. et al., The CyberKnife: A frameless robotic system for radiosurgery. *Stereotact Funct Neurosurg*, 1997. **69**(1–4 Pt 2): 124–8.
33. Ramakrishna, N. et al., A clinical comparison of patient setup and intra-fraction motion using frame-based radiosurgery versus a frameless image-guided radiosurgery system for intracranial lesions. *Radiother Oncol*, 2010. **95**(1): 109–15.
34. Amer, A. et al., Imaging doses from the Elekta Synergy X-ray cone beam CT system. *Br J Radiol*, 2007. **80**(954): 476–82.
35. Bissonnette, J.P., Quality assurance of image-guidance technologies. *Semin Radiat Oncol*, 2007. **17**(4): 278–86.

36. Dietrich, L. et al., Linac-integrated 4D cone beam CT: First experimental results. *Phys Med Biol*, 2006. **51**(11): 2939–52.
37. Fave, X. et al., Can radiomics features be reproducibly measured from CBCT images for patients with non-small cell lung cancer? *Med Phys*, 2015. **42**(12): 6784.
38. Nardi, C. et al., Motion artefacts in cone beam CT: An in vitro study about the effects on the images. *Br J Radiol*, 2016. **89**(1058): 20150687.
39. Li, J. et al., Evaluation of Elekta 4D cone beam CT-based automatic image registration for radiation treatment of lung cancer. *Br J Radiol*, 2015. **88**(1053): 20140620.
40. Kalogeridi, M.A. et al., Challenges and choices in prostate cancer irradiation: From the three dimensional conformal radiotherapy to the era of intensity modulated, image-guided and adaptive radiation treatment. *Urol J*, 2014. **11**(6): 1925–31.
41. Zhong, Q. et al., Significance of image guidance to clinical outcomes for localized prostate cancer. *Biomed Res Int*, 2014. 2014: 860639.
42. Kunkler, I.H. et al., Review of current best practice and priorities for research in radiation oncology for elderly patients with cancer: The International Society of Geriatric Oncology (SIOG) task force. *Ann Oncol*, 2014. **25**(11): 2134–46.
43. Sermeus, A. et al., Advances in radiotherapy delivery for rectal cancer: A European perspective. *Expert Rev Gastroenterol Hepatol*, 2015. **9**(4): 393–7.
44. McCloskey, P. et al., Radical treatment of non-small cell lung cancer during the last 5 years. *Eur J Cancer*, 2013. **49**(7): 1555–64.
45. Humphrey, P., P. Cornes, and H. Al-Booz, Vaginal vault brachytherapy in endometrial cancer: Verifying target coverage with image-guided applicator placement. *Br J Radiol*, 2013. **86**(1023): 20120428.
46. Hajj, C. and K.A. Goodman, Role of radiotherapy and newer techniques in the treatment of GI cancers. *J Clin Oncol*, 2015. **33**(16): 1737–44.
47. Van De Voorde, L. et al., Image-guided stereotactic ablative radiotherapy for the liver: A safe and effective treatment. *Eur J Surg Oncol*, 2015. **41**(2): 249–56.
48. Bhatt, A.D. et al., Tumor volume change with stereotactic body radiotherapy (SBRT) for early-stage lung cancer: Evaluating the potential for adaptive SBRT. *Am J Clin Oncol*, 2015. **38**(1): 41–6.
49. Wu, C. et al., Re-optimization in adaptive radiotherapy. *Phys Med Biol*, 2002. **47**(17): 3181–95.
50. Fletcher, G.H., Hypofractionation: Lessons from complications. *Radiother Oncol*, 1991. **20**(1): 10–5.
51. Laughlin, J.S., Physical aspects of radiation treatment. Some past and present developments with implications for the future. *Am J Clin Oncol*, 1986. **9**(6): 463–75.
52. Bucci, M.K., A. Bevan, and M. Roach, Advances in radiation therapy: Conventional to 3D, to IMRT, to 4D, and beyond. *CA Cancer J Clin*, 2005. **55**(2): 117–34.
53. Mohan, R. et al., A comprehensive three-dimensional radiation treatment planning system. *Int J Radiat Oncol Biol Phys*, 1988. **15**(2): 481–95.
54. Brahme, A., J.E. Roos, and I. Lax, Solution of an integral equation encountered in rotation therapy. *Phys Med Biol*, 1982. **27**(10): 1221–9.
55. Kong, C. et al., A new index comparable to BED for evaluating the biological efficacy of hypofractionated radiotherapy schemes on early stage non-small cell lung cancer: Analysis of data from the literature. *Lung Cancer*, 2014. **84**(1): 7–12.
56. Nahum, A.E., The radiobiology of hypofractionation. *Clin Oncol (R Coll Radiol)*, 2015. **27**(5): 260–9.
57. Timmerman, R.D., C. Park, and B.D. Kavanagh, The North American experience with stereotactic body radiation therapy in non-small cell lung cancer. *J Thorac Oncol*, 2007. **2**(7 Suppl 3): S101–12.
58. Chang, B.K. and R.D. Timmerman, Stereotactic body radiation therapy: A comprehensive review. *Am J Clin Oncol*, 2007. **30**(6): 637–44.
59. Kavanagh, B.D., R. Timmerman, and J.L. Meyer, The expanding roles of stereotactic body radiation therapy and oligofractionation:toward a new practice of radiotherapy. *Front Radiat Ther Oncol*, 2011. **43**: 370–81.
60. Rombouts, S.J. et al., Systematic review of innovative ablative therapies for the treatment of locally advanced pancreatic cancer. *Br J Surg*, 2015. **102**(3): 182–93.

61. Tipton, K. et al., Stereotactic body radiation therapy: Scope of the literature. *Ann Intern Med*, 2011. **154**(11): 737–45.
62. Onishi, H. and T. Araki, Stereotactic body radiation therapy for stage I non-small-cell lung cancer: A historical overview of clinical studies. *Jpn J Clin Oncol*, 2013. **43**(4): 345–50.
63. Timmerman, R.D., J. Herman, and L.C. Cho, Emergence of stereotactic body radiation therapy and its impact on current and future clinical practice. *J Clin Oncol*, 2014. **32**(26): 2847–54.
64. Shirvani, S.M., J.Y. Chang, and J.A. Roth, Can stereotactic ablative radiotherapy in early stage lung cancers produce comparable success as surgery? *Thorac Surg Clin*, 2013. **23**(3): 369–81.
65. Rusthoven, C.G., B.D. Kavanagh, and S.D. Karam, Improved survival with stereotactic ablative radiotherapy (SABR) over lobectomy for early stage non-small cell lung cancer (NSCLC): Addressing the fallout of disruptive randomized data. *Ann Transl Med*, 2015. **3**(11): 149.
66. Chang, J.Y. and J.A. Roth, Stereotactic body radiation therapy for stage I non-small cell lung cancer. *Thorac Surg Clin*, 2007. **17**(2): 251–9.
67. Chi, A. et al., What would be the most appropriate α/β ratio in the setting of stereotactic body radiation therapy for early stage non-small cell lung cancer. *Biomed Res Int*, 2013. **2013**: 391021.
68. Hiraoka, M. and Y. Nagata, Stereotactic body radiation therapy for early-stage non-small-cell lung cancer: The Japanese experience. *Int J Clin Oncol*, 2004. **9**(5): 352–5.
69. Chang, J.Y. et al., Stereotactic ablative radiotherapy for centrally located early stage non-small-cell lung cancer: What we have learned. *J Thorac Oncol*, 2015. **10**(4): 577–85.
70. Li, Q. et al., Stereotactic ablative radiotherapy (SABR) using 70 Gy in 10 fractions for non-small cell lung cancer: Exploration of clinical indications. *Radiother Oncol*, 2014. **112**(2): 256–61.
71. Welsh, J. et al., Obesity increases the risk of chest wall pain from thoracic stereotactic body radiation therapy. *Int J Radiat Oncol Biol Phys*, 2011. **81**(1): 91–6.
72. Evans, J.D. et al., Cardiac ^{18}F-fluorodeoxyglucose uptake on positron emission tomography after thoracic stereotactic body radiation therapy. *Radiother Oncol*, 2013. **109**(1): 82–8.
73. Chang, J. et al., Stereotactic ablative radiotherapy for centrally located early stage non-small-cell lung cancer what we have learned. *J Thorac Oncol*, 2015. **10**(4): 577–585.
74. Potters, L. et al., American Society for Therapeutic Radiology and Oncology (ASTRO) and American College of Radiology (ACR) practice guideline for the performance of stereotactic body radiation therapy. *Int J Radiat Oncol Biol Phys*, 2010. **76**(2): 326–32.
75. Benedict, S.H. et al., Stereotactic body radiation therapy: The report of AAPM Task Group 101. *Med Phys*, 2010. **37**(8): 4078–101.
76. Klein, E.E. et al., Task Group 142 report: quality assurance of medical accelerators. *Med Phys*, 2009. **36**(9): 4197–212.
77. Bissonnette, J.P. et al., Quality assurance for image-guided radiation therapy utilizing CT-based technologies: A report of the AAPM TG-179. *Med Phys*, 2012. **39**(4): 1946–63.
78. Foote, M. et al., Guidelines for safe practice of stereotactic body (ablative) radiation therapy. *J Med Imaging Radiat Oncol*, 2015. **59**(5):646-53.
79. Sahgal, A. et al., The Canadian Association of Radiation Oncology scope of practice guidelines for lung, liver and spine stereotactic body radiotherapy. *Clin Oncol (R Coll Radiol)*, 2012. **24**(9): 629–39.
80. Solberg, T.D. et al., Quality assurance of immobilization and target localization systems for frameless stereotactic cranial and extracranial hypofractionated radiotherapy. *Int J Radiat Oncol Biol Phys*, 2008. **71**(1 Suppl): S131–5.
81. Solberg, T., TH-CD-BRB-04: ASTRO/AAPM Guidance On Quality and Safety in SRS and SBRT. *Med Phys*, 2015. **42**(6): 3725.
82. Timmerman, R. et al., Accreditation and quality assurance for Radiation Therapy Oncology Group: Multicenter clinical trials using Stereotactic Body Radiation Therapy in lung cancer. *Acta Oncol*, 2006. **45**(7): 779–86.
83. Williamson, J.F. et al., Quality assurance needs for modern image-based radiotherapy: Recommendations from 2007 interorganizational symposium on "quality assurance of radiation therapy: Challenges of advanced technology". *Int J Radiat Oncol Biol Phys*, 2008. **71**(1 Suppl): S2–12.

84. Nagafuchi, K. et al., Development of an automated method for analysis of Winston-Lutz test results using digital radiography and photostimulable storage phosphor. *Nihon Hoshasen Gijutsu Gakkai Zasshi*, 2013. **69**(11): 1266–73.
85. Lutz, W., K.R. Winston, and N. Maleki, A system for stereotactic radiosurgery with a linear accelerator. *Int J Radiat Oncol Biol Phys*, 1988. **14**(2): 373–81.
86. Du, W. et al., A quality assurance procedure to evaluate cone-beam CT image center congruence with the radiation isocenter of a linear accelerator. *J Appl Clin Med Phys*, 2010. **11**(4): 3297.
87. Gao, S. et al., Evaluation of IsoCal geometric calibration system for Varian linacs equipped with on-board imager and electronic portal imaging device imaging systems. *J Appl Clin Med Phys*, 2014. **15**(3): 4688.
88. Geyer, P. et al., Filmless evaluation of the mechanical accuracy of the isocenter in stereotactic radiotherapy. *Strahlenther Onkol*, 2007. **183**(2): 76–80.
89. Grimm, J. et al., A quality assurance method with submillimeter accuracy for stereotactic linear accelerators. *J Appl Clin Med Phys*, 2011. **12**(1): 3365.
90. Peace, T., B. Subramanian, and P. Ravindran, An experimental study on using a diagnostic computed radiography system as a quality assurance tool in radiotherapy. *Australas Phys Eng Sci Med*, 2008. **31**(3): 226–34.
91. Rowshanfarzad, P. et al., Verification of the linac isocenter for stereotactic radiosurgery using cine-EPID imaging and arc delivery. *Med Phys*, 2011. **38**(7): 3963–70.
92. Tatsumi, D. et al., Quality assurance procedure for assessing mechanical accuracy of a radiation field center in stereotactic radiotherapy. *Nihon Hoshasen Gijutsu Gakkai Zasshi*, 2012. **68**(10): 1333–9.
93. Killoran, J.H. et al., A numerical simulation of organ motion and daily setup uncertainties: Implications for radiation therapy. *Int J Radiat Oncol Biol Phys*, 1997. **37**(1): 213–21.
94. Muren, L. et al., Testing the new ICRU 62 'Planning Organ at Risk Volume' concept for the rectum. *Radiother Oncol*, 2005. **75**(3): 293–302.
95. Stroom, J. and B. Heijmen, Geometrical uncertainties, radiotherapy planning margins, and the ICRU-62 report. *Radiother Oncol*, 2002. **64**(1): 75–83.
96. McCann, C. et al., Lung sparing and dose escalation in a robust-inspired IMRT planning method for lung radiotherapy that accounts for intrafraction motion. *Med Phys*, 2013. **40**(6): 061705.
97. Rit, S. et al., Quantification of the variability of diaphragm motion and implications for treatment margin construction. *Int J Radiat Oncol Biol Phys*, 2012. **82**(3): e399–407.
98. Sonke, J.J., J. Lebesque, and M. van Herk, Variability of four-dimensional computed tomography patient models. *Int J Radiat Oncol Biol Phys*, 2008. **70**(2): 590–8.
99. Wolthaus, J.W. et al., Comparison of different strategies to use four-dimensional computed tomography in treatment planning for lung cancer patients. *Int J Radiat Oncol Biol Phys*, 2008. **70**(4): 1229–38.
100. Hurkmans, C.W. et al., Quality assurance of 4D-CT scan techniques in multicenter phase III trial of surgery versus stereotactic radiotherapy (radiosurgery or surgery for operable early stage (stage 1A) non-small-cell lung cancer [ROSEL] study). *Int J Radiat Oncol Biol Phys*, 2011. **80**(3): 918–27.
101. Low, D.A. et al., A method for the reconstruction of four-dimensional synchronized CT scans acquired during free breathing. *Med Phys*, 2003. **30**(6): 1254–63.
102. Persson, G.F. et al., Deviations in delineated GTV caused by artefacts in 4DCT. *Radiother Oncol*, 2010. **96**(1): 61–6.
103. Purdie, T.G. et al., Respiration correlated cone-beam computed tomography and 4DCT for evaluating target motion in Stereotactic Lung Radiation Therapy. *Acta Oncol*, 2006. **45**(7): 915–22.
104. Watkins, W.T. et al., Patient-specific motion artifacts in 4DCT. *Med Phys*, 2010. **37**(6): 2855–61.
105. Chang, Z. et al., Evaluation of integrated respiratory gating systems on a Novalis Tx system. *J Appl Clin Med Phys*, 2011. **12**(3): 3495.
106. Guana, H., Time delay study of a CT simulator in respiratory gated CT scanning. *Med Phys*, 2006. **33**(4): 815–9.
107. Kini, V.R. et al., Patient training in respiratory-gated radiotherapy. *Med Dosim*, 2003. **28**(1): 7–11.
108. Glide-Hurst, C.K. et al., Evaluation of two synchronized external surrogates for 4D CT sorting. *J Appl Clin Med Phys*, 2013. **14**(6): 4301.

109. Noel, C.E. and P.J. Parikh, Effect of mid-scan breathing changes on quality of 4DCT using a commercial phase-based sorting algorithm. *Med Phys*, 2011. **38**(5): 2430–8.
110. Thomas, D. et al., A novel fast helical 4D-CT acquisition technique to generate low-noise sorting artifact-free images at user-selected breathing phases. *Int J Radiat Oncol Biol Phys*, 2014. **89**(1): 191–8.
111. White, B. et al., Distribution of lung tissue hysteresis during free breathing. *Med Phys*, 2013. **40**(4): 043501.
112. White, B.M. et al., Physiologically guided approach to characterizing respiratory motion. *Med Phys*, 2013. **40**(12): 121723.
113. White, B.M. et al., Quantification of the thorax-to-abdomen breathing ratio for breathing motion modeling. *Med Phys*, 2013. **40**(6): 063502.
114. Liu, P., J. Dong, and S. Wang, Method for sorting ct image slices and method for constructing 3d ct image. 2013, Waukesha, WI: GE Medical Systems Global Technology Company. p. 11.
115. Keall, P.J. et al., The management of respiratory motion in radiation oncology report of AAPM Task Group 76. *Med Phys*, 2006. **33**(10): 3874–900.
116. Piermattei, A. et al., Real time transit dosimetry for the breath-hold radiotherapy technique: An initial experience. *Acta Oncol*, 2008. **47**(7): 1414–21.
117. Sager, O. et al., Evaluation of active breathing control-moderate deep inspiration breath-hold in definitive non-small cell lung cancer radiotherapy. *Neoplasma*, 2012. **59**(3): 333–40.
118. Wang, R. et al., High-dose-rate three-dimensional conformal radiotherapy combined with active breathing control for stereotactic body radiotherapy of early-stage non-small-cell lung cancer. *Technol Cancer Res Treat*, 2014. **14**(6): 677–82.
119. Balter, J.M. et al., Uncertainties in CT-based radiation therapy treatment planning associated with patient breathing. *Int J Radiat Oncol Biol Phys*, 1996. **36**(1): 167–74.
120. Peng, Y. et al., A new respiratory monitoring and processing system based on Wii remote: Proof of principle. *Med Phys*, 2013. **40**(7): 071712.
121. Brock, J. et al., The use of the Active Breathing Coordinator throughout radical non-small-cell lung cancer (NSCLC) radiotherapy. *Int J Radiat Oncol Biol Phys*, 2011. **81**(2): 369–75.
122. Bouilhol, G. et al., Is abdominal compression useful in lung stereotactic body radiation therapy? A 4DCT and dosimetric lobe-dependent study. *Phys Med*, 2013. **29**(4): 333–40.
123. Banki, F. et al., Stereotactic radiosurgery for lung cancer. *Minerva Chir*, 2009. **64**(6): 589–98.
124. Distefano, G. et al., Survey of stereotactic ablative body radiotherapy in the UK by the QA group on behalf of the UK SABR Consortium. *Br J Radiol*, 2014. **87**(1037): 20130681.
125. Hodge, W. et al., Feasibility report of image guided stereotactic body radiotherapy (IG-SBRT) with tomotherapy for early stage medically inoperable lung cancer using extreme hypofractionation. *Acta Oncol*, 2006. **45**(7): 890–6.
126. Hof, H., K. Herfarth, and J. Debus, Stereotactic irradiation of lung tumors. *Radiologe*, 2004. **44**(5): 484–90.
127. Lo, S.S. et al., Stereotactic body radiation therapy: A novel treatment modality. *Nat Rev Clin Oncol*, 2010. **7**(1): 44–54.
128. Gasinska, A. et al., Influence of overall treatment time and radiobiological parameters on biologically effective doses in cervical cancer patients treated with radiation therapy alone. *Acta Oncol*, 2004. **43**(7): 657–66.
129. Ding, G.X. et al., Impact of inhomogeneity corrections on dose coverage in the treatment of lung cancer using stereotactic body radiation therapy. *Med Phys*, 2007. **34**(7): 2985–94.
130. Hurkmans, C.W. et al., Dosimetric evaluation of heterogeneity corrections for RTOG 0236: Stereotactic body radiotherapy of inoperable Stage I-II non-small-cell lung cancer. In reply to Dr. Xiao et al. *Int J Radiat Oncol Biol Phys, 2009.* **75**(1): 318; author reply 318.
131. Seppala, J. et al., A dosimetric phantom study of dose accuracy and build-up effects using IMRT and RapidArc in stereotactic irradiation of lung tumours. *Radiat Oncol*, 2012. **7**: 79.
132. Huang, B. et al., Dose calculation of Acuros XB and Anisotropic Analytical Algorithm in lung stereotactic body radiotherapy treatment with flattening filter free beams and the potential role of calculation grid size. *Radiat Oncol*, 2015. **10**: 53.
133. Khan, R.F. et al., Effect of Acuros XB algorithm on monitor units for stereotactic body radiotherapy planning of lung cancer. *Med Dosim*, 2014. **39**(1): 83–7.

134. Ojala, J.J. et al., Performance of dose calculation algorithms from three generations in lung SBRT: Comparison with full Monte Carlo-based dose distributions. *J Appl Clin Med Phys*, 2014. **15**(2): 4662.
135. Tsuruta, Y. et al., Dosimetric comparison of Acuros XB, AAA, and XVMC in stereotactic body radiotherapy for lung cancer. *Med Phys*, 2014. **41**(8): 081715.
136. Rauschenbach, B.M., L. Mackowiak, and H.K. Malhotra, A dosimetric comparison of three-dimensional conformal radiotherapy, volumetric-modulated arc therapy, and dynamic conformal arc therapy in the treatment of non-small cell lung cancer using stereotactic body radiotherapy. *J Appl Clin Med Phys*, 2014. **15**(5): 4898.
137. Hazell, I. et al., Automatic planning of head and neck treatment plans. *J Appl Clin Med Phys*, 2016. **17**(1): 5901.
138. Quan, E.M. et al., Automated volumetric modulated Arc therapy treatment planning for stage III lung cancer: How does it compare with intensity-modulated radio therapy? *Int J Radiat Oncol Biol Phys*, 2012. **84**(1): e69–76.
139. Dickey, M. et al., A planning comparison of 3-dimensional conformal multiple static field, conformal arc, and volumetric modulated arc therapy for the delivery of stereotactic body radiotherapy for early stage lung cancer. *Med Dosim*, 2015. **40**(4): 347–51.
140. Court, L.E. et al., Use of a realistic breathing lung phantom to evaluate dose delivery errors. *Med Phys*, 2010. **37**(11): 5850–7.
141. Brock, J. et al., Optimising stereotactic body radiotherapy for non-small cell lung cancer with volumetric intensity-modulated arc therapy–a planning study. *Clin Oncol (R Coll Radiol)*, 2012. **24**(1): 68–75.
142. Sapkaroski, D., C. Osborne, and K.A. Knight, A review of stereotactic body radiotherapy - is volumetric modulated arc therapy the answer? *J Med Radiat Sci*, 2015. **62**(*2): 142–51.*
143. Teoh, M. et al., Volumetric modulated arc therapy: A review of current literature and clinical use in practice. *Br J Radiol*, 2011. **84**(1007): 967–96.
144. Register, S.P. et al., Proton stereotactic body radiation therapy for clinically challenging cases of centrally and superiorly located stage I non-small-cell lung cancer. *Int J Radiat Oncol Biol Phys*, 2011. **80**(4): 1015–22.
145. Berman, A.T., S.S. James, and R. Rengan, Proton beam therapy for non-small cell lung cancer: Current clinical evidence and future directions. *Cancers (Basel)*, 2015. **7**(3): 1178–90.
146. Grant, J.D. and J.Y. Chang, Proton-based stereotactic ablative radiotherapy in early-stage non-small-cell lung cancer. *Biomed Res Int*, 2014. **2014**: 389048.
147. Ahn, S.H. et al., Treatment of stage I non-small cell lung cancer with CyberKnife, image-guided robotic stereotactic radiosurgery. *Oncol Rep*, 2009. **21**(3): 693–6.
148. Bahig, H. et al., Predictive parameters of CyberKnife fiducial-less (XSight Lung) applicability for treatment of early non-small cell lung cancer: A single-center experience. *Int J Radiat Oncol Biol Phys*, 2013. **87**(3): 583–9.
149. Bahig, H. et al., Excellent Cancer Outcomes Following Patient-adapted Robotic Lung SBRT But a Case for Caution in Idiopathic Pulmonary Fibrosis. *Technol Cancer Res Treat*, 2014. **14**(6): 667–76.
150. Bibault, J.E. et al., Image-guided robotic stereotactic radiation therapy with fiducial-free tumor tracking for lung cancer. *Radiat Oncol*, 2012. **7**: 102.
151. Brown, W.T. et al., CyberKnife radiosurgery for stage I lung cancer: Results at 36 months. *Clin Lung Cancer*, 2007. **8**(8): 488–92.
152. Ding, C. et al., Optimization of normalized prescription isodose selection for stereotactic body radiation therapy: Conventional vs robotic linac. *Med Phys*, 2013. **40**(5): 051705.
153. Gibbs, I.C. and B.W. Loo, CyberKnife stereotactic ablative radiotherapy for lung tumors. *Technol Cancer Res Treat*, 2010. **9**(6): 589–96.
154. Ding, C. et al., A dosimetric comparison of stereotactic body radiation therapy techniques for lung cancer: Robotic versus conventional linac-based systems. *J Appl Clin Med Phys*, 2010. **11**(3): 3223.
155. Hu, Y. et al., Characterization of the onboard imaging unit for the first clinical magnetic resonance image guided radiation therapy system. *Med Phys*, 2015. **42**(10): 5828–37.

156. Mutic, S. and J.F. Dempsey, The ViewRay system: Magnetic resonance-guided and controlled radiotherapy. *Semin Radiat Oncol*, 2014. **24**(3): 196–9.
157. Saenz, D.L. et al., Characterization of a 0.35T MR system for phantom image quality stability and in vivo assessment of motion quantification. *J Appl Clin Med Phys*, 2015. **16**(6): 5353.
158. Yorke, E.D., P. Keall, and F. Verhaegen, Anniversary paper: Role of medical physicists and the AAPM in improving geometric aspects of treatment accuracy and precision. *Med Phys*, 2008. **35**(3): 828–39.
159. Rekers, N.H. et al., Stereotactic ablative body radiotherapy combined with immunotherapy: Present status and future perspectives. *Cancer Radiother*, 2014. **18**(5–6): 391–5.
160. Sharabi, A.B. et al., Stereotactic radiation therapy combined with immunotherapy: Augmenting the role of radiation in local and systemic treatment. *Oncology (Williston Park)*, 2015. **29**(5): 331–40.
161. Wang, Y.S. et al., Early efficacy of stereotactic body radiation therapy combined with adoptive immunotherapy for advanced malignancies. *Mol Clin Oncol*, 2013. **1**(5): 925–929.

12

Uncertainties of IGRT for lung cancer

IRINA VERGALASOVA, GUANG LI, CHRIS R. KELSEY,
HONG GE, LONG HUANG, AND JING CAI

12.1 INTRODUCTION

Radiation therapy is an integral treatment modality in the management of all stages and types of lung cancer. In many circumstances, radiation therapy is the primary modality necessary for a cure. Thus, careful treatment planning and execution are critical to achieve optimal clinical outcomes. Furthermore, radiation therapy can lead to side effects based on the amount of normal tissue that is exposed. This is particularly relevant for stereotactic body radiation therapy (SBRT), where large daily doses are utilized. Accurate dose delivery is critical to achieve an optimal risk/benefit profile. Complicating this, are many uncertainties present throughout the process of staging (i.e., determining the extent of disease), treatment planning, and implementation. An understanding and appreciation of these uncertainties will help guide radiation oncologists in the management of this common malignancy.

12.2 UNCERTAINTIES IN IMAGING SIMULATION

12.2.1 Uncertainties in 3D simulation/planning CT

Three-dimensional computed tomography (3D-CT), which detects tissue attenuation coefficients of patient tissue to kilovoltage (kV) x-ray beams, is the clinical standard imaging modality for treatment planning. It provides precise patient anatomy at simulated treatment conditions, and the tissue attenuation coefficient, which can be converted to tissue electron density, for radiation dose calculation using therapeutic beams with megavoltage (MV) energy.

CT images contains various artifacts, which can be caused by patients and by scanners. Common patient-related artifacts include body motion, metal implants, beam hardening and out-of-field artifacts, while common scanner-related artifacts are partial volume effects, aliasing, low-statistics and staircase. These artifacts may appear as streaks, shading, bands and rings, and can be minimized using various methods. Voluntary and involuntary body motions can cause image blurring and distortion, as a point in tissue may appear at different place in time during gantry rotation. Breath-hold CT or four dimensional CT (4D-CT) reduces motion artifacts [1,2]. Metal artifacts are caused by strong scattering and photon absorption from implanted metal devices, such as dental crowns and metallic bone prostheses, and commercial CT scanners can now correct the metal artifacts [3,4]. Beam hardening (or cupping) and out-of-field artifacts can be overcome by increasing kVp and field of view, respectively. Compared with patient-related artifacts, Scanner-related artifacts have smaller scales of uncertainties and can be minimized by using location-specific scanning protocols and performing regular machine QA.

An accurate conversion from linear attenuation coefficient to electron density is required for accurate planning dose calculation. Tissue heterogeneity correction is almost always used based on tissue electron density. Small tissue density variation within the same tissue type may only contribute negligible dose uncertainties, which allow tissue-type-based MRI-to-CT density conversion for potential MRI-based treatment planning [5].

12.2.2 Uncertainties in 3D MRI and PET/CT

Magnetic resonance imaging (MRI), which detects tissue nuclear interactions, such as spin-spin or spin-lattice relaxation upon radiofrequency excitation, is a powerful and versatile 3D imaging modality, offering soft-tissue high contrast without ionizing radiation. MRI images are often used with CT to define the treatment target, such as brain, head and neck and abdominal tumors. Because of MRI diversified capabilities, many types of artifacts are expected [6]. Fortunately, most clinical scan protocols are optimized and MRI scanner QA is regularly performed so minimal scanner-related artifacts appear in clinical patient images. In radiotherapy, the most concerning uncertainty is geometric distortion artifact, caused by inhomogeneity of the magnetic field, susceptibility change at tissue interfaces, and tissue-dependent chemical shift. Magnetic field inhomogeneity can be examined and corrected based on a large grid phantom, while the patient-related artifacts due to tissue inhomogeneity at interfaces are difficult to correct.

Positron emission tomography (PET) detects a paired photon traveling in opposite direction and their origin, where a new-born positron emitted from a biological tracer, such as ^{18}F-FDG, annihilates with a surrounding electron. Because the biological tracers involve cancer metabolic or proliferative activities, therefore PET images tumor activity and location. Patient anatomy is often obtained from CT in a PET/CT scanner, where the activity and anatomy are co-registered [7]. As PET images have low spatial resolution limited by the detector size, partial volume effect is one of major uncertainties. PET imaging is also slow so that motion blurring is pronounced [8]. In addition, as the co-registered CT is used for attenuation correction, any CT artifacts (motion, metal or out-of-field) increase PET uncertainties. In addition, the biological specificity and dynamic uptake-removal equilibrium of a tumor tracer affect the PET image. Non-specific uptakes, such as the brown fat, are known and may cause uncertainties [9].

When using multimodal images in treatment simulation, image registration to simulation CT is essential. Registration uncertainty mostly comes from tissue deformation, which cannot be accommodated by rigid registration. Recently, deformable image registration has become available in commercial systems for treatment planning [10]. With integrated PET/CT and PET/MRI scanners [11], image registration uncertainty in treatment simulation is minimized and multimodality simulation has been widely applied in radiotherapy [12,13].

12.2.3 Uncertainties in 4D-CT imaging

4D-CT has been developed to overcome severe motion artifacts observed in 3D-CT image of tumors with respiration-induced motion [14,15]. In 2003, 4D-CT was reported independently by four different institutions, including Virginia Commonwealth University [16], Memorial Sloan Kettering Cancer Center [17], Washington University [18], and Massachusetts General Hospital [19]. Assuming a periodic breathing motion, image projections around the patient are sorted into different respiratory phase bins based on a respiratory signal from an external breathing surrogate, such as RPM (real-time positioning management), bellows (a tension sensor), or spirometry. The projections within a bin are used to reconstruct a 3D-CT representing the corresponding respiratory phase, and the 3D-CT images in all phases are combined as a 4D-CT image. Ten respiratory phase bins are used in commercial CT scanners and both helical [16,17] and cine [18,19] CT scanning can be used to acquire 4D-CT.

Although 4D-CT is designed to quantify patient-specific respiratory motion with improved image quality, substantial motion artifacts—the binning artifacts—can be found in 4D-CT owing to breathing irregularities, which violates the periodic motion assumption. In cine mode, motion artifacts have distinct patterns at the image junction between two adjacent bed scans [20,21] (as shown in Figure 12.1), while in helical mode, the artifacts are spread out among slices [22]. The motion artifact can cause gross tumor volume (GTV) within a breathing cycle to vary by up to 90%–110% mostly due to motion artifacts present in phase-binned

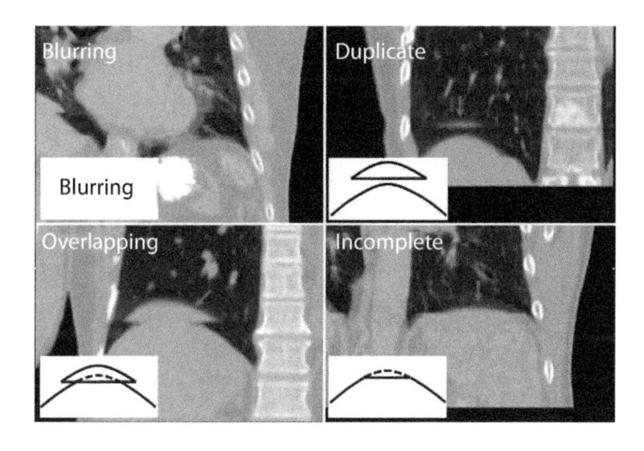

Figure 12.1 Four typical motion artifacts in cine 4D-CT scans. (From Yamamoto, T. et al., *Int J Radiat Oncol Biol Phys*, 72, 1250–1258, 2008. Courtesy of Dr. Paul Keall.)

4D-CT image [23,24]. The true variation of tumor volume may be as high as 20%–30% when relatively large tumors (>100 cc) are imaged using 4D-CT with negligible motion artifacts [25]. Despite of these shortcomings due to breathing irregularities, 4D-CT has become the clinical standard for tumor motion assessment for treatment planning and delivery.

The severity of motion artifacts in 4D-CT may also be affected by the respiratory surrogate used for binning. An internal surrogate, such the diaphragm, would be ideal since a strong correlation ($c \approx 0.98$) between tumor motion and the surrogate has been reported [26–28]. External surrogates, such as RPM and bellows, are commonly used in 4D-CT binning in major commercial CT scanners. As the external-internal correlation is inferior to internal correlation, the quality of 4D-CT image can be affected. Uncertainty in surrogate placements can also affect the external-internal correlation. Recently, a novel marker-less external surrogate is reported with accurate measurements of spirometry and breathing pattern from the torso surface motion using optical surface imaging [29]. Since the mean diaphragm motion can be accurately predicted by tidal volume and breathing pattern [28,30], this method is potentially useful as a more reliable external surrogate for 4D-CT binning and organ motion prediction at treatment.

12.2.4 Uncertainties of phase/amplitude binning

The residual motion artifacts in 4D-CT are resulted from the periodic binning method in the presence of common breathing irregularities. Various approaches have been studied to reduce or eliminate such artifacts. In contrast to phase binning, amplitude binning method has demonstrated reduced motion artifacts. This is because amplitude-binning reduces the residual motion within a bin, whereas phase-binning cannot translate phase into amplitude consistently in the presence of breathing irregularities [31], as demonstrated in Figure 12.2.

As all commercial 4D-CT scanning protocols (helical or cine) perform 4D scans continuously for a little over one breathing cycle without pause-and-reassume functionality, a certain respiratory stage may be missed when severe breathing irregularity occur. For instance, a low amplitude cycle may occur and cannot reach the averaged full-inhalation amplitude (Figure 12.2c) and thus the corresponding stage is not available. In this case, a patient-specific respiratory model can be built and used to fill the gap [32,33].

Breathing irregularities are dynamic and vary from time to time. Therefore, there is uncertainty if a motion model derived from simulation 4D-CT is directly applied in treatment, including 4D cone beam CT (4D-CBCT) to reduce scan time [34] or predict tumor motion using single cone beam projection image [35]. A breathing model with real-time update from measured tidal volume and airflow provides adaption [36].

As the motion artifact is rooted from breathing irregularities, a "bad" 4D-CT scan may build in too many-artifacts to correct. In contrast to post-imaging correction, motion irregularity could be minimized in the first place during 4D-CT scanning. It has been suggested that real-time periodicity assessment of the breathing trace could provide guidance to gate the scan, minimizing irregularities [21]. Alternatively, a prospective 4D-CT can minimize the binning artifacts. Coolens et al. [37] have applied 320-slice CBCT to directly acquire prospective 4D-CT or $4D_{vol}$ CT, minimizing motion artifacts, as shown in Figure 12.3.

12.2.5 Uncertainties of 4D-MRI and 4D-PET

Four-dimensional positron emission tomography (4D-PET) [38,39] and 4D magnetic resonance imaging (4D-MRI) [40,41] have also been reported. 4D-PET adopted the retrospective respiratory binning strategy [42–45] while 4D-MRI applied prospective multi-channel imaging strategy with or without binning [46–49]. PET scans take 3–5 minutes per one bed position (16–22 cm), much slower than CT or MRI. The uncertainties of 4D-PET in target delineation comes mostly from low image resolution ($4 \times 4 \times 4$ mm^3), residual motion blurring, partial volume effects, high quantum noise, as well as controversial tumor delineation owing to lack of ground truth in patients [45]. To reduce the prolonged 4D acquisition time, a patient motion model from 4D-CT can be applied to derive a motion-compensated PET image [39].

MRI provides versatile 4D scanning techniques, including cine 2D(t) MRI, prospective 3D(t) ($4D_{vol}$) -MRI, and retrospective 4D-MRI. Each technique contains method-specific uncertainties, in addition to the

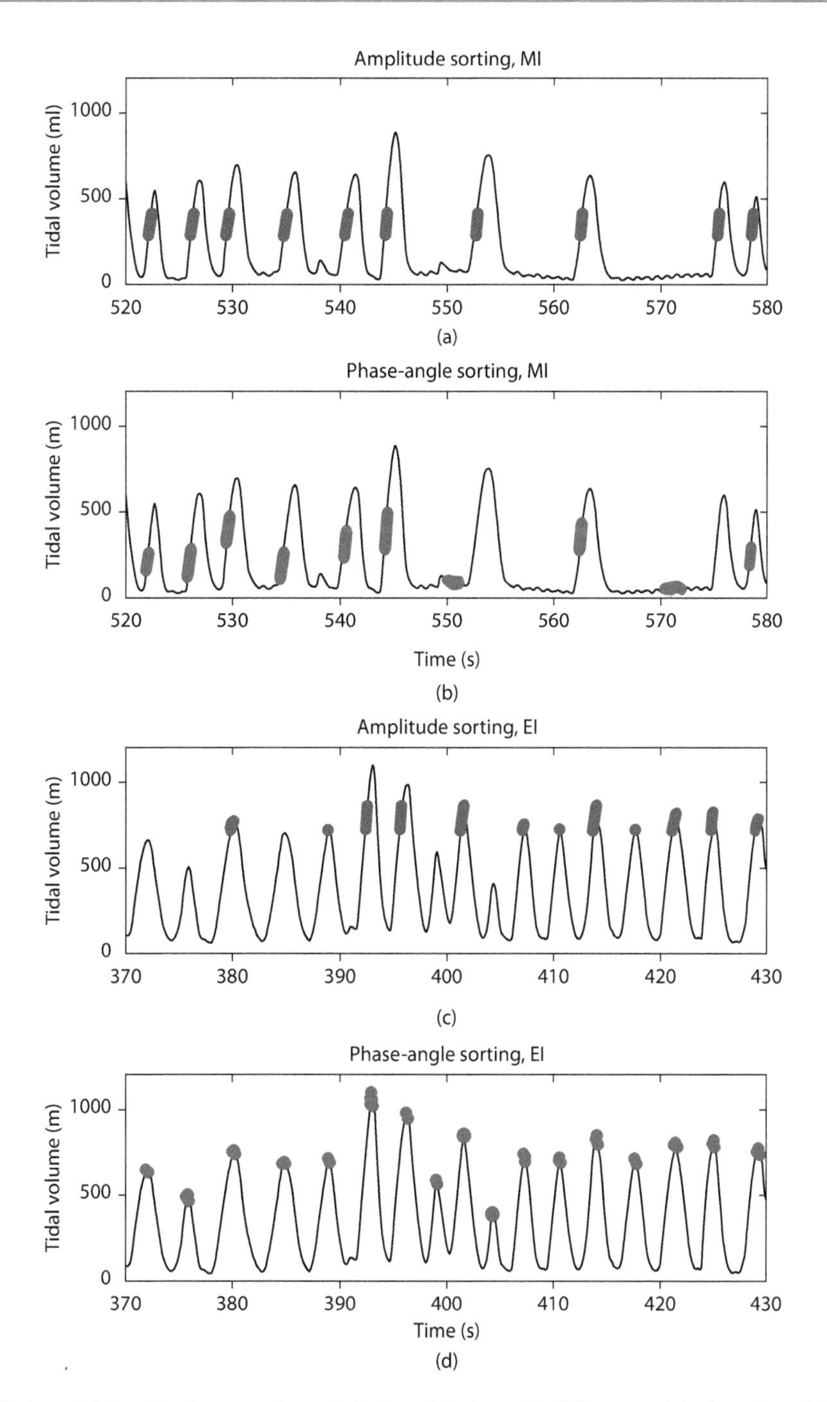

Figure 12.2 (a and c) Amplitude versus (b and d) phase binning with different residual motions. (From Lu, W. et al., *Med Phy*, 33, 2964–2974, 2006. Courtesy of Dr. Daniel Low.)

common uncertainties in 3DMR imaging; including image distortion caused by non-uniformity of magnetic field, non-linearity of magnetic gradient, and variation of susceptibility at tissue interfaces. For cine 2D(t) MRI, out-of-plane motion can cause large uncertainty in tumor motion trajectory: a tracking point could partially or completely move out of the cine 2D image. For prospective 3D(t) MRI, the compromised spatial-temporal resolutions lead to uncertainties in these dimensions, affecting imaging quality or speed of a moving tumor. Uncertainties for retrospective 4D-MRI primarily result from the binning method due to

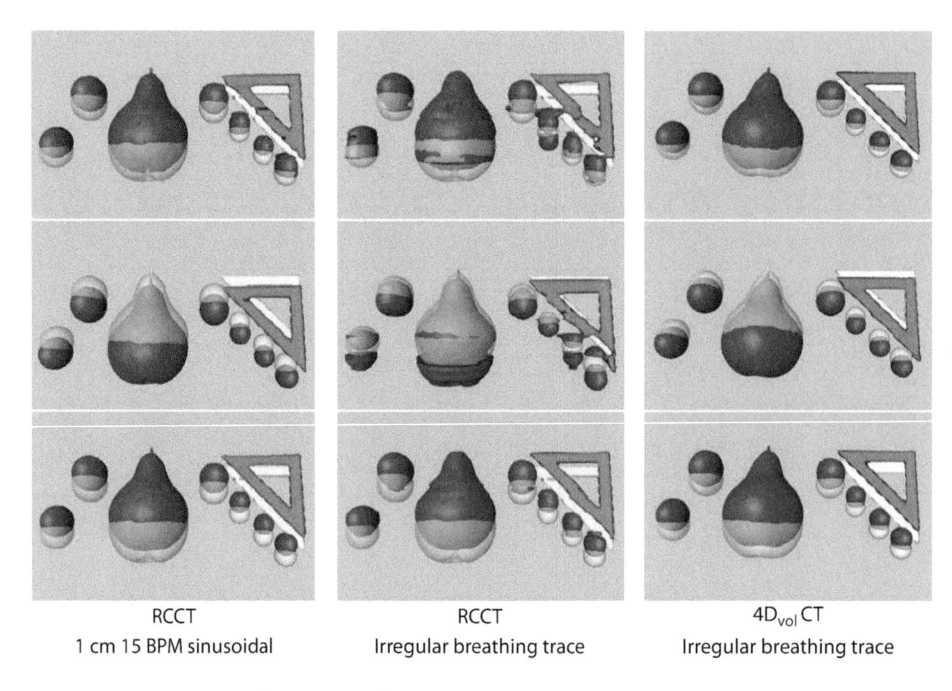

Figure 12.3 Demonstration of motion artifacts in respiratory correlated CT (RCCT) caused by breathing irregularities and a solution to address this problem using $4D_{vol}$ CT. (From Coolens, C. et al., *Med Phys*, 39, 2669–2681, 2012.) Courtesy by Dr. Catherine Coolens.

breathing irregularities. Since MR imaging is slice based, motion artifacts appear to be zigzag edges in the stacking neighbor slices. 4D-MRI is an active research area, considering clinical use of MRI-Cobalt treatment units and active development of MRI-Linac units.

12.2.6 Breathing variations and management strategies

As breathing irregularities are the primary cause of motion artifacts, and associated uncertainties in internal target volume (ITV) delineation, efforts have been made toward improving the regularity of patient respiration during 4D simulation and treatment. A commonly employed technique is the biofeedback approach using audio-video (AV) coaching signals to instruct patients to breathe in and out [50]. The method can improve the regularity for many patients but may not for all [51]. AV coaching also tends to induce patient breathe deeper than free breathing. The coaching also requires patients to comply throughout the entire treatment, in which patients may fall asleep with shallow breathing, deviating from coached 4D-CT simulation. A different approach has been suggested to use 4D-MRI in treatment simulation so that patient breathing irregularities could be better characterized and represented in treatment planning and delivery [48]. By far, respiratory motion management remains a challenge to radiotherapy clinic and demands a large margin to combat high motion uncertainty caused by breathing irregularities.

Various motion management techniques have been applied in treatment of lung cancer to reduce tumor motion and sparing normal tissue, including active breathing control (ABC) [52–54], deep inhalation breath hold (DIBH) [55,56], abdominal compression [57,58], and mechanical ventilation [45,59]. Proper patient body immobilization is also necessary, since voluntary body motion is inevitable, causing baseline drift during a 20-minute treatment. The uncertainty of baseline drift in simulation is often small because simulation scan is short. However, the baseline drift and adjustment during treatment are important to avoid a systematic targeting error [60].

In summary, the uncertainty in treating lung cancer is primarily associated with the patient factors—the breathing irregularities, which cause the binning artifacts and affect ITV delineation. The imaging factor alone is secondary and the uncertainty is lower in 4D-CT than in 4D-MRI and 4D-PET. With recent advancements in MR-guided radiation therapy, we expect to see motion uncertainty decreasing in the coming years as the result of clinical research on real-time image guidance during treatment.

12.3 UNCERTAINTIES IN TARGET VOLUME DETERMINATION

12.3.1 Gross tumor volume (GTV)

Variability in GTV definition is a major source of systematic error and persists over the course of treatment,and can potentially have a large impact on the dose delivered to the lung tumor. The shape, size, and location of a tumor may be determined by different imaging methods such as CT, PET/CT, and less commonly MRI. Therefore, adequate imaging or image fusion studies should be obtained for diagnosis, staging, and planning prior to lung cancer treatment. CT-based treatment planning is standard in lung cancer. The appearance of the primary tumor is highly dependent on the windowing of the CT scan [61]. It is recommended to use standard lung windows when contouring a parenchymal lesion. Several clinical scenarios can complicate clear identification of a parenchymal lesion including atelectasis, pleural effusions, and adjacent blood vessels for more central lesions. Intravenous contrast is usually not necessary to accurately delineate a parenchymal lesion unless it is located near the hilum. The GTV is defined as all macroscopically identifiable tumor manifestations [62]. Several factors will impact GTV size variations including delineation uncertainty, tumor deformation due to breathing, and image artifacts. The GTV definition is usually carried out by radiation oncologists, sometimes with the help of radiologists to interpret uncertainties in the imaging. However, due to these uncertainties and characteristics of lung tumors, variation in GTV delineation is observed among physicians. Previous research has shown that different physicians interpret GTVs differently and that oncologists and radiologists often define different volumes [63–66]. Large target delineation variability of up to 10 mm has been observed in conventional lung cancer external-beam radiotherapy planning for larger or locally advanced tumors, as shown in Figure 12.4 [67]. An earlier study found that a change of up 10.6% in volume could be caused by delineation uncertainty [23]. These changes were a result of (a) differentiation of tumor from atelectasis or ground glass shadowing, (b) separation of tumor from vasculature, and (c) defining the mediastinal extent of tumor [66].

PET imaging has been used as a guide to the physician during GTV delineation. Since their introduction, PET/CT scanners have become widely prevalent in oncology and are crucial for the diagnosis and staging of lung cancer [68]. PET can be particularly helpful to delineate gross disease from atelectasis, though the spatial resolution with PET is limited. Some lung cancer histology's, particularly adenocarcinoma in situ, often appear as ground glass opacities that are only mildly FDG-avid on PET. These are often more challenging to delineate given their less discrete borders. Identification of involved lymph nodes in the mediastinum is challenging and is ideally assessed both clinically (e.g., PET-CT) and pathologically (e.g., mediastinoscopy or endobronchial ultrasound). PET-CT, while more accurate than CT alone, has limitations related to histologic subtype, type of PET-CT scanner, dose of ^{18}F-2-fluoro-deoxy-D-glucose (FDG), and so forth [69]. Lymph nodes known or suspected of harboring disease should be contoured using soft tissue (chest/abdomen) windows. Most mediastinal lymph node stations, except for the AP window (level 5), are easily visualized without intravenous contrast. On the other hand, involved lymph nodes in the hilum are often very difficult to distinguish from blood vessels on non-contrasted scans. Utilizing IV contrast is suggested when hilar lymph nodes are involved.

However, there are uncertainties associated with relying on PET imaging for treatment planning purposes of mobile tumors. First, there are a several methods to determine the GTV, ranging from simple visual assessment, to automated methods, standard uptake value (SUV)-based contouring, SUV-based thresholding, background cut-off, and segmentation based on signal-to-background ratios [70]. Each of these methods has its corresponding challenges—with the most common being the lack of reproducibility—mainly due to the degree of image noise present in PET acquisition. Currently, none of these methods is deemed superior to the others and thus it is important to be aware of the potential inaccuracies associated with the chosen

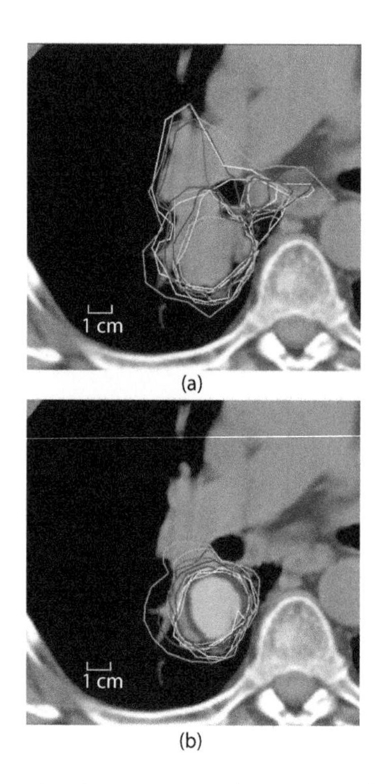

Figure 12.4 Computed tomography slice of a patient with delineations of (a) first phase and (b) second phase. Color wash represents overlay of matched 2-[18F] fluoro-2-deoxy-D-glucose positron emission tomography. Note that sub carinal lymph node and some blood vessels delineated in first phase did not have increased 2-[18F] fluoro-2-deoxy-D-glucose uptake in second phase and therefore were excluded by all radiation oncologists. (From Steenbakkers, R.J. et al., *Int J Radiat Oncol Biol Phys*, 64, 435–448, 2006.)

technique. The more pressing concern of using PET to guide GTV delineation is that the length of acquisition (around 15–20 minutes) produces an image that is essentially an integral over the whole range of tumor motion. This can be problematic when the corresponding CT is used for breath-hold or gated treatment, as it will only represent a snippet of the respiratory motion. An example of this is illustrated in Figure 12.5. Therefore, one must recognize that the PET may show an increased lesion size, decreased maximum activity concentration and less intense FDG-uptake at the extremes of the motion range, which may lead to potential mis-registration and difficulty in accurately characterizing PET-avid disease [71].

If a fused FDG-PET-CT is available for delineation of stage I–III non-small cell lung cancer (NSCLC), it has been shown that delineation variability can be decreased by up to 6 mm, which is most pronounced in case of atelectasis (Figure 12.4) [67]. However, FDG PET has a poor spatial resolution [72], and much uncertainty exists regarding the most appropriate threshold cutoff that should be used to define a PET target volume in NSCLC therapy planning. CT scan with contrast is preferred to demonstrate blood vessels and guide clinical treating physicians to delineate active disease, particularly for the mediastinum lymph nodes.

Respiration-induced tumor motion can cause target volumetric deformation with conventional CT scans [73]. The choice of CT method significantly influences the delineated GTV size. The GTV size in a breath-hold CT scan (BHCT) is considered closest to that of the true tumor volume, considering the breathing-related tumor deformation is minimal. GTV sizes for free breathing 3D-CT and 4D-CT are expected to be larger than those in the BHCT scans. Substantial variation in GTV size throughout the phases of 4D-CT has been observed, and was significantly correlated to larger breathing-related tumor motion [23].

Artifacts in CT images will impact the imaged tumor volume in the planning CT scan and introduce a systematic error in the following treatment course. The magnitude of image artifacts in CT images is impacted by several factors such as slice thickness, beam width (collimation), gantry rotation time, interpolation, and

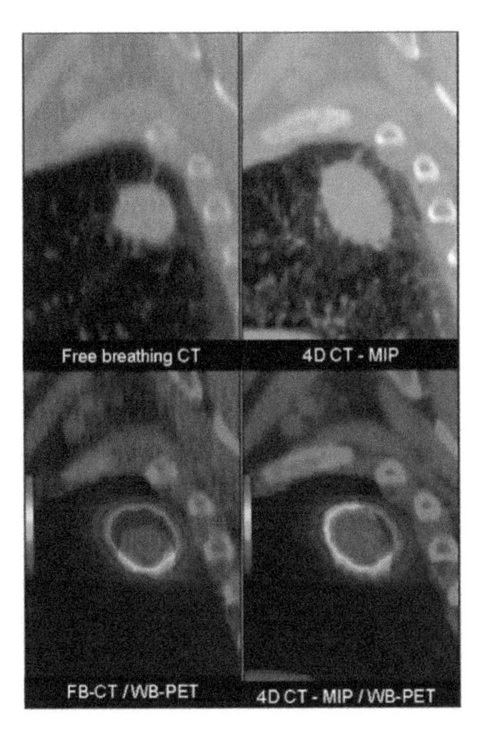

Figure 12.5 This figure shows the blurring effect of respiration on ungated whole-body PET imaging. The top left shows the appearance of a lung lesion on a free-breathing CT and the top right shows the lesions when the scan is reconstructed and a MIP reconstruction from a 4D-CT. The 4D-CT MIP reconstruction is generated by using the maximum pixel values across all 4D-CT frames. The bottom left,shows the ungated whole-body PET fused with the free-breathing CT and the PET lesion appears larger than the CT lesions. However, when the ungated whole-body PET is fused with the MIP reconstruction, there is much better agreement in the lesion size.

breathing motion. The magnitude of GTV volume changes appeared more reliable for larger as opposed to smaller tumors due to the lower susceptibility to artifacts of larger volumes [62]. A more formal approach to GTV definition could lead to greater agreement between physicians and a reduction in the systematic error.

12.3.2 Clinical target volume (CTV)

It has been well documented that microscopic disease frequently extends outside the primary margin of a parenchymal pulmonary malignancy [74–76]. In most patients, this does not exceed 6–8 mm, but in a minority of patients, it can extend up to 1 cm or more. It has been reported that adenocarcinomas and well differentiated tumors are more likely to have greater microscopic extension. However, there is much uncertainty how to apply this to clinical practice where patients are being planned using CT imaging. How a gross primary tumor as visualized on CT correlates with a gross primary tumor that has been resected is unclear, especially when the latter is assessed after laboratory processing that can lead to tissue shrinkage. In any case, it may be prudent to apply a small expansion to a gross tumor volume to account for microscopic disease extension. Similarly, extracapsular extensions of disease through the capsule and into the surrounding soft tissues occurs in about 33% of lymph nodes. The extent is typically minimal (<1 mm on average) with 95% of cases ≤3 mm [77]. Therefore, a small margin around clinically evident lymph nodes is appropriate.

Elective nodal irradiation for both NSCLC and small-cell lung cancer (SCLC) is controversial [78]. Most national lung cancer trials mandate no elective nodal irradiation and many oncologists currently treat gross disease only. To many, elective nodal irradiation is considered an all-or-none phenomenon. In some circumstances, a selective approach to treating elective lymph node regions is rational. When pursued in select patients, a simple understanding of lobe-specific lymphatic spread [79,80] and patterns of failure after surgery [81] can be employed to develop a strategy whereby those lymph node regions at *highest* risk are adequately covered.

12.3.3 Internal target volume (ITV)

Breathing irregularities are one of the biggest uncertainties when treating pulmonary malignancies with radiation. Most patients have chronic obstructive pulmonary disease (COPD) and poor pulmonary function. Many are current smokers. Patients are sometimes anxious during the treatment planning process and/or actual treatments. These factors and others lead to increased work with breathing and chronic dyspnea, which contributes to irregular breathing patterns.

There are several methods to account for respiratory motion, all of which are plagued by irregular breathing patterns. One method is to perform a 4D-CT scan and create an internal target volume using a maximum intensity projection (MIP) dataset. A free-breathing 3D dataset is often obtained during the same planning session. Theoretically, the disease apparent on the free-breathing CT should be encompassed completely in the MIP dataset. However, it has been observed that the MIP dataset frequently fails to include all the tumor appreciated on the free-breathing dataset (Figure 12.6) [82–85]. This is presumably due to different breathing patterns between the two scans as well as outlying tumor positions from respiratory extremes that are discarded when the MIP is generated. Deep inspiratory breath-hold techniques are theoretically appealing, because the lungs are expanded and the tumor is stationary, both decreasing normal tissue exposure. However, the extent of breath-hold, and the patient's ability to hold at a certain position without drifting, leads to significant uncertainty. Many patients with COPD are simply unable to hold their breath adequately. Gating is another appealing methodology but isn't a good choice with irregular breathing patterns. Further, the many complexities inherent in gating a radiation treatment often prompt radiation oncologists to use larger margins to account for the uncertainties which can defeat the purpose of gating (decreasing normal tissue exposure).

Uncertainties in tumor motion assessment for treatment planning relate to the method for ITV delineation and treatment choice. For ITV delineation, there are two widely applied methods: (1) to contour the ITV using the MIP image synthesized from 4D-CT and (2) to contour the ITV based on all phase images of a 4D-CT using the union of the clinical tumor volume CTV (= GTV, gross tumor volume, + margin). The all-phase ITV is almost always greater than the MIP ITV, primarily owing to the short duration at the extreme

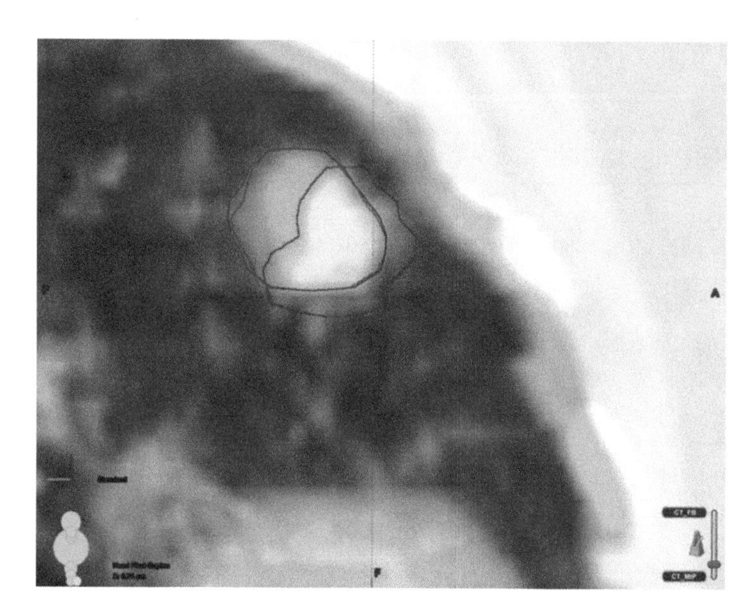

Figure 12.6 Example of different target volumes in a lung cancer patient, illustrating the differences between GTV_{3D} (*red line*) and ITV_{MIP} (*green line*) and $ITV_{10phase}$ (*blue line*). Here ITV_{COMB} is the Boolean addition of GTV_{3D} + ITV_{MIP}. Note that $ITV_{10phase}$ was not completely overlapped with ITV_{MIP} and ITV_{COMB}.

phases, such as full inhalation [86]. A study of five different ITV delineation methods in 20 lung patients concluded that combining the MIP ITV and free-breathing 3D-CT would provide a suitable treatment target [82]. Although MIP method is convenient as only one contour is needed for ITV, there is a concern on whether MIP method would be sufficient to represent the entire tumor motion trajectory considering breathing irregularities.

In tumor tracking approach, the tumor delineation should be performed based on individual phase, and a reduced ITV can be applied to account for the variation in size and shape within a breathing cycle [87]. Frequently 4D-CTs consist of motion artifacts, which could lead the GTV vary up to 90% [23] or 110% [24] for small peripheral lesions with large motion range. Using 4D-CT with minimal motion artifacts, it has been found that the tumor volume variation is about 20% for large tumors (V>100cc) [25]. Although these reports are not directly comparable, it implies that uncertainties from motion artifact can be substantial. For real-time tumor tracking, uncertainties using external surrogates are high since the correlation and linear relationship can be altered by breathing irregularities. Uncertainties in internal surrogates lies in the latency between imaging and beam tracking, which can be improved by anticipated positioning [88,89].

MIP-based ITVs have been widely implemented, being that they encompass much more of the respiratory motion than FB-CT and AIP, without the hassle of contouring the GTV ten different times [83–85,90–93]. However, subsequent studies have demonstrated that MIP-based ITVs as well as ITVs generated from all ten 4D-CT phases can both potentially underestimate or overestimate the true ITV due to the variability in patient respiration [83,94–96]. Similar uncertainties were also demonstrated for AIP-based ITVs due to patient's respiratory variability, as well as tumor size [97]. After all, the 4D-CT only captures several cycles of a patient's breathing pattern, which can be affected by a multitude of external factors such as anxiety, pain, etc., compounded with an acquisition that occurs at least a week before actual treatment delivery. Furthermore, there is increased uncertainty in MIP-based ITVs for tumors located near high-intensity structures, such as the liver or spleen cupola [98]. While these studies highlight the difficulty of obtaining the true total extent of the tumor from any of the available sets of images, a different study investigated ways to quantify and minimize the degree of uncertainty present in ITVs [82]. Multiple methods were employed to generate ITVs for phantom and patient data and quantitative comparisons illustrated that ITV uncertainty can be minimized by combining ITVs generated from the FB-CT, 4D-CT, and MIP. Since the results also showed that an ITV combined from both the MIP and FB-CT was comparable to that of the 4D-CT (see Figure 12.6), the authors recommended the use of that technique if delineating the ITV on the entire 4D-CT is deemed unfeasible. The largest difference between all ITV methods was noted for cases where the tumor volume was small and the extent of motion was large. Another possible solution to minimize ITV uncertainties from 4D-CT proposed the combination of 4D-CT and modified slow CT techniques to generate the ITV [99].

In fact, one study [100] proposed using the PET to determine the ITV instead of the 4D-CT MIP, despite finding large differences in ITVs generated between the two (likely due to respiration variability), like others' results also demonstrating their inequality [101]. To correct this, several motion-management techniques have been investigated for PET/CT with tracking of the respiratory signal in order to bin the data according to phase or amplitude (single or multiple), or applying motion corrections either pre- or post-reconstruction. [102] Multiple studies have highlighted the superiority of 4D PET/CT in terms of achieving more accurate image co-registration, reduced blurring, and increased SUV measurements [38,42,103–106]. 4D or gated PET/CT procedures have yet to see mass integration into the clinical atmosphere, likely due to the increased time required for patient setup, scanning and data processing. In the meantime, it is important to be aware of the shortcomings of PET's current role in treatment planning.

12.3.4 Planning target volume (PTV)

A planning target volume expansion is utilized to account for uncertainties in daily set-up. There are two relevant aspects. The first,is differences in internal anatomy that affect accurate daily targeting. This includes all the factors that contribute to shifts in tumor position from day to day and over the course of treatment (e.g., differences in daily respiration, tumor shrinkage, changes in surrounding effusions and atelectasis). The second,are factors that affect external setup and consistency (e.g., weight changes, obesity, body rotations in immobilization devices). These factors are primarily related to interfractional uncertainties. Intrafractional uncertainties require consideration also. This would include discomfort in the immobilization device due to back, neck, or shoulder ailments, anxiety, tremors, and so forth, all of which can lead to movement.

12.4 UNCERTAINTIES IN TREATMENT PLANNING

12.4.1 Uncertainties in motion management strategy

Patients with tumors affected by respiratory motion will typically first receive a 4D-CT, which has quickly become the standard of care. This scan aids in the decision of whether the treatment delivery will be free-breathing, breath-hold or gated to specific phases of the respiration. In the case of free-breathing or breath-hold, the patient will then be scanned in the corresponding state (FB-CT or BH-CT). For those patients that will be treated free-breathing, the question that immediately arises is which scan(s) should be used for determining the ITV and subsequent treatment planning. Naturally, the FB-CT scan alone cannot represent the true ITV, as it only captures a snippet of the patient's respiration. Conversely, the 4D-CT scan provides time-resolved images of the respiratory-induced target motion and an ITV can be created by combining GTV contours from each phase, but this is extremely labor-intensive. To significantly reduce this workload, an ITV can be generated from a maximum intensity projection (MIP) scan, which collapses the highest pixel intensities of the ten 4D-CT phase sets into one volume image. Additionally, an AIP scan can also be created, by taking the average instead of the maximum intensities.

For patients that experience large respiratory-induced tumor motion, but are unable to hold their breath, gated treatments are the most viable option to treat the patient comfortably, while sparing a greater amount of healthy lung tissue than a free-breathing treatment. For these cases, 4D-CT simulation is fundamental in the selection of an appropriate gating window to be used for treatment. Typically, a window with less than 5mm of motion is chosen, as recommended by the American Association of Physicists in Medicine (AAPM) Task Group 76 report. [107] However, it has been demonstrated that the gating window ITV can be significantly underestimated because of irregular breathing, compounded with the low temporal resolution of 4D-CT acquisition [108]. To account for the potential underestimation, the authors recommend incorporating an additional margin associated with the breathing variation, whose size would be influenced by not only the degree of irregularity but by the target size and motion extent, as well. Aside from the images generated by 4D-CT, there is additional uncertainty demonstrated in the correlation between the external surrogate used to track the respiratory motion and the actual internal motion of the tumor [109–113]. This doubt ultimately translates into the delivery phase of treatment, as there is concern whether the position of the external marker truly reflects the location of the tumor exactly where it was planned.

Upon proper determination of the ITV and subsequent planning target volume (PTV), the next important decision lies in determining which scan should be used for the actual treatment planning. Of course, prior to the advent of 4D-CT, everything was contoured and calculated on the free-breathing 3D helical scan. Generic margins were then applied to compensate for the lack of patient-specific information, while still providing adequate dose coverage. We know that this is likely to lead to large inaccuracies, ranging from geometric miss to excessive treatment of healthy lung tissue. There has been a variety of 4D-CT-based planning strategies proposed to dosimetrically account for the presence of anatomical motion. True 4D planning approaches involve 3D planning on each phase set combined with deformable image registration (DIR) (and in some cases Monte Carlo) to generate a warped dose distribution, representing the dose delivered to the target because of respiratory motion [91,114–119]. However, the large increase in workload coupled with the uncertainties associated with deformable registration mark these strategies impractical for clinical translation.

12.4.2 Uncertainties in planning image

To simplify this workflow, other studies investigated the accuracy of planning on a specific set of the 4D-CT, such as the mid-ventilation CT [120,121] or end-exhalation CT [122], as well as the average 4D-CT [123]. The consensus comparing 4D planning to 3D planning on a 4D-CT-based image agreed that they were similar enough to recommend the latter option. Proceeding with this notion, one group performed a dosimetric comparison of FB-CT versus AIP versus MIP and found no significant differences between FB-CT versus AIP for both PTV and normal structures, whereas the MIP plans gave slightly better PTV coverage and a much smaller low-dose region to lung, only because of a smaller total lung volume [124]. They recommended the use of the AIP instead of the FB-CT due to the decreased presence of image artifacts. Another study, utilizing the term 3.5D-CT planning, proposed aligning the centers of delineated GTVs in all phases of 4D-CT and then creating the average to synthesize a 3.5D-CT image, which displays a motionless target with motion-blurred anatomical structures [24]. Their comparison against 4D planning also found 3.5D to be equivalent, resulting in <1% dose difference in PTV coverage and negligible dose differences among normal structures. Of course, it is key to remember that since treatment planning is only one link in a long chain of processes, its accuracy is only as strong as the previous link, ITV delineation.

12.4.3 Uncertainties in planning technique

Lastly, the technique used for planning will also impose its own corresponding uncertainties onto the accuracy of the treatment. The selection of Three-Dimensional Conformal Radiation Therapy (3D-CRT) versus IMRT and VMAT involves consideration of the different advantages/disadvantages specific to each method. For example, IMRT and VMAT are known to better dosimetrically spare surrounding critical structures whereas 3D-CRT is less likely to be impacted by patient motion. Furthermore, 3D-CRT is entirely insensitive to the interplay effect, which is the interaction between multi-leaf collimator (MLC) motion and the respiratory-induced tumor motion. The interplay effect has been shown to dosimetrically average out over the course of many fractions, but may potentially be more significant for SBRT treatments [125]. Recent investigations of employing SBRT treatment with IMRT and VMAT have found minimal dosimetric differences relative to 3D-CRT for the studied patient cohort [126,127]. Another benefit of using 3D-CRT is the ability to acquire cine MV images during treatment, which provide for real-time verification of the tumor position. Additionally, these images provided information to pave the way toward implementation of more accurate 4D dose calculation, probability-based treatment planning, tumor trailing and adaptive radiation therapy [24,128–130]. Nevertheless, the ultimate decision is case and patient specific, with each technique containing its own proponents [131].

It is evident that there are several uncertainties prevalent in the treatment planning of moving tumors. The first leap of faith lies in the idea that a patient's respiration remains identical between simulation and delivery, especially since it is unmonitored during free-breathing treatments. The second, being that the 4D-CT scan accurately captures the entire range of tumor motion, which many studies have already shown to not always be the case. Using PET-CT as a guide for GTV delineation imposes different degrees of uncertainties depending on whether the treatment will be gated, breath-hold or free-breathing. For gated and breath-hold treatments, there is also the uncertainty of ITV generation and whether the target is where you planned it to be, based on the amplitude of the external surrogate. Last and certainly not least, is the planning technique's variable impact on the accuracy of treatment. Thus, thoracic and abdominal tumors will continue to require PTV margins that encompass these uncertainties until more improvements are made in the way of accurately and reproducibly defining the range of target motion.

In intensity-modulated radiotherapy (IMRT) and volumetric-modulated radiotherapy (VMAT), multileaf collimator motion may interplay with the tumor motion; however, the uncertainty caused by the interplay effect has been demonstrated to be minimal in multifraction treatment [125,132].

12.5 UNCERTAINTIES IN IMAGE GUIDANCE

The advent of on-board image guidance has revolutionized the achievable accuracy of radiation treatment delivery. Present day imaging technology has the capability of localizing the patient within millimeter accuracy. Even sub-millimeter accuracy can be achieved in conjunction with certain immobilization techniques.

However, targets affected by respiratory motion introduce a slew of uncertainties that may complicate the achievement of that level of accuracy, even with the readily available imaging capabilities. One such example is demonstrated with CBCT [133].

12.5.1 Uncertainties in CBCT

CBCT images, acquired with a kilovoltage (kV) x-ray tube and amorphous silicon detector mounted orthogonally to the linac head, provide the highest degree of volumetric information and soft tissue contrast (excluding CT-on-rails) currently available in the treatment room. However, the reconstruction algorithm that creates the 3D dataset from a set of radially acquired projections assumes the imaged object is static. This assumption is inherently violated during image acquisition of a free-breathing lung cancer patient. The resultant image displays blurred anatomy with contrast that is dependent upon both the relationship between the patient's respiratory cycle and the rate of image acquisition. Vergalasova [133] et al. demonstrated that due to the nature of CBCT imaging and reconstruction, the ITV generated for patients with irregular breathing patterns may be underestimated and lead to potential misalignment with the ITV corresponding to the simulation CT. The irregularity focused on was the disproportionality between time spent in the inspiration phase versus the expiration phase. As the irregularity becomes more severe, the underestimation of the ITV increases, as illustrated in Figure 12.7. This phenomenon is explained by the fact that much fewer projections are acquired in the inspiration phase relative to the expiration phase and therefore results in much less contrast of the target at the inspiration phase. A patient example (Figure 12.8) exhibited ITV underestimation of 40.1% for a small tumor and as much as 24.2% for a large tumor, also demonstrating that the potential for underestimation becomes more severe with decreasing tumor size. The concern arises when matching the fraudulent center of the underestimated ITV (which will be shifted superior to that of the actual center) with the ITV from the planning CT. The consequential dosimetric impact remains to be investigated, but it is important to be vigilant for patients exhibiting such an irregularity, particularly for small tumors, so that appropriate adjustments can be incorporated at the planning stage to minimize uncertainties.

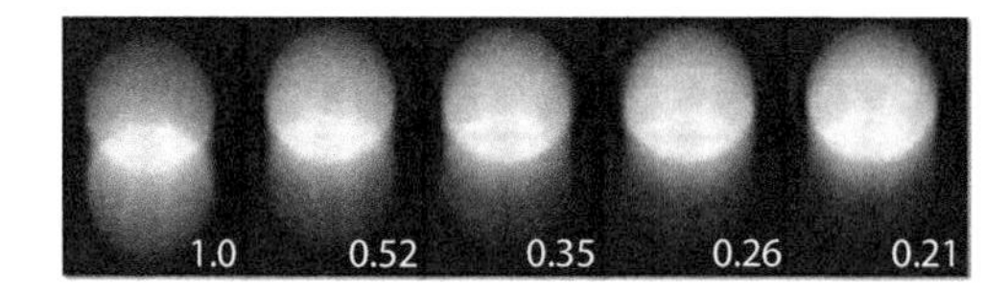

Figure 12.7 CBCT images of a free-breathing phantom with five simulated respiratory profiles. The ratio of time spent in inspiration versus expiration is indicated on the bottom right corner of each FB-CBCT.

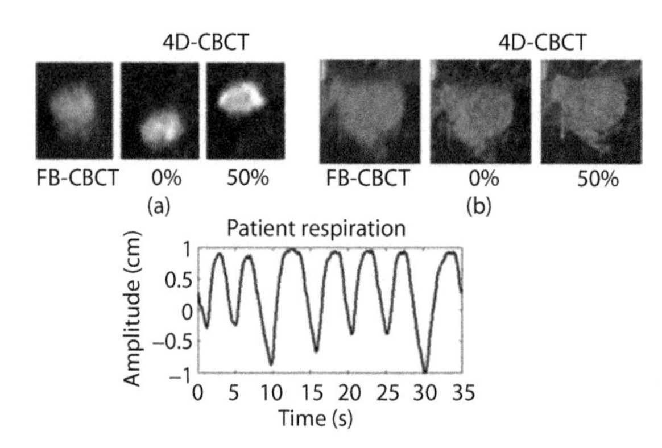

Figure 12.8 Reconstructed FB-CBCT and 4D-CBCT images of two tumors within one lung cancer patient and the corresponding respiratory profile.

12.5.2 Uncertainties in matching

Aside from cases of irregular respiration, uncertainties still exist for routine matching of the planning CT to the CBCT, in terms of which CT better serves this purpose. Should the FB-CT or the AIP dataset be matched with the CBCT? Theoretically, since the CBCT represents an average of the tumor position over multiple respiratory cycles, it should be matched with the AIP, which is also generated as an average from the 4D-CT (acquired over a series of patient breaths) as opposed to the much shorter acquisition of the FB-CT. Being that the AIP is a synthetically generated image volume from the 4D-CT acquisition, not every simulation scanner is currently capable of creating this dataset and thus additional software is required. This implies that as of now, different clinics institute different practices for matching ITVs. Dosimetrically, the results have been shown to be similar between SBRT planning with the FB-CT versus AIP, with a preference for AIP due to the decreased presence of image artifacts [124]. Another analysis was performed comparing couch shifts between FB-CBCT and MIP versus AIP image volumes (Figure 12.9) for asymmetrical respiratory cycles, like those studied by Vergalasova et al. For phantom data, differences of 0.1 mm (AIP) versus 1.5–1.9 mm (MIP) in the inferior direction were reported. For the studied patients, differences ranged from 1.7 mm (superior) to 3.5 mm (inferior) between MIP versus AIP as can be seen in Figure 12.10. Thus, the investigators recommended that AIP be used for target alignment with FB-CBCT for the studied respiratory patterns [134].

Further uncertainties in the localization matching process may arise during treatment, if any anatomical changes occur due to a positive response. Significant changes would of course warrant re-simulation and re-planning, on a case-by-case basis. However, ignoring the possibility of these changes and assuming all aspects (anatomy, respiration, etc.) remain the same between planning and delivery still does not eliminate all uncertainties. It is important to realize that some degree of inter-observer variability will always exist when visually registering two datasets. One study on RTOG clinical trial credentialing compared the shifts recorded by several different institutions versus that of the reviewers for a total of 92 lung cases and revealed differences on the order of 2 mm in all three directions—superior/inferior, left/right and anterior/posterior [135]. A different study focusing specifically on delineating lung SBRT GTVs compared inter-observer variability between CT and CBCT and as a function of target size [136]. The results demonstrated a 17% inter-observer variability for CT and 21% for CBCT (among the different radiation oncologists) with an overall lower agreement for smaller tumors, as would be expected. Although the statistics dictated that contouring on CT versus CBCT was not significantly different from each other, inter-observer variability has a presence and plays a role in the overall treatment process. Therefore, not only does the localization accuracy depend on the patient's respiration and type of planning CT used, it most certainly also depends on the user performing the registration.

12.5.3 Uncertainties in imaging techniques

Additional uncertainties are associated with the variety of image guidance techniques that are clinically available today. Instead of the kV-CBCT, megavoltage (MV) CBCT is also used for localization of lung targets. This higher energy results in less contrast relative to kV images, and thus can be more challenging to use during localization. This is reflected by the larger mean absolute difference in superior/inferior shifts that was reported in the previously described study for MV-CBCT (3.7 ± 1.7 mm) versus kV-CBCT (1.6 ± 0.9 mm) when comparing registration differences between different institutions versus reviewers. [135] Another

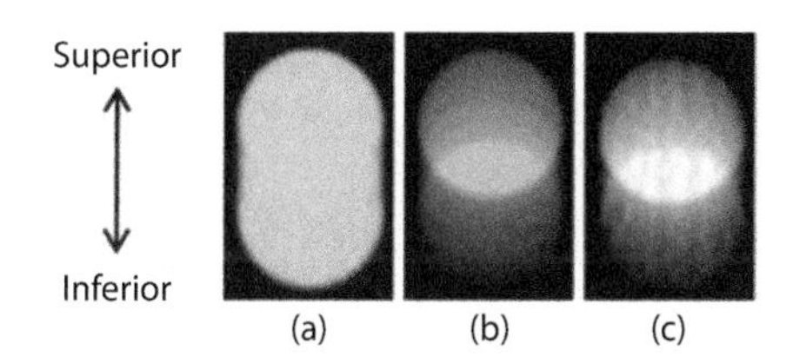

Figure 12.9 Coronal images for registration. (a) MIP, (b) AIP, and (c) dynamic CBCT of the target moving with a 2-cm amplitude. AIP = average intensity projection; CBCT = cone beam computed tomography; MIP = maximum intensity projection.

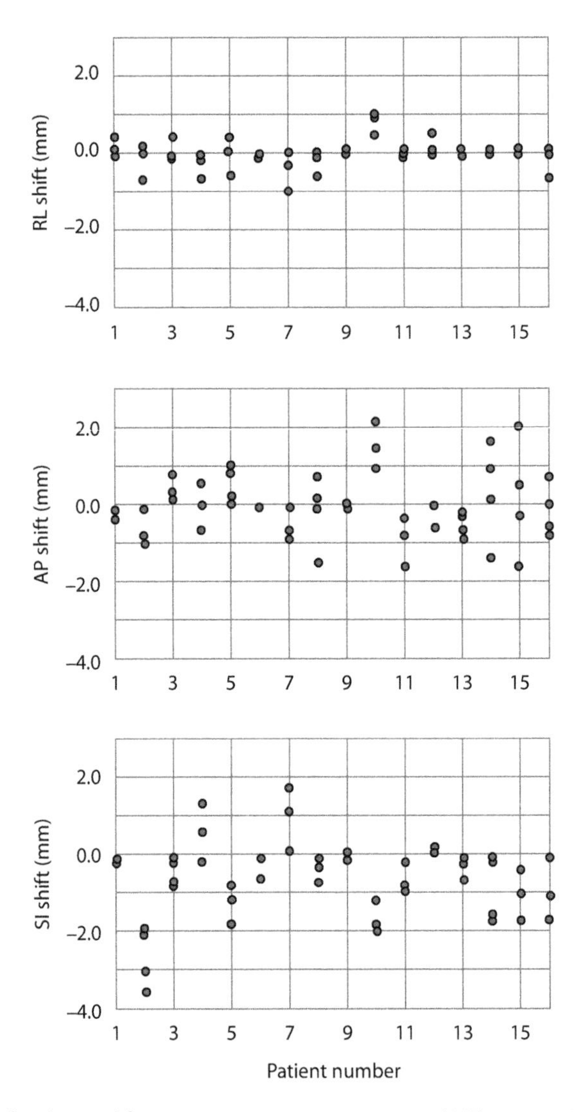

Figure 12.10 Couch shifts obtained from average intensity projection (AIP) registration to maximum intensity projection (MIP) registration for each of the 16 patients. Negative values indicate the couch shift on the right, posterior, and inferior sides. AP = anterior–posterior; RL = right–left; SI = superior–inferior.

kV technology, ExacTrac®, consisting of two diagonal x-ray tubes mounted in the ceiling with opposing detectors underneath the treatment room floor, is mainly used for localization of stereotactic targets due to its ability to achieve sub-millimeter accuracy. It complements existing image guidance tools because it can image (and thus track potential motion) at any couch or gantry angle. In fact, one study evaluating the shifts dictated by ExacTrac 6 Degrees-of-Freedom (6D) versus kV-CBCT found moderate discrepancies between the two for retrospective patient studies (<2 mm translational and <1.5° rotational), but still recommended caution when solely relying on ExacTrac [137]. Lastly, a relatively modern optical tracking system, AlignRT®, has proven to be effective at repositioning patients undergoing gated breast radiotherapy. It employs multiple camera pods that project patterns onto the patient's surface, which are then reflected and detected to reconstruct a 3D model of that surface [138,139]. This system has the potential to be applied to lung and it is important to be aware of the uncertainties that may be associated with this technology. First and foremost, it would be crucial to establish a correlation between the internal moving target and the surface contour, which may require synchronization with a radiographic system. Aside from this, the accuracy of the signal may be affected by poorly reflective surfaces, such as hair and clothing.

It is evident that there is still a spectrum of uncertainties prevalent in the realm of image guided radiation therapy for lung cancer. Those associated with ITV generation and matching ITVs between simulation and treatment can certainly be eradicated with the eventual implementation of 4D-CBCT into the treatment room. Addressing the other described issues will take more research and development. In the meantime, however, it is important to be aware of the present uncertainties and maintain some room for setup errors in PTV margins, so as not blindly rely on image guidance techniques as the unwavering truth. After all, the cardinal rule of a successful treatment is to first and foremost irradiate the target.

12.6 UNCERTAINTIES IN TREATMENT DELIVERY

12.6.1 4D DOSE ACCUMULATION

Treatment delivery accuracy is critical for lung cancer treatment. Due to the presence of lung motion, any static-based assumptions made during treatment planning, inevitably face the dilemma of accurate treatment delivery. Interfractional motion, setup error and anatomical changes also contribute to the uncertainty of delivery. To avoid this problem, a large margin (1.5 cm to 2.5 cm) for lung tumor is required in traditional lung treatment. A much smaller margin (0.5 cm) is applied for SBRT lung treatment. However, the challenge is the lung motion and tumor motion. One simple solution is 4D-CT which can help to build ITV either by phase images or MIP images. AIP images from 4D-CT used for dose calculation are common and popular [123,140,141]. Huang et al. [58] reported that a dosimetric evaluation in phantoms to simulate tumor motions from patient's breathing patient showed good agreement between the measured and computed dose distributions when tumor motion was under 7.0 ± 1.8 mm. However, the accuracy of this method is challenged by the accuracy of 4D-CT images when tumor motion becomes large [58,96]. Several studies [82,96,142,143] showed the 4D-CT images can underestimate or overestimate the tumor motion which can translate to AIP/MIP images. Phase-based dose calculation from 4D-CT is another method to generate 4D dose [144]. The 4D-CT plan was derived from multiple 3D plans based on all phase CT images, each of which used the same conformal beam configuration but with an isocenter shift to aim at the moving tumor and a minor beam aperture and weighting adjustment to maintain plan conformality [24].

4D treatment delivery is defined as continuous delivery of the designed 4D treatment plan throughout the entire breathing cycle [119]. Linear accelerators with multileaf collimators (MLCs) are capable, in principle, of delivering 4D treatments with knowledge patient's respiratory signal or tumor motion. However, due to motion speed and difficulty of detection of lung tumor, current accelerators require predictive software and feedback from the patient's respiratory signal in 200 ms [145]. Robotic linear accelerators such as CyberKnife® are also well suited for 4D treatment delivery. It provides a real-time track of breathing cycle and fluorescence verification of bony or tumor location.

12.6.2 TUMOR VARIATIONS

Lung tumor volumes can be from less than 1 cc up to 200 cc. For SBRT protocols, lung tumor size is limited up to 7 cm or 162.6 cc (PTV). Based on the tumor location to bronchial tree, RTOG 236 and RTOG 813 are designed for peripheral and central located tumors. Liu et al. reported tumor motion analysis of patients who have Stage III or IV non-small-cell lung cancer. They found that tumors that moved >0.5 cm along the superior–inferior (SI), lateral, and anterior–posterior (AP) axes during normal breathing were 39.2%, 1.8%, and 5.4%, respectively, only 10.8% of tumors moving on SI direction more than 1.0 cm [146]. For traditional radiotherapy, lung tumor size is not limited to size and location. A larger size tumor can easily attach to rigid tissue which shows less motion range compared with smaller-size tumor.

Lung tumors can be located on any lobe of the lung. Based on location of the lung, tumor motion can vary from 0.3 cm to 2–3 cm. Tumor located on upper lobe or attached to chest wall show much less motion than the tumor locating on lower lobe. Tumor in hilum region showed an average lateral movement of 9 ± 6 mm (± 1SD), with a range from 0 mm to 16 mm [147]. Diaphragm motion is critical for lung cancer due to its large motion and location. It is around 0.8 cm to 1.6 cm for normal breathing and 4.0 cm to 10.3 cm for deep breathing.

12.6.3 Tracking accuracy, gating correlations, and breath-hold reproducibility

Shirato et al. reported the development of a real-time tumor-tracking system with a gated accelerator. The system detects the location of a 2.0-mm gold marker with an accuracy of better than 1.5 mm in a pelvic phantom using diagnostic x-ray [148]. They also showed that real-time tumor-tracking radiotherapy (RTRT) is feasible for performing 4D radiotherapy with the aid of a fiducial marker near the tumor [149]. CyberKnife can track and localize internal lung tumor position very precise by x-ray and does not depend on patient positioning errors [150]. During the treatment, it continuously checks the relation between internal and external motion by x-ray and fluorescence images [151]. However, 2D projection images are limited in their ability to resolve the motion along the imaging beam axis. There is an uncertainty by using 2D images to find 3D motions. Suh et al. showed 0.18 cm for the treatment fractions for a patient whose breathing range is over 0.5 cm by using 2D projection images [152]. To eliminate this uncertainty, a simultaneous two oblique imager system in CyberKnife or Brainlab EXTRAC is an easy solution. A combination of KV and MV imager on linac can complete the 3D real-time tracking during treatment [153,154]. Rottmann et al. demonstrate using MV-EPID images alone to track a marker-less lung tumor in real time with a motion phantom [155]. They also presented their algorithm that can show errors of 1 mm or smaller in phantom studies and a patient data sample. However, the combination of KV and MV on tracking still has some questions to address, such as the image dose from multiple MV images and continuous KV images, as well as the time lag between MV and KV imagers [156,157].

Gating of moving tumors has the potential to reduce treatment uncertainties, better than dose margins [158]. Keall et al. reported to reduce a 2–11 mm in the CTV to PTV margin with gating [159]. Saito et al. reported that patients treated with respiratory gating showed greater respiratory tumor motion during treatment, but tumor position variability was lower than patients treated without gating [160]. However, Burnett et al. showed that gating provides only a modest advantage unless the tumor is highly mobile [161].

Cheung et al. reported that reproducibility of lung tumor position by using ABC device [54]. They use a standard 1.5-cm PTV margin around the GTV and found the displacement of GTV centers with ABC breath hold applied was 0.3 ± 1.8 mm, 1.2 ± 2.3 mm, and 1.1 ± 3.5 mm in the lateral direction, anterior-posterior direction, and superior-inferior direction, respectively.

REFERENCES

1. Li, G. et al., Advances in 4D medical imaging and 4D radiation therapy. *Technol Cancer Res Treat*, 2008. **7**(1): 67–81.
2. Li, G. et al., Image-guided radiation therapy, in Treatment Planning in Radiation Oncology, F.M. Khan and B.J. Gerbi, Editors. 2016, Philadelphia, PA: Lippincott Williams & Wilkins. pp. 229–258.
3. Bal, M. and L. Spies, Metal artifact reduction in CT using tissue-class modeling and adaptive prefiltering. *Med Phys*, 2006. **33**(8): 2852–9.
4. Li, H. et al., Clinical evaluation of a commercial orthopedic metal artifact reduction tool for CT simulations in radiation therapy. *Med Phys*, 2012. **39**(12): 7507–17.
5. Kapanen, M. and M. Tenhunen, T1/T2*-weighted MRI provides clinically relevant pseudo-CT density data for the pelvic bones in MRI-only based radiotherapy treatment planning. *Acta Oncol*, 2013. **52**(3): 612–8.
6. Graves, M.J. and D.G. Mitchell, Body MRI artifacts in clinical practice: A physicist's and radiologist's perspective. *J Magn Reson Imaging*, 2013. **38**(2): 269–87.
7. Townsend, D.W., Positron emission tomography/computed tomography. *Semin Nucl Med*, 2008. **38**(3): 152–66.
8. Nehmeh, S.A. et al., Reduction of respiratory motion artifacts in PET imaging of lung cancer by respiratory correlated dynamic PET: Methodology and comparison with respiratory gated PET. *J Nucl Med*, 2003. **44**(10): 1644–8.
9. Rosenbaum, S.J. et al., False-positive FDG PET uptake—the role of PET/CT. *Eur Radiol*, 2006. **16**(5): 1054–65.

10. Kadoya, N. et al., Evaluation of various deformable image registration algorithms for thoracic images. *J Radiat Res*, 2014. **55**(1): 175–82.
11. Disselhorst, J.A. et al., Principles of PET/MR Imaging. *J Nucl Med*, 2014. **55**(Suppl. 2): 2S–10S.
12. Gregoire, V. et al., PET-based treatment planning in radiotherapy: A new standard? *J Nucl Med*, 2007. **48**(Suppl 1): 68S–77S.
13. Zaidi, H. and I. El Naqa, PET-guided delineation of radiation therapy treatment volumes: A survey of image segmentation techniques. *Eur J Nucl Med Mol Imaging*, 2010. **37**(11): 2165–87.
14. Jiang, S.B. et al., An experimental investigation on intra-fractional organ motion effects in lung IMRT treatments. *Phys Med Biol*, 2003. **48**(12): 1773–84.
15. Chen, G.T., J.H. Kung, and K.P. Beaudette, Artifacts in computed tomography scanning of moving objects. *Semin Radiat Oncol*, 2004. **14**(1): 19–26.
16. Vedam, S.S. et al., Acquiring a four-dimensional computed tomography dataset using an external respiratory signal. *Phys Med Biol*, 2003. **48**(1): 45–62.
17. Ford, E.C. et al., Respiration-correlated spiral CT: A method of measuring respiratory-induced anatomic motion for radiation treatment planning. *Med Phy*, 2003. **30**(1): 88–97.
18. Low, D.A. et al., A method for the reconstruction of four-dimensional synchronized CT scans acquired during free breathing. *Med Ph*, 2003. **30**(6): 1254–63.
19. Pan, T. et al., 4D-CT imaging of a volume influenced by respiratory motion on multi-slice CT. *Med Phys*, 2004. **31**(2): 333–40.
20. Yamamoto, T. et al., Retrospective analysis of artifacts in four-dimensional CT images of 50 abdominal and thoracic radiotherapy patients. *Int J Radiat Oncol Biol Phys*, 2008. **72**(4): 1250–8.
21. Li, G. et al., Rapid estimation of 4DCT motion-artifact severity based on 1D breathing-surrogate periodicity. *Med Phys*, 2014. **41**(11): 111717.
22. Lewis, J.H. and S.B. Jiang, A theoretical model for respiratory motion artifacts in free-breathing CT scans. *Phys Med Biol*, 2009. **54**(3): 745–55.
23. Persson, G.F. et al., Deviations in delineated GTV caused by artefacts in 4DCT. *Radiother Oncol*, 2010. **96**(1): 61–6.
24. Li, G. et al., A novel four-dimensional radiotherapy planning strategy from a tumor-tracking beam's eye view. *Phys Med Biol*, 2012. **57**(22): 7579–98.
25. Senthi, S. et al., Investigating strategies to reduce toxicity in stereotactic ablative radiotherapy for central lung tumors. *Acta Oncol*, 2013. **53**: 330–5.
26. Cervino, L.I. et al., The diaphragm as an anatomic surrogate for lung tumor motion. *Phys Med Biol*, 2009. **54**(11): 3529–41.
27. Yang, J. et al., Is diaphragm motion a good surrogate for liver tumor motion? *Int J Radiat Oncol Biol Phys*, 2014. **90**(4): 952–8.
28. Li, G. et al., A novel analytical approach to the prediction of respiratory diaphragm motion based on external torso volume change. *Phys Med Biol*, 2009. **54**(13): 4113–30.
29. Li, G. et al., Novel spirometry based on optical surface imaging. *Med Phys*, 2015. **42**(4): 1690.
30. Li, G. et al., Quantitative prediction of respiratory tidal volume based on the external torso volume change: A potential volumetric surrogate. *Phys Med Biol*, 2009. **54**(7): 1963–78.
31. Lu, W. et al., A comparison between amplitude sorting and phase-angle sorting using external respiratory measurement for 4D CT. *Med Phy*, 2006. **33**(8): 2964–74.
32. Hertanto, A. et al., Reduction of irregular breathing artifacts in respiration-correlated CT images using a respiratory motion model. *Med Phys*, 2012. **39**(6): 3070–9.
33. Low, D.A. et al., A novel CT acquisition and analysis technique for breathing motion modeling. *Phys Med Biol*, 2013. **58**(11): L31–6.
34. Rit, S. et al., On-the-fly motion-compensated cone-beam CT using an a priori model of the respiratory motion. *Med Phy*, 2009. **36**(6): 2283–96.
35. Li, R. et al., Single-projection based volumetric image reconstruction and 3D tumor localization in real time for lung cancer radiotherapy. *Med Image Comput Comput-Assist Interv*, 2010. **13**(Pt 3): 449–56.
36. Low, D.A. et al., Novel breathing motion model for radiotherapy. *Int J Radiat Oncol Biol Phys*, 2005. **63**(3): 921–9.

37. Coolens, C. et al., Dynamic volume vs respiratory correlated 4DCT for motion assessment in radiation therapy simulation. *Med Phys*, 2012. **39**(5): 2669–81.
38. Nehmeh, S.A. et al., Four-dimensional (4D) PET/CT imaging of the thorax. *Med Phys*, 2004. **31**(12): 3179–86.
39. Li, T. et al., Model-based image reconstruction for four-dimensional PET. *Med Phys*, 2006. **33**(5): 1288–98.
40. Plathow, C. et al., Evaluation of lung volumetry using dynamic three-dimensional magnetic resonance imaging. *Invest Radiol*, 2005. **40**(3): 173–9.
41. Sodickson, D.K. et al., Rapid volumetric MRI using parallel imaging with order-of-magnitude accelerations and a 32-element RF coil array: Feasibility and implications. *Acad Radiol*, 2005. **12**(5): 626–35.
42. Park, S.J. et al., Evaluation of the combined effects of target size, respiratory motion and background activity on 3D and 4D PET/CT images. *Phys Med Biol*, 2008. **53**(13): 3661–79.
43. Bettinardi, V. et al., Detection and compensation of organ/lesion motion using 4D-PET/CT respiratory gated acquisition techniques. *Radiother Oncol*, 2010. **96**(3): 311–6.
44. Bowen, S.R. et al., Imaging and dosimetric errors in 4D PET/CT-guided radiotherapy from patient-specific respiratory patterns: A dynamic motion phantom end-to-end study. *Phys Med Biol*, 2015. **60**(9): 3731–46.
45. Li, G. et al., Assessing and accounting for the impact of respiratory motion on FDG uptake and viable volume for liver lesions in free-breathing PET using respiration-suspended PET images as reference. *Med Phys*, 2014. **41**(9): 091905.
46. Hu, Y. et al., Respiratory amplitude guided 4-dimensional magnetic resonance imaging. *Int J Radiat Oncol Biol Phys*, 2013. **86**(1): 198–204.
47. Cai, J. et al., Four-dimensional magnetic resonance imaging (4D-MRI) using image-based respiratory surrogate: A feasibility study. *Med Phys*, 2011. **38**(12): 6384–94.
48. Tryggestad, E. et al., Respiration-based sorting of dynamic MRI to derive representative 4D-MRI for radiotherapy planning. *Med Phys*, 2013. **40**(5): 051909.
49. Tokuda, J. et al., Adaptive 4D MR imaging using navigator-based respiratory signal for MRI-guided therapy. *Magn Reson Med*, 2008. **59**(5): 1051–61.
50. Neicu, T. et al., Synchronized moving aperture radiation therapy (SMART): Improvement of breathing pattern reproducibility using respiratory coaching. *Phys Med Biol*, 2006. **51**(3): 617–36.
51. Lu, W. et al., Audio-visual biofeedback does not improve the reliability of target delineation using maximum intensity projection in 4-dimensional computed tomography radiation therapy planning. *Int J Radiat Oncol Biol Phys*, 2014. **88**(1): 229–35.
52. Wong, J.W. et al., The use of active breathing control (ABC) to reduce margin for breathing motion. *Int J Radiat Oncol Biol Phys*, 1999. **44**(4): 911–9.
53. Dawson, L.A. et al., The reproducibility of organ position using active breathing control (ABC) during liver radiotherapy. *Int J Radiat Oncol Biol Phys*, 2001. **51**(5): 1410–21.
54. Cheung, P.C. et al., Reproducibility of lung tumor position and reduction of lung mass within the planning target volume using active breathing control (ABC). *Int J Radiat Oncol Biol Phys*, 2003. **57**(5): 1437–42.
55. Hanley, J. et al., Deep inspiration breath-hold technique for lung tumors: The potential value of target immobilization and reduced lung density in dose escalation. *Int J Radiat Oncol Biol Phys*, 1999. **45**(3): 603–11.
56. Rosenzweig, K.E. et al., The deep inspiration breath-hold technique in the treatment of inoperable non-small-cell lung cancer. *Int J Radiat Oncol Biol Phys*, 2000. **48**(1): 81–7.
57. Timmerman, R. et al., Lung cancer: A model for implementing stereotactic body radiation therapy into practice. *Front Radiat Ther Oncol*, 2007. **40**: 368–85.
58. Huang, L. et al., A study on the dosimetric accuracy of treatment planning for stereotactic body radiation therapy of lung cancer using average and maximum intensity projection images. *Radiother Oncol*, 2010. **96**(1): 48–54.
59. Fritz, P. et al., High-frequency jet ventilation for complete target immobilization and reduction of planning target volume in stereotactic high single-dose irradiation of stage I non-small cell lung cancer and lung metastases. *Int J Radiat Oncol Biol Phys*, 2010. **78**(1): 136–42.
60. McNamara, J.E. et al., Toward correcting drift in target position during radiotherapy via computer-controlled couch adjustments on a programmable Linac. *Med Phys*, 2013. **40**(5): 051719.

61. Harris, K.M. et al., The effect on apparent size of simulated pulmonary nodules of using three standard CT window settings. *Clin Radiol*, 1993. **47**(4): 241–4.
62. Weiss, E. et al., Tumor and normal tissue motion in the thorax during respiration: Analysis of volumetric and positional variations using 4D CT. *Int J Radiat Oncol Biol Phys*, 2007. **67**(1): 296–307.
63. Giraud, P. et al., Conformal radiotherapy for lung cancer: Different delineation of the gross tumor volume (GTV) by radiologists and radiation oncologists. *Radiother Oncol*, 2002. **62**(1): 27–36.
64. Van de Steene, J. et al., Definition of gross tumor volume in lung cancer: Inter-observer variability. *Radiother Oncol*, 2002. **62**(1): 37–49.
65. Roy, A.E. and P. Wells, Volume definition in radiotherapy planning for lung cancer: How the radiologist can help. *Cancer Imaging*, 2006. **6**: 116–23.
66. Hollingdale, A.E. et al., Multidisciplinary collaborative gross tumour volume definition for lung cancer radiotherapy: A prospective study. *Cancer Imaging*, 2011. **11**: 202–8.
67. Steenbakkers, R.J. et al., Reduction of observer variation using matched CT-PET for lung cancer delineation: A three-dimensional analysis. *Int J Radiat Oncol Biol Phys*, 2006. **64**(2): 435–48.
68. Ung, Y.C. et al., 18Fluorodeoxyglucose positron emission tomography in the diagnosis and staging of lung cancer: A systematic review. *J Natl Cancer Inst*, 2007. **99**(23): 1753–67.
69. Schmidt-Hansen, M. et al., PET-CT for assessing mediastinal lymph node involvement in patients with suspected resectable non-small cell lung cancer. *Cochrane Database Syst Rev*, 2014. **11**: CD009519.
70. MacManus, M. et al., Use of PET and PET/CT for Radiation Therapy Planning: IAEA expert report 2006–2007. *Radiother Oncol*, 2009. **91**(1): 85–94.
71. Callahan, J. et al., The clinical significance and management of lesion motion due to respiration during PET/CT scanning. *Cancer Imaging*, 2011. **11**(1): 224–236.
72. van Loon, J. et al., Microscopic disease extension in three dimensions for non-small-cell lung cancer: Development of a prediction model using pathology-validated positron emission tomography and computed tomography features. *Int J Radiat Oncol Biol Phys*, 2012. **82**(1): 448–56.
73. Watkins, W.T. et al., Patient-specific motion artifacts in 4DCT. *Med Phys*, 2010. **37**(6): 2855–61.
74. Chan, R. et al., Computed tomographic-pathologic correlation of gross tumor volume and clinical target volume in non-small cell lung cancer: A pilot experience. *Arch Pathol Lab Med*, 2001. **125**(11): 1469–72.
75. Giraud, P. et al., Evaluation of microscopic tumor extension in non-small-cell lung cancer for three-dimensional conformal radiotherapy planning. *Int J Radiat Oncol Biol Phys*, 2000. **48**(4): 1015–24.
76. Grills, I.S. et al., Clinicopathologic analysis of microscopic extension in lung adenocarcinoma: Defining clinical target volume for radiotherapy. *Int J Radiat Oncol Biol Phys*, 2007. **69**(2): 334–41.
77. Yuan, S. et al., Determining optimal clinical target volume margins on the basis of microscopic extracapsular extension of metastatic nodes in patients with non-small-cell lung cancer. *Int J Radiat Oncol Biol Phys*, 2007. **67**(3): 727–34.
78. Kelsey, C.R., L.B. Marks, and E. Glatstein, Elective nodal irradiation for locally advanced non-small-cell lung cancer: It's called cancer for a reason. *Int J Radiat Oncol Biol Phys*, 2009. **73**(5): 1291–2.
79. Hata, E. et al., Rationale for extended lymphadenectomy for lung cancer. *Theor Surg*, 1990. **5**: 19–25.
80. Nohl-Oser, H.C., An investigation of the anatomy of the lymphatic drainage of the lungs as shown by the lymphatic spread of bronchial carcinoma. *Ann R Coll Surg Engl*, 1972. **51**(3): 157–76.
81. Kelsey, C.R., K.L. Light, and L.B. Marks, Patterns of failure after resection of non-small-cell lung cancer: Implications for postoperative radiation therapy volumes. *Int J Radiat Oncol Biol Phys*, 2006. **65**(4): 1097–105.
82. Ge, H. et al., Quantification and minimization of uncertainties of internal target volume for stereotactic body radiation therapy of lung cancer. *Int J Radiat Oncol Biol Phys*, 2013. **85**(2): 438–43.
83. Cai, J. et al., Estimation of error in maximal intensity projection-based internal target volume of lung tumors: A simulation and comparison study using dynamic magnetic resonance imaging. *Int J Radiat Oncol Biol Phys*, 2007. **69**(3): 895–902.
84. Muirhead, R. et al., Use of Maximum Intensity Projections (MIPs) for target outlining in 4DCT radiotherapy planning. *J Thorac Oncol*, 2008. **3**(12): 1433–8.

85. Underberg, R.W. et al., Use of maximum intensity projections (MIP) for target volume generation in 4DCT scans for lung cancer. *Int J Radiat Oncol Biol Phys*, 2005. **63**(1): 253–60.
86. Wolthaus, J.W. et al., Comparison of different strategies to use four-dimensional computed tomography in treatment planning for lung cancer patients. *Int J Radiat Oncol Biol Phys*, 2008. **70**(4): 1229–38.
87. Kyriakou, E. and D.R. McKenzie, Changes in lung tumor shape during respiration. *Phys Med Biol*, 2012. **57**(4): 919–35.
88. Vedam, S. et al., Dosimetric impact of geometric errors due to respiratory motion prediction on dynamic multileaf collimator-based four-dimensional radiation delivery. *Med Phys*, 2005. **32**(6): 1607–20.
89. Ruan, D., J.A. Fessler, and J.M. Balter, Real-time prediction of respiratory motion based on local regression methods. *Phys Med Biol*, 2007. **52**(23): 7137–52.
90. Ezhil, M. et al., Determination of patient-specific internal gross tumor volumes for lung cancer using four-dimensional computed tomography. *Radiat Oncol*, 2009. **4**: 4.
91. Rietzel, E. et al., Four-dimensional image-based treatment planning: Target volume segmentation and dose calculation in the presence of respiratory motion. *Int J Radiat Oncol Biol Phys*, 2005. **61**(5): 1535–50.
92. Rietzel, E. et al., Design of 4D treatment planning target volumes. *Int J Radiat Oncol Biol Phys*, 2006. **66**(1): 287–95.
93. Bradley, J.D. et al., Comparison of helical, maximum intensity projection (MIP), and averaged intensity (AI) 4D CT imaging for stereotactic body radiation therapy (SBRT) planning in lung cancer. *Radiother Oncol*, 2006. **81**(3): 264–8.
94. Simon, L. et al., Initial evaluation of a four-dimensional computed tomography system using a programmable motor. *J Appl Clin Med Phys*, 2006. **7**(4): 50–65.
95. St James, S. et al., Quantifying ITV instabilities arising from 4DCT: A simulation study using patient data. *Phys Med Biol*, 2012. **57**(5): L1–L7.
96. Park, K. et al., Do maximum intensity projection images truly capture tumor motion? *Int J Radiat Oncol Biol Phys*, 2009. **73**(2): 618–25.
97. Cai, J., P.W. Read, and K. Sheng, The effect of respiratory motion variability and tumor size on the accuracy of average intensity projection from four-dimensional computed tomography: An investigation based on dynamic MRI. *Med Phys*, 2008. **35**(11): 4974–81.
98. Mancosu, P. et al., Semiautomatic technique for defining the internal gross tumor volume of lung tumors close to liver/spleen cupola by 4D-CT. *Med Phys*, 2010. **37**(9): 4572–6.
99. Jang, S.S. et al., Reconstitution of internal target volumes by combining four-dimensional computed tomography and a modified slow computed tomography scan in stereotactic body radiotherapy planning for lung cancer. *Radiat Oncol*, 2014. **9**: 106.
100. Chang, G. et al., Determination of internal target volume from a single positron emission tomography/computed tomography scan in lung cancer. *Int J Radiat Oncol Biol Phys*, 2012. **83**(1): 459–66.
101. Duan, Y. et al., Comparison of primary tumour volumes delineated on four-dimensional computed tomography maximum intensity projection and F-fluorodeoxyglucose positron emission tomography computed tomography images of non-small cell lung cancer. *J Med Imaging Radiat Oncol*, 2015. **59**(5): 623–30.
102. Pepin, A. et al., Management of respiratory motion in PET/computed tomography: The state of the art. *Nucl Med Commun*, 2014. **35**(2): 113–22.
103. Aristophanous, M. et al., Clinical utility of 4D FDG-PET/CT scans in radiation treatment planning. *Int J Radiat Oncol Biol Phys*, 2012. **82**(1): e99–105.
104. Callahan, J. et al., Motion effects on SUV and lesion volume in 3D and 4D PET scanning. *Australas Phys Eng Sci Med*, 2011. **34**(4): 489–95.
105. Nehmeh, S.A. et al., Quantitation of respiratory motion during 4D-PET/CT acquisition. *Med Phys*, 2004. **31**(6): 1333–8.
106. Guerra, L. et al., Comparative evaluation of CT-based and respiratory-gated PET/CT-based planning target volume (PTV) in the definition of radiation treatment planning in lung cancer: Preliminary results. *Eur J Nucl Med Mol Imaging*, 2014. **41**(4): 702–10.
107. Keall, P.J. et al., The management of respiratory motion in radiation oncology report of AAPM Task Group 76. *Med Phys*, 2006. **33**(10): 3874–900.

108. Cai, J. et al., Effects of breathing variation on gating window internal target volume in respiratory gated radiation therapy. *Med Phys*, 2010. **37**(8): 3927–34.
109. Beddar, A.S. et al., Correlation between internal fiducial tumor motion and external marker motion for liver tumors imaged with 4D-CT. *Int J Radiat Oncol Biol Phys*, 2007. **67**(2): 630–8.
110. Gierga, D.P. et al., The correlation between internal and external markers for abdominal tumors: Implications for respiratory gating. *Int J Radiat Oncol Biol Phys*, 2005. **61**(5): 1551–8.
111. Hoisak, J.D. et al., Correlation of lung tumor motion with external surrogate indicators of respiration. *Int J Radiat Oncol Biol Phys*, 2004. **60**(4): 1298–306.
112. Koch, N. et al., Evaluation of internal lung motion for respiratory-gated radiotherapy using MRI: Part I—Correlating internal lung motion with skin fiducial motion. *Int J Radiat Oncol Biol Phys*, 2004. **60**(5): 1459–72.
113. Yan, H. et al., The correlation evaluation of a tumor tracking system using multiple external markers. *Med Phys*, 2006. **33**(11): 4073–84.
114. Huang, T.C. et al., Four-dimensional dosimetry validation and study in lung radiotherapy using deformable image registration and Monte Carlo techniques. *Radiat Oncol*, 2010. **5**: 45.
115. Starkschall, G. et al., Potential dosimetric benefits of four-dimensional radiation treatment planning. *Int J Radiat Oncol Biol Phys*, 2009. **73**(5): 1560–5.
116. Engelsman, M., E. Rietzel, and H.M. Kooy, Four-dimensional proton treatment planning for lung tumors. *Int J Radiat Oncol Biol Phys*, 2006. **64**(5): 1589–95.
117. Rosu, M. et al., How extensive of a 4D dataset is needed to estimate cumulative dose distribution plan evaluation metrics in conformal lung therapy? *Med Phys*, 2007. **34**(1): 233–45.
118. Keall, P.J. et al., Monte Carlo as a four-dimensional radiotherapy treatment-planning tool to account for respiratory motion. *Phys Med Biol*, 2004. **49**(16): 3639–48.
119. Keall, P., 4-dimensional computed tomography imaging and treatment planning. *Semin Radiat Oncol*, 2004. **14**(1): 81–90.
120. Wolthaus, J.W. et al., Mid-ventilation CT scan construction from four-dimensional respiration-correlated CT scans for radiotherapy planning of lung cancer patients. *Int J Radiat Oncol Biol Phys*, 2006. **65**(5): 1560–71.
121. Mexner, V. et al., Effects of respiration-induced density variations on dose distributions in radiotherapy of lung cancer. *Int J Radiat Oncol Biol Phys*, 2009. **74**(4): 1266–75.
122. Guckenberger, M. et al., Four-dimensional treatment planning for stereotactic body radiotherapy. *Int J Radiat Oncol Biol Phys*, 2007. **69**(1): 276–85.
123. Glide-Hurst, C.K. et al., A simplified method of four-dimensional dose accumulation using the mean patient density representation. *Med Phys*, 2008. **35**(12): 5269–77.
124. Tian, Y. et al., Dosimetric comparison of treatment plans based on free breathing, maximum, and average intensity projection CTs for lung cancer SBRT. *Med Phys*, 2012. **39**(5): 2754–60.
125. Berbeco, R.I., C.J. Pope, and S.B. Jiang, Measurement of the interplay effect in lung IMRT treatment using EDR2 films. *J Appl Clin Med Phy*, 2006. **7**(4): 33–42.
126. Merrow, C.E., I.Z. Wang, and M.B. Podgorsak, A dosimetric evaluation of VMAT for the treatment of non-small cell lung cancer. *J Appl Clin Med Phy*, 2013. **14**(1): 228–238.
127. Rao, M. et al., Dosimetric impact of breathing motion in lung stereotactic body radiotherapy treatment using image-modulated radiotherapy and volumetric modulated arc therapy. *Int J Radiat Oncol Biol Phys*, 2012. **83**(2): E251–E6.
128. Ueda, Y. et al., Craniocaudal safety margin calculation based on interfractional changes in tumor motion in lung SBRT assessed with an EPID in cine mode. *Int J Radiat Oncol Biol Phys*, 2012. **83**(3): 1064–9.
129. Zhang, F. et al., Reproducibility of tumor motion probability distribution function in stereotactic body radiation therapy of lung cancer. *Int J Radiat Oncol Biol Phys*, 2012. **84**(3): 861–6.
130. McQuaid, D. and T. Bortfeld, 4D planning over the full course of fractionation: Assessment of the benefit of tumor trailing. *Phys Med Biol*, 2011. **56**(21): 6935–49.
131. Cai, J., H.K. Malhotra, and C.G. Orton, Point/Counterpoint. A 3D-conformal technique is better than IMRT or VMAT for lung SBRT. *Med Phys*, 2014. **41**(4): 040601.

132. Chui, C.S., E. Yorke, and L. Hong, The effects of intra-fraction organ motion on the delivery of intensity-modulated field with a multileaf collimator. *Med Phys*, 2003. **30**(7): 1736–46.
133. Vergalasova, I., J. Maurer, and F.F. Yin, Potential underestimation of the internal target volume (ITV) from free-breathing CBCT. *Med Phys*, 2011. **38**(8): 4689–99.
134. Shirai, K. et al., Phantom and clinical study of differences in cone beam computed tomographic registration when aligned to maximum and average intensity projection. *Int J Radiat Oncol Biol Phys*, 2014. **88**(1): 189–94.
135. Cui, Y. et al., Implementation of remote 3-dimensional image guided radiation therapy quality assurance for radiation therapy oncology group clinical trials. *Int J Radiat Oncol Biol Phys*, 2013. **85**(1): 271–7.
136. Altorjai, G. et al., Cone-beam CT-based delineation of stereotactic lung targets: The influence of image modality and target size on interobserver variability. *Int J Radiat Oncol Biol Phys*, 2012. **82**(2): e265–72.
137. Chang, Z. et al., 6D image guidance for spinal non-invasive stereotactic body radiation therapy: Comparison between ExacTrac X-ray 6D with kilo-voltage cone-beam CT. *Radiother Oncol*, 2010. **95**(1): 116–21.
138. Gierga, D.P. et al., Comparison of target registration errors for multiple image-guided techniques in accelerated partial breast irradiation. *Int J Radiat Oncol Biol Phys*, 2008. **70**(4): 1239–46.
139. Schoffel, P.J. et al., Accuracy of a commercial optical 3D surface imaging system for realignment of patients for radiotherapy of the thorax. *Phys Med Biol*, 2007. **52**(13): 3949–63.
140. Kang, Y. et al., 4D Proton treatment planning strategy for mobile lung tumors. *Int J Radiat Oncol Biol Phys*, 2007. **67**(3): 906–14.
141. Keall, P.J. et al., Four-dimensional radiotherapy planning for DMLC-based respiratory motion tracking. *Med Phys*, 2005. **32**(4): 942–51.
142. Spadea, M.F. et al., Uncertainties in lung motion prediction relying on external surrogate: A 4DCT study in regular vs. irregular breathers. *Technol Cancer Res Treat*, 2010. **9**(3): 307–16.
143. Persson, G.F. et al., Artifacts in conventional computed tomography (CT) and free breathing four-dimensional CT induce uncertainty in gross tumor volume determination. *Int J Radiat Oncol Biol Phys*, 2011. **80**(5): 1573–80.
144. Admiraal, M.A., D. Schuring, and C.W. Hurkmans, Dose calculations accounting for breathing motion in stereotactic lung radiotherapy based on 4D-CT and the internal target volume. *Radiother Oncol*, 2008. **86**(1): 55–60.
145. Fledelius, W. et al., Tracking latency in image-based dynamic MLC tracking with direct image access. *Acta Oncol*, 2011. **50**(6): 952–9.
146. Liu, H.H. et al., Assessing respiration-induced tumor motion and internal target volume using four-dimensional computed tomography for radiotherapy of lung cancer. *Int J Radiat Oncol Biol Phys*, 2007. **68**(2): 531–40.
147. Langen, K.M. and D.T. Jones, Organ motion and its management. *Int J Radiat Oncol Biol Phys*, 2001. **50**(1): 265–78.
148. Shirato, H. et al., Physical aspects of a real-time tumor-tracking system for gated radiotherapy. *Int J Radiat Oncol Biol Phys*, 2000. **48**(4): 1187–95.
149. Shirato, H. et al., Organ motion in image-guided radiotherapy: Lessons from real-time tumor-tracking radiotherapy. *Int J Clin Oncol*, 2007. **12**(1): 8–16.
150. Seppenwoolde, Y. et al., Accuracy of tumor motion compensation algorithm from a robotic respiratory tracking system: A simulation study. *Med Phys*, 2007. **34**(7): 2774–84.
151. Shiomi, H. et al., [CyberKnife]. *Igaku Butsuri*, 2001. **21**(1): 11–6.
152. Suh, Y., S. Dieterich, and P.J. Keall, Geometric uncertainty of 2D projection imaging in monitoring 3D tumor motion. *Phys Med Biol*, 2007. **52**(12): 3439–54.
153. Rozario, T. et al., An accurate algorithm to match imperfectly matched images for lung tumor detection without markers. *J Appl Clin Med Phys*, 2015. **16**(3): 5200.
154. Liu, W. et al., Real-time 3D internal marker tracking during arc radiotherapy by the use of combined MV-kV imaging. *Phys Med Biol*, 2008. **53**(24): 7197–213.
155. Rottmann, J., P. Keall, and R. Berbeco, Real-time soft tissue motion estimation for lung tumors during radiotherapy delivery. *Med Phys*, 2013. **40**(9): 091713.

156. Yan, H. et al., Hybrid MV-kV 3D respiratory motion tracking during radiation therapy with low imaging dose. *Phys Med Biol*, 2012. **57**(24): 8455–69.
157. Wiersma, R.D., W. Mao, and L. Xing, Combined kV and MV imaging for real-time tracking of implanted fiducial markers. *Med Phys*, 2008. **35**(4): 1191–8.
158. Wurm, R.E. et al., Image guided respiratory gated hypofractionated Stereotactic Body Radiation Therapy (H-SBRT) for liver and lung tumors: Initial experience. *Acta Oncol*, 2006. **45**(7): 881–9.
159. Keall, P.J. et al., Potential radiotherapy improvements with respiratory gating. *Australas Phys Eng Sci Med*, 2002. **25**(1): 1–6.
160. Saito, T. et al., Respiratory gating during stereotactic body radiotherapy for lung cancer reduces tumor position variability. *PLOS ONE*, 2014. **9**(11): e112824.
161. Burnett, S.S. et al., A study of tumor motion management in the conformal radiotherapy of lung cancer. *Radiother Oncol*, 2008. **86**(1): 77–85.

PART 4

ADVANCES IN IGRT FOR LUNG CANCER

13

Advances in imaging simulation for lung cancer IGRT

JING CAI, DANIEL LOW, TINSU PAN, YILIN LIU, ZHENG CHANG, AND WEI LU

13.1 INTRODUCTION

Radiation therapy of lung cancer is among the most common and important areas of image-guided radiation therapy. Imaging simulations including computed tomography (CT), magnetic resonance imaging (MRI), positron emission tomography with 2-fluorine-18 fluoro-2-deoxy-D-glucose (FDG-PET) and FDG-PET combined with CT (FDG-PET/CT) are currently being used for clinical assessment of lung cancer. Recent technological advances in these imaging systems hold great promises to produce marked improvements toward more precise treatment of lung cancer. In this chapter, we will focus on recent advances in CT, MRI, PET, and other imaging methods in lung cancer applications, and discuss their potentials and limitations for use in clinical practice.

13.2 ADVANCES IN CT SIMULATION

CT is an essential imaging technology in radiation therapy for patient simulation and treatment planning. In recent years, there have been several notable advances in CT technology, including radiation dose reduction, iterative reconstruction, dual-energy CT, improved 4D-CT techniques, etc.

New CT systems have been introduced in the past few years, featuring innovative scanner technology to reduce radiation dose, increase speed, and improve image quality. For example, GE Healthcare Revolution platform offers 256 detector rows and features an 80 cm bore and a gantry rotation speed of 0.28 seconds. It can reduce metal artifacts, offering the potential for sedation-free CT scanning. The Revolution system also contains technology to allow spectral imaging in the future, which is enabled via a very fast kV switching system, changing the scanning energy level back and forth between 40–140 kV during the scan using the same detector and x-ray tube. Another example is Siemens' Somatom Force system, which is the company's next generation dual-source CT system. It has a gantry speed of 0.25 ms, enabling imaging of an adult chest in about one second, eliminating the need for breath hold. Usage of different energy levels can enhance the contrasts-to-noise ratio and lower patient radiation dose.

Several commercial software packages of iterative reconstruction are now available for CT application, including IRIS (Siemens, Erlangen, Germany), ASiR (GE Healthcare, Milwaukee, WI), Adaptive Iterative Dose Reduction (Toshiba, Tochigi, Japan), and iDose (Philips Healthcare, Best, Netherlands) [1]. A filtered Fourier back-projection image reconstruction is initially performed in the raw data domain to generate a master reconstruction which is an approximate reconstruction. The discordance between the measured and calculated projections is used to derive correction projections, reconstruct a correction image, and update the original image. This process is repeated until the deviation between measured and calculated projections is smaller than a predefined limit. Implementation of iterative reconstruction can yield diagnostic-quality images at 20%–66% lower volume CT dose index values than those obtained with filtered Fourier back-projection techniques for CT of the chest and abdomen [2,3].

4D-CT has become the clinical standard for patient specific respiratory motion imaging for radiation therapy. Despite its wide use, it often suffers motion artifacts owing to patient's breathing irregularities, which has been shown to adversely impact treatment planning. Recently, progress has been made to improve the image quality of 4D-CT using novel image sorting methods and respiratory motion modeling. This following section will detail these developments, motion modeling based on 4D-CT, as well as the implementation of derivative products of 4D-CT, average CT and maximum intensity projection (MIP) CT, in PET/CT applications.

13.2.1 Improved 4D-CT

4D-CT is used to account for respiratory motion in radiation treatment planning, but artifacts resulting from the acquisition and post-processing limit its accuracy. Artifacts of 4D-CT are mainly due to breathing irregularities or incorrect breathing phase identification. Various methods have been proposed to improve

4D-CT by reducing motion artifacts, using novel post processing/sorting algorithms, or new image acquisition schemes.

Ehrhardt et al. developed an optical flow based method for improved reconstruction of 4D-CT datasets from multi-slice CT scans [4]. The optical flow between scans at neighboring respiratory states is estimated by a nonlinear registration method. The calculated velocity field is then used to reconstruct a 4D-CT dataset by interpolating data at exactly the predefined respiratory phase. Evaluation results show a relevant reduction of reconstruction artifacts by this technique. Zhang et al. derived a mathematical model to represent the regular respiratory motion from a patient-specific 4D-CT set and have demonstrated its application in reducing irregular motion artifacts in 4D-CT images [5]. This approach can mitigate shape distortions of anatomy caused by irregular breathing motion during 4D-CT acquisition. Bernatowicz et al. [6] developed a novel simulation framework incorporating a realistic deformable digital phantom driven by patient tumor motion patterns. Based on this framework, the authors tested the hypothesis that respiratory-gated 4D-CT can significantly reduce lung imaging artifacts. Respiratory-gated 4D-CT can reduce image artifacts affecting up to 90 cm^3 of normal lung tissue compared to conventional acquisition. Gianoli et al. developed a method to reduce 4D-CT artifacts by using multiple respiratory related signals to reduce uncertainties and increase robustness in breathing phase identification [7]. Multiple respiratory-related signals were provided by infrared 3D localization of a configuration of markers placed on the thoracoabdominal surface. Multidimensional K-means clustering was used for retrospective 4D-CT image sorting, which was based on multiple marker variables, to identify clusters representing different breathing phases. The implemented multiple point method demonstrated the ability to reduce artifacts in 4D-CT imaging. Thomas et al. developed a novel 4D-CT technique that exploits standard fast-helical acquisition, a simultaneous breathing surrogate measurement, deformable image registration, and a breathing motion model to remove sorting artifacts [8]. This method is robust in the presence of irregular breathing and allows the entire imaging dose to contribute to the resulting image quality, providing sorting artifact-free images at a patient dose similar to or less than current 4D-CT techniques.

Different acquisition methods have also been developed to reduce 4D-CT image artifacts. Castillo et al. [9] investigated the efficacy of three experimental 4D-CT acquisition methods to reduce artifacts in a prospective institutional review board approved study. In their study, 18 lung cancer patients received standard clinical 4D-CT scans followed by each of the alternative 4D-CT acquisitions: 1) data oversampling, 2) beam gating with breathing irregularities, and 3) rescanning the clinical acquisition acquired during irregular breathing. Relative values of a validated correlation-based artifact metric (CM) determined the best acquisition method per patient. Each 4D-CT was processed by an extended phase sorting approach that optimizes the quantitative artifact metric (CM sorting). The clinical acquisitions were also post processed by phase sorting for artifact comparison of our current clinical implementation with the experimental methods. The results showed that the oversampling acquisition reduced artifact presence from the current clinical 4D-CT implementation to the largest degree and provided the simplest and most reproducible implementation. The rescan acquisition increased artifact presence significantly, compared to all acquisitions, and suffered from combination of data from independent scans over which large internal anatomic shifts occurred.

13.2.2 Motion modeling based on 4D-CT

Early works of motion modeling studied the motion of a single point, usually the tumor center of mass [10,11]. Based on fluoroscopic video images of implanted markers in several patients, they determined that the motion had an elliptic pattern [10]. They elected to parameterize the elliptic motion into components aligned with the elliptic axes. Figure 13.1 shows a schematic of the motion model for cases without and with hysteresis. The method for including hysteresis was to add a phase angle between the different directional components. The variation in time spent at specific phases, such as spending more time at exhalation than inhalation, were managed by taking the sinusoidal function to an even power, with tunable period and amplitude. Figure 13.2 shows an example of the model for regular and irregular breathing patients. While this model worked for regular breathing patients, it broke down for irregular breathing patients because the model could not predict changes in breathing period.

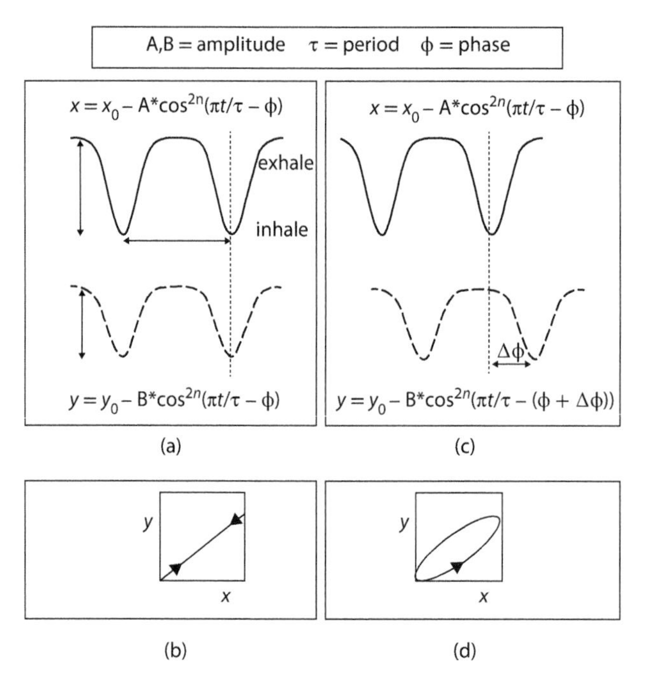

Figure 13.1 Breathing motion model proposed by Seppenwolde et al. [10] to describe tissue motion. The model describes the spatial coordinates as periodic functions in time. (a) Breathing motion without hysteresis (two dimensional). These traces are shown as functions of time. (b) Breathing motion without hysteresis shown in space. (c) Breathing motion with hysteresis (two dimensional). These traces are shown as functions of time. The *x* coordinate is the same as in (a), but the *y* coordinate has a phase offset. (d) Breathing motion with hysteresis shown in space.

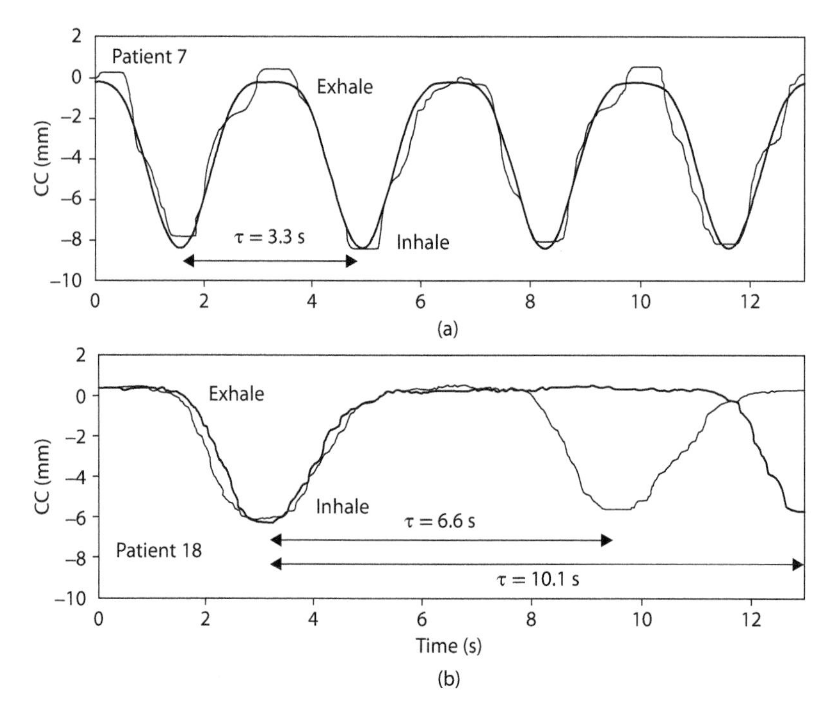

Figure 13.2 Example of breathing motion model results from Seppenwoolde et al. [10] for (a) a regular-breathing patient and (b) irregular breathing patient. The model works well when the breathing frequency and amplitude are stable, but breaks down if the breathing frequency changes.

In view of addressing these modeling inadequacies, patient-specific breathing motion models [5,12–14] have been proposed to provide more accurate spatio-temporal positions and trajectories in the entire lung volume. Ideally, a breathing motion model should consider patient organ physiology and supply mechanical and functional information. Breathing motion models have commonly been constructed by correlating the external surrogate signals to the acquired image data. The surrogate data should be easily measureable and have a strong correlation with the motion of interest. If the correspondence model can be successfully established between the two sets of data, the surrogate signal can then be used to estimate or predict the motion of interest. A survey of the breathing motion models can be found in McClelland et al. [15]. Figure 13.3 [16] shows an example schematic of a motion model generation by McClelland et al.

Recently, principal component analysis (PCA) based approaches have also been proposed [5,17]. The PCA was used to analyze the underlying data structure of the deformation vector fields obtained from deformable image registration processing of the 4D-CT image data between a reference phase and other phases. The authors found that three principal components were sufficient to describe the respiratory motion based on 4D-CT data, with the first principal component basis characterizing the regular respiratory motion, while the rest of the bases account for the variation caused by image noise, registration error, or image reconstruction errors.

13.2.2.1 5D MOTION MODELING

In addition to the semi-voluntary tidal volume changes associated with breathing, an important physiological phenomenon in lung motion is tissue hysteresis behavior, or the observation that many lung tissues do not follow the same trajectories from inhalation to exhalation as the reverse. This motion hysteresis was observed in Seppenwoolde et al. [10] where real-time fluoroscopic imaging was implemented to monitor implanted radio-opaque markers. In their study of 21 monitored tumors, many expressed hysteresis-like trajectories. Vedam et al. [18] treated breathing as a cyclic process and designated eight phases in the breathing cycle: peak exhalation, early, mid-, and late inhalation, peak inhalation, and early and late exhalation. This scheme was used to bin acquired CT scans into breathing phases and worked well in describing regular breathing motion.

To address irregular breathing, Low et al. proposed a technique that described breathing based on tidal volume as the measured breathing amplitude surrogate and directly incorporated the hysteretic motion

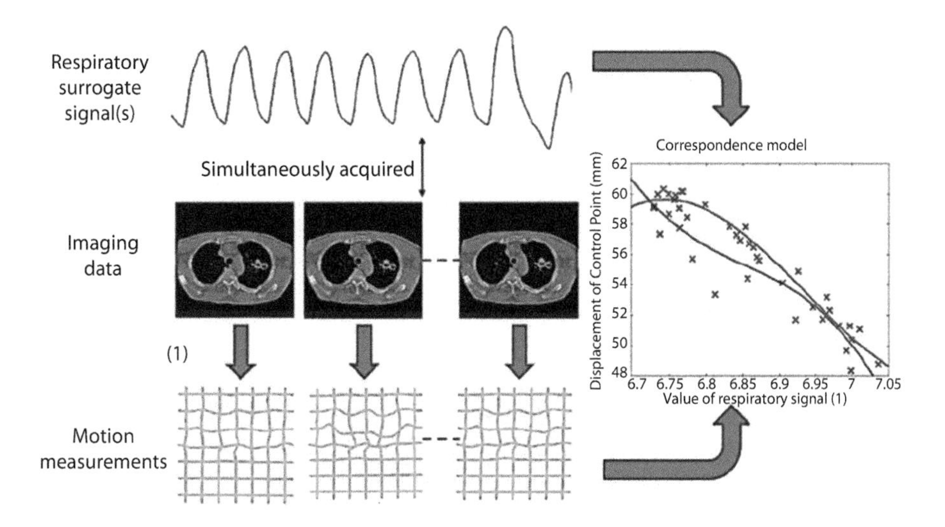

Figure 13.3 Workflow of general breathing motion model development. A breathing surrogate is acquired in real time and is synchronized to 4D-CT image data. The CT scans are deformably registered to measure the relative motion of each piece of tissue within the scans. The relationship between the motion and the surrogate is evaluated to determine the motion model parameters. (From McClelland, J.R., B.A.S. Champion, and D.J. Hawkes, Combining image registration, respiratory motion modelling, and motion compensated image reconstruction, *in Biomedical Image Registration: 6th International Workshop, WBIR*, S. Ourselin and M. Modat, Editors. July 7–8, 2014. London, Cham: Springer International Publishing. pp. 103–13.)

trajectory into the model formulation [14]. Hysteresis motion was assumed to be caused by pressure imbalances in the lungs during respiration. For quiet respiration, whether regular or irregular, the pressure imbalances were assumed to be proportional to the excess or deficit pressure in the trachea, and that excess or deficit pressure was approximated to be proportional to the airflow in and out of the mouth. Therefore, the time-dependent surrogates were tidal volume and airflow, which when combined with the three spatial dimensions, led to the term "5D." The relationship between tissue displacement and the surrogates was assumed to be linear; tissue displacement was modeled as vectors whose lengths were linear functions of the tidal volume and airflow. When written in the form of an equation, the displacement of a piece of tissue X when the patient had tidal volume v and airflow f was

$$\vec{X} = \overrightarrow{X_o} + \vec{\alpha} \cdot v + \vec{\beta} \cdot f, \tag{13.1}$$

where $\overrightarrow{X_o}$ was the tissue position at 0 volume and airflow, and, $\vec{\alpha}$ and $\vec{\beta}$ were the linear vector approximations to the motion as functions of the surrogates volume and airflow, respectively. The meaning of an airflow of 0 was clear, but the meaning of a tidal volume of 0 was not defined in the literature. Therefore, Low et al. elected to use tidal volume percentiles to define the tidal volume of 0. Typically, they defined the 5th percentile tidal volume as 0, with the percentile computed from the breathing traces during the CT session. In Low et al. [14], the validity of the motion model in Equation 13.1 was evaluated by tracking 76 tissue positions in four patients at 15 different breathing phases.

One challenge of employing tidal volume as the time-dependent surrogate was that spirometers often drifted during their measurements. Werner et al. [19] investigated this issue and found that the use of abdominal pressure belts as breathing surrogates led to tidal volume measurements that were highly correlated with those obtained through spirometry acquisitions. This finding allowed for the replacement of a spirometer with a more straightforward abdominal bellows signal measurement. Either the bellows signal would be converted to tidal volume using the image data, or the analysis conducted by evaluating percentiles rather than the bellows signal directly. In either case, since airflow was the time derivative of tidal volume in Equation 13.1, any surrogate proportional to tidal volume could be employed as the replacement for airflow by taking its time derivative.

The group used multiple cine scans, acquiring up to 25 low-mAs scans at each couch position. They employed deformable image registration to measure the tissue motion and provide the necessary data to fit the motion model. The greatest challenge of this approach was in registering tissues near the craniocaudal boundaries of the cine images. In 2013, Low et al. [20] changed the method they used to acquire the CT data needed to generate the breathing motion model. Rather than acquire all images at a single location sequentially, they elected to use fast-helical CT scanning. They employed both a Siemens Flash and a Siemens AS64. The scanners operated with rotation rates of 0.28 s and 0.33 s, employing pitch values of 1.2 and 1.5, respectively. This meant that a single location was scanned for only approximately 0.22 s, fast enough that most motion blurring was eliminated. Similar to the cine scans, the fast-helical scans were acquired using low mAs to restrict the radiation dose.

The fast-helical CT scans required between 1.5 s and 2.5 s to acquire, so the patient was breathing for up to a half a breath during the CT scan acquisition. Therefore, the scans were not representative of any single breathing phase. Instead, each slice was assigned a breathing phase since the breathing surrogate was synchronized with the CT scan acquisition.

The fast-helical CT scans often looked like breath-hold scans. The breathing motion artifacts were minor and each scan included the entire lungs. Therefore, deformable image registration was quite straightforward. The workflow started with selecting one CT scan as the reference scan (typically the first scan), segmenting the lungs, conducting deformable image registration separately inside and outside the lungs to measure the motion of the voxels relative to the reference scan, determining the motion model parameters based on that motion, the surrogate amplitude and rate, and averaging the CT scans in the reference scan geometry to reduce image noise. The averaged image could be deformed to any breathing phase (amplitude and rate) based on the motion model. For treatment planning, scans were reconstructed at user-selected breathing phases. Figure 13.4 shows an example of the clinical 4D-CT protocol and the 5D protocol with fast-helical CT scan acquisition for 5 of the first 10 patients [8].

Dou et al. showed that the original helical CT scans could be used to determine the accuracy of the process 5D-CT by reconstructing the original fast-helical CT scans [21]. Figure 13.5a shows an example of the reference and a second fast-helical CT scan. Figure 13.5b shows the same CT scans with the second scan deformed using the motion model to the reference CT scan geometry. Figure 13.6a summarizes the error histograms

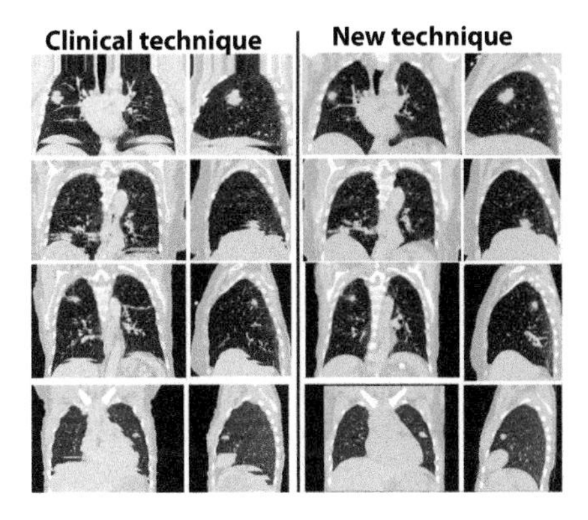

Figure 13.4 Examples of the commercial 4D-CT technique and the 5D-CT technique using fast-helical CT scan acquisitions. Note the elimination of sorting artifacts and the improved noise characteristics of the 5D protocol scans. (From Thomas, D. et al., *Int J Radiat Oncol Biol Phys*, 89, 191–198, 2014.)

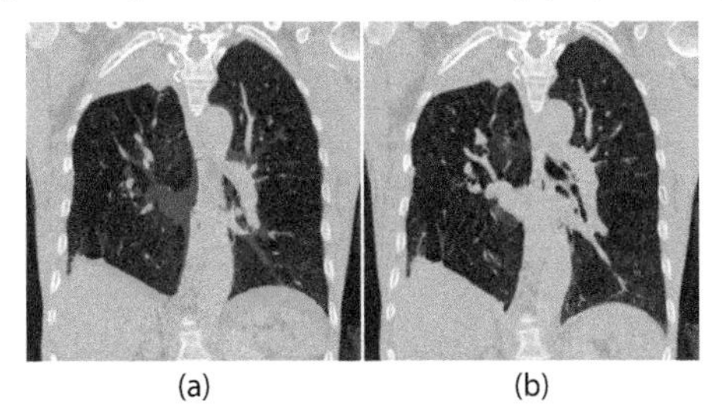

(a) (b)

Figure 13.5 (a) The reference and a second fast-helical CT scan superimposed showing the discrepancies of the tissue positions. (b) The same two scans with the reference scan deformed to the second CT scan geometry using the 5D model. The reconstructed and original scans look nearly identical. (Figure generated from same dataset as published by Dou et al.)

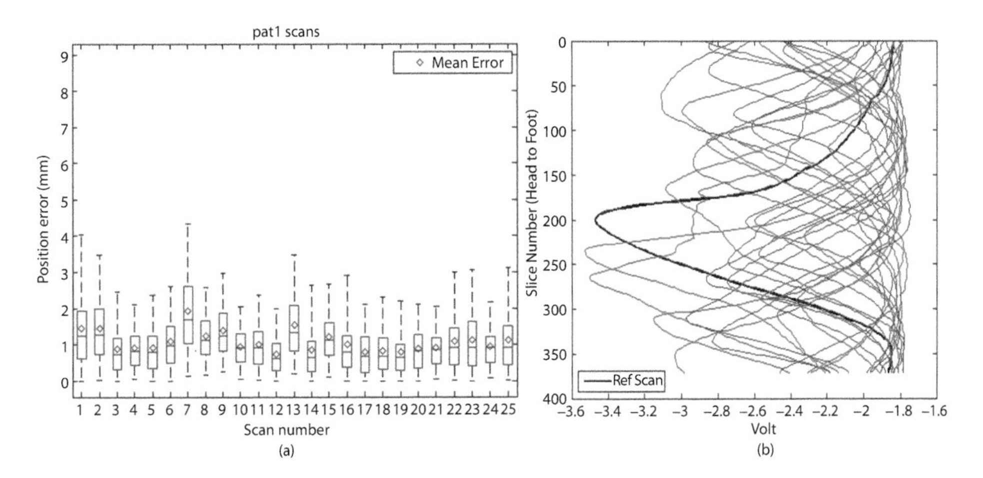

Figure 13.6 (a) Whisker plot of differences between reconstructed and original helical CT scans in the 5D process. The whiskers correspond to the 5th, 25th, 50th (red line), 75th, and 95th percentiles and the diamond is the mean error. (b) The breathing pattern for the 25 fast-helical CT scans. The black trace is the reference scan. Red and blue traces indicate opposing scanning directions. The ratio of the deepest to shallowest breaths is a factor of 8.

comparing the reconstructed and original CT scans and Figure 13.6b shows the breathing traces of these scans. The results show that the 5D process accurately reconstructs the original scans within 3 mm (95th percentile) for all the CT scans. This is despite the factor of 8 difference between the deepest and shallowest breaths of this patient.

13.3 ADVANCES IN MRI SIMULATION

In recent years, radiation oncology departments have begun to more routinely use MRI to aid radiotherapy treatment planning. MRI is often used in areas of poor tissue discrimination with CT scans, such as the brain, abdomen and pelvis, but not historically in the lungs. Numerous advances in MRI have been developed in the past decade, such as fast MR sequences, powerful gradients and coils, parallel imaging, novel contrast agents, etc. Some innovative MR sequences are specifically designed to improve lung imaging by effectively manage the challenges associated with lung MRI: short T2*, low proton density, and respiratory motion. For instance, recent developments allow 3D spatial resolution of MR images on the order of a cubic millimeter to be achieved in the lung [22]. These advances have markedly improved the quality of lung MR imaging, making MRI an emerging tool for imaging lung diseases, including lung cancer. This section will focus on the recent advances in MRI for anatomical and functional lung imaging, and their applications in radiotherapy of lung cancer.

13.3.1 MRI-BASED ANATOMICAL IMAGING OF HUMAN LUNG

A lung MRI protocol usually consists of a combination of T1-weighted (T1-w) and T2-weighted (T2-w) MR images. T1-w MR images show high-signal pulmonary nodules and masses, and T2-w MR images highlight tumor infiltration and nodular lesions or masses with high fluid content. T1-w 3D spoiled gradient echo (GRE) MR sequence with volumetric interpolated breath-hold (VIBE) has a pulmonary nodule-detection rate comparable with CT [23]. When delineating lung tumors that are close to structures with similar electron densities, MRI can enable differentiation between them owning to its excellent soft-tissue contrast. For instance, T2-w single-shot fast-spin echo (SSFSE) MR image can clearly differentiate between tumor mass and mediastinum, while the boundary between tumor and consolidation is less clear, as shown in example in Figure 13.7 [24]. Short inversion time inversion recovery (STIR) turbo SE was recently introduced as promising MR sequences for pulmonary nodule assessment. Koyama et al. [19] demonstrated that STIR turbo SE imaging was significantly better than T1-w or T2-w for differentiating malignant from benign solitary pulmonary nodules [25].

Ultrashort echo-time (UTE) MRI is a pulse-sequence specifically designed to image short T2* tissues, such as lung parenchyma, and thus particularly useful for lung imaging. It can be used to generate 3D images of the whole-lung with extraordinary spatial resolution and signal-to-noise ratio (SNR), revealing structural features such as airway walls, lobar fissures, and patterns of pulmonary fibrosis with a level of detail not typically seen in 2D spin-echo acquisitions [22]. Another pulse-sequence development for lung imaging is balanced steady-state free precession (SSFP) [26,7], which can yield higher steady-state MR signal than an equivalent spoiled GRE acquisition [28]. Using ultrafast repetition times (TR) approaching 1 ms, which is shorter than the typical T2* value of lung parenchyma at 1.5 Tesla, balanced SSFP acquisition with 3D Cartesian k-space encoding can be used to acquire lung images with significantly enhanced parenchyma signal in a single-breath-hold [24]. Furthermore, Miller et al. recently demonstrated an ultra-resolution pulse sequence which combines a TrueFISP (a.k.a. balanced SSFP) excitation scheme with 3D spoke-radial *k*-space sampling. This technique enables very fine isotropic voxel resolution to be achieved while maintaining extremely short repetition times (TR ~ 1 ms), as shown in Figure 13.8 [29]. The extremely short TR makes the resulting images immune to banding artifacts that can plague conventional TrueFISP acquisitions. The anatomical imaging techniques improve the spatial resolution, SNR, and spatial coverage achievable in the

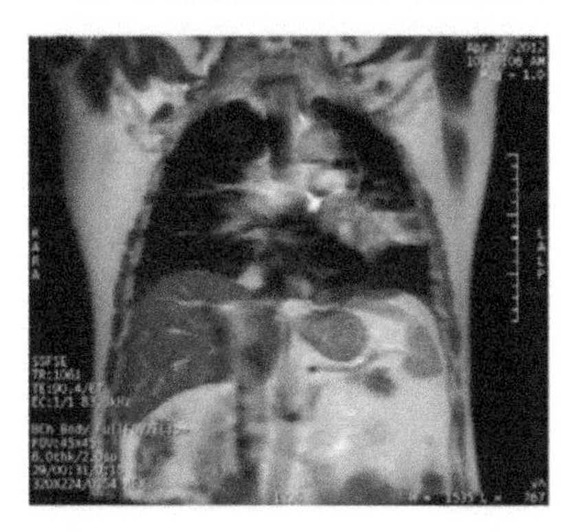

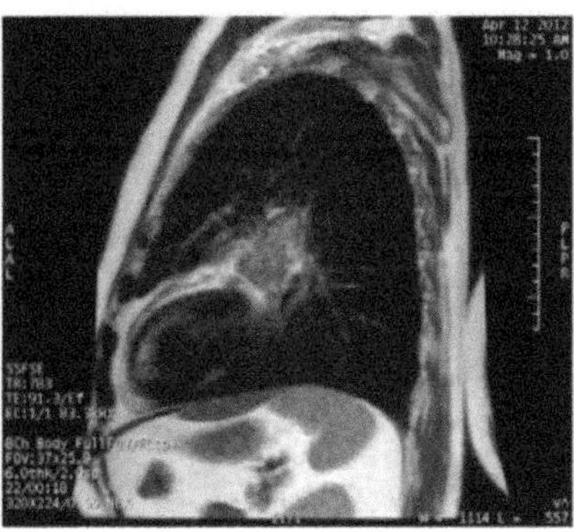

Figure 13.7 Axial plane of a T2-w single-shot fast-spin echo (SSFSE) image of a small-cell lung cancer for a 64-year-old male with T4 N2 M0 disease. There is excellent differentiation between the mediastinum and tumor mass, although the boundary between the tumor and the consolidation is unclear. (Images done on 1.5T GE scanner, with inspiration breath-hold.) (From Metcalfe, P. et al., *Technol Cancer Res Treat*, 12, 429–446, 2013.)

lung, without requiring contrast injection or difficult breath-hold maneuvers, which greatly enhances their potential clinical usefulness.

13.3.2 MRI-BASED FUNCTIONAL IMAGING OF HUMAN LUNG

Exciting advances in functional lung MRI have been achieved in recent years in both technical development and clinical application. Functional MR imaging is defined loosely here as any MRI technique capable of revealing information in addition to anatomical images, such as ventilation MRI, dynamic contrast-enhanced MRI (DEC-MRI), and diffusion-weighted MRI (DWI). Functional information of the lungs can be extracted from these MR images and potentially used to improve radiotherapy of lung cancer.

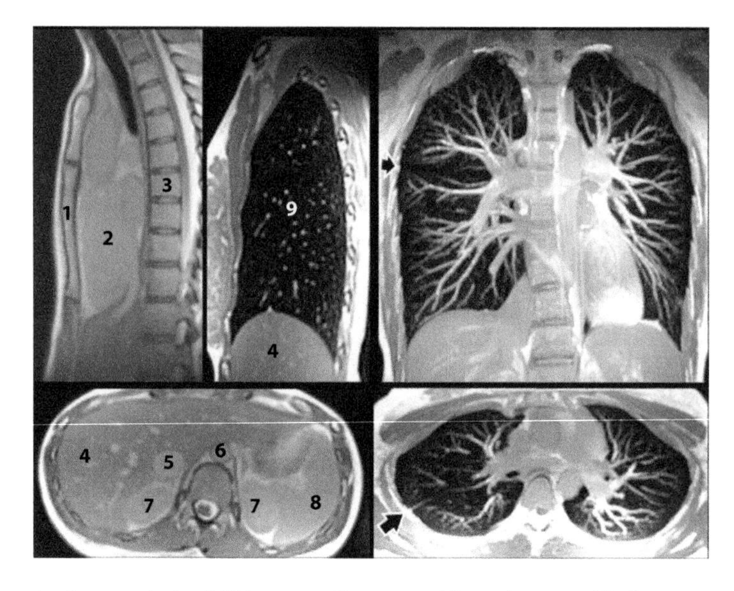

Figure 13.8 Sample ultra-resolution MR images, all extracted from the same 3D dataset acquired at 1.7 mm isotropic resolution. The 1.7-mm-thick sagittal and axial slices on the left show the artifact-free depiction of the sternum (1), heart (2), spine (3), liver (4), inferior vena cava (5), aorta (6), kidneys (7), and spleen (8), along with the numerous high-signal features (mostly vessels) in the lung (9). (Courtesy of Dr. G. Wilson Miller of the University of Virginia. From Miller, G.W. et al., *NMR Biomed*, 27, 1542–1556, 2014.)

13.3.2.1 VENTILATION MRI

Lung ventilation is usually measured by introducing a contrast agent into the inspired gas mixture and over its accumulation in the lung. Oxygen-enhanced MRI is a proton-based technique that uses pure oxygen as an exogenous contrast agent to image pulmonary ventilation [30,31]. The presence of oxygen in the lung airspaces shortens the T1 of the surrounding tissue, allowing oxygen accumulation in the air spaces to be detected indirectly by measuring its effect on the MR signal in the parenchyma. An alternative approach for lung ventilation imaging is using inhaled hyperpolarized gas (e.g., helium-3 and xenon-129) as the contrast agent to directly image lung ventilation by measuring the accumulation of the hyperpolarized gas [32–35]. A third approach is a Fourier decomposition technique [36,37], which instead of measuring the wash-in of a contrast agent, directly measures the movement of the lung airspaces during breathing by detecting the resulting variation in local water density [38]. This is accomplished by acquiring a series of proton-density weighted images of the same slice. After registering each of these images to a common reference image, the time-domain Fourier transform is computed at each voxel location, and the amplitude of the Fourier component corresponding to the respiratory frequency is taken as a relative measure of the local ventilation.

Lung ventilation MR imaging has been explored to improve lung cancer radiotherapy by identifying and sparing healthy, functional lung tissues in treatment planning. Cai et al. demonstrated that by incorporating lung ventilation information into treatment planning of lung cancer, radiation dose to highly functional lungs can be reduced [39]. Small, but significant improvements in sparing functional lungs could be achieved when lung tumor sits close to both healthy and diseased lung volumes. Bates et al. [40] and Ireland et al. [41] have also separately observed benefits in healthy tissue sparing of functional-based treatment planning utilizing the functional information derived from lung ventilation MRI. Lung ventilation MRI has also been used to monitor radiation induced lung function changes before and after radiotherapy of lung cancers [42,43]. This study showed the feasibility of detecting ventilation changes between pre and post-treatment using hyperpolarized gas MRI for patients with lung cancer. Pre-treatment, the degree of emphysema and MRI ventilation were correlated. MRI ventilation changes between pre- and post-treatment imaging were consistent with CT evidence of radiation-induced lung injury.

13.3.2.2 DYNAMIC CONTRAST-ENHANCED MRI (DCE-MRI)

DCE-MRI is a promising method for tumor characterization and therapy monitoring [44]. Studies have shown that DCE-MRI has diagnostic value in various tumors, and correlates with therapy effect of radiotherapy [45]. Studies have shown that DCE-MRI can be used to differentiate lung tumor subtypes [46]. Information about pulmonary perfusion and blood volume can be extracted from DCE-MRI. An important example of DCE-MRI for lung cancer is the assessment of lung cancer treatments. It can be used to estimate the postoperative lung function for patients with non-small cell lung cancer (NSCLC) [47]. DCE-MRI is usually performed by sequential imaging following the injection of a suitable paramagnetic contrast agent. There are currently three major methods for DCE-MRI of the lung. These broad categories include 2D SE or turbo SE sequences and various types of 2D and 3D GRE sequences. The use of DCE-MRI with the 3D GRE sequence and UTE is more likely to be effective than other methods and may lead to improved diagnostic performance of DCE-MRI. This method has the potential to play a complementary role in the characterization of pulmonary nodules. Efforts are being made to investigate the role of DCE-MRI in therapy monitoring of NSCLC.

13.3.2.3 DIFFUSION-WEIGHTED MRI (DWI)

DWI is sensitive to tissue microstructure on the cellular level and may therefore help to define biological tumor subvolumes and add complementary information to morphology-based cancer treatment and therapy monitoring. DWI has been shown to have superior tumor-to-tissue contrast for cancer detection compared to other MRI sequences and CT. Studies have shown that DWI can be used to differentiate lung cancer from consolidations [48,49]. DWI is increasingly used in clinic in conjunction with other imaging modalities to help with target delineation, treatment planning and assessing/monitoring of tumor treatment. Uto et al. conducted a patient study that showed DWI is useful for differentiating between benign and malignant lung nodules [50]. Kosucu et al. drew the same conclusion for mediastinal lymph nodes [51]. Kanauchi et al. demonstrated that DWI helps to predict tumor invasiveness for NSCLC [52]. Furthermore, the apparent diffusion coefficient (ADC) map derived from DWI images can help to differentiate different cancer types. For example, Matoba et al. showed that ADC of adenocarcinoma is significantly higher compared to squamous cell carcinoma and large-cell carcinoma [53]. These findings indicate that DWI may represent a complex interplay of several processes and strongly depends on treatment and histological tumor type. Moreover, changes over time must be observed to draw the right conclusions for a dedicated therapy. Studies have shown that ADC is a potential biomarker for tumor response during radiochemotherapy of NSCLC [54–56]. Significant ADC value increases during radiochemotherapy for NSCLC were observed. ADC value change during treatment appears to be an independent marker of lung cancer treatment outcome and warrants further investigation [56,57].

13.3.3 MRI-BASED RESPIRATORY MOTION MEASUREMENT

While 4D-CT is the current standard for imaging respiratory motion in radiotherapy, MRI techniques have been explored for this purpose and shown to have unique advantages over 4D-CT for respiratory motion measurement: 1) MRI has no radiation hazard, allowing for prolonged imaging time and subsequently more accurate measurement of breathing variations and statistical features; and 2) MRI has flexibility in imaging plane selection, leading to far more accurate and efficient measurement of respiratory motion in its dominant directions.

Fast MRI sequences such as 2D GRE or 2D fast steady-state GRE, often called cine MRI, allow for lung-motion imaging with a temporal resolution between 3 and 10 images per second. Using cine MRI, Plathow et al. found that the tumor mobility caused by respiratory motion is prominent in the superior-inferior direction and significantly impacted by tumor location [58–60]. Blackall et al. investigated intra- and intercycle tumor motion variabilities using cine MRI and showed that the variability could introduce mean errors over 5 mm in definition of the tumor and lung boundaries [61]. Cai et al. investigated the effects of imaging scan time and sampling rate on the lung tumor probability density function (PDF) reproducibility using cine MRI [62,63]. Owning to its noninvasive and non-ionizing nature, MRI is suited for studies that require prolonged and repeating imaging acquisition. The high temporal resolution of cine MRI allows the study of the dependency of PDF reproducibility on the imaging frame rate. Cine MRI has a limitation that it measures only 2D motion. To overcome that, Tryggestad et al. developed a practical dynamic MRI technique employing two orthogonal planes acquired in a continuous, interleaved fashion to characterize 3D tumor motion and associated variability [64]. In addition, Paganelli et al. quantified lung tumors' rotation by using an automatic feature extraction method in combination with the acquisition of fast orthogonal cine MRI images [65]. Compared with 4D-CT, cine MRI is not affected by the time resolved imaging resorting and provides a more accurate tumor motion trajectory in the superior-inferior direction, particularly when the respiratory pattern is irregular [66]. In addition, cine MRI does not require dedicated hardware and can be easily implemented with standard sequences in most clinics equipped with a MRI unit.

More recently, four-dimensional MRI (4D-MRI) techniques have been developed for more comprehensive evaluation of respiratory motion. Mainly developed for abdominal applications owning to its superior soft-tissue contrast, 4D-MRI also has a potential role for lung applications. For instance, 4D-MRI has been used to investigate the complex breathing patterns in patients with hemi-diaphragmatic paralysis due to malignant infiltration [67]. The study concluded that 4D-MRI is a promising tool to analyze complex breathing patterns in patients with lung tumors, and it should be considered for use in planning of radiotherapy to account for individual tumor motion. Blackall et al. implemented a T1-w 3D real-time MRI using Fast Field Echo-Echo Planar Imaging (FFE-EPI) sequence with sensitivity encoding (SENSE) technique [59]. It has achieved a high frame rate (330 ms/volume) and spatial resolution ($1.8 \times 1.8 \times 7$ mm). However, significant compromises in signal to noise ratio and image quality in general [68] must be made to achieve real-time imaging, result in inadequate image quality for radiotherapy application. Hu et al. developed T2-w 4D-MRI technique with a respiratory amplitude based triggering system to prospectively gate image acquisition [69]. Besides image acquisition gating applied on images, Akçakaya et al. investigated a k-Space-dependent respiratory gating technique. With this technique, a respiratory navigator is used as the surrogate to gate the acquisition of the k-space center data [70]. In addition, von Siebenthal et al. developed a method using an MR navigator for retrospectively stacking dynamic 2D images to generate time-resolved 3D images [68]. Multiple image contrasts and respiratory surrogates were explored for application. Cai et al. proposed a T2/T1-w 4D-MRI phase sorting technique that used body area (BA) extracting from images as the respiratory surrogate for sorting [71,72]. Tryggestad et al. and Liu et al. separately developed a T2-w 4D-MRI phase sorting technique for sequential MRI image acquisition mode with external respiratory surrogate physiologic monitoring unit (PMU) system [73,74]. Furthermore, Liu et al. implemented a diffusion-weighted 4D-MRI technique (4D-DWI), which has the potential to assist differentiating lung cancer from consolidations [75]. Furthermore, the ADC maps derived from 4D-DWI can be further developed to be a potential biomarker for tumor response of NSCLC [76]. Most recently, Liu et al. also implemented retrospective reordering of k-space based on respiratory phase to generate T2-w 4D-MRI [77].

In addition to the abovementioned proton MRI techniques, hyperpolarized gas MR tagging is a novel, unique technique capable of direct *in vivo* measurement of respiratory lung motion on a regional basis [78–82]. Figure 13.9 illustrates the principle and fundamental of hyperpolarized gas tagging MRI. Compared to the proton MRI techniques, tagging MRI has unique features for lung motion measurement: 1) it directly measures regional lung deformation *in vivo* in real human beings, providing a physiological ground-truth of lung motion; 2) the hyperpolarized tagging MR images embed a large number (~500) of uniformly distributed landmarks within the lungs, allowing for complete study of the entire lung. Conversely, current methods have difficulty identifying landmarks in low-featured, peripheral lung regions [83,84]; and 3) the tag elements have high signal-to-noise ratio (~60), minimizing errors in landmark identification.

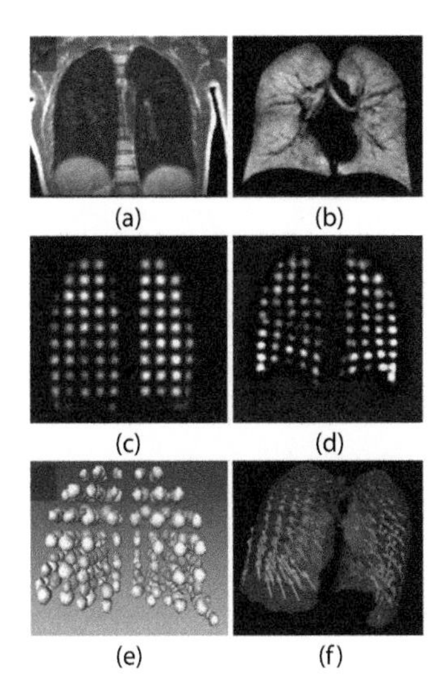

Figure 13.9 Hyperpolarized gas tagging MRI: (a) conventional proton MRI shows no signal in the lungs; (b) non-tagged hyperpolarized gas MRI shows high signal of hyperpolarized gas distribution within the lungs; (c) Inhalation and (d) exhalation 2D hyperpolarized gas tagging MR images revealed regional lung motion during breathing; (e) surface-rendered 3D hyperpolarized gas tagging MR images of the lungs, where gold and blue indicate inhalation and exhalation respectively; and (f) the corresponding 3D lung motion displacement vector fields.

13.4 ADVANCES IN PET SIMULATION

As a noninvasive imaging technique, ^{18}F-fluorodeoxyglucose positron emission tomography (FDG-PET) has been widely used for tumor staging and restaging [85], and it is the most useful modality for detecting distant metastasis [86]. The level of FDG uptake in tumor cells is a reliable marker of tumor cell glycolysis or metabolic activity and is linearly related to tumor cell proliferative activity or aggressiveness [87]. The overall sensitivity, specificity, and accuracy of FDG-PET for lung cancers are very high for primary, residual, and recurrent lung cancer diagnosis [88]. Applications of PET/CT in radiation oncology can be categorized into two major groups: for treatment planning and for response evaluation.

FDG-PET/CT has been proved to be an important modality in lung cancer radiotherapy for both treatment planning and response evaluation. Further technical developments will yield better image resolution and image quality, making PET/CT more accurate and precise. PET/MRI will benefit some specific diseases and when simultaneous data acquisition or high spatial precision is important. Non-FDG tracers have great potential to be integrated into radiation oncology.

13.4.1 PET/CT FOR TREATMENT PLANNING

13.4.1.1 TARGET VOLUME SELECTION/STAGING

FDG-PET/CT has been demonstrated in many studies to be important in disease staging and target volume selection for lung cancers. Mac Manus et al. [89] studied 153 patients with NSCLC who were candidates for radical radiotherapy (RT). They found that FDG-PET detected unsuspected distant metastasis in 28 patients or extensive loco regional disease in 18 patients thus changed their treatment strategy from radical/curative radiation therapy to palliative radiation therapy. In a study of 24 patients with NSCLC, Bradley et al. [90] found that FDG-PET (1) detected unsuspected distant metastatic disease in 2 patients; (2) helped to distinguish tumor from atelectasis in all 3 patients with atelectasis (Figure 13.10); and (3) detected unsuspected nodal disease in 10 patients, and a separate tumor focus in 1 patient. A multi-center trial showed that the elective nodal failure rate for GTVs derived by PET/CT is low at 2%, suggesting that nodal GTVs should be limited to PET/CT-defined tumor volumes,

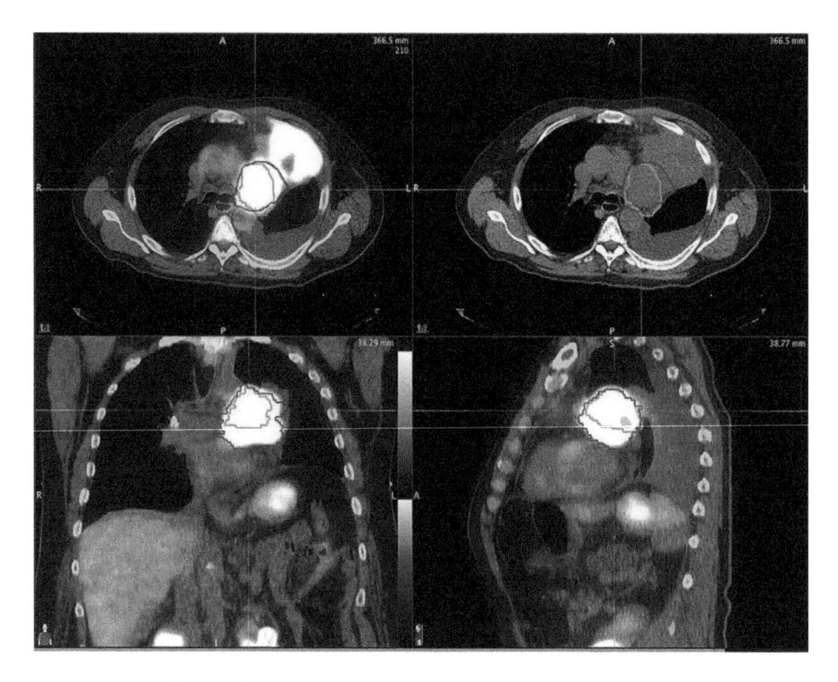

Figure 13.10 An example of the difference between the defined gross tumor volume (GTV) between PET/CT (red contour) and CT alone (green contour) in a patient with left upper lobe atelectasis. PET/CT images are displayed in axial, sagittal, and coronal planes through the tumor. The corresponding CT alone axial image is displayed on the upper right. (From Bradley, J. et al., *Int J Radiat Oncol Biol Phys*, 82, 435–441, e1, 2012.)

i.e. involved nodes [91]. FDG-PET was found to alter target volume selection in about 30%–50% of patients, with an overall impact in terms of change in RT planning from 34% to 100% [91].

13.4.1.2 TARGET VOLUME DELINEATION

FDG-PET/CT has been shown to have an added role to CT only in delineating gross target volume (GTV) in lung cancers. GTV sizes were increased or decreased in various studies using PET/CT compared to CT only. Larger differences in GTV sizes were often because different target volumes were selected as discussed above. Studies showed a significant reduction in inter-observer contouring variation with the use of PET/CT [92].

Nevertheless, one needs to be cautious when using FDG-PET/CT for delineation of GTV, due to several limitations of this imaging modality. The spatial resolution of PET is poor at 5–8 mm compared to 1 mm of CT. As FDG is not tumor specific, adjacent normal tissues often have above-background FDG-uptake, making it difficult to draw a boundary between the tumor and normal tissues. Though PET and CT in a combined PET/CT scanner are hardware-registered, misalignments between PET and CT (due to patient motion, respiratory motion and cardiac motion) can be problematic for GTV delineation. Leong et al. described a rigorous manual delineation protocol in PET/CT for esophageal cancer [93]. GTV was defined using the complementary features of PET and CT—a visual interpretation of the PET image was used to determine the nature of a lesion and the CT image to determine its anatomical boundary. In cases where no boundary was visible on CT (e.g., cranial or caudal extent of primary tumor), the FDG-avid tumor volume was defined using a qualitative visual assessment of the PET image displayed on a liver-SUV-normalized gray scale.

13.4.1.3 SELECTIVE DOSE ESCALATION

Radiation dose escalation has been shown to improve local control and survival in lung cancer [94,95]. FDG-PET is the most widely used molecular imaging in attempts to identify "higher-risk" subvolumes within the GTV [96,97]. Because of the smaller target volumes, the dose to these "higher-risk" subvolumes may be escalated considerably while the dose to the organs-at-risk (OAR) may be kept the same as the standard techniques.

For effective dose escalation to "higher-risk" subvolumes based on FDG-PET pre-therapy, two conditions are required: (1) the locations of these subvolumes remain stable during RT; and (2) FDG-PET can identify these subvolumes pre-therapy. For (1), Aerts et al. found that in 23 NSCLC patients, the high uptake areas (60%) remained stable during RT with mean overlap fraction (OF = max (AinB, BinA)) of 72.3% and 71.3% at Day 0 with Days 7 and 14, respectively [98]. For (2), Aerts et al. found that 22 of 55 NSCLC patients had residual FDG uptake post-therapy that highly corresponded (OF > 91%) with GTV pre-therapy [96]. They concluded that pre-therapy FDG PET/CT allows for identification of "higher-risk" subvolumes. These studies led to a randomized phase II trial whose feasibility has been shown [99]. However, the OF overestimated the volume overlap and resulted in unreliable value (1.0) for progressive disease [100]. Lu et al. suggested that Volume Overlap by Dice Coefficient and BinA should be used instead of OF for such studies [100].

Considering the significant changes in the volume and location of high FDG-uptake areas during RT and the heterogeneity in tumor response, an adaptive dose escalation strategy (re-imaging, response evaluation, and re-planning during RT) is more advantageous over dose escalation pre-therapy. Feng et al. demonstrated in a pilot study that using during-RT PET/CT, tumor dose can be significantly escalated or normal tissue complication probability reduced in NSCLC [101]. A similar RTOG 1106 trial is ongoing.

13.4.1.4 TECHNICAL ASPECT OF USING PET/CT SIMULATION FOR RT PLANNING

Many clinics fuse a PET/CT (for target delineation) with a planning CT (for RT planning), acquired on two scanners. In principle, it is more efficient and more precise to use just the PET/CT acquired on a single scanner for both target delineation and RT planning. A few technical modifications on the PET/CT system are necessary or desired: 1) a flat couch top that mimics RT treatment couch, 2) large bore PET/CT for certain bulky RT immobilization devices, 3) ceiling and side external lasers for patient positioning and marking, and 4) CT protocols for both RT planning and PET attenuation correction. These modifications allow reproducible patient position, target delineation and dose calculation with a single PET/CT simulation session.

13.4.2 PET/CT FOR RESPONSE EVALUATION

There are large differences in tumor response to current population-based therapy. This warrants the development of personalized therapy in which early, accurate assessment of tumor response is important. Traditionally, tumor response is evaluated visually or measured with anatomic changes in tumor diameters using CT imaging. FDG-PET imaging has shown advantages over anatomic imaging as a response evaluation tool in many malignancies [102–107]. Metabolic response is evaluated in PET visually and measured semi-quantitatively with changes in tumor standard uptake value (SUV) [102]. The optimal SUV cutoff values defining response varied considerably for different diseases as well as for the same disease. For NSCLC, criteria for tumor response included 50% [108] or 80% decrease in SUV_{max} [109], and SUV thresholds ranging from 2.5 to 4.5 post therapy [110].

In recent years, many studies proposed the use of computerized PET/CT image analysis to improve the evaluation of tumor response. Lu et al. [111], summarized these studies in the four steps of the analysis: image registration, tumor segmentation, image feature extraction, and response evaluation. Registering the baseline PET/CT and evaluation PET/CT images provides new opportunities to quantify changes at the original tumor site and to model changes as a function of spatial location. Segmenting the tumors allows measurements on the entire tumor rather than at single point or in small "peak" region. Various image features (recently termed radiomics), including volumetric, attenuation or uptake, geometric, and textural descriptors, allows comprehensive quantification of tumor characteristics and their changes due to therapy [112]. Finally, advanced response predictive models that are based on various clinical and image features show higher accuracy than traditional response evaluation [113].

13.4.3 RESPIRATORY-GATED PET AND 4D PET/CT

Tumors in the lungs and upper abdomen are impacted by respiratory motion, which may cause blurring of the tumor and breathing artifacts in both CT and PET, as well as disturbance of uptake level and distribution in PET.

This leads to inaccurate tumor measurement and inaccurate PET quantification [114]. Typically, a free-breathing CT is acquired for attenuation correction on a PET/CT scanner. Since the CT is acquired in a few seconds while the PET is acquired in a few minutes, they represent a snapshot of and an average over many breathing cycles, respectively. Therefore, misalignment between CT and PET may be frequent and large [115]. Pan et al. showed that using average CT for attenuation correction significantly reduced breathing artifacts and led to more accurate PET quantification [115]. A further development for respiratory motion correction is 4D PET/CT, in which CT and PET data were sorted into 10 respiration phases and then correlated per the respiration phase [116]. Nehmeh et al. showed that in four patients, the 4D PET/CT improved accuracy in PET-CT image co-registration, reduced blurring of tumor and thus the observed tumor volume, yielding an increase in the measured SUV by up to 16% over the clinical measured SUV. However, one disadvantage of this 4D PET/CT is the increased noise due to the lower (1/10) counts in each respiratory phase. Several groups applied image registration to "sum" PET images of all phases into a single phase, and thus keeping all counts for each phase [117–119]. Lamare et al. showed further improvements by applying image registration in raw data (list mode data) prior to reconstruction [119] or in local regions [118].

Although respiratory-gated PET and 4D PET/CT are hot research topics; they have achieved limited clinical use in radiation oncology. 4D-CT remains as the major modality for respiratory motion correction in delineating GTV for RT planning. Though many reported that the measured SUVs in 4D PET/CT were statistically different from those measured in clinical PET/CT, the differences were rarely clinically significant. Another limiting factor of 4D PET/CT is its longer acquisition time.

13.4.4 Average CT and MIP CT images for PET/CT simulation

The advent of PET/CT scanners made it possible that a single imaging table transporting the patient between PET and CT to hardware-fuse the PET and CT data without a repeat of patient setup. Application of PET/CT is over 90% on oncology with ^{18}F-FDG. PET/CT plays an important role in image-guided radiation therapy [120] and treatment response assessment [121]. Integration of functional PET data with anatomical CT data is critical in radiation therapy [122]. However, it remains a challenge to quantify the improvement of simulation with PET/CT over CT in treatment planning for radiation treatment as conclusive clinical data are not yet available. Early studies have found PET/CT has advantages over CT in standardization of volume delineation [123,124], in reduction of the risk for geometrical misses [125], and in minimization of radiation dose to the non-target organs [126–128]. Utilization of PET/CT is expected to grow as more molecular targeted imaging agents are being developed [129].

Average (or average intensity) and maximum intensity projection (MIP) CT images are by-products of 4D-CT because the average CT and MIP CT images can be derived from averaging the pixel values and finding the maximum pixel value of the multiple phases of 4D-CT, respectively. Mis-registration between the CT and PET data is typically identified by a curvilinear white band or photon-penic region near the diaphragm in the PET images (Figure 13.11). A tumor may become smaller (or larger) than it appears due to the interplay of

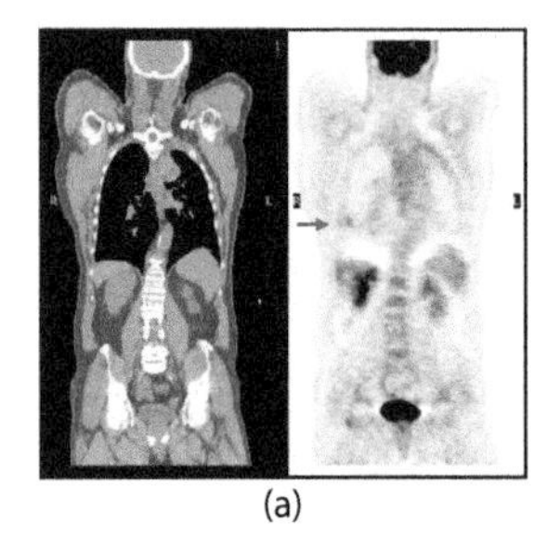

(a)

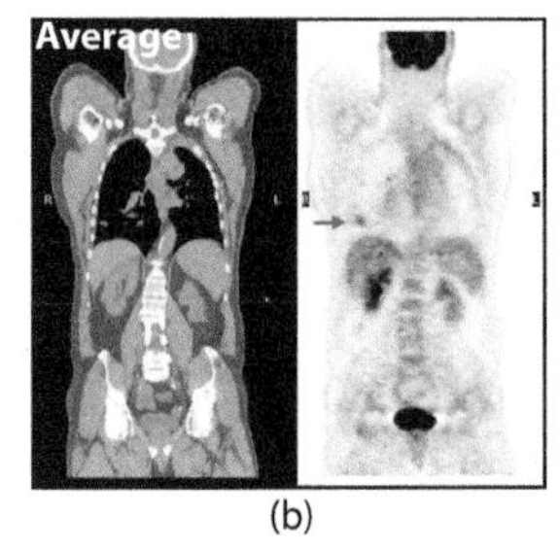

(b)

Figure 13.11 (a) A clinical PET/CT study with the photo penic or under-attenuation correction artifact, which was removed by average CT in (b). The max SUV of the lung lesion is changed from 2.3 in (a) to 3.6 in (b), an increase of 59%.

the CT scan and the tumor motion direction and speed. Since we spend more time in expiration than inspiration, the PET data averaged over 2–3 mins is closer to the end-expiration than the end-inspiration. If the CT data can be acquired near the end-expiration, then the CT and PET data will register with each other. On the other hand, if the CT data is acquired in or near the end-inspiration, the inflated lungs from inspiration will be larger than the deflated lungs at expiration. The larger area of the inflated lungs in CT renders less attenuation correction in the reconstruction of the PET data near the diaphragm. The result is a white band region identified as a mis-registered region or a photon-penic region.

Coaching the patient to hold-breath at mid-expiration during the CT acquisition was suggested as an alternative to improve the registration between the CT and PET data [130]. However, the outcomes were mixed because coaching a patient to breath-hold at a certain state during the CT acquisition is not very reliable from both the patient and the technologist, operating the PET/CT scanner, perspectives. It may not be easy to train a patient or technologist that the breath-hold CT to best match with PET should be taken at the mid-expiration in light-breathing not in deep respiration.

If the CT scan is conducted when the patient is free-breathing, there is possibility that the CT and the PET data may misalign with each other because some CT slices are taken at the inspiration, and some at the expiration whereas the PET data is averaged over 2–3 mins. The distance between two consecutive end expiration phases can become longer (or shorter) with a faster (or slower) speed helical CT scan. Figure 13.12 [131] shows an example of the CT images taken when the patient was free breathing during a CT scan at the speed of 1.72 cm/s. There were skin-fold artifacts at the abdomen and cardiac pulsation artifacts at the heart, which might not be identified in the review of each individual CT slice. By measuring the distance between the adjacent peaks of the respiratory (cardiac pulsation) artifacts, and dividing the distance by the table translation speed of the CT scan, one can estimate the breathing cycle and the heat rate of the patient to be about 4.7 s and 50 beats per minute, respectively. These artifacts were due to the respiration and the heart beatings of the patient.

A study of 216 patients in quantification with SUV and gross target volume (GTV) delineation was reported [132]. There were 68% of the patients with at least one respiratory artifact and 10% of the mis-registrations in PET/CT could cause an SUV change of over 25%, which can be a threshold indicating a partial response to therapy [133]. The small tumors of < 50 cm^3 in size near the diaphragm could have a shift of the centroid tumor location of 2.4 mm and a GTV change of over 154% and an SUV change of 21%. Clearly, whole-body PET/CT exams are with mis-registration between the CT and PET data, but only a small portion of the scans with small tumors near the diaphragm could be impacted by mis-registration.

Acquiring the cine CT images for average CT can be accomplished by scanning at the same location with a fast gantry rotation of subsecond over a breath cycle of 3–5 seconds and without a respiratory monitoring device on the GE scanner [132–136]. However, all vendors require the purchase of 4D-CT to derive average CT. There are two key components in the implementation of the average CT: one is to scan at a fast gantry rotation to achieve high temporal resolution and to minimize motion artifacts in each CT image; the other one is to scan over one breath cycle of 3–5 seconds to produce sufficient samples of the CT images across the multiple phases of a respiratory cycle to achieve a similar averaging effect like PET. The slow-scan CT acquires data over one CT gantry rotation of 4 secs, could cause severe reconstruction artifacts. Figure 13.13 shows a clinical example of a patient scanned with the slow-scan CT of 4 secs per gantry rotation and the average CT by the cine CT of fast gantry rotation of 0.5 seconds for 4 sec. There were severe reconstruction artifacts caused by the respiratory motion in the images of the slow 4-sec gantry rotation because the projection data of the slow 4-sec CT were not consistent over one revolution of the CT scan due to breathing motion, in violation of the basic tomographic image reconstruction principle which requires the imaged object stationary during data acquisition. Except some expected blurring at the boundary of the liver, there were no artifacts in the averaged CT over a breath cycle of the CT images of high temporal resolution. The average CT and PET data are similar in temporal resolution and the average CT is without the reconstruction artifacts as shown in the slow CT.

Scans with either cine CT on the GE scanner or low-pitch helical CT (pitch < 0.1) on the PET/CT scanners of the other manufacturers can be adopted to obtain average CT, and has been available in 4D-CT imaging [137–139]. In a whole-body PET/CT scan, the CT images are typically acquired before PET. The technologist can determine if an average CT scan is needed when the CT and PET images of the thorax and abdomen, which are more likely to be impacted by the mismatch of the CT and PET images, are available for review before completion of the PET scan. Radiation therapy has embraced the use of average CT for dose calculation in conventional radiation therapy [140], and for proton beam therapy [66] when the respiratory motion can alter the dose calculation. Average CT has also been shown to benefit the alignment with the cone beam CT images taken right before radiation treatment in image-guided radiation therapy [141]. Average CT can be generated from the cine CT scan by averaging the cine CT images without a respiratory gating device [132–135], for the purposes of attenuation correction of PET images, dose calculation for radiation therapy with photon and proton and alignment with cone beam CT for image-guided radiation therapy.

MIP CT images are effective in depicting the extent of tumor motion [142,143]. For peripheral lung tumors (surrounded by the lower density air in the lungs), MIP CT images can be used to determine the tumor target volume and to avoid ambiguity in using a threshold of SUV to determine the target volume in

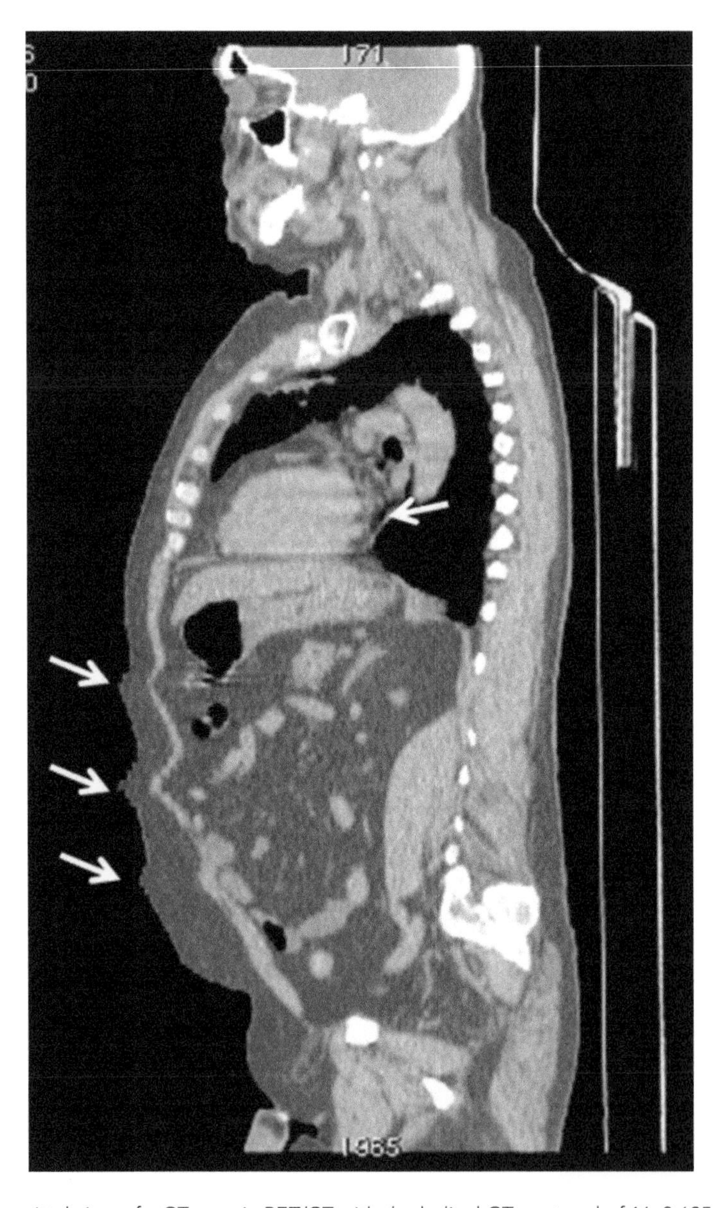

Figure 13.12 A sagittal view of a CT scan in PET/CT with the helical CT protocol of 16x0.625 mm, 0.8 s gantry rotation, pitch 1.375:1. There were three skinfold artifacts on the abdomen and some pulsating artifacts on the heart. The speed of CT scan in the table direction is 17.2 mm/s. (Reproduced from Zaid, H. and T. Pan., *PET Clin*, 6, 207–226, 2011; with permission.)

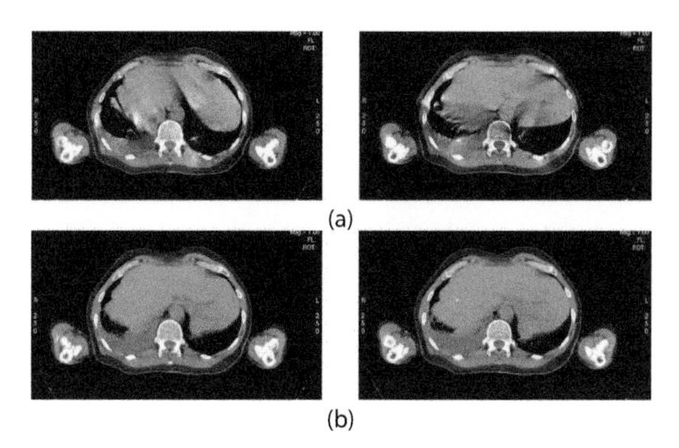

Figure 13.13 The average CT and the slow scan CT images of a patient with an average breath cycle of 4 s. The slow scan CT images in (a) were taken with one single CT gantry rotation of 4 s, and the two images were 2.5 mm apart and 2.5 mm thick. The corresponding average CT images in (b), obtained by averaging the cine CT images, were averaged from 4 s of data collection over 8 gantry rotations. The average CT images were almost free of reconstruction artifacts, which were observed in the SSCT images. (Reproduced from Pan T. et al., *Med Phys*, 33, 3931–3938, 2006; with permission.)

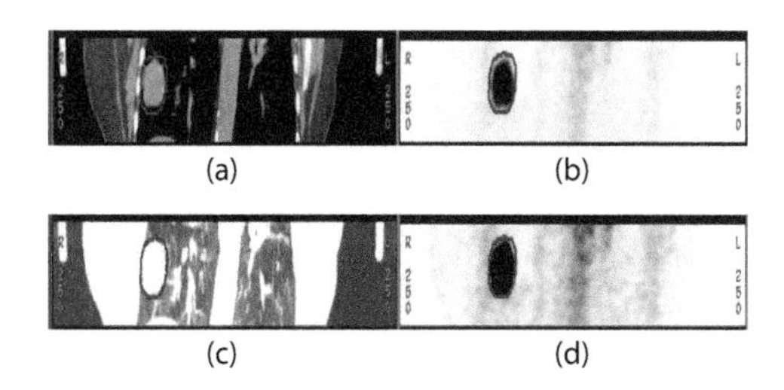

Figure 13.14 The MIP CT and PET images of a patient. The MIP CT in (a) is displayed with (window, level) = (400,40) and PET in (b) with a threshold of 40% of the maximum SUV of the tumor. The images of (a) and (b) are displayed again with (1000, –700) in (c) and the threshold of 20% in (d), respectively. The tumor contour in (c) is superimposed in (a), (b) and (d) to demonstrate the effect on tumor size by display parameters.

PET. Any ^{18}F-FDG uptake in the lungs should be supported by the soft tissues depicted in the MIP images. Any PET GTV determined with an SUV threshold should not exceed the soft-tissue boundary in the MIP images. Their application for treatment planning for stereotactic body radiation therapy has been demonstrated in [144]. The MIP CT images can help determine the tumor volume in the thorax. Figure 13.14 shows an example of determining the extent of PET GTV with MIP CT to avoid the uncertainty of thresholding a functional tumor with SUV. A similar concept has been attempted with the regular helical CT data for peripheral non-small cell lung cancer (NSCLC) by Biehl et al. [145], when the boarder of the tumor can be identified by the CT data.

Figure 13.15 [146] shows an example of mis-registration that caused a false-negative diagnosis, and a change of the gross target volume for radiation therapy when the mis-registration was removed with average CT. In the era of image-guided radiation therapy to deliver a very high dose of radiation at a great precision, it is very important to pay attention to any mis-registration between the CT and the PET images during tumor delineation when PET/CT images are used in the treatment planning.

13.4.5 PET/MRI

Recent technical developments have realized integrated PET/MRI scanners. PET/MRI combines the superb sensitivity of PET and excellent soft tissue contrast and spatial resolution of MRI, providing unique opportunities to simultaneously imaging multiple characteristics of a tumor. Additional advantages of PET/MRI compared to PET/CT include that, unlike CT, MRI does not include ionizing radiation; and better PET/MRI co-registration

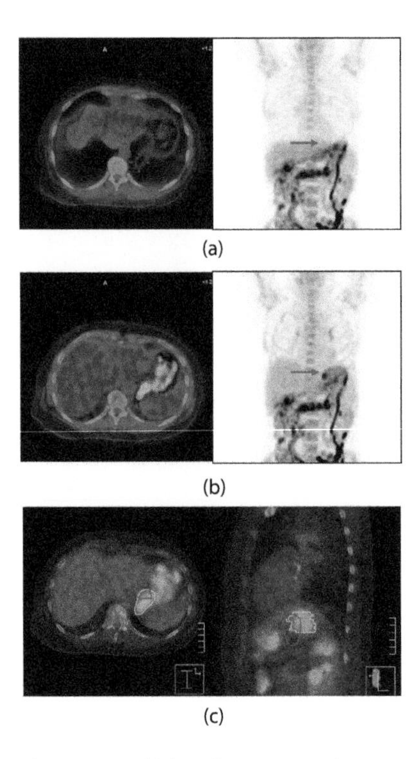

Figure 13.15 The PET/CT images of a 69-year-old female patient with an esophageal tumor after an induction chemotherapy. (a) shows an axial slice of the fused clinical CT and PET image at the level of the esophageal tumor (left) and the PET image in coronal view (right). The radiology report indicated the patient had a positive response to the chemotherapy. After removal of misalignment by the average CT, the tumor reappeared in the same PET dataset in (b). The arrows pointed to the tumor location. The gross target volumes drawn in the images of (a) and (b) are shown in blue and in green, respectively in (c). The patient was treated with the tumor volume in green, and the radiology report was corrected by the average CT. (Reproduced from Pan, T. and O. Mawlawi, *Med. Phys*, 35, 4955–4966, 2008; with permission.)

(for fully integrated system) due to its simultaneous data acquisition versus sequential data acquisition in PET/CT. The major challenges of implementing PET/MRI are to avoid or lower the mutual interferences between the two modalities. Wehrl et al. [147] reviewed a few PET/MRI designs including: (1) using two separated PET and MR scanners with a common patient positioning system allowing minimal movement between the two modalities; (2) using long light fibers that transfer the light from scintillator detectors in PET out of the magnet in MR; (3) using split magnet and short light fibers; (4) using short light fibers and replacing photomultiplier tubes (PMTs) with avalanche photo diodes (APDs) in PET. APDs are compact silicon semiconductors and can be operated without interferences in high magnetic fields; (5) coupling scintillator to APDs without light fibers; (6) using solid-state photomultipliers (SSPM) as light detectors; and (7) field cycling: switching off the magnetic field during PET data acquisition and on during MR data acquisition. There are three current clinical PET/MR systems: GE SIGNA PET/MR system features design (6), Philips Ingenuity TF PET/MR system features design (1), and Siemens Biograph mMR PET/MR system features design (5). Pilot studies so far suggested that FDG PET/CT and FDG PET/MRI were of equal diagnostic accuracy for TNM staging in NSCLC [148] and several other solid tumors [149]. PET/MR is expected to have advantages over PET/CT in studies that (1) MR is much more useful than CT, like in brain imaging; (2) simultaneous data acquisition is preferred, like in multi-parametric imaging that yield morphologic, functional, and molecular information; and (3) high spatial precision is required, like in delineating tumors affected by motion (patient motion, respiratory and cardiac motion).

Another technical challenge of PET/MR systems is how to perform attenuation correction necessary for PET quantification. In PET/CT the attenuation map is measured directly by CT, while in PET/MR no information related to attenuation is directly available. Bezrukov et al. [150] reviewed the state-of-the-art methods for MR-based attenuation correction (MRAC). These include (1) segmentation-based methods segment the patient image into tissue classes that are assigned uniform linear attenuation coefficients, (2) methods based on atlas and machine learning deform an attenuation atlas template to obtain the patient's attenuation map or learn a mapping function to predict continuous attenuation maps from the MR data, and (3) combine PET emission data and anatomical information from MR images to compute the attenuation maps.

PET/MR has high potential in achieving higher level of accuracy and precision in GTV delineation for RT planning. Thorwarth et al. [151] evaluated step-and-shoot IMRT in a meningioma patient with PET/MR. They showed that a small infiltrative tumor region was better visualized in integrated PET/MR than in fused PET/CT and MR. Though the volume difference was small, both the dose distribution and the dose-volume histogram showed that this infiltrative tumor region would not receive the full prescribed the dose with the GTV delineated based on the fused PET/CT and MR. Causes of this difference could be improved PET resolution of 3 mm in PET/MR versus a PET resolution of 6 mm in fused PET/CT and MR, longer uptake time in PET/MR, and/or the MRI-based attenuation correction.

13.4.6 New PET/CT imaging techniques

13.4.6.1 Image reconstruction with time-of-flight and point spread function

Current PET/CT systems use 3D data acquisition and iterative image reconstruction with ordered-subsets expectation maximization (OSEM) algorithm for PET. Recent development in fast detectors provides the temporal resolution required for time-of-flight (TOF) reconstruction. TOF PET use the measured time difference between the detection of the two coincidence events to more accurately determine the location of the positron annihilation point along the line of response (LOR). This is better than conventional PET, in which this information is not measured and thus equal weights are used for all points along the LOR. TOF PET improves image signal-to-noise ratio (SNR), particularly in large patients [152]. The better the time resolution of the PET scanner, the higher level of improvement in SNR. Another recent development is using a point-spread function (PSF) measured at many points in the FOV to compensate for the geometric distortion when the photons are not from the center [153,154]. Figure 13.16 shows a comparison of these image reconstruction methods, where both TOF and PSF improved significantly the image quality and SNR.

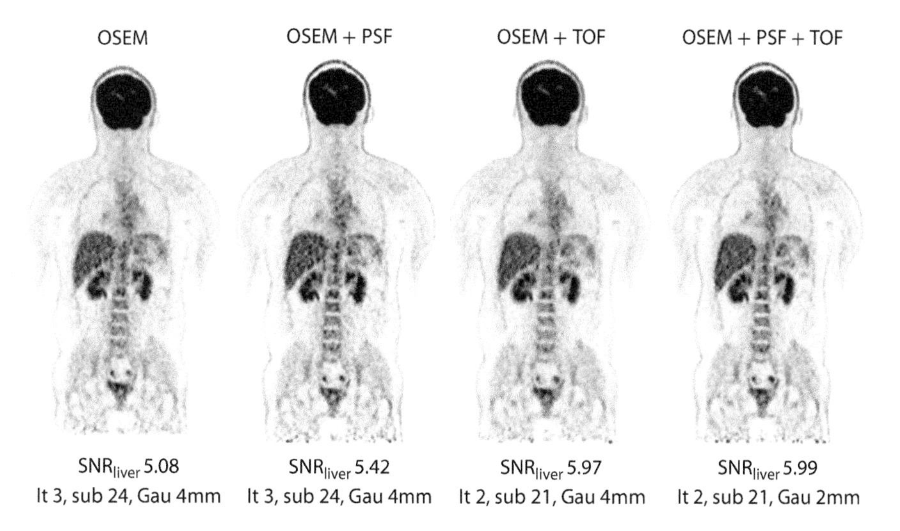

Figure 13.16 Patient images reconstructed by different algorithms. Patient with postsurgical state of colorectal cancer (BMI, 25.2; body weight, 71 kg; injected dose, 296.8 MBq; NECliver, 2.91 mega counts). It, sub, and Gau represent iteration, subsets, and Gaussian filter FWHM width, respectively. TOF clearly improved uniformity of liver and sharpness of edge of vertebral body. Uptake in physiologically low-uptake areas, such as perirenal fat, lung, and intervertebral disks, was decreased by TOF correction. Combination of PSF and TOF markedly improved image quality. (From Akamatsu, G. et al., *J Nucl Med*, 53, 1716–1722, 2012.)

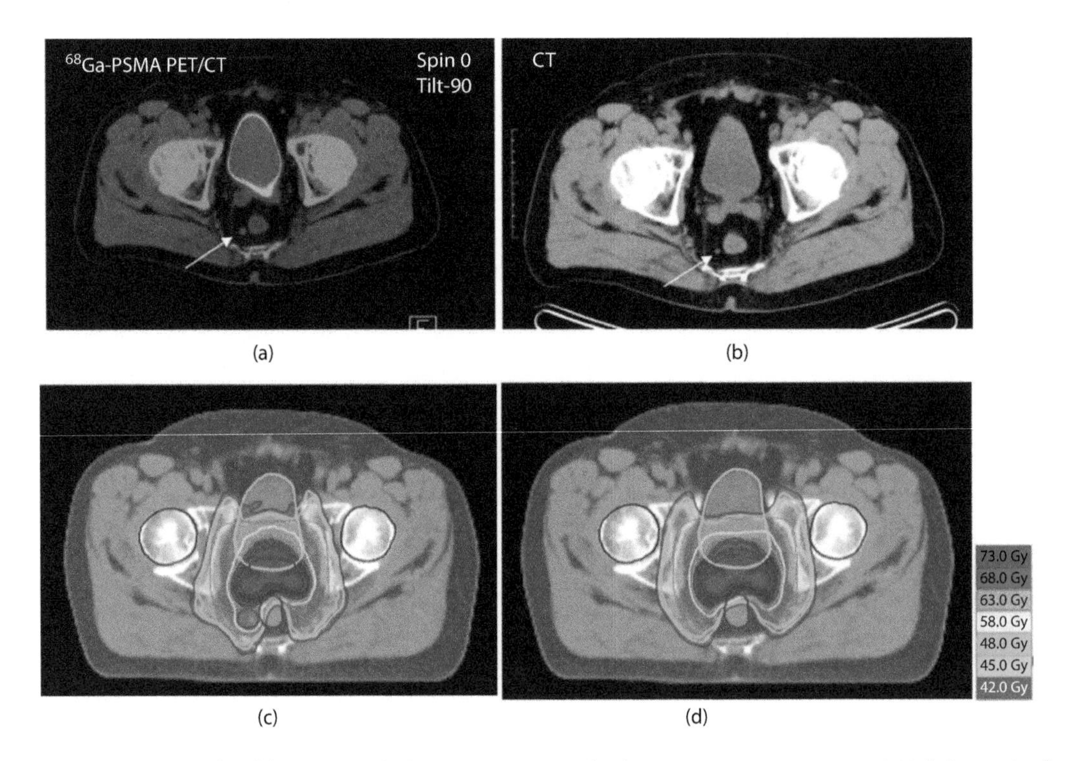

Figure 13.17 Example of the impact of PSMA imaging on radio therapeutic management at initial diagnosis of intermediate-risk prostate cancer. (a) A PSMA PET/CT with tracer uptake in a pararectal lymph node (SUVmax 3.1; arrow) which was not clearly pathological in conventional CT (b). Accordingly, the irradiation plan was changed with coverage of perirectal space and a simultaneous boost to the lymph node (c): IMRT in 34 fractions with 51 Gy to lymphatic pathways, 76.5 Gy to the prostate, and 61.2 Gy to the pathological lymph node). (d) IMRT plan prior to PSMA PET information without sufficient coverage of the pathological lymph node. (From Sterzing, F. et al., *Eur J Nucl Med Mol Imaging*, 43, 34–41, 2015.)

13.4.6.2 NON-FDG TRACERS

Quite a few new PET tracers, including FLT that measures cell proliferation [155,156], FMISO that measures hypoxia [157,158], and others [159–161]_ENREF_61 have brought enthusiasm in oncology. Yang et al. showed that FLT PET/CT had a lower sensitivity (74% versus 94%) than FDG PET/CT for diagnosis of primary lesion, but higher specificity (98% versus 84%) for lymph nodes in NSCLC [162]. Trigonis et al. [163] found that during early course of RT for NSCLC, FLT uptake decreased significantly, in the primary tumor in the absence of volume change, and in the lymph nodes with volume regression. These studies supported the potential of FLT PET/CT as a supplemental diagnostic modality and an early response marker for NSCLC.

Recently, Sterzing et al. [164] demonstrated dramatic impact of prostate-specific membrane antigen (PSMA) PET/CT on RT of prostate cancer. In a cohort of 57 patients, 18 patients received an additional lymph node boost due to a change from N0–N1 (regional metastases), 8 patients received an enlarged lymphatic field irradiation due to a change from M0–M1a (soft-tissue metastases), RT was cancelled and systemic therapy was given for 4 patients due to a change from M0–M1b (bone metastases). An example is shown in Figure 13.17.

REFERENCES

1. Ginat, D.T. and R. Gupta, Advances in computed tomography imaging technology. *Annu Rev Biomed Eng*, 2014. **16**: 431–53.
2. Hara, A.K. et al., Iterative reconstruction technique for reducing body radiation dose at CT: Feasibility study. *Am J Roentgenol*, 2009. **193**(3): 764–71.

3. Prakash, P. et al., Diffuse lung disease: CT of the chest with adaptive statistical iterative reconstruction technique. *Radiology*, 2010. **256**(1): 261–9.
4. Ehrhardt, J. et al., An optical flow based method for improved reconstruction of 4D CT data sets acquired during free breathing. *Med Phys*, 2007. **34**(2): 711–21.
5. Zhang, Y.B. et al., Modeling respiratory motion for reducing motion artifacts in 4D CT images. *Med Phys*, 2013. **40**(4): 041716.
6. Bernatowicz, K. et al., Quantifying the impact of respiratory-gated 4D CT acquisition on thoracic image quality: A digital phantom study. *Med Phys*, 2015. **42**(1): 324–34.
7. Gianoli, C. et al., A multiple points method for 4D CT image sorting. *Med Phys*, 2011. **38**(2): 656–67.
8. Thomas, D. et al., A novel fast helical 4D CT acquisition technique to generate low-noise sorting artifact-free images at user-selected breathing phases. *Int J Radiat Oncol Biol Phys*, 2014. **89**(1): 191–8.
9. Castillo, S.J. et al., Evaluation of 4D CT acquisition methods designed to reduce artifacts. *J Appl Clin Med Phys*, 2015. **16**(2): 4949.
10. Seppenwoolde, Y. et al., Precise and real-time measurement of 3D tumor motion in lung due to breathing and heartbeat, measured during radiotherapy. *Int J Radiat Oncol Biol Phys*, 2002. **53**(4): 822–34.
11. Lujan, A.E. et al., A method for incorporating organ motion due to breathing into 3D dose calculations. *Med Phys*, 1999. **26**(5): 715–20.
12. McClelland, J.R. et al., A continuous 4D motion model from multiple respiratory cycles for use in lung radiotherapy. *Med Phys*, 2006. **33**(9): 3348–58.
13. Hertanto, A. et al., Reduction of irregular breathing artifacts in respiration-correlated CT images using a respiratory motion model. *Med Phys*, 2012. **39**(6): 3070–9.
14. Low, D.A. et al., Novel breathing motion model for radiotherapy. *Int J Radiat Oncol Biol Phys*, 2005. **63**(3): 921–9.
15. McClelland, J.R. et al., Respiratory motion models: A review. *Med Image Anal*, 2013. **17**(1): 19–42.
16. McClelland, J.R., B.A.S. Champion, and D.J. Hawkes, Combining image registration, respiratory motion modelling, and motion compensated image reconstruction, in *Biomedical Image Registration: 6th International Workshop, WBIR*, S. Ourselin and M. Modat, Editors. July 7–8, 2014. London, Cham: Springer International Publishing. pp. 103–13.
17. Zhang, Q.H. et al., A patient-specific respiratory model of anatomical motion for radiation treatment planning. *Med Phys*, 2007. **34**(12): 4772–81.
18. Vedam, S.S. et al., Acquiring a four-dimensional computed tomography dataset using an external respiratory signal. *Phys Med Biol*, 2003. **48**(1): 45–62.
19. Werner, R. et al., Technical Note: Development of a tidal volume surrogate that replaces spirometry for physiological breathing monitoring in 4D CT. *Med Phys*, 2010. **37**(2): 615–9.
20. Low, D.A. et al., A novel CT acquisition and analysis technique for breathing motion modeling. *Phys Med Biol*, 2013. **58**(11): L31–L6.
21. Dou, T.H. et al., A method for assessing ground-truth accuracy of the 5DCT technique. *Int J Radiat Oncol Biol Phys*, 2015. **93**(4): 925–33.
22. Johnson, K.M. et al., Optimized 3D ultrashort echo time pulmonary MRI. *Magn Reson Med*, 2013. **70**(5): 1241–50.
23. Biederer, J. et al., Lung morphology: Fast MR imaging assessment with a volumetric interpolated breath-hold technique: Initial experience with patients. *Radiology*, 2003. **226**(1): 242–9.
24. Metcalfe, P. et al., The potential for an enhanced role for MRI in radiation-therapy treatment planning. *Technol Cancer Res Treat*, 2013. **12**(5): 429–46.
25. Koyama, H. et al., Quantitative and qualitative assessment of non-contrast-enhanced pulmonary MR imaging for management of pulmonary nodules in 161 subjects. *Eur Radiol*, 2008. **18**(10): 2120–31.
26. Bieri, O., Ultra-fast steady state free precession and its application to in vivo (1)H morphological and functional lung imaging at 1.5 tesla. *Magn Reson Med*, 2013. **70**(3): 657–63.
27. Failo, R. et al., Lung morphology assessment using MRI: A robust ultra-short TR/TE 2D steady state free precession sequence used in cystic fibrosis patients. *Magn Reson Med*, 2009. **61**(2): 299–306.
28. Scheffler, K. and S. Lehnhardt, Principles and applications of balanced SSFP techniques. *Eur Radiol*, 2003. **13**(11): 2409–18.

29. Miller, G.W. et al., Advances in functional and structural imaging of the human lung using proton MRI. *NMR Biomed*, 2014. **27**(12): 1542–56.
30. Mai, V.M. et al., MR ventilation-perfusion imaging of human lung using oxygen-enhanced and arterial spin labeling techniques. *J Magn Reson Imaging*, 2001. **14**(5): 574–9.
31. Molinari, F. et al., Navigator-triggered oxygen-enhanced MRI with simultaneous cardiac and respiratory synchronization for the assessment of interstitial lung disease. *J Magn Reson Imaging*, 2007. **26**(6): 1523–9.
32. de Lange, E.E. et al., Lung air spaces: MR imaging evaluation with hyperpolarized 3He gas. *Radiology*, 1999. **210**(3): 851–7.
33. Salerno, M. et al., Hyperpolarized noble gas MR imaging of the lung: Potential clinical applications. *Eur J Radiol*, 2001. **40**(1): 33–44.
34. Moller, H.E. et al., MRI of the lungs using hyperpolarized noble gases. *Magn Reson Med*, 2002. **47**(6): 1029–51.
35. Mata, J.F. et al., Evaluation of emphysema severity and progression in a rabbit model: Comparison of hyperpolarized 3He and 129Xe diffusion MRI with lung morphometry. *J Appl Physiol (1985)*, 2007. **102**(3): 1273–80.
36. Bauman, G. et al., Non-contrast-enhanced perfusion and ventilation assessment of the human lung by means of fourier decomposition in proton MRI. *Magn Reson Med*, 2009. **62**(3): 656–64.
37. Bauman, G. et al., Lung ventilation- and perfusion-weighted Fourier decomposition magnetic resonance imaging: In vivo validation with hyperpolarized 3He and dynamic contrast-enhanced MRI. *Magn Reson Med*, 2013. **69**(1): 229–37.
38. Zapke, M. et al., Magnetic resonance lung function—A breakthrough for lung imaging and functional assessment? A phantom study and clinical trial. *Respir Res*, 2006. **7**: 106.
39. Cai, J. et al., Helical tomotherapy planning for lung cancer based on ventilation magnetic resonance imaging. *Med Dosim*, 2011. **36**(4): 389–96.
40. Bates, E.L. et al., Functional image-based radiotherapy planning for non-small cell lung cancer: A simulation study. *Radiother Oncol*, 2009. **93**(1): 32–6.
41. Ireland, R.H. et al., Feasibility of image registration and intensity-modulated radiotherapy planning with hyperpolarized helium-3 magnetic resonance imaging for non-small-cell lung cancer. *Int J Radiat Oncol Biol Phys*, 2007. **68**(1): 273–81.
42. Allen, A.M. et al., Can Hyperpolarized Helium MRI add to radiation planning and follow-up in lung cancer? *J Appl Clin Med Phys*, 2011. **12**(2): 3357.
43. Ireland, R.H. et al., Detection of radiation-induced lung injury in non-small cell lung cancer patients using hyperpolarized helium-3 magnetic resonance imaging. *Radiother Oncol*, 2010. **97**(2): 244–8.
44. Henzler, T. et al., Diffusion and perfusion MRI of the lung and mediastinum. *Eur J Radiol*, 2010. **76**(3): 329–36.
45. Hunter, G.J. et al., Dynamic T1-weighted magnetic resonance imaging and positron emission tomography in patients with lung cancer: Correlating vascular physiology with glucose metabolism. *Clin Cancer Res*, 1998. **4**(4): 949–55.
46. Pauls, S. et al., The role of dynamic, contrast-enhanced MRI in differentiating lung tumor subtypes. *Clin Imaging*, 2011. **35**(4): 259–65.
47. de Langen, A.J. et al., Monitoring response to antiangiogenic therapy in non-small cell lung cancer using imaging markers derived from PET and dynamic contrast-enhanced MRI. *J Nucl Med*, 2011. **52**(1): 48–55.
48. Yang, R.M. et al., Differentiation of central lung cancer from atelectasis: Comparison of diffusion-weighted MRI with PET/CT. *PLOS ONE*, 2013. **8**(4): e60279.
49. Wang, L.L. et al., Intravoxel incoherent motion diffusion-weighted MR imaging in differentiation of lung cancer from obstructive lung consolidation: Comparison and correlation with pharmacokinetic analysis from dynamic contrast-enhanced MR imaging. *Eur Radiol*, 2014. **24**(8): 1914–22.
50. Uto, T. et al., Higher sensitivity and specificity for diffusion-weighted imaging of malignant lung lesions without apparent diffusion coefficient quantification. *Radiology*, 2009. **252**(1): 247–54.

51. Kosucu, P. et al., Mediastinal lymph nodes: Assessment with diffusion-weighted MR imaging. *J Magn Reson Imaging*, 2009. **30**(2): 292–7.
52. Kanauchi, N. et al., Role of diffusion-weighted magnetic resonance imaging for predicting of tumor invasiveness for clinical stage IA non-small cell lung cancer. *Eur J Cardiothorac Surg*, 2009. **35**(4): 706–10; discussion 710–1.
53. Matoba, M. et al., Lung carcinoma: Diffusion-weighted mr imaging—Preliminary evaluation with apparent diffusion coefficient. *Radiology*, 2007. **243**(2): 570–7.
54. Ohno, Y. et al., Diffusion-weighted MRI versus 18F-FDG PET/CT: Performance as predictors of tumor treatment response and patient survival in patients with non-small cell lung cancer receiving chemoradiotherapy. *Am J Roentgenol*, 2012. **198**(1): 75–82.
55. Chang, Q. et al., Diffusion-weighted magnetic resonance imaging of lung cancer at 3.0 T: A preliminary study on monitoring diffusion changes during chemoradiation therapy. *Clin Imaging*, 2012. **36**(2): 98–103.
56. Iizuka, Y. et al., Prediction of clinical outcome after stereotactic body radiotherapy for non-small cell lung cancer using diffusion-weighted MRI and (18)F-FDG PET. *Eur J Radiol*, 2014. **83**(11): 2087–92.
57. Iizuka, Y. et al., Preliminary analysis of pretreatment diffusion-weighted MRI and (18)F-FDG PET/CT as prognostic factors in patients with non-small cell lung cancer receiving stereotactic body radiation therapy. *Pract Radiat Oncol*, 2013. **3**(2 Suppl. 1): S13.
58. Plathow, C. et al., Measurement of tumor diameter-dependent mobility of lung tumors by dynamic MRI. *Radiother Oncol*, 2004. **73**(3): 349–54.
59. Plathow, C. et al., Quantitative analysis of lung and tumour mobility: Comparison of two time-resolved MRI sequences. *Br J Radiol*, 2005. **78**(933): 836–40.
60. Plathow, C. et al., Analysis of intrathoracic tumor mobility during whole breathing cycle by dynamic MRI. *Int J Radiat Oncol Biol Phys*, 2004. **59**(4): 952–9.
61. Blackall, J.M. et al., MRI-based measurements of respiratory motion variability and assessment of imaging strategies for radiotherapy planning. *Phys Med Biol*, 2006. **51**(17): 4147–69.
62. Cai, J. et al., Evaluation of the reproducibility of lung motion probability distribution function (PDF) using dynamic MRI. *Phys Med Biol*, 2007. **52**(2): 365–73.
63. Cai, J. et al., Reproducibility of interfraction lung motion probability distribution function using dynamic MRI: Statistical analysis. *Int J Radiat Oncol Biol Phys*, 2008. **72**(4): 1228–35.
64. Tryggestad, E. et al., 4D tumor centroid tracking using orthogonal 2D dynamic MRI: Implications for radiotherapy planning. *Med Phys*, 2013. **40**(9): 091712.
65. Paganelli, C. et al., Quantification of lung tumor rotation with automated landmark extraction using orthogonal cine MRI images. *Phys Med Biol*, 2015. **60**(18): 7165–78.
66. Cai, J. et al., Estimation of error in maximal intensity projection-based internal target volume of lung tumors: A simulation and comparison study using dynamic magnetic resonance imaging. *Int J Radiat Oncol Biol Phys*, 2007. **69**(3): 895–902.
67. Dinkel, J. et al., 4D-MRI analysis of lung tumor motion in patients with hemidiaphragmatic paralysis. *Radiother Oncol*, 2009. **91**(3): 449–54.
68. von Siebenthal, M. et al., 4D MR imaging of respiratory organ motion and its variability. *Phys Med Biol*, 2007. **52**(6): 1547–64.
69. Hu, Y. et al., Respiratory amplitude guided 4-dimensional magnetic resonance imaging. *Int J Radiat Oncol Biol Phys*, 2013. **86**(1): 198–204.
70. Akcakaya, M. et al., Free-breathing phase contrast MRI with near 100% respiratory navigator efficiency using k-space-dependent respiratory gating. *Magn Reson Med*, 2014. **71**(6): 2172–9.
71. Cai, J. et al., Four-dimensional magnetic resonance imaging (4D-MRI) using image-based respiratory surrogate: A feasibility study. *Med Phys*, 2011. **38**(12): 6384–94.
72. Liu, Y. et al., Investigation of sagittal image acquisition for 4D-MRI with body area as respiratory surrogate. *Med Phys*, 2014. **41**(10).
73. Tryggestad, E. et al., Respiration-based sorting of dynamic MRI to derive representative 4D-MRI for radiotherapy planning. *Med Phys*, 2013. **40**(5): 051909.

74. Liu, Y. et al., T2-weighted four dimensional magnetic resonance imaging with result-driven phase sorting. *Med Phys*, 2015. **42**(8): 4460–71.
75. Liu, Y. et al., Four-dimensional diffusion-weighted MR imaging (4D-DWI): A feasibility study. *Med Phys*, 2016. **44**: 397–406.
76. Liu, Y., F. Yin, and J. Cai, SU-F-R-29: The influence of four dimensional diffusion-weighted MRI (4D-DWI) on feature analysis of time-resolved apparent diffusion coefficient (ADC) measurement: Initial evaluation. *Med Phys*, 2016. **43**(6): 3379.
77. Liu, Y. et al., Four dimensional magnetic resonance imaging with retrospective k-space reordering: A feasibility study. *Med Phys*, 2015. **42**(2): 534–41.
78. Cai, J. et al., Dynamic MRI of grid-tagged hyperpolarized helium-3 for the assessment of lung motion during breathing. *Int J Radiat Oncol Biol Phys*, 2009. **75**(1): 276–84.
79. Fain, S. et al., Imaging of lung function using hyperpolarized helium-3 magnetic resonance imaging: Review of current and emerging translational methods and applications. *J Magn Reson Imaging*, 2010. **32**(6): 1398–408.
80. Tustison, N.J. et al., Pulmonary kinematics from tagged hyperpolarized helium-3 MRI. *J Magn Reson Imaging*, 2010. **31**(5): 1236–41.
81. Cai, J. et al., MR grid-tagging using hyperpolarized helium-3 for regional quantitative assessment of pulmonary biomechanics and ventilation. *Magn Reson Med*, 2007. **58**(2): 373–80.
82. Cai, J. et al., Direct measurement of lung motion using hyperpolarized helium-3 MR tagging. *Int J Radiat Oncol Biol Phys*, 2007. **68**(3): 650–3.
83. Yeo, U.J. et al., Performance of 12 DIR algorithms in low-contrast regions for mass and density conserving deformation. *Med Phys*, 2013. **40**(10): 101701.
84. Liu, F. et al., Evaluation of deformable image registration and a motion model in CT images with limited features. *Phys Med Biol*, 2012. **57**(9): 2539–54.
85. Wanet, M. et al., Gradient-based delineation of the primary GTV on FDG-PET in non-small cell lung cancer: A comparison with threshold-based approaches, CT and surgical specimens. *Radiother Oncol*, 2011. **98**(1): 117–25.
86. Flamen, P. et al., Utility of positron emission tomography for the staging of patients with potentially operable esophageal carcinoma. *J Clin Oncol*, 2000. **18**(18): 3202–10.
87. Czernin, J. and C. Yap, From FDG-PET to FDG PET/CT imaging, in Atlas of PET/CT Imaging in *Oncology*, J. Czernin et al., Editors. 2004, Berlin and New York, NY: Springer p.8, 315 p.
88. Zhu, A., D. Lee, and H. Shim, Metabolic positron emission tomography imaging in cancer detection and therapy response. *Semin Oncol*, 2011. **38**(1): 55–69.
89. Mac Manus, M.P. et al., F-18 fluorodeoxyglucose positron emission tomography staging in radical radiotherapy candidates with nonsmall cell lung carcinoma. *Cancer*, 2001. **92**(4): 886–95.
90. Bradley, J. et al., Impact of FDG-PET on radiation therapy volume delineation in non–small-cell lung cancer. *Int J Radiat Oncol Biol Phys*, 2004. **59**(1): 78–86.
91. Bradley, J. et al., A phase II comparative study of gross tumor volume definition with or without PET/CT fusion in dosimetric planning for non-small-cell lung cancer (NSCLC): Primary analysis of Radiation Therapy Oncology Group (RTOG) 0515. *Int J Radiat Oncol Biol Phys*, 2012. **82**(1): 435–41, e1.
92. Lee, P. et al., Current concepts in F18 FDG PET/CT-based radiation therapy planning for lung cancer. *Front Oncol*, 2012. **2**: 71.
93. Leong, T. et al., A prospective study to evaluate the impact of FDG-PET on CT-based radiotherapy treatment planning for oesophageal cancer. *Radiother Oncol*, 2006. **78**(3): 254–61.
94. Kong, F.M. et al., High-dose radiation improved local tumor control and overall survival in patients with inoperable/unresectable non-small-cell lung cancer: Long-term results of a radiation dose escalation study. *Int J Radiat Oncol Biol Phys*, 2005. **63**(2): 324–33.
95. Martel, M.K. et al., Estimation of tumor control probability model parameters from 3-D dose distributions of non-small cell lung cancer patients. *Lung Cancer*, 1999. **24**(1): 31–7.
96. Aerts, H.J. et al., Identification of residual metabolic-active areas within individual NSCLC tumours using a pre-radiotherapy (18)Fluorodeoxyglucose-PET-CT scan. *Radiother Oncol*, 2009. **91**(3): 386–92.

97. Abramyuk, A. et al., Is pre-therapeutical FDG-PET/CT capable to detect high risk tumor subvolumes responsible for local failure in non-small cell lung cancer? *Radiother Oncol*, 2009. **91**(3): 399–404.
98. Aerts, H.J.W.L. et al., Stability of F-18-deoxyglucose uptake locations within tumor during radiotherapy for NSCLC: A prospective study. *Int J Radiat Oncol Biol Phys*, 2008. **71**(5): 1402–7.
99. van Elmpt, W. et al., The PET-boost randomised phase II dose-escalation trial in non-small cell lung cancer. *Radiother Oncol*, 2012. **104**(1): 67–71.
100. Lu, W. et al., Pre-chemoradiotherapy FDG PET/CT cannot identify residual metabolically-active volumes within individual esophageal tumors. *J Nucl Med Radiat Ther*, 2015. **6**. doi:10.4172/2155-9619.1000226.
101. Feng, M. et al., Using fluorodeoxyglucose positron emission tomography to assess tumor volume during radiotherapy for non-small-cell lung cancer and its potential impact on adaptive dose escalation and normal tissue sparing. *Int J Radiat Oncol Biol Phys*, 2009. **73**(4): 1228–34.
102. Wahl, R.L. et al., From RECIST to PERCIST: Evolving considerations for PET response criteria in solid tumors. *J Nucl Med.*, 2009. **50** (Suppl. 1): 122S–50S.
103. Mac Manus, M.P. et al., Positron emission tomography is superior to computed tomography scanning for response-assessment after radical radiotherapy or chemoradiotherapy in patients with non-small-cell lung cancer. *J Clin Oncol*, 2003. **21**(7): 1285–92.
104. Benz, M.R. et al., FDG-PET/CT imaging predicts histopathologic treatment responses after the initial cycle of neoadjuvant chemotherapy in high-grade soft-tissue sarcomas. *Clin Cancer Res*, 2009. **15**(8): 2856–63.
105. Krause, B.J. et al., 18F-FDG PET and 18F-FDG PET/CT for assessing response to therapy in esophageal cancer. *J Nucl Med*, 2009. **50**(Suppl. 1): 89S–96S.
106. Heron, D.E. et al., PET-CT in radiation oncology: The impact on diagnosis, treatment planning, and assessment of treatment response. *Am J Clin Oncol*, 2008. **31**(4): 352–62.
107. Brindle, K., New approaches for imaging tumour responses to treatment. *Nat Rev Cancer*, 2008. **8**(2): 94–107.
108. Vansteenkiste, J.F. et al., Potential use of FDG-PET scan after induction chemotherapy in surgically staged IIIa-N2 non-small-cell lung cancer: A prospective pilot study. The Leuven Lung Cancer Group. *Ann Oncol*, 1998. **9**(11): 1193–8.
109. Cerfolio, R.J. et al., Repeat FDG-PET after neoadjuvant therapy is a predictor of pathologic response in patients with non-small cell lung cancer. *Ann Thorac Surgery*, 2004. **78**(6): 1903–9.
110. de Geus-Oei, L.F. et al., Predictive and prognostic value of FDG-PET in nonsmall-cell lung cancer: A systematic review. *Cancer*, 2007. **110**(8): 1654–64.
111. Lu, W., J. Wang, and H.H. Zhang, Computerized PET/CT image analysis in the evaluation of tumor response to therapy. *Br J Radiol*, 2015. **88**: 20140625.
112. Tan, S. et al., Spatial-temporal [(18)F]FDG-PET features for predicting pathologic response of esophageal cancer to neoadjuvant chemoradiation therapy. *Int J Radiat Oncol Biol Phys*, 2013. **85**(5): 1375–82.
113. Zhang, H. et al., Modeling pathologic response of esophageal cancer to chemoradiation therapy using spatial-temporal (18)F-FDG PET features, clinical parameters, and demographics. *Int J Radiat Oncol Biol Phys*, 2014. **88**(1): 195–203.
114. Nehmeh, S.A. and Y.E. Erdi, Respiratory motion in positron emission tomography/computed tomography: A review. *Semin Nucl Med*, 2008. **38**(3): 167–76.
115. Pan, T. et al., Attenuation correction of PET images with respiration-averaged CT images in PET/CT. *J Nucl Med*, 2005. **46**(9): 1481–7.
116. Nehmeh, S.A. et al., Four-dimensional (4D) PET/CT imaging of the thorax. *Med Phys*, 2004. **31**(12): 3179–86.
117. Dawood, M. et al., Respiratory motion correction in 3-D PET data with advanced optical flow algorithms. *IEEE Trans Med Imaging*, 2008. **27**(8): 1164–75.
118. Lamare, F. et al., Local respiratory motion correction for PET/CT imaging: Application to lung cancer. *Med Phys*, 2015. **42**(10): 5903.
119. Lamare, F. et al., List-mode-based reconstruction for respiratory motion correction in PET using non-rigid body transformations. *Phys Med Biol*, 2007. **52**(17): 5187–204.

120. Stewart, R.D. and X.A. Li, BGRT: Biologically guided radiation therapy—the future is fast approaching. *Med Phys*, 2007. **34**(10): 3739–51.
121. Gregory, D.L. et al., Effect of PET/CT on management of patients with non-small cell lung cancer: Results of a prospective study with 5-year survival data. *J Nucl Med*, 2012. **53**(7): 1007–15.
122. Mah, K. et al., The impact of (18)FDG-PET on target and critical organs in CT-based treatment planning of patients with poorly defined non-small-cell lung carcinoma: A prospective study. *Int J Radiat Oncol Biol Phys*, 2002. **52**(2): 339–50.
123. Steenbakkers, R.J. et al., Reduction of observer variation using matched CT-PET for lung cancer delineation: A three-dimensional analysis. *Int J Radiat Oncol Biol Phys*, 2006. **64**(2): 435–48.
124. Ashamalla, H. et al., The contribution of integrated PET/CT to the evolving definition of treatment volumes in radiation treatment planning in lung cancer. *Int J Radiat Oncol Biol Phys*, 2005. **63**(4): 1016–23.
125. Erdi, Y.E. et al., Radiotherapy treatment planning for patients with non-small cell lung cancer using positron emission tomography (PET). *Radiother Oncol*, 2002. **62**(1): 51–60.
126. Ciernik, I.F. et al., Radiation treatment planning with an integrated positron emission and computer tomography (PET/CT): A feasibility study. *Int J Radiat Oncol Biol Phys*, 2003. **57**(3): 853–63.
127. Schwartz, D.L. et al., FDG-PET/CT-guided intensity modulated head and neck radiotherapy: A pilot investigation. *Head Neck*, 2005. **27**(6): 478–87.
128. van Baardwijk, A. et al., The current status of FDG-PET in tumour volume definition in radiotherapy treatment planning. *Cancer Treat Rev*, 2006. **32**(4): 245–60.
129. Chao, K.S. et al., A novel approach to overcome hypoxic tumor resistance: Cu-ATSM-guided intensity-modulated radiation therapy. *Int J Radiat Oncol Biol Phys*, 2001. **49**(4): 1171–82.
130. Goerres, G.W. et al., PET/CT of the abdomen: Optimizing the patient breathing pattern. *Eur Radiol*, 2003. **13**(4): 734–9.
131. Zaid, H. and T. Pan, Recent advances in hybrid imaging for radiation therapy planning: The cutting edge. *PET Clin*, 2011. **6**: 207–26.
132. Chi, P.C.M. et al., Effects of respiration-averaged computed tomography on positron emission tomography/computed tomography quantification and its potential impact on gross tumor volume delineation. *Int J Radiat Oncol Biol Phys*, 2008. **71**(3): 890–9.
133. Young, H. et al., Measurement of clinical and subclinical tumour response using [18F]-fluorodeoxyglucose and positron emission tomography: Review and 1999 EORTC recommendations. European Organization for Research and Treatment of Cancer (EORTC) PET Study Group. *Eur J Cancer, 1999.* **35**(13): 1773–82.
134. Pan, T., X. Sun, and D. Luo, Improvement of the cine-CT based 4D-CT imaging. *Med Phys*, 2007. **34**(11): 4499–503.
135. Riegel, A.C. et al., Cine computed tomography without respiratory surrogate in planning stereotactic radiotherapy for non-small-cell lung cancer. *Int J Radiat Oncol Biol Phys*, 2009. **73**(2): 433–41.
136. Pan, T. et al., Attenuation correction of PET cardiac data with low-dose average CT in PET/CT. *Med Phys*, 2006. **33**(10): 3931–8.
137. Low, D.A. et al., A method for the reconstruction of four-dimensional synchronized CT scans acquired during free breathing. *Med Phys*, 2003. **30**(6): 1254–63.
138. Pan, T. et al., 4D-CT imaging of a volume influenced by respiratory motion on multi-slice CT. *Med Phys*, 2004. **31**(2): 333–40.
139. Keall, P.J. et al., Acquiring 4D thoracic CT scans using a multislice helical method. *Phys Med Biol*, 2004. **49**(10): 2053–67.
140. Riegel, A.C. et al., Dose calculation with respiration-averaged CT processed from cine CT without a respiratory surrogate. *Med Phys*, 2008. **35**(12): 5738–47.
141. Shirai, K. et al., Phantom and clinical study of differences in cone beam computed tomographic registration when aligned to maximum and average intensity projection. *Int J Radiat Oncol Biol Phys*, 2014. **88**(1): 189–94.
142. Underberg, R.W. et al., Use of maximum intensity projections (MIP) for target volume generation in 4DCT scans for lung cancer. *Int J Radiat Oncol Biol Phys*, 2005. **63**(1): 253–60.

143. Bradley, J.D. et al., Comparison of helical, maximum intensity projection (MIP), and averaged intensity (AI) 4D CT imaging for stereotactic body radiation therapy (SBRT) planning in lung cancer. *Radiother Oncol*, 2006. **81**(3): 264–8.
144. Riegel, A.C. et al., Cine CT without a respiratory surrogate in planning of stereotactic radiotherapy for non-small cell lung cancer. *Int J Radiat Oncol Biol Phys (accepted for publication)*, 2009. **73**(2): 433–41.
145. Biehl, K.J. et al., 18F-FDG PET definition of gross tumor volume for radiotherapy of non-small cell lung cancer: Is a single standardized uptake value threshold approach appropriate? *J Nucl Med*, 2006. **47**(11): 1808–12.
146. Pan, T. and O. Mawlawi, PET/CT in radiation oncology. *Med Phys*, 2008. **35**(11), 4955–66.
147. Wehrl, H.F. et al., Combined PET/MR imaging—Technology and applications. *Technol Cancer Res Treat*, 2010. **9**(1): 5–20.
148. Heusch, P. et al., Thoracic staging in lung cancer: Prospective comparison of 18F-FDG PET/MR imaging and 18F-FDG PET/CT. *J Nucl Med*, 2014. **55**(3): 373–8.
149. Heusch, P. et al., Diagnostic accuracy of whole-body PET/MRI and whole-body PET/CT for TNM staging in oncology. *Eur J Nucl Med Mol Imaging*, 2015. **42**(1): 42–8.
150. Bezrukov, I. et al., MR-Based PET attenuation correction for PET/MR imaging. *Semin Nucl Med*, 2013. **43**(1): 45–59.
151. Thorwarth, D. et al., Simultaneous 68Ga-DOTATOC-PET/MRI for IMRT treatment planning for meningioma: First experience. *Int J Radiat Oncol Biol Phys*, 2011. **81**(1): 277–83.
152. Lois, C. et al., An assessment of the impact of incorporating time-of-flight information into clinical PET/CT imaging. *J Nucl Med*, 2010. **51**(2): 237–45.
153. Akamatsu, G. et al., Improvement in PET/CT image quality with a combination of point-spread function and time-of-flight in relation to reconstruction parameters. *J Nucl Med*, 2012. **53**(11): 1716–22.
154. Panin, V.Y. et al., Fully 3-D PET reconstruction with system matrix derived from point source measurements. *IEEE Trans Med Imaging*, 2006. **25**(7): 907–21.
155. Herrmann, K. et al., Imaging gastric cancer with PET and the radiotracers 18F-FLT and 18F-FDG: A comparative analysis. *J Nucl Med*, 2007. **48**(12): 1945–50.
156. Yue, J., et al., Measuring tumor cell proliferation with 18F-FLT PET during radiotherapy of esophageal squamous cell carcinoma: A pilot clinical study. *J Nucl Med*, 2010. **51**(4): 528–34.
157. Chang, J.H. et al., Hypoxia-targeted radiotherapy dose painting for head and neck cancer using (18) F-FMISO PET: A biological modeling study. *Acta Oncol*, 2013. **52**: 1723–9.
158. Hicks, R.J. et al., Utility of FMISO PET in advanced head and neck cancer treated with chemoradiation incorporating a hypoxia-targeting chemotherapy agent. *Eur J Nucl Med Mol Imaging*, 2005. **32**(12): 1384–91.
159. Lehtio, K. et al., Imaging perfusion and hypoxia with PET to predict radiotherapy response in head-and-neck cancer. *Int J Radiat Oncol Biol Phys*, 2004. **59**(4): 971–82.
160. Wieder, H. et al., PET imaging with [11C]methyl—L-methionine for therapy monitoring in patients with rectal cancer. *Eur J Nucl Med Mol Imaging*, 2002. **29**(6): 789–96.
161. Allen, A.M. et al., Assessment of response of brain metastases to radiotherapy by PET imaging of apoptosis with 18F-ML-10. *Eur J Nucl Med Mol Imaging*, 2012. **39**(9): 1400–8.
162. Yang, W. et al., Imaging of proliferation with 18F-FLT PET/CT versus 18F-FDG PET/CT in non-small-cell lung cancer. *Eur J Nucl Med Mol Imaging*, 2010. **37**(7): 1291–9.
163. Trigonis, I. et al., Early reduction in tumour [18F]fluorothymidine (FLT) uptake in patients with non-small cell lung cancer (NSCLC) treated with radiotherapy alone. *Eur J Nucl Med Mol Imaging*, 2014. **41**(4): 682–93.
164. Sterzing, F. et al., Ga-PSMA-11 PET/CT: A new technique with high potential for the radiotherapeutic management of prostate cancer patients. *Eur J Nucl Med Mol Imaging*, 2015. **43**: 34–41.

14

Advances in treatment planning

MEI LI, RUIJIANG LI, AND LEI XING

14.1 INTRODUCTION

Lung cancer, with non-small-cell lung cancer (NSCLC) accounting for 80% of these cases, is the leading cause of cancer death all over the world. In 2015, an estimated 221,200 new cases (115,610 in men and 105,590 in women) of lung and bronchial cancer will be diagnosed, and 158,040 deaths (86,380 in men and 71,660 in women) are estimated to occur because of this disease in the United States [1]. From 2004 to 2010, the overall 5-year relative survival rate for lung cancer was 16.8% in the United States [2]. Radiation therapy, (RT) which is an important treatment modality, has a potential role in all stages of NSCLC, as either definitive or palliative therapy. An estimated 40% of NSCLC patients will be treated with RT, as part of the multidisciplinary therapy. For stage I and II NSCLC, RT is an alternative curative option to surgery for patients who are medically inoperable or refuse surgery. Newer techniques such as stereotactic ablative radiotherapy (SABR), also denominated as stereotactic body radiotherapy (SBRT), for selected stage I NSCLC are showing survival control rates equivalent to surgery at short follow-up [3–5]. Radiotherapy, in combination with chemotherapy, remains the main curative modality for patients with stage III NSCLC. It can be used preoperatively for

Pancoast tumors [6] and postoperatively for pN2 cancers [7]. Finally, radiotherapy is an important palliative treatment modality to treat symptoms from the primary or bone or brain metastases and improve patients' quality of life [8].

Current radiation therapy treatment planning techniques for lung cancer, including 3D conformal (3D-CRT), intensity modulated radiation therapy (IMRT), and volumetric modulated radiation therapy (VMAT), have been well described in previous chapters. Recently, there have been introduced several new treatment planning techniques for more precise tumor target coverage and better organ-at-risk (OAR) sparing, including 4D planning, functional-based planning, etc. These advanced techniques have been increasingly used in the radiation therapy for lung cancer [9]. This chapter will provide an overview of the recent advances in treatment planning techniques for lung cancer in the IGRT era.

14.2 MONTE CARLO DOSE CALCULATION

The use of an accurate dose calculation model is a crucial step to the success of treatment planning for lung cancer. Pencil beam dose calculation algorithms perform poorly in the thorax region due their poor ability in handling heterogeneity correction. Convolution algorithms, such as analytical anisotropic algorithm and collapsed cone convolution implemented in the Eclipse treatment planning system (TPS), have improved dose calculation accuracy but may still be insufficient for lung planning, where the effects of electron transport disequilibrium cannot be accurately handled with conventional, deterministic dose algorithms due to the presence of heterogeneous patient tissues, especially when high-energy phone beams are used. A consequence of electronic disequilibrium is the under dosage of the planning target volume (PTV), as shown in Figure 14.1. The penumbral widening in the dose distribution because of the increased electron scattering in the lung is illustrated for a conformal lung plan in Figure 14.2. Monte Carlo (MC)-based dose calculation is a statistical method capable of accurately modeling the tissue density inhomogeneity and thus desirable for high-precision lung RT. The model is, however, rather complex and computationally demanding. Issues such as statistical uncertainties, the use of variance reduction, and clinical implementation of Monte Carlo–based photon and electron external beam treatment planning were discussed in the report of the AAPM Task Group No. 105 [10]. Recent advances in high-performance computing [11–13] and cloud infrastructure [11,13] are changing the landscape of dose calculation techniques and may make routine use of MC calculation a reality.

Depending on the location and size of the tumor, and beam energy, under dosage of the PTV in lung planning could be significant. In addition to this, doses to normal tissues, particularly the normal lung, may also be affected. Studies have shown substantial differences (10%–20%) could exist between conventional and

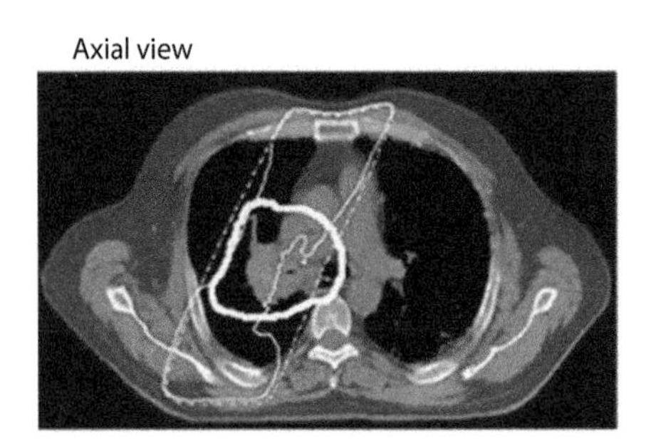

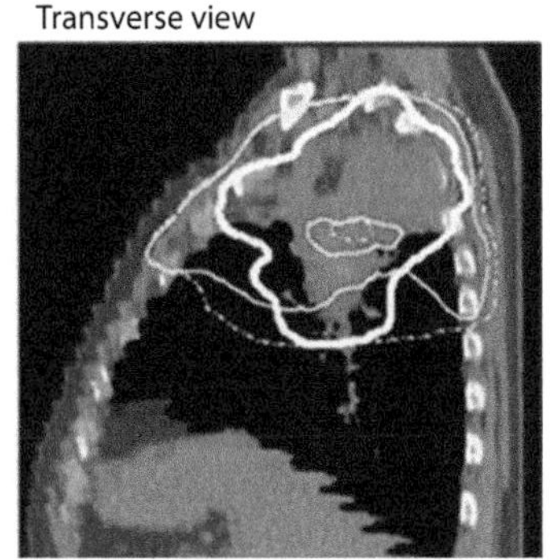

Figure 14.1 A lung RT plan demonstrates the under dosage of the PTV because of electronic disequilibrium. The opposed, oblique field treatment plan (15 MV photons) shows the 100% isodose coverage for MC calculation (modified DPM) in the solid line, and an EPL algorithm in the dashed line. The PTV is demarcated in white. Abbreviations: MC, Monte Carlo; DPM, dose planning method; EPL, equivalent path length. (Reprinted from Chetty, I.J. et al., *Med Phys*, 34, 4818–53, 2007. With permission.)

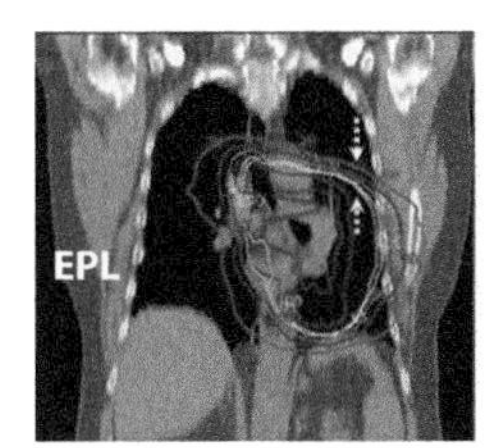

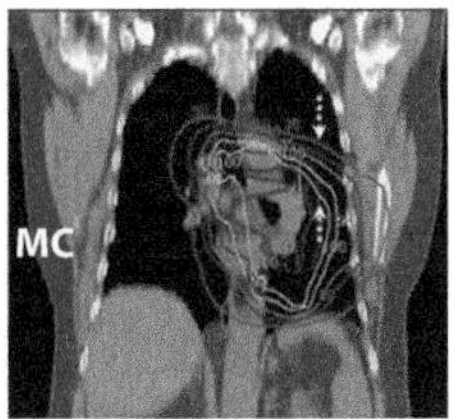

Figure 14.2 A 3D conformal lung plan (15 MV photons) illustrates the penumbral broadening in the MC-based (modified DPM) dose distribution (on the right) because of the increased electron scattering in the lung tissue. This effect is not as pronounced in the EPL-calculated dose distribution. Abbreviations: MC, Monte Carlo; DPM, dose planning method; EPL, equivalent path length. (Reprinted from Chetty, I.J. et al., *Med Phys*, 34, 4818–53, 2007. With permission.)

MC algorithms [14–17]. MC method is particularly suitable for lung RT, especially with sophisticated dose delivery schemes such as IMRT/VMAT. These advanced RT modalities often involve high levels of intensity modulation and are generated by using a sequence of small static or dynamically shaped MLC segments. Under these circumstances, the assumptions used in conventional algorithms regarding scatter equilibrium and output ratio variation with field size often break down [18]. Additionally, in IMRT a significant fraction of dose to the OARs is due to radiation scattered from or transmitted through the MLC [19]. MC simulation can include these effects accurately [20–25].

In the past three decades, many general-purpose MC algorithms have been developed for simulating the transport of electrons and photons including EGS code system [26,27], GEANT 4 [28], ITS [29] and MCNP systems [30,31], et al. While the accuracy of these general-purpose codes can be roughly the same if they are carefully used, these codes are considered too slow for routine treatment planning purposes. Several groups have published reports on the use of parallelization of MC techniques over multiple computers to provide more reasonable turn-around times for simulation in clinical research [32]. Specific to RT, there have been a variety of MC codes developed to improve the calculation efficiency, among which the PEREGRINE system™ (North American Scientific: Nomos Division) was the first MC algorithm to receive FDA 510-K approval and represents the first commercially available photon beam treatment planning system in the US. PEREGRINE uses the random hinge approach [33] for electron transport mechanics with several efficiencies enhancing and variance reduction techniques implemented including source particle reuse, range rejection, Russian roulette and photon splitting [34,35]. Parallelizing the calculation on several computer processors is also implemented to reduce the overall dose calculation time. Other MC codes that have reached commercial implementation including Voxel Monte Carlo (VMC) series of codes [36] and the subsequently developed XVMC code and VMC++ code. XVMC code is incorporated into the Monaco™ (CMS, Elekta, Stockholm, Sweden), PrecisePlan™ (Elekta, Stockholm, Sweden), and iPlan™ (BrainLab, Munich, Germany) treatment planning systems [37]. VMC++ code is the basis for the first commercial electron MC algorithm from Nucletron and is being incorporated into the Masterplan™ (Nucletron, the Netherland) and Eclipse™ (Varian, Palo Alto, CA) treatment planning systems for photon beam dose calculations [38]. Treatment planning applications and experimental verification of VMC-based systems have been reported in several articles [38–40]. Some other developed MC codes and their implementation were detailed described in the report of the AAPM Task Group No. 105 [10]: Macro MC (MMC) code [41,42] and eMC™ (Eclipse, Varian, Palo Alto, CA) [43,44]; MCV (Monte Carlo Vista) code [45] and Pinnacle™ (Philips Radiation Oncology Systems, Madison, WI).

Lindsay et al. performed retrospective MC-based recalculations of 218 NSCLC treatment plans, and showed significant differences in dose indices V20, maximum lung dose and mean GTV dose between plans without heterogeneity correction and MC calculations. Moreover, correlations between V20 and observed radiation pneumonitis in this study were found to be different between plans without heterogeneity correction and MC-based treatment plans [46]. Fregoso et al. reported their work on the dosimetric verifications, and initial clinical evaluations of a commercial MC-based photon beam dose calculation algorithm (iPlan™ v.4.1 TPS). Significant differences between the MC and one-dimensional pencil beam (PB) algorithms were observed, especially for small lesions in the lung, where electronic disequilibrium effects are emphasized. For typical lung treatment plans, the computation time was found to be less than 10 min for 1%–2% mean variance [47]. The clinical evidence thus far, although preliminary and retrospective, supports the notion that MC-based dose calculation and delivery may lead to clinically significant changes in treatment outcome. Kong et al. have shown that the accuracy of radiation dose significantly impacts the local control and overall survival for NSCLC. Local control was found to increase at a rate of 1.3% per gray above the conventional dose fractionation scheme (63–69 Gy in 2.0-Gy fractions) [48], suggesting that even a small change in dose distribution because of inaccurate dose calculation, is likely to affect local control and survival.

Previous studies demonstrated the feasibility of the MC method in IMRT optimization [49–52]. But a full-fledged MC-based plan optimization has yet to be accomplished despite of many attractive features offered by the approach. MC simulation during optimization would allow the optimizer to account for heterogeneity induced dose perturbations, as well as for MLC leakage and scattered radiation. Inaccurate dose algorithms used during optimization can result in convergence errors [50], in which the optimized fluency pattern differs from that corresponding to the optimal dose distribution.

14.3 BEAM ORIENTATION SELECTION FOR LUNG IMRT

IMRT treatment planning starts with the selection of suitable beam angles. Traditionally, the selection is done manually, possibly with trial-and-error adjustment. Considerable time and effort is required to come up with a set of acceptable beams. Also, the results may strongly depend on the planner's experience and understanding of the planning system. Alternatively, a class-solution approach may be adopted, where a predefined set of beam angles are used for similar clinical cases. However, this population-based approach does not take patient-specific anatomy into account, and thus could compromise the treatment plan quality. A better approach is to automate beam placement and incorporate beam orientation optimization into the treatment planning process.

The simplest method to find the optimal beam placement is exhaustive search, which optimizes IMRT plans for all combinations of M beams out of a pool of N equi-spaced beams. This method, although simple, is often computationally prohibitive. For example, for a coplanar pool of n=36 beams uniformly distributed over 360°, all possible combinations of the m=7 beams would require generation and evaluation of C_n^m =8,347,680 IMRT plans. Some approximation to accelerate the search process is needed to make this approach practical. Wang et al. reported a multiresolution search strategy and its application in IMRT for NSCLC [53]. An "influence vector" (IV) approximation technique for high-speed estimation of IMRT dose distributions combined with a fast gradient search algorithm was used for IMRT optimization. First, they determine the most and the least preferred angles using the exhaustive search approach for configurations containing a small number of beams (e.g., three) in a pool of a given number of equi-spaced beams (e.g., 24). The small number of beams greatly reduces the magnitude of the search space, and hence, the optimization time. If the number of the most preferred directions indicated by the results of the previous step is less than the desired number of beams in the optimum configuration, fix the most preferred directions and search for additional directions in the space that includes the remaining beams but excludes the least preferred directions. If the number of the most preferred directions found is greater than the desired number of beams, then search for the optimum angles in the search space of only the most preferred angle subset. This two-step process is considerably faster than full exhaustive search, and yet produces similar treatment plans.

Several sophisticated optimization algorithms have been adopted in radiotherapy planning, mostly using a global search mechanism [54], such as simulated annealing (SA) [55–59] and genetic algorithm (GA) [54,60–63]. SA was among the first to be introduced to solve the radiotherapy treatment optimization problem, but it has many parameters to be optimized and is time consuming in clinical routine. GA is demonstrated to feasibly solve the beam angle optimization (BAO) problem [60,63]. However, this approach is prone to local minimums and a true global minimum is often not attainable. Previous studies have highlighted the limitations of different BAO approaches for IMRT [64,65].

Methods that incorporate prior knowledge into beam orientation optimization are emerging. Recently, Magome et al. reported the similar-case-based optimization (SCBO) of beam arrangements in SBRT for NSCLC [66,67]. Figure 14.3 showed the overall scheme of the method which consisted mainly of three steps.

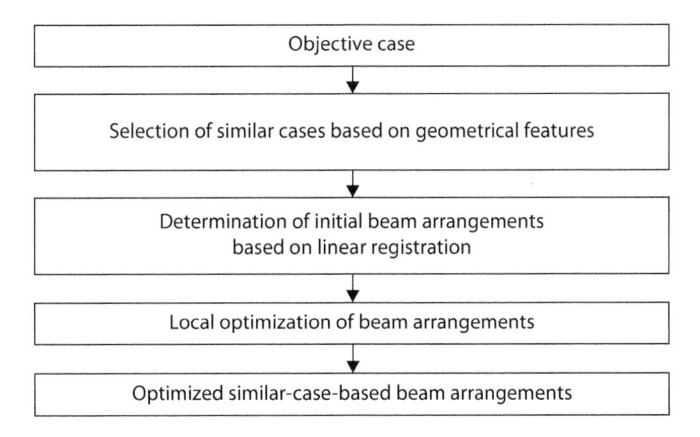

Figure 14.3 Overall scheme of the similar-case-based optimization method for beam arrangements in SBRT. (Reprinted from Magome, T. et al., *Biomed Res Int*, 2013, 309534, 2013.)

Firstly, cases that are like an objective case were automatically selected based on geometrical features related to structures such as the location, size, and shape of the PTV, lung, and spinal cord. Secondly, the initial beam arrangements of the objective case were determined by registering cases that are like the objective case in terms of lung regions, using a linear registration technique, that is, an affine transformation [68]. Finally, the beam directions of the objective case were locally optimized based on the cost function, which considers the radiation absorption in normal tissues and OAR. They concluded that method could be used as a computer-aided treatment planning tool for the determination of beam arrangements in SBRT, with the result that the procedure for the local optimization of beam arrangements improved the quality of treatment plans with significant differences ($P < .05$) in the homogeneity index and conformity index for the PTV, V10, V20, mean dose, and NTCP for the lung.

14.4 AUTOMATED PLANNING AND ITS POTENTIAL FOR LUNG CANCER TREATMENT

Wang and Xing developed an application programming method in C# environment with recorded interactions of planner-TPS and implemented an autopilot VMAT/IMRT planning scheme in the platform [69,70]. Some commonly used planner-TPS interactions as subroutines using Microsoft Visual Studio Coded UI are recorded first. A recorded action is called back in C# application programming, when the corresponding task needs to be accomplished. A strategy was developed to autopilot Eclipse™ (Varian Medical Systems, Palo Alto, CA) VMAT/IMRT plan selection process, which was done in the C# program and in the Eclipse optimization invoked by the C# program. In this approach, the dosimetric characteristics of a reference treatment plan (e.g. DVHs and/or other dosimetric characteristics such as mean/max/min doses) are used to guide the search for a clinically optimal treatment plan through iteratively evaluation and modification of the Eclipse plan. The process mimics a planner's planning process and can provide clinically sensible treatment plans that would otherwise require a large amount of manual trial-and-errors of a planner. Figure 14.4 presents a specific implementation of an auto piloted VMAT/IMRT planning. Practicability and efficiency of the proposed approach was confirmed by application in planning two clinical cases, a head and neck case with VMAT and a prostate case with IMRT.

MDACC also developed their own auto plan system "mdaccAutoPlan system" and adopted in a clinical trial that randomized proton and photon treatments for patients with stage III non-small-cell lung cancer in which the clinical value of passive-scattering proton therapy (PSPT) were compared with that of IMRT [65].

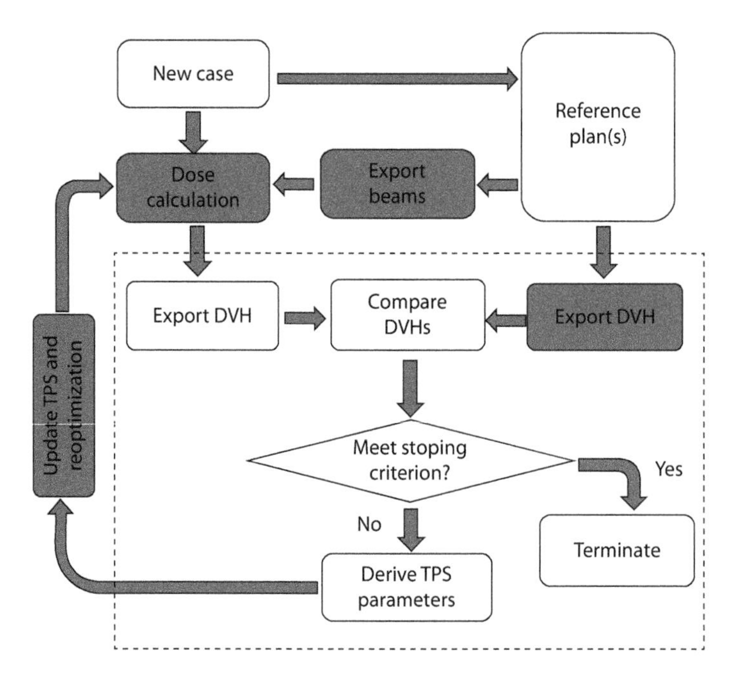

Figure 14.4 An architectural overview of the auto piloted VMAT/IMRT plan optimization scheme. Inner-loop plan optimization is done using the Eclipse™ planning system, whereas an outer-loop calculation analyzes the generated Eclipse plan and feeds the Eclipse optimizer with updated parameters for improved dose distribution. The gray boxes are realized using recorded Eclipse actions stored in a library. (Reprinted from Wang, H. and L. Xing, *J Appl Clin Med Phys*,.17, 6425, 2016.)

14.5 4D TREATMENT PLANNING

Lung tumors tend to move during treatment due to respiratory motion. To account for this, an additional margin for tumor motion is typically added to the gross tumor volume (GTV), leading to a greater volume of healthy tissues irradiated [71,72]. With widespread implementation of 4D imaging techniques, such as 4D-CT [73–75], 4D-PET [76–78], 4D cone beam CT [79–81], and MRI [82–84], and image guided dynamic delivery, 4D planning and treatment is becoming increasingly possible [85–87].

Because the lung density and shape change during the different phases of respiration, it is advantageous to calculate dose on each of breathing phases, and accumulate the dose to a reference phase. To accomplish this, deformable image registration (DIR) is necessary to generate the displacement vector field (DVF) between the source and reference images [85,88,89]. DVFs describe the voxel-by-voxel correlation across multiple CT sets, and can be used to map the doses deposited during other phases back to the reference phase. The most straightforward, although not efficient, implementation of 4D dose accumulation is to perform a full 4D dose calculation and calculate the weighted average over the breathing course [90]. To simplify 4D dose calculation and computational expense, reduction in datasets have been proposed such as coupling the DVFs with the average computed tomography (AVG-CT) to estimate cumulative dose [91], using fewer breathing phases [90], or using the mid-ventilation phase [86,92]. These approaches have revealed close approximations to a full 4D dose accumulation, thereby supporting integration of cumulative dose into clinical treatment planning. For example, in a patient case that was the worst-case scenario (tumor abutted the diaphragm with ~2 cm of superior-inferior motion), the largest deviation observed between DIR coupled with full 4D dose accumulation or the AVG-CT was 2% for the maximum dose and dose to 1% of the gross target volume [91] as shown in Figure 14.5.

The direct dose mapping (DDM) and energy/mass transfer (EMT) mapping are two essential algorithms for accumulating the dose from different anatomic phases to the reference phase when there is organ motion or tumor/tissue deformation during the delivery of radiation therapy. DDM is based on interpolation of the dose values from one dose grid to another and thus lacks rigor in

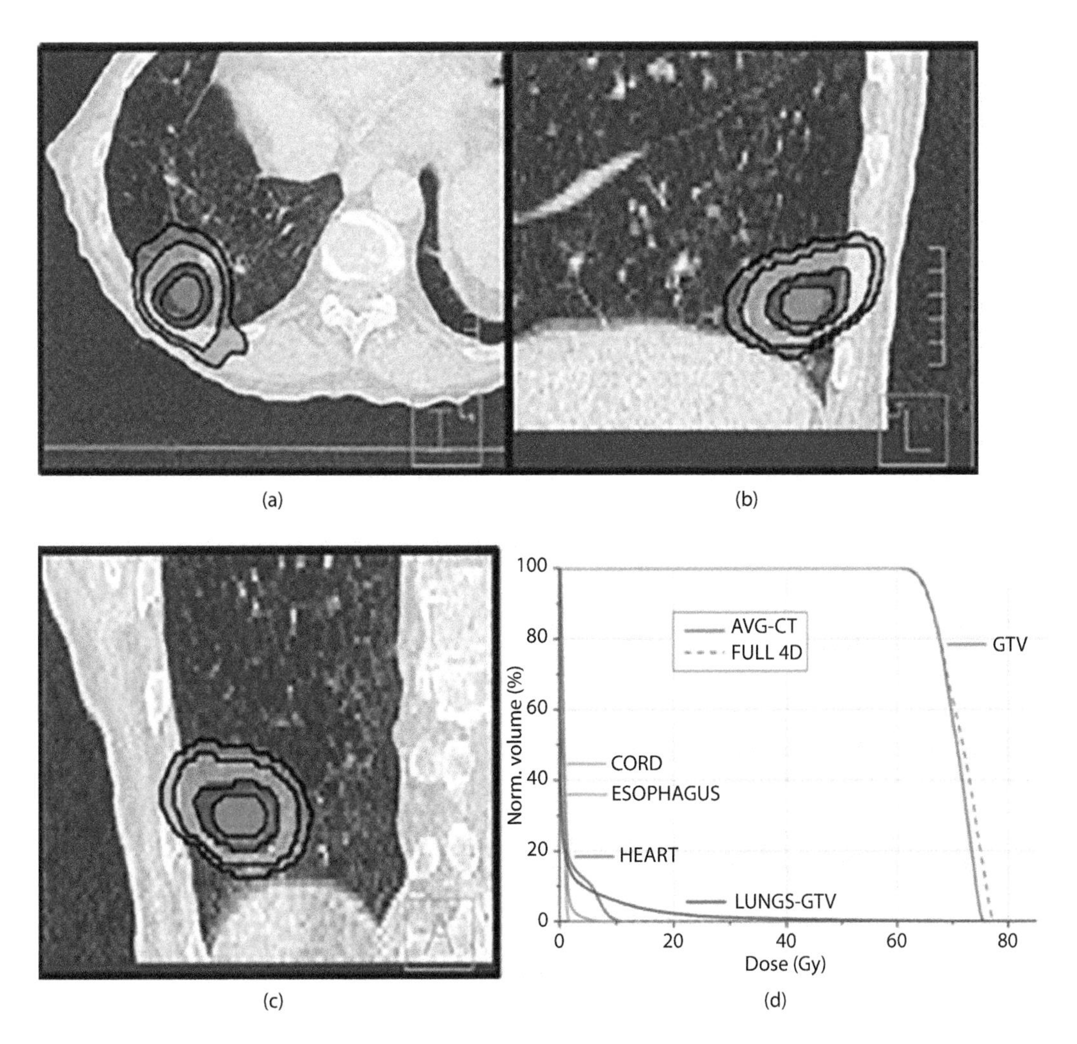

Figure 14.5 Transverse (a), sagittal (b), coronal (c) 4D-CT dataset and dose volume histogram (d) demonstrate the close association between DIR coupled with full 4D dose summation or using the AVG-CT as an approximation for a patient with 2 cm superior-inferior tumor excursion. Isodose washes represent the AVG-CT approximation while the black isodose lines represent the corresponding full 4D dose summation [91]. Abbreviations: 4D-CT, four-dimensional computed tomography; 4D, four-dimensional; DIR, deformable image registration; AVG-CT, average computed tomography. (Reprinted from Glide-Hurst, C.K. et al., *Med Phys*, 35, 5269–5277, 2008. With permission.)

defining the dose when there are multiple dose values mapped to one dose voxel in the reference phase due to tissue/tumor deformation [93]. On the other hand, EMT counts the total energy and mass transferred to each voxel in the reference phase and calculates the dose by dividing the energy by mass (termed energy/mass transfer mapping). Therefore, it is based on fundamentally sound physics principles [94–97]. A comparison of DDM and EMT mapping in 10 lung SBRT patients with the largest lung-motion amplitudes revealed similar cumulative doses to the ITV and PTV, although minimum dose differences of up to 11% in the PTV and 4% in the ITV were observed between the two dose-mapping algorithms with treatment plans computed with anisotropic analytical algorithm (AAA). The authors suggested that DDM might not be adequate for obtaining an accurate dose distribution of the cumulative plan and instead, EMT should be considered [93].

Chin et al. compared 4D VMAT, gated VMAT and 3D VMAT for SBRT in three NSCLC patients [98]. Tumor motion ranged from 1.4 to 3.4 cm. The dose and fractionation scheme was 48 Gy in 4 fractions. 4D-CT data used in this study was divided into 10 respiratory phases. A B-spline transformation model registered the 4D-CT

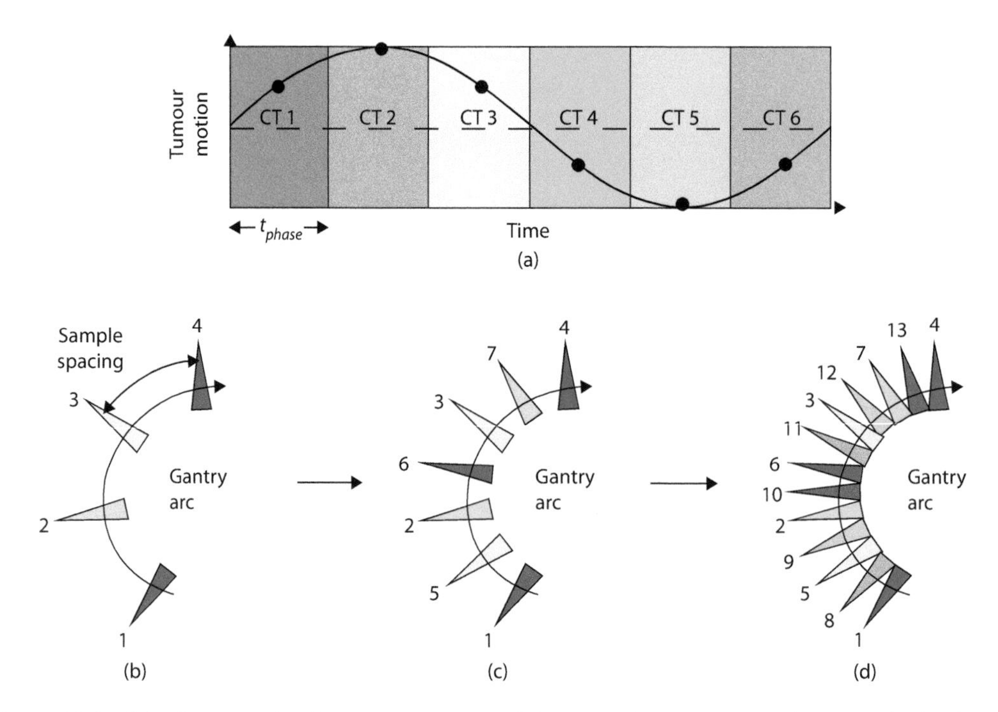

Figure 14.6 (a) A schematic plot shows segmentation of the patient's respiratory cycle into multiple phases. Colors represent specific CT phases 1 through 6. (b) At the start of treatment plan optimization, the arc is coarsely sampled with few beam apertures. (c) As optimization progresses, more beams are inserted. Numbers represent the order in which beam apertures are introduced into the optimization process. (d) By the end of optimization, the arc is fully sampled and sequentially delivered beams correlate to sequential CT phases. The 4D-CT data is sampled multiple times over the arc. Note that (a)–(d) are simplified illustrations. Real plan optimizations used 4D-CT data with 10 respiratory phases, 360° arcs, at least 177 beam apertures per arc, and 1–3 arcs. (Reprinted from Chin, E. et al., *Phys Med Biol*, 58, 749–770, 2013. With permission.)

images. The continuous arc rotation of the radiation source is approximated by multiple static beam apertures using a 4D-VMAT algorithm written in Matlab™ [99], and a cost function guiding treatment plan optimization based on dose-volume constraints [100]. At the start of optimization, the arc is sampled by only a few evenly spaced beam apertures (e.g. 9–13) and the flexibility to alter the beam weights and MLC leaf positions is high. Eventually, more beam apertures are added to the optimization, and the flexibility to change machine parameters decreases until the arc is fully sampled (e.g. 177–289 beams/arc). The addition of new beam apertures always occurs halfway between two existing apertures. While other radiation therapy techniques such as gated VMAT and 3D-VMAT rely on a static representation of the patient based on 3D-CT data, the key characteristic of the 4D-VMAT algorithm is its integration of the patient's 4D-CT data into the optimization process. This is achieved by correlating consecutive beam apertures to consecutive CT phases (Figure 14.6). Only one CT phase is assigned per beam, generating treatment plans with respiratory phase-optimized apertures whose deliveries are synchronized to the patient's breathing motion. For most OARs, gated VMAT achieved the most radiation sparing but treatment times were 77%–148% longer than 3D-VMAT. 4D-VMAT plan qualities were comparable to gated VMAT, but, much more efficient delivery treatment times were found to be only 11%–25% longer than 3D-VMAT.

14.6 BIOLOGY-GUIDED TREATMENT OPTIMIZATION

Treatment optimization based on dose-volume constraints is routinely used in the clinical setting for treatment planning. It appears unlikely that this practice will change significantly soon, especially since there is a wealth of clinical experience relating organ volumes above specific dose thresholds to the incidence of complications. Furthermore, quantitative analysis of normal tissue effects in the clinic (QUANTEC) has led to updated dose-volume constraints for different organs, including the lung [99–102]. These recommendations of updated data are likely to be widely adopted, potentially implying even greater future clinical reliance on dose-volume constraints.

Although dose-volume optimization (DVO) is a mainstay of current clinical practice, incorporating additional information into the treatment optimization process, such as important biological properties of the tumor and critical organs, could potentially enhance the efficacy of radiotherapy in general. Specifically, adding biological optimization after DVO, without destroying the "important" dose-volume characteristics achieved by DVO, which would be identified by the planner/clinician on the dose-volume optimized dose-volume histograms (DVH). While this method necessarily limits the efficacy of biological optimization, it would be acceptable within the current clinical paradigm. Biological information may be obtained by, for example, biological or functional imaging (e.g. PET/CT, ventilation and/or perfusion (V/Q) imaging) as opposed anatomical imaging with CT, normal tissue complication probability models (NTCP)/tumor control probability (TCP) models, such as Lyman-probit [103] and relative-seriality [104], phenomenological models such as the equivalent uniform dose (EUD) [105–107], or hybrid physio-biological models [108–112].

14.6.1 NTCP-based optimization in SBRT for NSCLC

Given that SBRT is a relatively new modality and doses are much more hypo-fractionated than traditionally used, established guidelines for dose selections do not exist. A variety of doses have been used, ranging from "radio surgical" single doses to hypo-fractionated regimens using multiple fractions ≤ 5. It is logical to assume that a dose-response relationship exists for tumors treated with SBRT, thus the optimal dose achieves a high level of tumor control without undue risks of normal tissue toxicity. Although predictive models of risk based on small-volume hypo-fractionated treatment such as SBRT do not exist, there are several generally accepted models for predicting lung NTCP based on conventionally fractionated external beam radiation therapy [113]. These models consider integral doses to the OARs, with radiation pneumonitis being the primary toxicity of concern. Compared with doses selected based on simpler parameters such as tumor size, NTCP models offer the potential for dose selection based on individual variations such as tumor location, organ volume, and conformity of the treatment plan.

Song et al. described their experience with SBRT on a pilot study in which a Lyman NTCP model was used to determine maximum allowable doses for treatment of lung tumors [114]. Twenty-five tumors in 17 patients were treated. All treatments were delivered in 3 daily fractions of 9–15 Gy per fraction. NTCP calculations (using the Lyman model) were performed to facilitate dose prescription, and doses were prescribed with a maximum allowable NTCP risk of pneumonitis of up to 20%, not to exceed 15 Gy per fraction [103]. Inhomogeneity within the dose distribution was accounted for using the dose volume histogram reduction method of Kutcher and Burman [115]. The median dose prescribed was 35 Gy (range, 24–45 Gy). Twenty-three of 25 tumors remained controlled at median follow-up of 14 months. Four patients experienced grade 1–2 acute toxicity. Late toxicity developed in 2 patients who received treatment to peri-hilar tumors and no patient had grade 3 or 4 radiation pneumonitis. Dosing based on NTCP calculations may be a rational way to safely select doses for a new modality without established dose guidelines. One limitation of this study was that complications of other adjacent organs, such as airways and esophagus, were not accounted for in the model.

14.6.2 PET/CT and its application in radiotherapy for NSCLC

Imaging with PET and PET/CT provides sensitive, quantifiable and accurate molecular information on the biology and extent of many tumors. The most commonly used radiopharmaceuticals as PET tracers in radiation oncology is fluorodeoxyglucose, of which a wide range of cancers have higher uptake than nearby normal tissues [116]. Noninvasive evaluation of hypoxia levels in NSCLC has been performed with F-18 fluoromisonidazole (FMISO) PET, copper-60-diacetylbis (N4-methylthiosemicarbazone; Cu-60 ATSM) and with (18) F-fluoroazomycin arabinoside ((18)F-FAZA)PET [117–120].

A combined PET/CT acquisition is now the standard method of acquiring FDG-PET images for the purposes of baseline staging and for radiotherapy treatment planning (RTP) in NSCLC [120]. Several staging studies have clearly demonstrated the superiority of PET/CT over CT for identification of involved mediastinal lymph nodes [121,122] and discriminating collapsed lungs from tumor [123]. Moreover, PET/CT-based target volume delineations are, on average, smaller than their CT counterpart, thereby reducing the dose to surrounding normal structures, which may open the possibility of dose escalation [121,124]. Ideally, FDG-PET staging scans for potential RT candidates should be performed in the RT treatment position, to enable dual use of PET images for staging and RT planning. Although an integrated PET/CT [125] acquisition is preferred, PET and CT image co-registration, ideally using fiducial markers, may also be used in practice [126].

The International Atomic Energy Agency (IAEA) published their consensus report on PET/CT imaging for target volume delineation (TVD) in curative intent radiotherapy of NSCLC in 2014 [127]. One thing to be noted is that, the definition of target volume should include the full motion path of all tumor locations to create a respiration expanded GTV (reGTV), which contains the tumor at all times of its excursion. 4D PET/CT imaging may overcome some of the inaccuracies associated with a free breathing PET/CT scan, by providing more accurate SUV quantification for moving lung tumors. A recent study using 4D PET/CT imaging has demonstrated that a 4D PET-based ITV closely approximates to a 4DCT [128]. Further investigation and clinical validation of the application of 4D PET/CT imaging are required.

Auto contours may provide consistent contours when compared with manual methods. However, there are several unresolved problems with PET-based auto contouring as follows: 1) there is some difficulty dealing with normal tissue adjacent to the tumor with high SUV uptake such as the heart; 2) there is no clear consensus on which method approximates to the tumor position, tumor edge, and pathological correlation has proven difficult [129]; 3) the variability of SUV values due to factors other than tumor activity such as patient biological factors and technical factors [130]; 4) the value of auto contours is without any supporting evidence when delineating a reGTV to include the full motion path of all tumor locations. The information obtained from the PET component of the scan is complementary to that contained within the CT scan and the use of information from both may lead to more reliable auto-contouring [131]. Nonetheless, automated PET-based contouring are worthy of further investigation, particularly in the era of 4D PET/CT imaging.

Besides glucose metabolism, regional tumor hypoxia has also been associated with increased radio resistance and treatment failure. Studies evaluating hypoxia imaging with FMISO have shown that it is possible to use this imaging technique to evaluate oxygenation status in tumors (Figure 14.7). This information can be potentially used to guide dose escalation to the hypoxic fraction of the tumor [118,119].

14.6.3 Lung functional imaging and its application in radiotherapy for NSCLC

Information on pulmonary function provided by ventilation and/or perfusion (V/Q) imaging has been shown to be important in evaluating lung toxicity after RT for NSCLC [132–143]. Several techniques exist for pulmonary

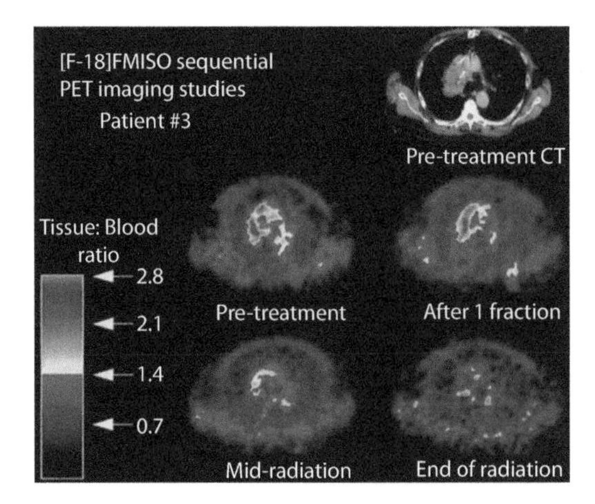

Figure 14.7 The serial (F-18) FMISO PET imaging studies for a patient of T2N3M0 NSCLC, who was treated with a 6.5-week course of photons, with corresponding pretreatment CT scan included. Serial scans with F-18 FMISO reveal decreasing hypoxia in the large tumor lesion of the right lung. (Reprinted from Koh, W.J. et al., *Int J Radiat Oncol Biol Phys*, 33, 391–398, 1995. With permission.)

V/Q imaging, including PET-CT [132], single photon emission computed tomography and x-ray CT (SPECT-CT) [134], hyperpolarized helium-3 magnetic resonance imaging (3He-MRI) [135,136,142], inert xenon CT (Xe-CT) [137,138, 143], and 4D-CT ventilation [139–141]. These imaging modalities can provide useful V/Q information.

Sivaassess et al. assessed the utility of IMRT optimization by incorporating information about lung function using 4D-V/Q-PET-CT acquisition technology in NSCLC (175). Planar scintigraphy using ^{99m}Tc-labelled macro aggregated albumin (MAA) is a long-established imaging standard for functional V/Q evaluation. In this study, ventilation imaging was performed following inhalation of Galligas, produced by substituting Gallium-68 instead of Technetium-99m. A contemporaneous low-dose chest 4D-CT acquisition was performed. The field of view for both 4D-PET and 4D-CT encompassed the entire lung fields. Ventilation-PET scan of the lungs was acquired. Subsequently, 4D-perfusion-PET was acquired over the same field-of-view with 68Ga-MAA administered intravenously. The ventilation and perfusion PET scans were reconstructed as both gated and un-gated images. Phase matched attenuation correction was used to reconstruct the 4D-PET/CT scan. The free-breathing PET acquisition was subsequently co-registered with the average intensity projection of the 4D-CT. Both "highly perfused" (HPLung) and "highly ventilated" (HVLung) lung volumes were delineated using a 70th centile SUV threshold, and a "ventilated lung volume" (VLung) was created using a 50th centile SUV threshold (Figure 14.8). For each patient four IMRT plans were created, optimized to the anatomical lung, HPLung, HVLung and VLung volumes, respectively. Plans optimized to HPLung resulted in a significant reduction of functional mean lung dose (MLD) and improved functional V5, V10 and V20 (Figure 14.9).

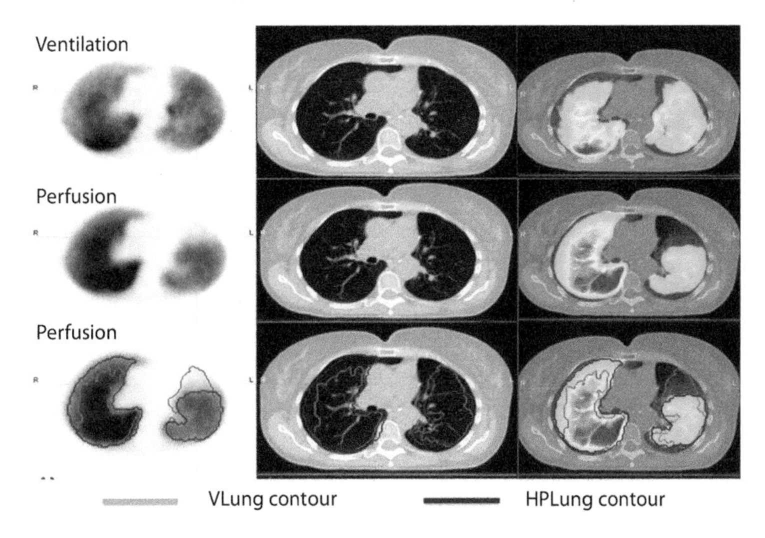

Figure 14.8 V/Q PET/CT scan in a patient with emphysema. PET images are displayed in the first column, co-registered PET/CT images in the second column showing both ventilation images (top row) and perfusion images (bottom row). There is markedly more artefact in the ventilation images with clumping of tracer in central airways. (Reprinted from Siva, S. et al., *Radiother Oncol*, 115, 157–162, 2015. With permission.)

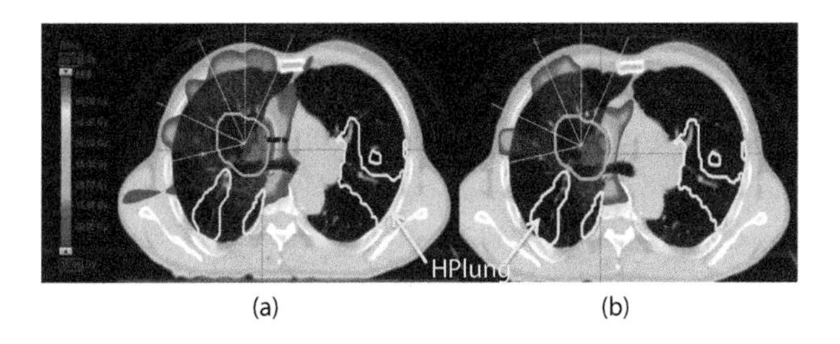

Figure 14.9 An IMRT plan of an NSCLC patient with severe emphysema. (a) Axial dose color wash shows a conventional IMRT plan optimized to anatomical lung. (b) The functionally adapted plan optimized to the HPLung volume demonstrates differences in dose distribution that may be observed due to functional dose painting. (Reprinted from Siva, S. et al., *Radiother Oncol*, 115, 157–162, 2015. With permission.)

Lung perfusion imaging using SPECT-CT provides 3D functional information on regional perfusion of lung in addition to anatomic information. Multiple previous studies have demonstrated that perfusion-weighted optimization might be useful in reducing radiation damage in patients with locally advanced NSCLC who had large perfusion defects [144–146]. It is conceivable that by combining IMRT, which has been shown to be more effective than 3D-CRT for focusing radiation dose to lung tumors while sparing normal lung tissue [147,148], with lung function imaging, dose distributions to normal lung may be tailored per its perfusion distribution to further minimize pulmonary toxicity [133,145,149,150].

Shioyama et al. assessed the feasibility of SPECT perfusion-based IMRT treatment planning in locally advanced NSCLC [133]. Sixteen patients underwent lung perfusion imaging with SPECT-CT, which was then registered with simulation CT and was used to segment the 50- and 90-centile hyper-perfusion lung (F50 lung and F90 lung; see Figure 14.10). Two IMRT plans were designed and compared in each patient: an anatomic plan using simulation CT alone and a functional plan, using SPECT-CT in addition to the simulation CT. In incorporating perfusion information in IMRT planning, the mean doses, and the percentage of volume irradiated with >5 Gy, >10 Gy, and >20 Gy to the F50 and F90 lungs in the functional plan were all reduced compared with those in the anatomic plans. They demonstrated that sparing of the functional lung was achieved for patients with large perfusion defects compared with those with relatively uniform perfusion distribution (see Figure 14.11).

Hyperpolarized noble gas MRI is a novel technique that enables quantitative analysis of pulmonary physiology [135,151]. With optical pumping techniques used before gas inhalation, extremely high nuclear-spin polarization levels can be produced that provide a signal size sufficient for MRI. By applying this method with the inert, non-radioactive isotope helium-3 (3He), MRI of lung ventilation and oxygen sensitivity can be obtained with unprecedented spatial and temporal resolution [152,153]. When applied in radiotherapy in NSCLC, 3He-MR images could tailor the radiation fields to limit the dose to the healthy regions of the lung, hence to reduce the incidence

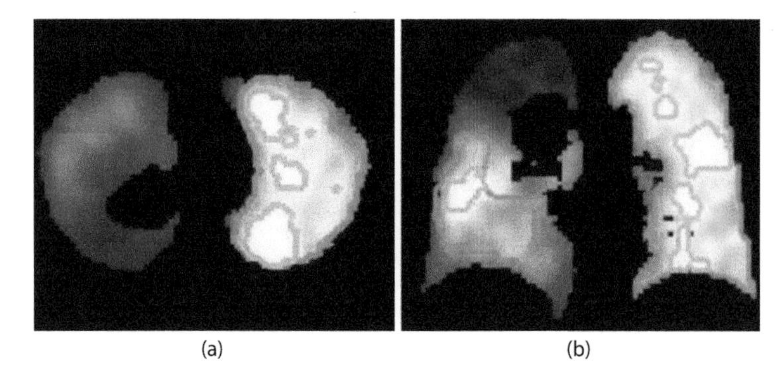

Figure 14.10 The centile SPECT images in a NSCLC case. The increase of the perfusion is represented by the intensity of the images. The F50 and F90 lung are highlighted in green and orange colors, respectively. (Reprinted from Shioyama, Y. et al., *Int J Radiat Oncol Biol Phys*, 68, 1349–1358, 2007. With permission.)

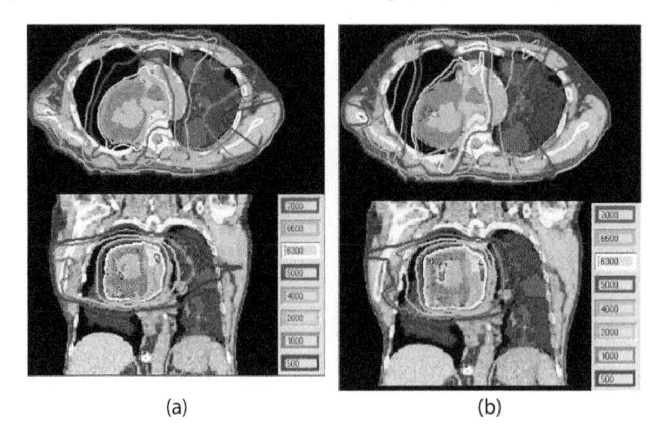

Figure 14.11 Comparison of the dose distributions between the anatomic plan (a) and functional plan (b) in the same case as that of Figure 14.10. (Reprinted from Shioyama, Y. et al., *Int J Radiat Oncol Biol Phys*, 68, 1349–1358, 2007. With permission.)

of radiation pneumonia. The study of Rob et al. demonstrated the feasibility of registering 3He-MRI to x-ray CT for functionally weighted IMRT planning [142]. Figure 14.12 shows improved superior functional and anatomic data of NSCLC patients, provided by 3He-MRI, fused with radiotherapy planning CT using rigid registration. Registration accuracy was sufficient, assessed using an overlap coefficient (Ω) (Figure 14.13). In comparison with the total lung IMRT plans, IMRT constrained with 3He-MRI reduced the V20 (i.e. the volume of lung receiving a dose >20 Gy) for the total and functional lung, in addition to the mean lung dose to the functional lung.

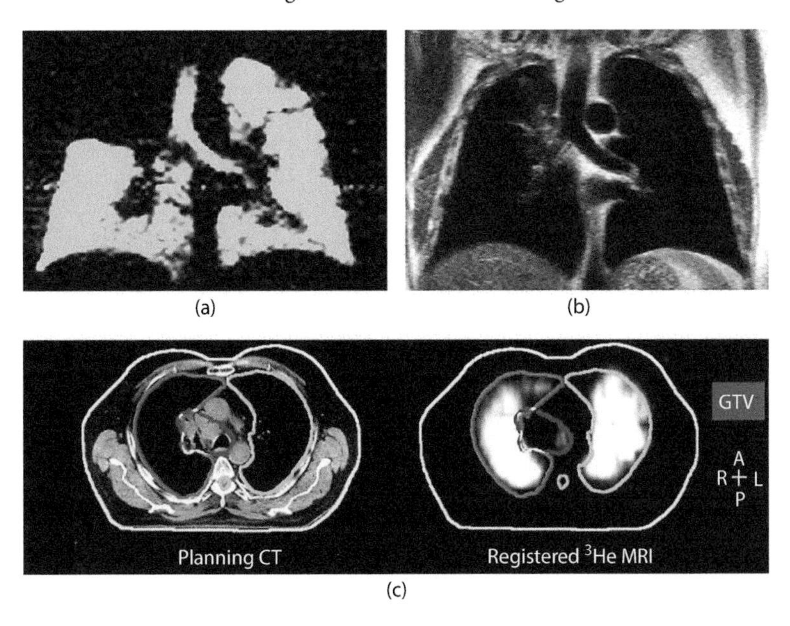

Figure 14.12 (a) Hyperpolarized 3He MRI exhibiting a complete ventilation obstruction in the upper right lobe in a NSCLC patient. (b) Corresponding 1H MRI. (c) Sample registered hyperpolarized 3He MRI (right) displayed with the external contour, left and right lung and GTV from the trans-axial radiotherapy treatment-planning CT (left). (Reprinted from Ireland, R.H. et al., *Int J Radiat Oncol Biol Phys*, 68, 273–281, 2007. With permission.)

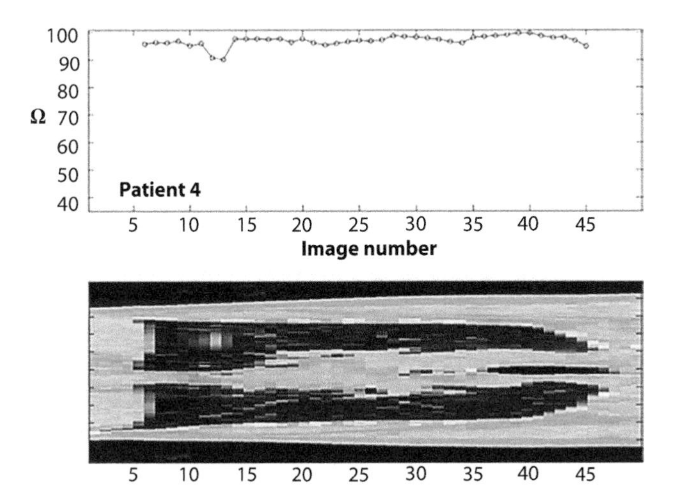

Figure 14.13 The overlap coefficient (Ω), which evaluates image registration for the same case of Figure 14.12 displayed with a sample coronal CT slice [142]. Ω calculated as the proportion of the segmented 3He-MR slice volume (V_{MRI}) that intersects the segmented CT lung slice volume (V_{CT}) expressed as a percentage of V_{MRI}:

$$\Omega = 100 \times \frac{V_{MRI} \cap V_{CT}}{V_{MRI}}$$

(Reprinted from Ireland, R.H. et al., *Int J Radiat Oncol Biol Phys*, 68, 273–281, 2007. With permission.)

4D-CT ventilation imaging is another emerging technique to assess lung function. 4D-CT consists of 3D-CT images resolved into different phases of the breathing cycle, and is widely used nowadays for radiation treatment planning of lung cancer. Calculating ventilation maps from 4D-CT data only involves additional image processing, which does not add any extra imaging dose or cost to the patient. Moreover, 4D-CT ventilation imaging has higher resolution, a shorter scan time and is more accessible than other existing techniques. 4D-CT ventilation image is created in two steps, first by spatial regional mapping of different respiratory phases of 4D-CT images using DIR, and second by quantitative analysis of the resultant displacement vector field [154–157]. Previous studies have investigated the incorporation of 4D-CT ventilation imaging into RT treatment planning [134,140,141,158]. Castillo et al. [134] examined different ways of calculating ventilation from 4D-CT data to estimate local volume changes, and compared the results with those obtained clinically from SPECT ventilation. Yamamoto et al. [140] and Yaremko et al. [141] discussed the idea of designing treatment plans to spare high-ventilation areas of the lung. Yamamoto et al. quantified the dosimetric impact of 4D-CT ventilation imaging-based functional IMRT/VMAT in NSCLC patients. For each patient, anatomic and functional plans were created for IMRT and VMAT with consistent beam angles and dose-volume constraints. Functional planning spared the high-functional lung, and anatomic planning treated the lungs as uniformly functional (Figure 14.14). It is demonstrated that functional planning led to significant reductions in the high-functional lung dose, without significantly increasing other critical organ doses, but at the expense of significantly degraded the PTV conformity and homogeneity (Figure 14.15). Significantly larger changes occurred in the metrics for patients with a larger amount of high-functional lung adjacent to the PTV.

14.7 DIGITAL LINEAR ACCELERATOR AND STATION PARAMETER OPTIMIZED RADIATION THERAPY (SPORT)

In meeting with the increased clinical demands for higher mechanical accuracy, improved intra-treatment image guidance, and faster dose delivery, a new generation of digital linear accelerator (linac) has been clinically implemented in several hospitals [159–163]. Some commercially available digital linacs include Varian TrueBeam™, Siemens ONCOR™, Elekta Synergy™ and Precise Treatment System™. A distinct feature of the digital linacs, is that parameters characterizing radiation delivery such as the gantry angle, collimator angle, couch angle, and dose rate are discretized and can be controlled easily in a programmable

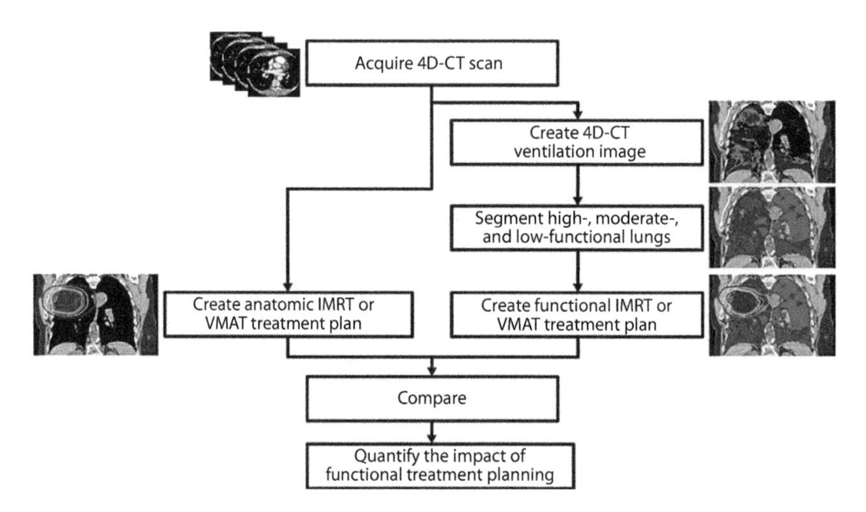

Figure 14.14 4D-CT-IMRT-VMAT schematic diagram for creating anatomic treatment plan and 4D-CT ventilation imaging-based functional plans and quantifying impact of functional planning. (Reprinted from Yamamoto, T. et al., *Int J Radiat Oncol Biol Phys*, 79, 279–288, 2011. With permission.)

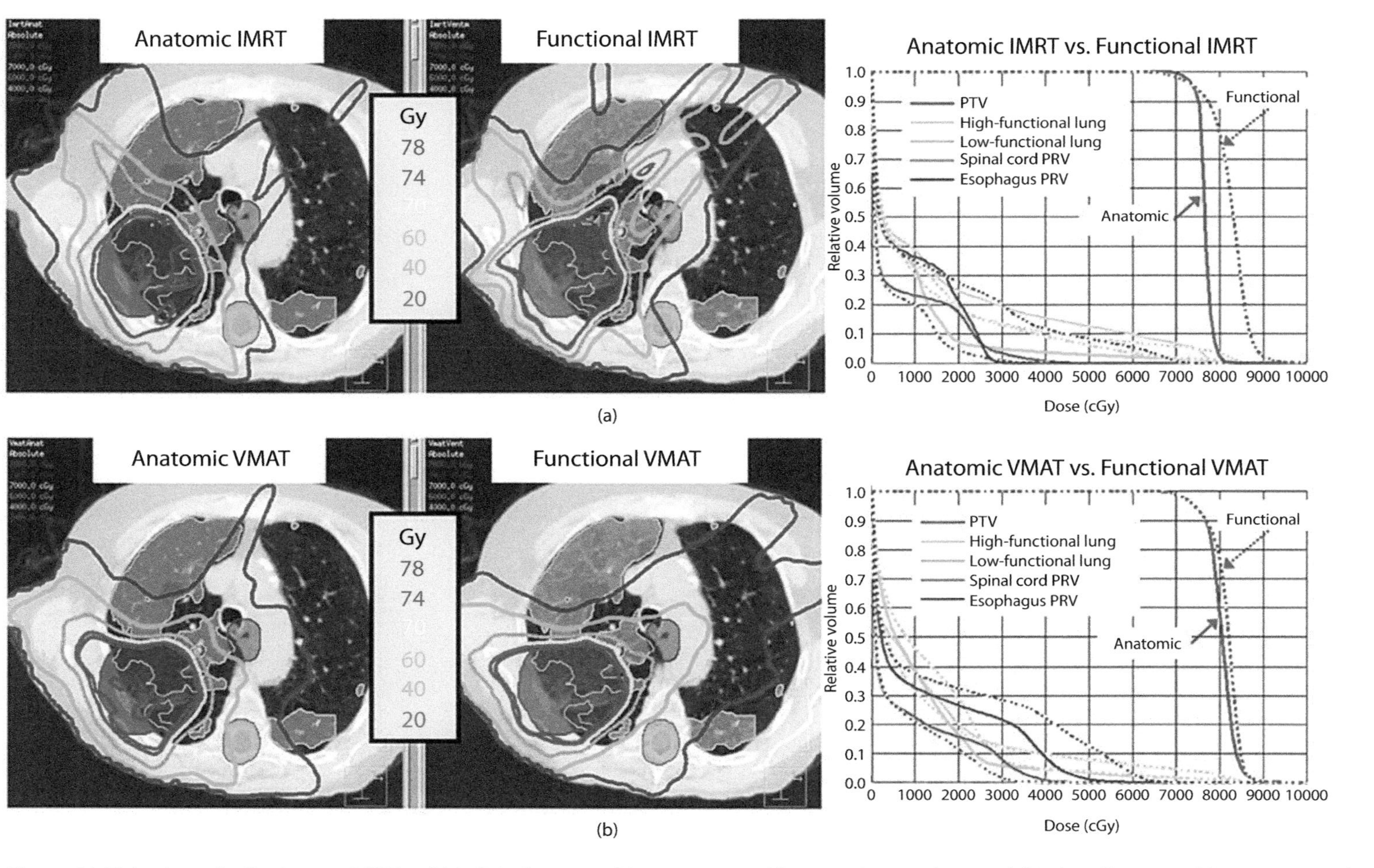

Figure 14.15 Isodose distributions and DVHs of (a) clinically acceptable anatomic and functional IMRT plans, and (b) clinically acceptable anatomic and functional VMAT plans. In isodose distributions, high-functional lung region is shaded orange; In DVHs, anatomic plans are represented by solid curves and functional plans by dashed lines. (Reprinted from Yamamoto, T. et al., *Int J Radiat Oncol Biol Phys*, 79, 279–288, 2011. With permission.)

fashion. The fundamental unit is a "station" point (a "station" can also be called a "node" in the CyberKnife® system).

In the emerging digital era of radiation therapy, a treatment will be done through the modulation of station parameters as the delivery is done "station by station" instead of "beam by beam." A "station" describes the state of delivery system (including LINAC configurations such as beam energy, aperture shape and weight, gantry/collimator/couch angle). Xing et al. of Stanford University named this emerged optimization of station parameters-station parameter optimized radiation therapy (SPORT) [164–166]. Intuitively, one may consider that SPORT is a scheme with increased angular beam sampling while eliminating dispensable segments of the incident fields. In digital linacs, efficient SPORT delivery is achieved by, 1) removing the redundant segments in the incident beams 2) concatenating the stations so that they can be delivered in sequence automatically (i.e., auto-field sequencing) and 3) using high-dose-rate beams (e.g. flattening filter free(FFF)) [162,163,167]. The promise of SPORT is that it will enable us to realize the enormous potential of digital linacs through optimal weighting and spatial distribution of the station points, including non-coplanar, non-isocentric distribution, and even multiple isocenters.

14.7.1 Specific implementations of SPORT

Treatment planning and delivery are generally intertwined. The actual delivery of SPORT can be realized in different ways. In the following section, we will describe two categories of SPORT delivery: rotational arc SPORT and fixed-station SPORT.

14.7.2 Rotational ARC SPORT

Conventional VMAT [168–170] such as Varian RapidArc™ discretizes the angular space into equally spaced station points during planning and then optimizes the apertures and weights of the stations. The aperture at an angle between two stations is obtained through interpolation. This wisdom tacitly ignores the differential need for intensity modulation of different angles. Unless the discretization is infinitely fine (which is computationally prohibitive and avoidably oversamples some angles), such an approach is incapable of providing sufficient modulation for some or all directions for many disease sites. To overcome the limitation, multiple arcs are often required to produce a clinically acceptable treatment plan.

In the one-arc SPORT implementation, the angular sampling rate (i.e. the number of stations per unit angle) is modulated per the need of individual angles for intensity modulation (see Figure 14.16 [171]). The essence is how to identify the need of an individual angle for intensity modulation and provide the necessary

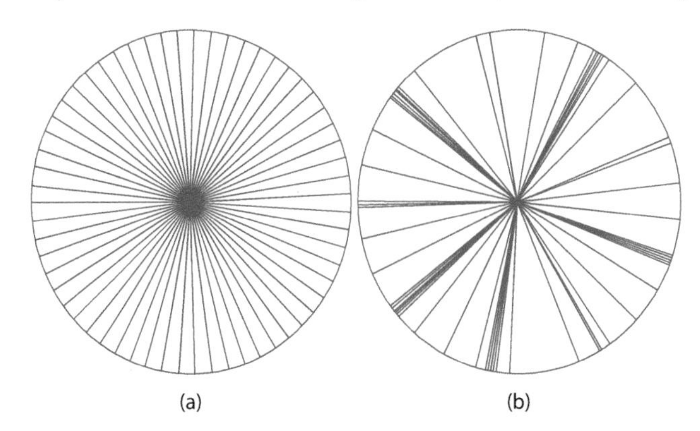

Figure 14.16 SPORT-1ARC Schematic plot of the beam angular distributions for two treatment schemes. The lines indicate the gantry angles of the station points or control points. (a) Conventional VMAT: the angular space is discretized into equally spaced station points and the apertures and weights of the stations are optimized; (b) SPORT: the proposed method provides angular modulation (modulation per unit angle) through optimal angular sampling of station points. (Reprinted from Li, R. and L. Xing, *Med Phys*, 40, 050701, 4912–4919, 2013. With permission.)

intensity modulation for those angles which need it. Obviously, treatment plans for the single arc SPORT can be obtained by a direct optimization of weights and aperture shapes of the station points and their coplanar distribution. For the ease of computation, the treatment is planned with a heuristic approach in an adaptive fashion by starting from a conventional 1-arc VMAT plan with equally spaced stations. The angles that need higher intensity modulation are identified with the help of a "demand metric." To boost an angle with a high "demand metric" value, several stations are added around the point. Additional segments are then added near the angles that require high-intensity modulation. The modified arc plan of the original one-arc VMAT with the added segments is optimized to provide the final segmented boost VMAT treatment plan.

14.7.3 Fixed-station SPORT

SPORT can also be delivered station by station, much like fixed-gantry IMRT delivery. The technique, which we termed as DASSIM-RT (dense angularly sampled and sparse intensity modulated radiation therapy) (see Figure 14.17) [159], presents a truly optimal RT scheme with optimal angular sampling (including non-coplanar beams), beam intensity modulation, and possible energy and collimator modulation when going from one gantry angle to another [172]. With the use of another inverse planning technique, which was proposed by Zhu and Xing [173,174] as compressed sensing (CS)-based strategy, it is straightforward to find fixed-station SPORT solutions that most effectively utilizes all the available station parameters. Dramatically different from simply increasing the number of beams for IMRT or increasing the arcs in VMAT, the dosimetric improvement is achieved by considering the interplay between the angular sampling and intensity modulation. The SPORT framework will enable us to harness the newly available features of digital linacs, and provide truly optimal patient treatment. A brute-force SPORT optimization can be computationally intractable because of many variables involved in the process. Hence knowledge-based planning technique, for example, a metric-named beam's-eye-view dosimetrics (BEVD) [57,58], is an effective way to reduce the complexity of the optimization [164].

The emergence of digital linac calls for new strategies for treatment plan optimization and delivery. In general, existing 3D-CRT, IMRT and VMAT represent special cases of SPORT. SPORT has several unique features and makes it possible to maximally utilize the technical capacity of digital linacs. Essentially, the benefit of SPORT stems from the better definition of search space and explicit incorporation of parameters characterizing the station points in inverse planning. SPORT enlarges the solution space through improved angular and intensity sampling of the stations. As indicated in numerous studies, conformal dose distribution is essential

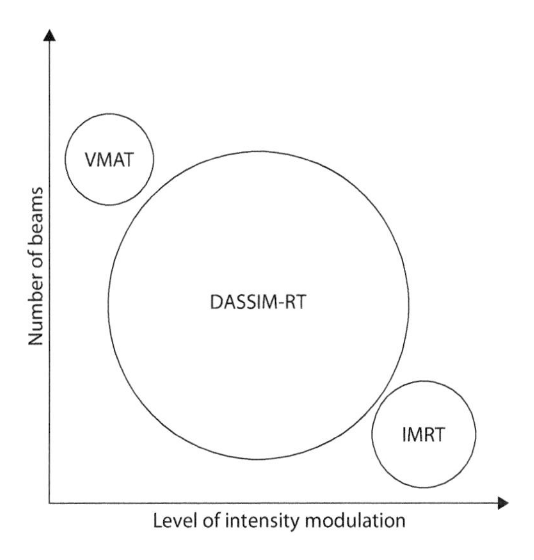

Figure 14.17 Schematic plot of DASSIM-RT, conventional IMRT, and VMAT in terms of the number of beams and level of intensity modulation. DASSIMRT completes the "phase space" extended by inter-beam and intra-beam modulation for radiotherapy. (Reprinted from Li, R. and L. Xing, *Med Phys*, 38, 4912–4919, 2013. With permission.)

to improved treatment outcome by maximizing tumor control and minimizing toxicity. Therefore, the SPORT formalism and tools should have a measurable clinical impact resulting in improved patient care in the future.

14.8 TREATMENT PLANNING IN LUNG CANCER WITH PARTICLE THERAPIES

14.8.1 Proton and carbon ion therapy in lung cancer

The combination of large tumor volumes in the chest, often invading critical vital organs such as the lungs, the large blood vessels, and the esophagus in patients with impaired organ function, poses a formidable challenge in lung cancer cases treated with radiotherapy. Escalating radiation doses with biologically enhancedt radiation can improve local control and overall survival [175,176]; whilst minimizing the dose to the surrounding normal tissue to decrease radiation-related toxicity, is a concept that has fueled research in both photons and particle therapies.

Charged particle therapies including proton and carbon ion therapy have unique physical properties that result in distinct advantages over conventional photon-based radiation [177]. Specifically, they typically have low entrance doses, and then display high-energy depositions as the charged particle reaches the end of its range in tissue, a phenomenon known as the Bragg peak. The dose falloff that ensues after the Bragg peak is much steeper than can be achieved with photon therapy. By modifying this Bragg peak per position and size of the tumor into a spread-out Bragg peak (SOBP) [178], it is possible to deliver high-dose radiation to a tumor while minimizing the dose delivered to the surrounding OARs [179] (Figure 14.18). In addition to minimal or no-exit dose, charged particle therapies typically result in total lower integral dose, which may translate into a lower risk of secondary malignancies.

Many dosimetric studies have demonstrated an improved dose distribution with protons compared to photons for different types of tumors including lung cancer [180]. This may allow a higher radiation dose to the tumor with the same risk of radiation-induced normal tissue toxicity with photons, or allow for reduction of adverse effects while keeping equivalent tumor-effective doses. Carbon ions have similar physical properties with protons but also deposit more energy along their tracks (i.e. high-LET radiation), resulting in a significantly higher radio biologic effect, which may lead to more effective treatment for radio-resistant and/or hypoxic tumors [179] (Figure 14.19, Table 14.1). Table 14.1 shows the comparison of the physical aspects of protons and carbons.

Proton therapy has been clinically used in both early- and advanced-stage NSCLC, and there are numerous ongoing trials exploring the role of proton therapy in NSCLC. Favorable results using proton therapy were reported compared with conventionally fractionated radiotherapy (CFRT), IMRT or SBRT [181–185]. In stage I NSCLC, protons achieved lower doses to OARs than SBRT [186–189]. This may be of interest in centrally located

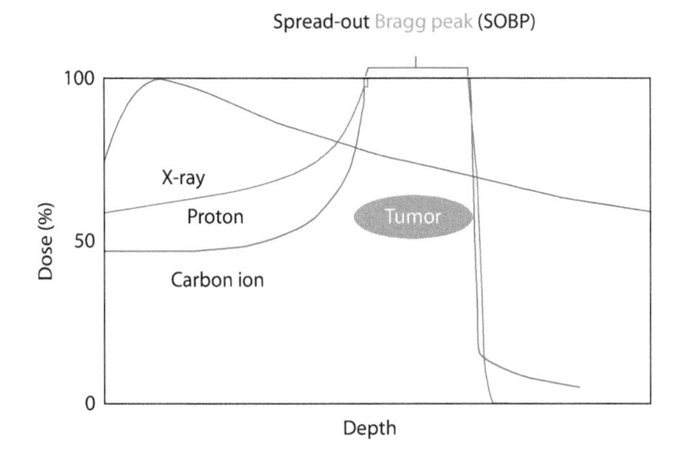

Figure 14.18 Dose distributions of x-rays, protons, and carbon ions. (Reprinted from Demizu, Y. et al., *Biomed Res Int*, 2014, 727962, 2014. with permission.)

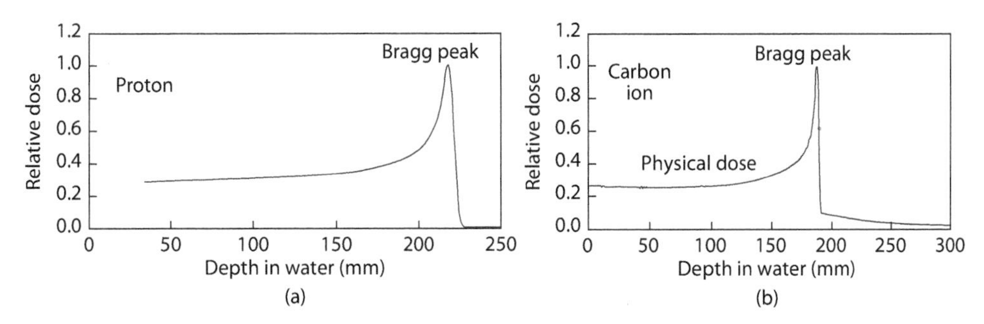

Figure 14.19 Differences in the dose distributions of proton (a) and carbon ion (b) mono energetic beams, shown in calculated and measured depth-dose curves. (Reprinted from Demizu, Y. et al., *Biomed Res Int*, 2014, 727962, 2014. With permission.)

Table 14.1 Comparison of the physical aspects of protons and carbons

	Protons	Carbon ions
Rotating gantry	Available	Not available (fixed portals only)
Penumbra	Inferior	Superior
Range	Longer	Shorter

Source: Demizu, Y. et al., *Biomed Res Int*, 2014, 727962, 2014.
Data with permission from Demizu et al., "Carbon ion therapy for early-stage non-small-cell lung cancer," BioMed research international (2014).

tumors where currently used hypofractionated schedules such as 3 fractions of 18 Gy may lead to severe chronic toxicity such as bleeding, perforation, and stenosis [190,191]. In a prospective phase I/II study in patients with stage IA, IB, and selected stage II (T3N0M0) NSCLC treated with protons to a dose of 87.5 cobalt Gray equivalent (CGE) delivered in 2.5-CGE fractions (biological effective dose (BED) =109.4 Gy, comparable with SABR BED dose using 48–50 Gy in 4 fractions regimen), no patient experienced grade 4 or 5 toxicity [191]. After a median follow-up time of 16 months, local control was achieved in 89% of the patients at 2 years. Chang et al. generated 3D-CRT, IMRT, and passive-scattering proton therapy (PSPT) plans in 25 patients with stage I–III NSCLC. In all cases, the radiation dose to the lungs, the spinal cord, the heart, and the esophagus and the integral dose were the lowest with proton beams [192]. For a mean tumor dose of 63 Gy with photons, the mean V20 (lung) was 34.8%, compared with a mean proton dose of 74 CGE to the tumor and a mean V20 (lung) of 31.6%. A planning study of 25 consecutive NSCLC patients, stage IA–IIIB, performed by the Radiation Oncology Collaborative Comparison consortium demonstrated that PSPT resulted in the lowest dose to the OARs, while keeping the dose to the target at 70 Gy [193]. The mean lung dose was 18.9 Gy for 3D-CRT, 16.4 Gy for IMRT, and 13.5 Gy for PSPT.

A meta-analysis has compared particle beam therapies and SBRT versus conventionally fractionated radiotherapy (CFRT) [194]. The meta-analysis included five studies with proton therapy and three studies with carbon ion therapy. No significant analyses could be made regarding the efficacy of the different types of treatment in locally advanced NSCLC given the lack of patient data. However, the authors could make statistical comparisons for stage I NSCLC. They found that CFRT had worse OS and disease-free survival compared to SBRT and particle beam therapies. There were no significant differences in survival noted between SBRT versus particle beam therapies. Lastly, there was a suggestion that particle therapies could also reduce adverse events.

14.8.2 Challenges in treatment planning of proton beam therapy (PBT) in NSCLC

Still, there are significant technical challenges in adequately delivering protons to a moving target surrounded by tissues with large in homogeneities. Specific challenges include, dose calculation algorithm uncertainties in inhomogeneous tissues, amplification of range uncertainties in low-density lung tissue (in 0.25-density lung tissue, the uncertainties are amplified by 1/0.25 = 4, so a 5-mm range uncertainty in soft tissue becomes a 2-cm uncertainty in lung tissue), range uncertainty [195] and range degradation effects [196]. Areas with a rapid change in tissue density, such as the lung, are more error-prone in terms of dose delivery. Compared with passive-scattering proton therapy, pencil-scanning technologies, such as intensity modulated proton therapy (IMPT), provide more flexibility in dose delivery and thus in principle can achieve higher conformality in dose distributions [197], particularly for tumors in difficult locations or adjacent to critical structures. Recent studies have demonstrated the superiority of IMPT in sparing surrounding critical structures compared to traditional proton therapy or IMRT, allowing for dose escalation for locally advanced NSCLC [198,199]. However, the greater precision achieved with IMPT implies that there is less room for errors, which can be a disadvantage for mobile targets. IMPT is thus recommended to be used for tumors with minimal motion (< 5 mm). It is critical to apply motion management techniques such as 4D-CT-based simulation and treatment planning, respiratory gating, to ensure an accurate dose delivery of PSPT.

PBT has been used in the treatment of stage I NSCLC although no clear clinical benefit over photon therapy has been shown. Data regarding the use of PBT in other clinical scenarios are limited and do not provide sufficient evidence to recommend PBT for lung cancer outside clinical trials. In addition, organ motion in the lung remains a critical issue. There is significant work to be done to improve treatment planning, dose delivery and verification in PBT for lung cancer [180].

14.9 SUMMARY

We have summarized recent works on treatment planning for lung RT. Treatment planning plays a critical role in RT and RT workflow. While the exiting approaches have led to clinical implementation of IMRT and VMAT, the planning process routinely used in the clinics is rather tedious and labor intensive. An underlying issue responsible is the involvement of multiple model parameters in the objective function, which is usually determined through manual trial-and-errors since their influence on the final dose distribution is unknown until an optimization is done. As described above, many researches in auto piloting the process with prior knowledge guidance and/or in using principle component analysis or learning algorithms are being done to facilitate the process. In not so distant future, automated planning should be accessible in clinical practice. For lung RT, because of respiratory motion, motion management and image guidance techniques constitute additional challenge for lung RT and treatment planning. A systematic approach seamlessly integrating all relevant components for optimal lung cancer management represents an area of active research.

ACKNOWLEDGMENTS

We wish to thank the grant supports from NIH (1R01 CA176553 and 1R01 EB016777), Varian Medical Systems and the supports from the Stanford University Asia–Medical Fund (SAMFUND), Ho Tim-Stanley Ho-Li Ka Shing Fellowship Training Fund, and Li Ka Shing Foundation.

REFERENCES

1. Siegel, R.L., K.D. Miller, and A. Jemal, Cancer statistics, 2015. *CA Cancer J Clin*, 2015. **65**(1): 5–29.
2. Howlader, N., A. Noone, and M. Krapcho, *SEER Cancer Statistics Review, 1975–2011, based on November 2013 SEER data submission, posted to the SEER web site.* April 2014, Bethesda, MD: National Cancer Institute.
3. Solda, F. et al., Stereotactic radiotherapy (SABR) for the treatment of primary non-small cell lung cancer; systematic review and comparison with a surgical cohort. *Radiother Oncol*, 2013. **109**(1): 1–7.
4. Chang, J.Y. et al., Stereotactic ablative radiotherapy versus lobectomy for operable stage I non-small-cell lung cancer: A pooled analysis of two randomised trials. *Lancet Oncol*, 2015. **16**(6): 630–7.
5. Timmerman, R.D. et al., Stereotactic body radiation therapy in multiple organ sites. *J Clin Oncol*, 2007. **25**(8): 947–52.

6. Rusch, V.W. et al., Induction chemoradiation and surgical resection for superior sulcus non-small-cell lung carcinomas: Long-term results of Southwest Oncology Group Trial 9416 (Intergroup Trial 0160). *J Clin Oncol*, 2007. **25**(3): 313–8.
7. Lally, B.E. et al., Postoperative radiotherapy for stage II or III non-small-cell lung cancer using the surveillance, epidemiology, and end results database. *J Clin Oncol*, 2006. **24**(19): 2998–3006.
8. Langendijk, J. et al., Quality of life after palliative radiotherapy in non-small cell lung cancer, a prospective study. *Int J Radiat Oncol Biol Phys*, 2000. **1**(47): 149–55.
9. Potters, L. et al., American Society for Therapeutic Radiology and Oncology (ASTRO) and American College of Radiology (ACR) practice guidelines for image-guided radiation therapy (IGRT). *Int J Radiat Oncol Biol Phys*, 2010. **76**(2): 319–25.
10. Chetty, I.J. et al., Report of the AAPM Task Group No. 105: Issues associated with clinical implementation of Monte Carlo-based photon and electron external beam treatment planning. *Med Phys*, 2007. 34(12): 4818–53.
11. Pratx, G. and L. Xing, Monte Carlo simulation of photon migration in a cloud computing environment with MapReduce. *J Biomed Opt*, 2011. **16**(12): 125003.
12. Pratx, G. and L. Xing, GPU computing in medical physics: A review. *Med Phys*, 2011. **38**(5): 2685–97.
13. Wang, H. et al., Toward real-time Monte Carlo simulation using a commercial cloud computing infrastructure. *Phys Med Biol*, 2011. **56**(17): N175–81.
14. Wang, L., E. Yorke, and C.-S. Chui, Monte Carlo evaluation of 6 MV intensity modulated radiotherapy plans for head and neck and lung treatments. *Med Phys*, 2002. **29**(11): 2705.
15. du Plessis, F.C.P. et al., Comparison of the Batho, ETAR and Monte Carlo dose calculation methods in CT based patient models. *Med Phys*, 2001. **28**(4): 582.
16. Knoos, T. et al., Comparison of dose calculation algorithms for treatment planning in external photon beam therapy for clinical situations. *Phys Med Biol*, 2006. **51**(22): 5785–807.
17. Yorke E.D. et al., Evaluation of deep inspiration breath-hold lung treatment plans with Monte Carlo dose calculation. *Int J Radiat Oncol Biol Phys*, 2002. **53**(4): 1058–70.
18. Siebers, J. et al., Trust, but verify: Comparison of MCNP and BEAM Monte Carlo codes for generation of phase space distributions for a Varian 2100C. *Med Phys*, 1998. **25**: A143.
19. Mohan, R. et al., The impact of fluctuations in intensity patterns on the number of monitor units and the quality and accuracy of intensity modulated radiotherapy. *Med Phys*, 2000. **27**(6): 1226.
20. Aaronson, R.F. et al., A Monte Carlo based phase space model for quality assurance of intensity modulated radiotherapy incorporating leaf specific characteristics. *Med Phys*, 2002. **29**(12): 2952.
21. Heath, E. and J. Seuntjens, Development and validation of a BEAMnrc component module for accurate Monte Carlo modelling of the Varian dynamic Millennium multileaf collimator. *Phys Med Biol*, 2003. **48**(24): 4045–63.
22. Kim, J.O. et al., A Monte Carlo study of radiation transport through multileaf collimators. *Med Phys*, 2001. **28**(12): 2497.
23. Liu, H.H., F. Verhaegen, and L. Dong, A method of simulating dynamic multileaf collimators using Monte Carlo techniques for IMRT. *Phys Med Biol*, 2001. **46**(9): 2283–98.
24. Keall, P.J. et al., Monte Carlo dose calculations for dynamic IMRT treatments. *Phys Med Biol*, 2001. **46**(4): 929–41.
25. Siebers, J.V. et al., Incorporating multi-leaf collimator leaf sequencing into iterative IMRT optimization. *Med Phys*, 2002. **29**(6): 952.
26. Kawrakow, I., Accurate condensed history Monte Carlo simulation of electron transport. I. EGSnrc, the new EGS4 version. *Med Phys*, 2000. **27**(3): 485.
27. Kawrakow, I., Accurate condensed history Monte Carlo simulation of electron transport. II. Application to ion chamber response simulations. *Med Phys*, 2000. **27**(3): 499.
28. Ulmer, W., J. Pyyry, and W. Kaissl, A 3D photon superposition/convolution algorithm and its foundation on results of Monte Carlo calculations. *Phys Med Biol*, 2005. **50**(8): 1767–90.
29. Jenkins, T.M. et al., *Monte Carlo Transport of Electrons and Photons, in International school of radiation damage and protection, Erice (Italy)*, 1988. New York, NY: Plenum Press. pp. 249–62.
30. Briesmeister, J.F., *MCNP—A General Monte Carlo N-Particle Transport Code-Version 4c, in LA-13709-M.* 2000, Los Alamos, NM: Los Alamos National Laboratory.

31. Brown, F.B., *MCNP—A general Monte Carlo-Particle Transport Code, Version 5, in Report LA-UR-03 1987.* 2003, Los Alamos, NM: Los Alamos National Laboratory.
32. Tyagi, N., A. Bose, and I.J. Chetty, Implementation of the DPM Monte Carlo code on a parallel architecture for treatment planning applications. *Med Phys*, 2004. **31**(9): 2721.
33. Fernandez-Varea, J.M. et al., On the theory and simulation of multiple elastic-scattering of electrons. *Nucl Instrum Methods Phys Res B*, 1993. **73**(4): 447–73.
34. Schach von Wittenau, A.E. et al., Correlated histogram representation of Monte Carlo derived medical accelerator photon-output phase space. *Med Phys*, 1999. **26**(7): 1196.
35. Schach von Wittenau, A.E., P.M. Bergstrom, and L.J. Cox, Patient-dependent beam-modifier physics in Monte Carlo photon dose calculations. *Med Phys*, 2000. **27**(5): 935.
36. Kawrakow, I., 3D electron dose calculation using a Voxel based Monte Carlo algorithm (VMC). *Med Phys*, 1996. **23**(4): 445.
37. Kawrakow, I. and M. Fippel, Investigation of variance reduction techniques for Monte Carlo photon dose calculation using XVMC. *Phys Med Biol*, 2000. **45**(8): 2163–83.
38. Doucet, R. et al., Comparison of measured and Monte Carlo calculated dose distributions in inhomogeneous. *Phys Med Biol*, 2003. **48**(15): 2339–54.
39. Fippel, M., Efficient particle transport simulation through beam modulating devices for Monte Carlo treatment planning. *Med Phys*, 2004. **31**(5): 1235.
40. Fippel, M., I. Kawrakow, and K. Friedrich, Electron beam dose calculations with the VMC algorithm and the verification data of the NCI working group. *Phys Med Biol*, 1997. **42**(3): 501–20.
41. Neuenschwander, H. and E.J. Born, A macro Monte Carlo method for electron beam dose calculations. *Phys Med Biol*, 1992. **37**(1): 107–25.
42. Neuenschwander, H., T. Mackie, and P.J. Reckwerdt, MMC-a high-performance Monte Carlo code for electron beam treatment planning. *Phys Med Biol*, 1995. **40**(4): 543–74.
43. Cris, C. et al., *A Scaling Method for Multiple Source Models. in 13th ICCR.* 2000, Heidelberg: Springer-Verlag.
44. Pemler, P. et al., Evaluation of a commercial electron treatment planning system based on Monte Carlo techniques (eMC). *Z Med Phys*, 2006. **16**(4): 313–29.
45. Siebers, J.V. et al., *Performance Benchmarks of the MCV Monte Carlo System, in 13th ICCR.* 2000, Heidelberg: Springer-Verlag.
46. Lindsay, P.E. et al., Retrospective Monte Carlo dose calculations with limited beam weight information. *Med Phys*, 2007. **34**(1): 334.
47. Fragoso, M. et al., Dosimetric verification and clinical evaluation of a new commercially available Monte Carlo-based dose algorithm for application in stereotactic body radiation therapy (SBRT) treatment planning. *Phys Med Biol*, 2010. **55**(16): 4445–64.
48. Kong, F.M. et al., High-dose radiation improved local tumor control and overall survival in patients with inoperable/unresectable non-small-cell lung cancer: Long-term results of a radiation dose escalation study. *Int J Radiat Oncol Biol Phys*, 2005. **63**(2): 324–33.
49. Jang, S.Y. et al., Dosimetric verification for intensity-modulated radiotherapy of thoracic cancers using experimental and Monte Carlo approaches. *Int J Radiat Oncol Biol Phys*, 2006. **66**(3): 939–48.
50. Jeraj, R., P. Keall, and J.V. Siebers, The effect of dose calculation accuracy on inverse treatment planning. *Phys Med Biol*, 2002. **47**(3): 391–407.
51. Laub, W. et al., Monte Carlo dose computation for IMRT optimization. *Phys Med Biol*, 2000. 45(7): 1741–54.
52. Siebers, J.V. et al., Reducing dose calculation time for accurate iterative IMRT planning. *Med Phys*, 2002. **29**(2): 231.
53. Wang, X. et al., Development of methods for beam angle optimization for IMRT using an accelerated exhaustive search strategy. *Int J Radiat Oncol Biol Phys*, 2004. **60**(4): 1325–37.
54. Lei, J. and Y. Li, An approaching genetic algorithm for automatic beam angle selection in IMRT planning. *Comput Methods Programs Biomed*, 2009. **93**(3): 257–65.
55. Pugachev, A.B., A.L. Boyer, and L. Xing, Beam orientation optimization in intensity-modulated radiation treatment planning. *Med Phys*, 2000. **27**(6): 1238.

56. Pugachev, A. et al., Role of beam orientation treatment planning. *Int J Radiat Oncol Biol Phys*, 2001. **50**(2): 551–60.
57. Pugachev, A. and L. Xing, Incorporating prior knowledge into beam orientation optimization in IMRT. *Int J Radiat Oncol Biol Phys*, 2002. **54**(5): 1565–74.
58. Pugachev, A. and L. Xing, Computer-assisted selection of coplanar beam orientations in intensity-modulated radiation therapy. *Phys Med Biol*, 2001. **46**(9): 2467–76.
59. Beaulieu, F. et al., Simultaneous optimization of beam orientations, wedge filters and field weights for inverse planning with anatomy-based MLC fields. *Med Phys*, 2004. **31**(6): 1546.
60. Li, Y., J. Yao, and D. Yao, Automatic beam angle selection in IMRT planning using genetic algorithm. *Phys Med Biol*, 2004. **49**(10): 1915–32.
61. Schreibmann, E. et al., Multiobjective evolutionary optimization of the number of beams, their orientations and weights for intensity-modulated radiation therapy. *Phys Med Biol*, 2004. **49**(5): 747–770.
62. Hou, Q. et al., Beam orientation optimization for IMRT by a hybrid method of the genetic algorithm and the simulated dynamics. *Med Phys*, 2003. **30**(9): 2360.
63. Li, Y. et al., A modified genetic algorithm for the beam angle optimization problem in intensity-modulated radiotherapy planning. *Lect Notes Comput Sci*, 2006. **3871**: 97–106.
64. Liu, H.H. et al., Beam angle optimization and reduction for intensity-modulated radiation therapy of non-small-cell lung cancers. *Int J Radiat Oncol Biol Phys*, 2006. **65**(2): 561–72.
65. Zhang, X. et al., A methodology for automatic intensity-modulated radiation treatment planning for lung cancer. *Phys Med Biol*, 2011. **56**(13): 3873–93.
66. Magome, T. et al., Similar-case-based optimization of beam arrangements in stereotactic body radiotherapy for assisting treatment planners. *Biomed Res Int*, 2013. **2013**: 309534.
67. Magome, T. et al., Computer-aided beam arrangement based on similar cases in radiation treatment-planning databases for stereotactic lung radiation therapy. *J Radiat Res*, 2013. **54**(3): 569–77.
68. Burger, W. and M.J. Burge, Digital Image Processing.
69. Wang, H. and L. Xing, Application programming in C# environment with recorded user software interactions and its application in autopilot of VMAT/IMRT treatment planning. *J Appl Clin Med Phys*, 2016. **17**(6): 6425. doi:10.1120/jacmp.v17i6.6425.
70. Wang, H. et al., Development of an autonomous treatment planning strategy for radiation therapy with effective use of population-based prior data. *Med Phys*, 2017. **44**(2): 389–96.
71. Trofimov, A. et al., Temporo-spatial IMRT optimization: Concepts, implementation and initial results. *Phys Med Biol*, 2005. **50**(12): 2779–98.
72. Keall, P.J. et al., The management of respiratory motion in radiation oncology report of AAPM Task Group 76. *Med Phys*, 2006. **33**(10): 3874–900.
73. Ford, E.C. et al., Respiration-correlated spiral CT: A method of measuring respiratory-induced anatomic motion for radiation treatment planning. *Med Phys*, 2003. **30**(1): 88–97.
74. Keall, P.J. et al., Acquiring 4D thoracic CT scans using a multislice helical method. *Phys Med Biol*, 2004. **49**(10): 2053–67.
75. Langner, U.W. and P.J. Keall, Accuracy in the localization of thoracic and abdominal tumors using respiratory displacement, velocity, and phase. *Med Phys*, 2009. **36**(2): 386.
76. Li, T. et al., Model-based image reconstruction for four-dimensional PET. *Med Phys*, 2006. **33**(5): 1288–98.
77. Thorndyke, B. et al., Reducing respiratory motion artifacts in positron emission tomography through retrospective stacking. *Med Phys*, 2006. **33**(7): 2632–41.
78. Thorndyke, B., E. Schreibmann, and L. Xing, Compensation for Respiratory Motion Artefacts in PET/CT Image Registration: A Hybrid Optimization Method. *in Biomedical Computation at Stanford*. 2004. Stanford, CA.
79. Dietrich, L. et al., Linac-integrated 4D cone beam CT: First experimental results. *Phys Med Biol*, 2006. **51**(11): 2939–52.
80. Sonke, J.J. et al., Respiratory correlated cone beam CT. *Med Phys*, 2005. **32**(4): 1176–86.
81. Li, T.F. et al., Four-dimensional cone-beam computed tomography using an on-board imager. *Med Phys*, 2006. **33**(10): 3825–33.

82. Liu, H.H. et al., Evaluation of internal lung motion for respiratory-gated radiotherapy using MRI: Part II-margin reduction of internal target volume. *Int J Radiat Oncol Biol Phys*, 2004. **60**(5): 1473–83.
83. Plathow, C. et al., Therapy monitoring using dynamic MRI: Analysis of lung motion and intrathoracic tumor mobility before and after radiotherapy. *Eur Radiol*, 2006. **16**(9): 1942–50.
84. Cervino, L.I., J. Du, and S.B. Jiang, MRI-guided tumor tracking in lung cancer radiotherapy. *Phys Med Biol*, 2011. **56**(13): 3773–85.
85. Flampouri, S. et al., Estimation of the delivered patient dose in lung IMRT treatment based on deformable registration of 4D-CT data and Monte Carlo simulations. *Phys Med Biol*, 2006. **51**(11): 2763–79.
86. Guckenberger, M. et al., Four-dimensional treatment planning for stereotactic body radiotherapy. *Int J Radiat Oncol Biol Phys*, 2007. **69**(1): 276–85.
87. Hugo, G.D. et al., Cumulative lung dose for several motion management strategies as a function of pre-treatment patient parameters. *Int J Radiat Oncol Biol Phys*, 2009. **74**(2): 593–601.
88. Keall, P.J. et al., Monte Carlo as a four-dimensional radiotherapy treatment-planning tool to account for respiratory motion. *Phys Med Biol*, 2004. **49**(16): 3639–48.
89. Orban de Xivry, J. et al., Tumour delineation and cumulative dose computation in radiotherapy based on deformable registration of respiratory correlated CT images of lung cancer patients. *Radiother Oncol*, 2007. **85**(2): 232–8.
90. Rosu, M. et al., How extensive of a 4D dataset is needed to estimate cumulative dose distribution plan evaluation metrics in conformal lung therapy? *Med Phys*, 2007. **34**(1): 233–45.
91. Glide-Hurst, C.K. et al., A simplified method of four-dimensional dose accumulation using the mean patient density representation. *Med Phys*, 2008. **35**(12): 5269–77.
92. Wolthaus, J.W. et al., Mid-ventilation CT scan construction from four-dimensional respiration-correlated CT scans for radiotherapy planning of lung cancer patients. *Int J Radiat Oncol Biol Phys*, 2006. **65**(5): 1560–71.
93. Li, H.S. et al., Direct dose mapping versus energy/mass transfer mapping for 4D dose accumulation: Fundamental differences and dosimetric consequences. *Phys Med Biol*, 2014. **59**(1): 173–88.
94. Zhong, H. and J.V. Siebers, Monte Carlo dose mapping on deforming anatomy. *Phys Med Biol*, 2009. **54**(19): 5815–30.
95. Zhong, H., E. Weiss, and J.V. Siebers, Assessment of dose reconstruction errors in image-guided radiation therapy. *Phys Med Biol*, 2008. **53**(3): 719–36.
96. Heath, E. and J. Seuntjens, A direct voxel tracking method for four-dimensional Monte Carlo dose calculations in deforming anatomy. *Med Phys*, 2006. **33**(2): 434.
97. Heath, E., F. Tessier, and I. Kawrakow, Investigation of voxel warping and energy mapping approaches for fast 4D Monte Carlo dose calculations in deformed geometries using VMC++. *Phys Med Biol*, 2011. **56**(16): 5187–202.
98. Chin, E. et al., 4D VMAT, gated VMAT, and 3D VMAT for stereotactic body radiation therapy in lung. *Phys Med Biol*, 2013. **58**(4): 749–70.
99. Chin, E. and K. Otto, Investigation of a novel algorithm for true 4D-VMAT planning with comparison to tracked, gated and static delivery. *Med Phys*, 2011. **38**(5): 2698.
100. Bortfeld, T, Optimized planning using physical objectives and constraints. *Semin Radiat Oncol*, 1999. **9**(1): 20–34.
101. Marks, L.B. et al., Use of normal tissue complication probability models in the clinic. *Int J Radiat Oncol Biol Phys*, 2010. **76**(Suppl. 3): S10–9.
102. Jackson, A. et al., The lessons of QUANTEC: Recommendations for reporting and gathering data on dose-volume dependencies of treatment outcome. *Int J Radiat Oncol Biol Phys*, 2010. **76**(Suppl. 3): S155–60.
103. Lyman, J.T., Complication probability as assessed from dose-volume histograms. *Radiat Res Suppl*, 1985. **8**: S13–9.
104. Kallman, P., A. Agren, and A. Brahme, Tumor and normal tissue responses to fractionated non-uniform dose delivery. *Int J Radiat Biol*, 1992. **62**(2): 249–62.
105. Niemierko, A., Reporting and analyzing dose distributions: A concept of equivalent uniform dose. *Med Phys*, 1997. **24**(1): 103.

106. Mohan, R., Clinically relevant optimization of 3-D conformal treatments. *Med Phys*, 1992. **19**(4): 933.
107. Kutcher, G.J. et al., Histogram reduction method for calculating complication probabilities for three-demensional treatment planning evaluations. *Int J Radiat Oncol Biol Phys*, 1991. **21**(1): 137–46.
108. Stavrev, P. et al., Inverse treatment planning by physically constrained minimization of a biological objective function. *Med Phys*, 2003. **30**(11): 2948.
109. Witte, M.G. et al., IMRT optimization including random and systematic geometric errors based on the expectation of TCP and NTCP. *Med Phys*, 2007. **34**(9): 3544.
110. Das, S., A role for biological optimization within the current treatment planning paradigm. *Med Phys*, 2009. **36**(10): 4672.
111. Semenenko, V.A. et al., Evaluation of a commercial biologically based IMRT treatment planning system. *Med Phys*, 2008. **35**(12): 5851.
112. Olafsson, A., R. Jeraj, and S.J. Wright, Optimization of intensity-modulated radiation therapy with biological objectives. *Phys Med Biol*, 2005. **50**(22): 5357–79.
113. Seppenwoolde, Y. and J.V. Lebesque, Partial irradiation of the lung. *Semin Radiat Oncol*, 2001. **11**(3): 247–58.
114. Song, D.Y. et al., Stereotactic body radiation therapy of lung tumors: Preliminary experience using normal tissue complication probability-based dose limits. *Am J Clin Oncol*, 2005. **28**(6): 591–6.
115. Burman, C. et al., Fitting of normal tissue tolerance data to an analytic function. *Int J Radiat Oncol Biol Phys*. **21**(1): 123–35.
116. Zasadny, K.R. et al., FDG-PET determination of metabolically active tumor volume and comparison with CT. *Clin Positron Imaging*, 1998. **1**(2): 123–9.
117. Dehdashti, F. et al., In vivo assessment of tumor hypoxia in lung cancer with 60Cu-ATSM. *Eur J Nucl Med Mol Imaging*, 2003. **30**(6): 844–50.
118. Bollineni, V.R. et al., PET imaging of tumor hypoxia using 18F-fluoroazomycin arabinoside in stage III-IV non-small cell lung cancer patients. *J Nucl Med*, 2013. **54**(8): 1175–80.
119. Koh, W.J. et al., Evaluation of oxygenation status during fractionated radiotherapy in human nonsmall cell lung cancers using [F-18]fluoromisonidazole positron emission tomography. *Int J Radiat Oncol Biol Phys*, 1995. **33**(2): 391–8.
120. Ung, J.C. et al., The lung cancer disease site group, positron emission tomography with 18Fluorodeoxyglucose in radiation treatment planning for non-small cell lung cancer. *J Thorac Oncol*, 2011. **6**: 86–97.
121. De Ruysscher, D. et al., Selective mediastinal node irradiation based on FDG-PET scan data in patients with non-small-cell lung cancer: A prospective clinical study. *Int J Radiat Oncol Biol Phys*, 2005. **62**(4): 988–94.
122. Belderbos, J.S. et al., Final results of a Phase I/II dose escalation trial in non-small-cell lung cancer using three-dimensional conformal radiotherapy. *Int J Radiat Oncol Biol Phys*, 2006. **66**(1): 126–34.
123. Nestle, U. et al., 18F-deoxyglucose positron emission tomography (FDG-PET) for the planning of radiotherapy in lung cancer, high impact in patients with atelectasis. *Int J Radiat Oncol Biol Phys*, 1999. **44**(3): 593–7.
124. van Elmpt, W. et al., The PET-boost randomised phase II dose-escalation trial in non-small cell lung cancer. *Radiother Oncol*, 2012. **104**(1): 67–71.
125. Messa, C. et al., PET/CT and radiotherapy. *Q J Nucl Med Mol Imaging*, 2006. **50**(1): 4–14.
126. Deniaud-Alexandre, E. et al., Impact of computed tomography and 18F-deoxyglucose coincidence detection emission tomography image fusion for optimization of conformal radiotherapy in non-small-cell lung cancer. *Int J Radiat Oncol Biol Phys*, 2005. **63**(5): 1432–41.
127. Konert, T. et al., PET/CT imaging for target volume delineation in curative intent radiotherapy of non-small cell lung cancer: IAEA consensus report 2014. *Radiother Oncol*, 2015. **116**: 27–34.
128. Callahan, J. et al., Validation of a 4D-PET maximum intensity projection for delineation of an internal target volume. *Int J Radiat Oncol Biol Phys*, 2013. **86**(4): 749–54.
129. van Loon, J. et al., Microscopic disease extension in three dimensions for non-small-cell lung cancer: Development of a prediction model using pathology-validated positron emission tomography and computed tomography features. *Int J Radiat Oncol Biol Phys*, 2012. **82**(1): 448–56.

130. Weiss GJ, K.R., Interpretation of PET scans, do not take SUVs at face value. *J Thorac Oncol*, 2012. **7**(12): 1744–6.
131. Wu, K. et al., PET CT thresholds for radiotherapy target definition in non-small-cell lung cancer: How close are we to the pathologic findings? *Int J Radiat Oncol Biol Phys*, 2010. **77**(3): 699–706.
132. Siva, S. et al., High-resolution pulmonary ventilation and perfusion PET/CT allows for functionally adapted intensity modulated radiotherapy in lung cancer. *Radiother Oncol*, 2015. **115**(2): 157–62.
133. Shioyama, Y. et al., Preserving functional lung using perfusion imaging and intensity-modulated radiation therapy for advanced-stage non-small cell lung cancer. *Int J Radiat Oncol Biol Phys*, 2007. **68**(5): 1349–58.
134. Castillo, R. et al., Ventilation from four-dimensional computed tomography: Density versus Jacobian methods. *Phys Med Biol*, 2010. **55**(16): 4661–85.
135. van Beek, E.J. et al., Functional MRI of the lung using hyperpolarized 3-helium gas. *J Magn Reson Imaging*, 2004. **20**(4): 540–54.
136. Fain, S. et al., Imaging of lung function using hyperpolarized helium-3 magnetic resonance imaging: Review of current and emerging translational methods and applications. *J Magn Reson Imaging*, 2010. **32**(6): 1398–408.
137. Gur, D. et al., Regional pulmonary ventilation measurements by xenon enhanced. *J Comput Assist Tomogr*, 1981. **5**(5): 678–83.
138. Tomiyama, N. et al., Mechanism of gravity-dependent atelectasis. Analysis by nonradioactive xenon-enhanced dynamic computed tomography. *Invest Radiol*, 1993. **28**(7): 633–8.
139. Wang, R. et al., Optimal beam arrangement for pulmonary ventilation image-guided intensity-modulated radiotherapy for lung cancer. *Radiat Oncol*, 2014. **9**: 184. doi:10.1186/1748-717X-9-184.
140. Yamamoto, T. et al., Impact of four-dimensional computed tomography pulmonary ventilation imaging-based functional avoidance for lung cancer radiotherapy. *Int J Radiat Oncol Biol Phys*, 2011. **79**(1): 279–88.
141. Yaremko, B.P. et al., Reduction of normal lung irradiation in locally advanced non-small-cell lung cancer patients, using ventilation images for functional avoidance. *Int J Radiat Oncol Biol Phys*, 2007. **68**(2): 562–71.
142. Ireland, R.H. et al., Feasibility of image registration and intensity-modulated radiotherapy planning with hyperpolarized helium-3 magnetic resonance imaging for non-small-cell lung cancer. *Int J Radiat Oncol Biol Phys*, 2007. **68**(1): 273–81.
143. Simon, B.A., Regional ventilation and lung mechanics using X-Ray CT. *Acad Radiol*, 2005. **12**(11): 1414–22.
144. Marks, L.B. et al., The utility of SPECT lung perfusion scans in minimizing and assessing the physiologic consequences of thoracic irradiation. *Int J Radiat Oncol Biol Phys*, 1993. **26**(4): 659–68.
145. Seppenwoolde, Y. et al., Optimizing radiation treatment plans for lung cancer using lung perfusion information. *Radiother Oncol*, 2002. **63**(2): 165–77.
146. Marks, L.B. et al., The role of three dimensional functional lung imaging in radiation treatment planning, the functional dose-volume histogram. *Int J Radiat Oncol Biol Phys*, 1995. **33**(1): 65–75.
147. Murshed, H. et al., Dose and volume reduction for normal lung using intensity-modulated radiotherapy for advanced-stage non-small-cell lung cancer. *Int J Radiat Oncol Biol Phys*, 2004. **58**(4): 1258–67.
148. Liu, H.H. et al., Feasibility of sparing lung and other thoracic structures with intensity-modulated radiotherapy for non-small-cell lung cancer. *Int J Radiat Oncol Biol Phys*, 2004. **58**(4): 1268–79.
149. Das, S.K. et al., Feasibility of optimizing the dose distribution in lung tumors using fluorine-18-fluorodeoxyglucose positron emission tomography and single photon emission computed tomography guided dose prescriptions. *Med Phys*, 2004. **31**(6): 1452.
150. Christian, J.A. et al., The incorporation of SPECT functional lung imaging into inverse radiotherapy planning for non-small cell lung cancer. *Radiother Oncol*, 2005. **77**(3): 271–7.
151. Wild, J.M. et al., Comparison between 2D and 3D gradient-echo sequences for MRI of human lung ventilation with hyperpolarized 3He. *Magn Reson Med*, 2004. **52**(3): 673–8.
152. Moller, H.E. et al., MRI of the lungs using hyperpolarized noble gases. *Magn Reson Med*, 2002. **47**(6): 1029–51.
153. Wild, J.M. et al., 3D volume-localized pO2 measurement in the human lung with 3He MRI. *Magn Reson Med*, 2005. **53**(5): 1055–64.

154. Kabus, S. et al., Lung ventilation estimation based on 4D-CT imaging, in *First International Workshop on Pulmonary Image Analysis*. 2008, New York, NY: MICCAI.
155. Guerrero, T. et al., Dynamic ventilation imaging from four-dimensional computed tomography. *Phys Med Biol*, 2006. **51**(4): 777–91.
156. Guerrero, T. et al., Quantification of regional ventilation from treatment planning CT. *Int J Radiat Oncol Biol Phys*, 2005. **62**(3): 630–4.
157. Christensen, G.E. et al., Tracking lung tissue motion and expansion/compression with inverse consistent image registration and spirometry. *Med Phys*, 2007. **34**(6): 2155.
158. Ding, K. et al., 4DCT-based measurement of changes in pulmonary function following a course of radiation therapy. *Med Phys*, 2010. **37**(3): 1261.
159. Li, R. and L. Xing, Bridging the gap between IMRT and VMAT: Dense angularly sampled and sparse intensity modulated radiation therapy. *Med Phys*, 2011. **38**(9): 4912–9.
160. Wang, L. et al., An end-to-end examination of geometric accuracy of IGRT using a new digital accelerator equipped with onboard imaging system. *Phys Med Biol*, 2012. **57**(3): 757–69.
161. Xing, L., M.H. Phillips, and C.G. Orton, Point/counterpoint. DASSIM-RT is likely to become the method of choice over conventional IMRT and VMAT for delivery of highly conformal radiotherapy. *Med Phys*, 2013. **40**(2): 020601.
162. Cho, W. et al., Development of a fast and feasible spectrum modeling technique for flattening filter free beams. *Med Phys*, 2013. **40**(4): 041721.
163. Cho, W. et al., Multisource modeling of flattening filter free (FFF) beam and the optimization of model parameters. *Med Phys*, 2011. **38**(4): 1931.
164. Kim, H. et al., Beam's-eye-view dosimetrics (BEVD) guided rotational station parameter optimized radiation therapy (SPORT) planning based on reweighted total-variation minimization. *Phys Med Biol*, 2015. **60**(5): N71–82.
165. Chen, X. et al., Independent calculation of monitor units for VMAT and SPORT. *Med Phys*, 2015. **42**(2): 918–24.
166. Zarepisheh, M. et al., Simultaneous beam sampling and aperture shape optimization for SPORT. *Med Phys*, 2015. **42**(2): 1012.
167. Georg, D., T. Knöös, and B. McClean, Current status and future perspective of flattening filter free photon beams. *Med Phys*, 2011. **38**(3): 1280.
168. Yu, C.X., Intensity-modulated arc therapy with dynamic multileaf collimation: An alternative to tomotherapy. *Phys Med Biol*, 1995. **40**(9): 1435–49.
169. Otto, K., Volumetric modulated arc therapy: IMRT in a single gantry arc. *Med Phys*, 2008. **35**(1): 310–7.
170. Crooks, S.M. et al., Aperture modulated arc therapy. *Phys Med Biol*, 2003. **48**(10): 1333–44.
171. Li, R. and L. Xing, An adaptive planning strategy for station parameter optimized radiation therapy (SPORT): Segmentally boosted VMAT. *Med Phys*, 2013. **40**(5): 050701, 4912–9.
172. Zhang, P. et al., Optimization of collimator trajectory in volumetric modulated arc therapy: Development and evaluation for paraspinal SBRT. *Int J Radiat Oncol Biol Phys*, 2010. **77**(2): 591–9.
173. Zhu, L. et al., Using total-variation regularization for intensity modulated radiation therapy inverse planning with field-specific numbers of segments. *Phys Med Biol*, 2008. **53**(23): 6653–72.
174. Zhu, L. and L. Xing, Search for IMRT inverse plans with piecewise constant fluence maps using compressed sensing techniques. *Med Phys*, 2009. **36**(5): 1895.
175. Aupérin, A. et al., Meta-analysis of concomitant versus sequential radiochemotherapy in locally advanced nonsmall-cell lung cancer. *J Clin Oncol*, 2010. **28**(13): 2181–90.
176. Machtay, M. et al., Higher biologically effective dose of radiotherapy is associated with improved outcomes for locally advanced non-small cell lung carcinoma treated with chemoradiation: An analysis of the Radiation Therapy Oncology Group. *Int J Radiat Oncol Biol Phys*, 2012. **82**(1): 425–34.
177. Williams, T.M. and A. Maier, Role of stereotactic body radiation therapy and proton/carbon nuclei therapies. *Cancer J*, 2013. **19**(3): 272–81.
178. Kanai, T. et al., Irradiation of mixed beam and design of spread-out Bragg peak for heavy—ion radiotherapy. *Radiat Res*, 1997. **147**(1): 78–85.

179. Demizu, Y. et al., Carbon ion therapy for early-stage non-small-cell lung cancer. *Biomed Res Int*, 2014. 2014: 727962.
180. Allen, A.M. et al., An evidence based review of proton beam therapy: The report of ASTRO's emerging technology committee. *Radiother Oncol*, 2012. **103**(1): 8–11.
181. Bush, D.A. et al., Hypofractionated proton beam radiotherapy for stage I lung cancer. *Chest*, 2004. 126: 1198–203.
182. Westover, K.D. et al., Proton SBRT for medically inoperable stage I NSCLC. *J Thorac Oncol*, 2012. **7**(6): 1021–5.
183. Chang, J.Y. et al., Toxicity and patterns of failure of adaptive/ablative proton therapy for early-stage, medically inoperable non-small cell lung cancer. *Int J Radiat Oncol Biol Phys*, 2011. **80**(5): 1350–7.
184. Chang, J.Y. et al., Phase 2 study of high-dose proton therapy with concurrent chemotherapy for unresectable stage III nonsmall cell lung cancer. *Cancer*, 2011. **117**(20): 4707–13.
185. Iwata, H. et al., Long-term outcome of proton therapy and carbon-ion therapy for large (T2a-T2bN0M0) non-small-cell lung cancer. *J Thorac Oncol*, 2013. **8**(6): 726–35.
186. Register, S.P. et al., Proton stereotactic body radiation therapy for clinically challenging cases of centrally and superiorly located stage I non-small-cell lung cancer. *Int J Radiat Oncol Biol Phys*, 2011. **80**(4): 1015–22.
187. Hoppe, B.S. et al., Double-scattered proton-based stereotactic body radiotherapy for stage I lung cancer: A dosimetric comparison with photon-based stereotactic body radiotherapy. *Radiother Oncol*, 2010. **97**(3): 425–30.
188. Macdonald, O.K. et al., Proton beam radiotherapy versus three-dimensional conformal stereotactic body radiotherapy in primary peripheral, early-stage non-small-cell lung carcinoma: A comparative dosimetric analysis. *Int J Radiat Oncol Biol Phys*, 2009. **75**(3): 950–8.
189. Welsh, J. et al., Evaluating proton stereotactic body radiotherapy to reduce chest wall dose in the treatment of lung cancer. *Med Dosim*, 2013. **38**(4): 442–7.
190. Timmerman, R. et al., Excessive toxicity when treating central tumors in a phase II study of stereotactic body radiation therapy for medically inoperable early-stage lung cancer. *J Clin Oncol*, 2006. **24**(30): 4833–9.
191. Chang, J.Y. et al., Stereotactic body radiation therapy in centrally and superiorly located stage I or isolated recurrent non-small-cell lung cancer. *Int J Radiat Oncol Biol Phys*, 2008. **72**(4): 967–71.
192. Chang, J.Y. et al., Significant reduction of normal tissue dose by proton radiotherapy compared with three-dimensional conformal or intensity-modulated radiation therapy in Stage I or Stage III non-small-cell lung cancer. *Int J Radiat Oncol Biol Phys*, 2006. **65**(4): 1087–96.
193. Roelofs, E. et al., Results of a multicentric in silico clinical trial (ROCOCO): Comparing radiotherapy with photons and protons for non-small cell lung cancer. *J Thorac Oncol*, 2012. **7**(1): 165–76.
194. Grutters, J.P. et al., Comparison of the effectiveness of radiotherapy with photons, protons and carbon-ions for non-small cell lung cancer: A meta-analysis. *Radiother Oncol*, 2010. **95**(1): 32–40.
195. Ahmad, M. et al., Theoretical detection threshold of the proton-acoustic range verification technique. *Med Phys*, 2015. **42**(10): 5735.
196. De Ruysscher, D. and J.Y. Chang, Clinical controversies: Proton therapy for thoracic tumors. *Semin Radiat Oncol*, 2013. **23**(2): 115–9.
197. Kase, Y. et al., A treatment planning comparison of passive-scattering and intensity-modulated proton therapy for typical tumor sites. *J Radiat Res*, 2012. **53**(2): 272–80.
198. Zhang, X. et al., Intensity-modulated proton therapy reduces the dose to normal tissue compared with intensity-modulated radiation therapy or passive scattering proton therapy and enables individualized radical radiotherapy for extensive stage IIIB non-small-cell lung cancer: A virtual clinical study. *Int J Radiat Oncol Biol Phys*, 2010. **77**: 357–66.
199. Chang, J.Y. and J.D. Cox, Improving radiation conformality in the treatment of non-small cell lung cancer. *Semin Radiat Oncol*, 2010. **20**(3): 171–7.

15

Advances in verification and delivery techniques

LEI REN, MARTINA DESCOVICH, AND JING WANG

15.1 INTRODUCTION

Target control and normal tissue complication probabilities are highly correlated to the target localization and treatment delivery accuracy in radiation therapy [1,2]. The goal of radiation therapy is to deliver the radiation dose to the target precisely with minimal radiation dose to the surrounding healthy tissues. The success of this goal heavily depends on the precision of the target verification techniques before and during the treatment, and the treatment delivery techniques to delivery radiation precisely based on the information obtained from verification. Several breakthroughs have been made in both areas in recent years to develop efficient, low-dose, high-quality imaging verification techniques and advanced delivery techniques to account for the respiratory motion of the lung tumor to minimize the target volume treated. In this chapter, recent advances in treatment verification and delivery techniques in radiation therapy of lung cancer are discussed.

15.2 ADVANCES IN IMAGING VERIFICATION TECHNIQUES

15.2.1 FAST LOW-DOSE LIMITED-ANGLE IMAGING

One major limitation of CBCT is its high-imaging dose and long scanning time due to the large scanning angle and number of projections acquired in a CBCT scan. Different x-ray-based imaging techniques are being developed to reconstruct images using only a limited angle scan, which can substantially reduce the imaging dose and scanning time.

15.2.1.1 DIGITAL TOMOSYNTHESIS (DTS)

DTS is a technique to reconstruct quasi-3D images using 2D cone beam x-ray projections acquired only within a limited scan angle [3]. By resolving overlying anatomy into slices, DTS greatly improves the visibility of both soft tissue and bone compared with kV or MV radiographic imaging. Furthermore, DTS requires less radiation exposure and unobstructed gantry rotation clearance, and can be acquired with a much shorter scan time than CBCT [4].

The DTS localization process includes the creation of reference DTS (RDTS) images from the digitally reconstructed radiograph (DRR) of the planning CT data, as well as the acquisition of on-board verification DTS images, acquired in the treatment room. Comparison of the two DTS image sets (reference and verification) allows for the determination of patient set-up error [5]. RDTS images are reconstructed from simulated limited angle cone beam projections through a planning CT image volume. On-board DTS (OBDTS) slices are acquired in the same fashion as full CBCT, but with limited gantry rotation. The *Feldkamp-Davis-Kress* (FDK) [6] back-projection algorithm is typically used to reconstruct reference and OBDTS images. Constraining the scan to 40° generally yields high-quality DTS slices with good soft-tissue visibility, while enabling the scan to be completed in less than 10 seconds with around one-ninth of the full-rotation CBCT imaging dose. Individual DTS slices exhibit high resolution in the viewing plane, but the resolution in the third (plane-to-plane) dimension is limited by the narrow scan angle. Thus, CT Hounsfield Unit (HU) values are not correctly reconstructed in DTS, and image contrast in DTS slices is inferior to that in full CBCT images. Although the effective slice profile of the DTS images is thicker than that of full CT/CBCT, soft-tissue visibility is reasonably good in the limited-angle DTS data and is markedly better than that provided by the traditional 2D radiographic fields with better localization accuracy for lung cancer treatments.

Phase-matched DTS has been developed recently to address the effect of respiratory motion on lung tumor localization using DTS [7]. Phase-matched DTS matches the motion-blurring pattern in reference and on-board DTS images by matching the phases of the DRRs used for RDTS reconstruction with those of the on-board projections used for OBDTS reconstruction.

Figure 15.1 shows the reconstructed DTS images using single-view 30° projections. In the left column are the mixed-phase OBDTS sets, which contained five consecutive respiratory phases. In the middle column are the conventional RDTS sets without phase matching. In the right column are the phase-matched RDTS sets with respiratory phase information matched to OBDTS sets. The tumor area on each DTS is pointed out

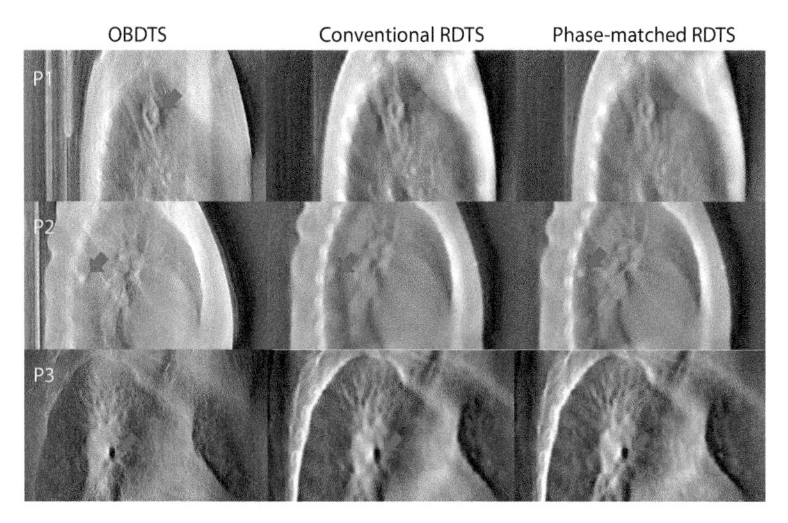

Figure 15.1 Comparison between the OBDTS, conventional RDTS, and phase-matched RDTS sets. All three DTS sets were reconstructed from single-view 30° projections. The OBDTS contained five consecutive respiratory phases. The arrows point to the tumor area. P1, P2 and P3 indicate patient 1, patient 2, and patient 3.

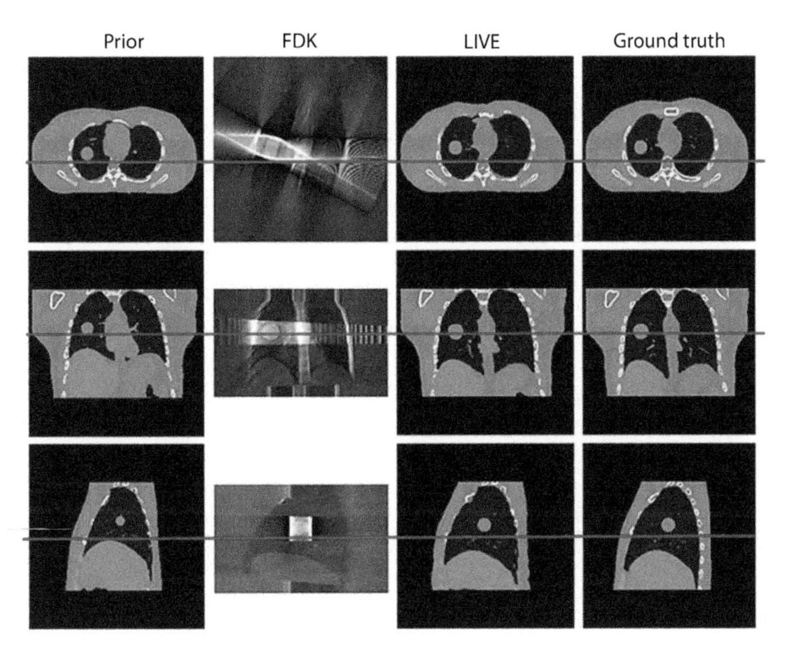

Figure 15.2 Comparison between images reconstructed by different methods using orthogonal 30° kV and BEV MV projections simulated from the XCAT phantom.

with an arrow. It is evident that the shape of the tumors in OBDTS sets matched better with those in phase-matched RDTS sets than conventional RDTS sets, especially for patient 2 and patient 3. Consequently, the registration between OBDTS and phase-matched RDTS will be more accurate than the registration between OBDTS and conventional RDTS. Preliminary studies showed that phase-matched DTS could localize the lung tumor with 1–2 mm accuracy, compared to 3–7 mm accuracy using 3D DTS [7].

15.2.1.2 LIMITED-ANGLE INTRAFRACTION VERIFICATION (LIVE) SYSTEM

Although DTS imaging improved anatomical visibility compared to 2D x-ray imaging, it doesn't provide full volumetric information of the patient due to the limited scan angle used in the acquisition. The lack of full 3D information may impair the localization accuracy of DTS when there is soft-tissue deformation of the patient. Novel image reconstruction techniques have been developed in recent years to reconstruct full volumetric images using limited number of projections acquired within a limited scan angle [8–13]. This method considers the on-board patient images as a deformation of prior images. So instead of solving the pixel values directly in reconstruction, it solves the deformation field that deforms the prior images to obtain the on-board images. The deformation field is usually solved iteratively using data fidelity constraint and motion modeling. Based on this method, a limited-angle intrafraction verification (LIVE) system was recently proposed to reconstruct patient intra fractional volumetric images based on limited-angle kV and MV projections acquired during the treatment [14]. Figure 15.2 shows the images reconstructed by the FDK back-projection method and the LIVE system using data from the 4D Digital Extended-cardiac-torso (XCAT) phantom. The LIVE system could reconstruct high-quality volumetric images using only orthogonal 30° scan angles.

15.2.2 Advances in 4D-CBCT

Limited by International Electrotechnical Commission (IEC) standards, the gantry rotation speed of on-board CBCT systems is slower than 60 seconds per rotation. Respiratory correlated CBCT, or four-dimensional (4D) CBCT [15–24], has been proposed to reduce motion artifacts in 3D-CBCT and to generate 4D patient motion model just prior to treatment. In 4D-CBCT, projection images are typically grouped into 8–10 phases per respiration signals. When an analytical image reconstruction algorithm, such as FDK, is used to reconstruct individual phase 4D-CBCT, strong streaking artifacts are presented due to the limited number of projections at each phase.

These artifacts make it difficult to identify the tumor boundary accurately for online guidance and decrease the subsequent registration accuracy. For example, from 4D-CBCT reconstructed by the standard FDK algorithm, the error of tumor motion trajectories extracted by deformation registration can be more than 7 mm [25,26].

Various strategies have been proposed to enhance the image quality of 4D-CBCT [27–38]. One strategy is based on the McKinnon-Bates (MKB) algorithm [30]. In MKB, an initial image is reconstructed from all projections. A correction image reconstructed from the difference between the measured data and forward projection of the initial image is then added to the initial image. The MKB algorithm can reduce the streaking artifacts to a certain extent. However, the motion artifacts in the initial image can still present in the final image. Another type of approach is through using iterative image reconstruction algorithms and a typical example is based on total variation (TV) minimization [27,28]. TV minimization only utilizes the projections from a phase, and independently reconstructs the individual phase image by assuming its inherent piecewise constancy. Such a solution often leads to over smoothness when the number of measurements is not sufficient, especially for small size or low-contrast objects [27]. Another type of algorithm [29] is called prior image constraint compressive sensing (PICCS) [29], which attempts to enhance 4D-CBCT by exploring the sparsity of the difference image between the target image and a prior image. In the application of PICCS for 4D-CBCT reconstruction, a motion-blurred 3D-CBCT is first reconstructed by using FDK from all projections and serves as the prior image. PICCS does not account for the deformation between different phases, where residue motion is still observed in the reconstructed 4D-CBCT [21].

Four-dimensional reconstruction strategies by utilizing all phase projections through a respiratory-motion model have also been explored [31–34]. When motion models between different phases are known, then projections from all respiration phases can be used to reconstruct a reference-phase 4D-CBCT through motion-compensated image reconstruction strategies. Image quality of 4D-CBCT can be greatly improved as the number of projection measurements available for any phase is substantially increased by effectively utilizing projections of other phases. These strategies [31–34] typically rely on the motion model built either from the planning 4D-CT [31,32] or reconstructed 4D-CBCT [33,34]. However, the assumption that the motion during 4D-CBCT data acquisition is identical to the prior motion could be violated [35,36] and the accuracy of motion model built from reconstructed 4D-CBCT is limited by the image quality. Strategies [37–39] to obtain 4D-CBCT by deforming planning CT with the update motion model have also been proposed. These strategies generate a synthetic 4D-CBCT (deformed planning CT) and it can be challenging for the algorithm when the image content changes between planning CT and CBCT.

Recently, a simultaneous motion estimation and image reconstruction (SMEIR) algorithm [26] has been developed for 4D-CBCT. The workflow of the SMEIR algorithm is illustrated in Figure 15.3. The SMEIR algorithm utilizes projections from all phases to simultaneously update both the inverse consistent motion model and the motion-compensated 4D-CBCT at any phase. Without using any prior image or prior motion model, the SMEIR algorithm relies only on the on-treatment CBCT data to improve the quality of image reconstruction and accuracy of motion estimation.

The SMEIR algorithm contains two alternating steps: 1) motion-compensated CBCT (mCBCT) reconstruction; and 2) motion modeling from the projections directly. In motion-compensated image reconstruction, projections from all phases are used to reconstruct a reference-phase 4D-CBCT (e.g., phase 0%) by explicitly considering the motion models between different phases. A modified simultaneous algebraic reconstruction technique (SART) is used to iteratively reconstruct the mCBCT at the reference phase. Mathematically, letting $\boldsymbol{p}^t = (p_1^t, p_2^t, \ldots, p_I^t)$ denote the log-transformed measured 4D-CBCT projections at phase t and $\boldsymbol{\mu}^t = (\mu_1^t, \mu_2^t, \ldots, \mu_J^t)$ denote the attenuation coefficients of the phase t image, the modified SART is given by the following formula:

$$\boldsymbol{\mu}_j^{0,(k+1)} = \boldsymbol{\mu}_j^{0,(k)} + \frac{\sum_{t,n} d_{jn}^{t\to 0} \sum_i \left[a_{in} \frac{p_i^t - \sum_n a_{in} \mu_n^{t,(k)}}{\sum_{n=1}^{J} a_{in}} \right]}{\sum_i a_{in}} \tag{15.1}$$

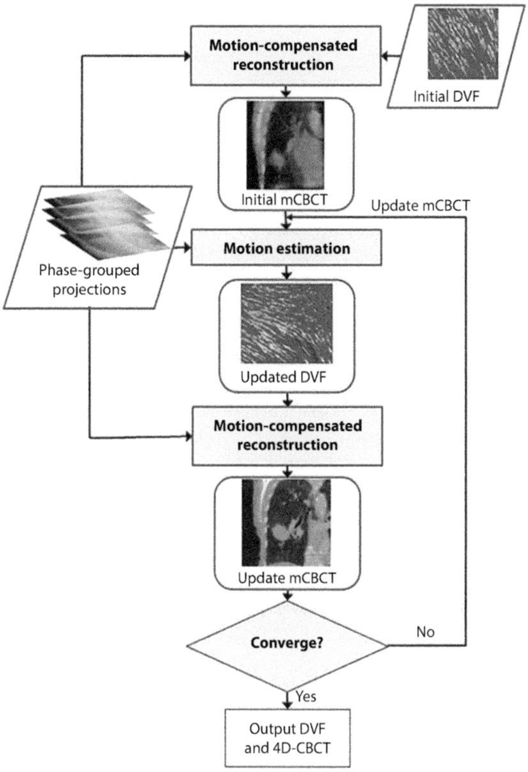

Figure 15.3 Flowchart of SMEIR for 4D-CBCT reconstruction: Image reconstruction and motion estimation are performed as two alternating steps until both accurate image and motion model are obtained.

$$\mu_n^{t,(k)} = \sum_j d_{jn}^{0\to t} \mu_j^{0,(k)} \tag{15.2}$$

Where k is the iteration step, and a_{in} is the intersection length of projection ray i with voxel n. $d_{jn}^{t\to 0}$ denotes the element of the inverse deformation vector fields (DVFs) that deform phase t to phase 0. j is the voxel index of phase 0 while n is the voxel index of phase t. The second term in Equation 15.1 describes the inverse deformation process that deforms the error image determined by projections at phase t to update the 4D-CBCT at phase 0. Equation 15.2 describes the forward deformation that deforms phase 0 4D-CBCT to phase t. $d_{jn}^{0\to t}$ denotes the element of the forward DVF map. To start the mCBCT reconstruction, the DVF initials are first obtained from registration between the total variation (TV) minimization reconstructed 4D-CBCT at other phases and phase 0. After SART reconstruction, the TV of the reconstructed mCBCT is minimized by the standard steepest descent method to suppress image noise.

Since Equations 15.1 and 15.2 are involved with both the forward and inverse DVF in updating μ^0, the DVF should be inversely consistent. In the motion model estimation step, the updated inverse consistent DVF between the reference phase 0 and other phases are obtained directly from the projections by matching the measured projections to the forward projection of the deformed mCBCT. To enforce the inverse consistency of the DVF, an interleaved optimization scheme is used to optimize a symmetric energy function under an inverse consistent constraint. The symmetric energy function is formulated as follows:

$$\begin{aligned} f_1\left(v^{0\to t}\right) &= \|\boldsymbol{p}^t - A\mu^0(x+\boldsymbol{v}^{0\to t})\|_{l_2}^2 + \beta\varphi(\boldsymbol{v}^{0\to t}) \\ f_2\left(v^{t\to 0}\right) &= \|\boldsymbol{p}^0 - A\mu^t(x+\boldsymbol{v}^{t\to 0})\|_{l_2}^2 + \beta\varphi(\boldsymbol{v}^{t\to 0}) \\ s.t.\ \ \boldsymbol{v}^{0\to t}\left(\boldsymbol{x}+\boldsymbol{v}^{t\to 0}\right)+\boldsymbol{v}^{t\to 0} &= \boldsymbol{v}^{t\to 0}\left(\boldsymbol{x}+\boldsymbol{v}^{0\to t}\right)+\boldsymbol{v}^{0\to t} = 0, \end{aligned} \tag{15.3}$$

where f_1 and f_2 denote the symmetric energy function. A is the projection matrix, with coefficients of a_{in}. $v^{0\to t}$ denotes the forward DVF and $v^{t\to 0}$ denotes the inverse DVF. The inverse consistent constraint is shown in the last line of Equation 15.3. The energy function contains a data fidelity term and a smoothness constraint term. β is a parameter that controls the tradeoff between the two terms. $\varphi(v)$ is a free-form energy of the deformation fields [40,41].

Both digital phantom and patient studies have demonstrated an excellent performance of the SMEIR algorithm. Figure 15.4 shows images of the 4D-NCAT phantom at the end-expiration phase, where left and right columns show trans-axial and coronal view images, respectively. Row (a) in Figure 15.4 shows the digital phantom images. Row (b) shows the 3D-CBCT reconstructed by FDK from all projections, where motion-blurring artifacts are presented. Row (c) in Figure 15.4 shows 4D-CBCT reconstructed by FDK, where severe view-aliasing images are presented. Row (d) shows 4D-CBCT reconstructed by TV. Bony structures and fine structures inside of the lung are severely blurred although view aliasing artifacts are suppressed. Row (e) shows images reconstructed by the SMEIR algorithm. Not only are view-aliasing artifacts suppressed, but the edges are also well preserved for both bone structures and inside of the lung. Evaluation studies were also performed on a limited number of lung cancer patients. To get a reference 4D-CBCT at each phase, patients underwent 4–6 minutes of scanning. With this large number of projections at each phase, high-quality 4D-CBCTs were obtained and used as references for the evaluation study. To investigate the dependence of the SMEIR algorithms on the number of projection views, fully sampled projections were down-sampled with different factors. These down-sampled projections were subsequently used for SMEIR, TV and FDK reconstructions. Figure 15.5 shows reconstructed images of one patient at phase 0 with an average projection number of 33. Results show that the SMEIR algorithm produces 4D-CBCT images that are closest to the reference image among the three investigated reconstruction methods. Moreover, SMEIR reconstruction

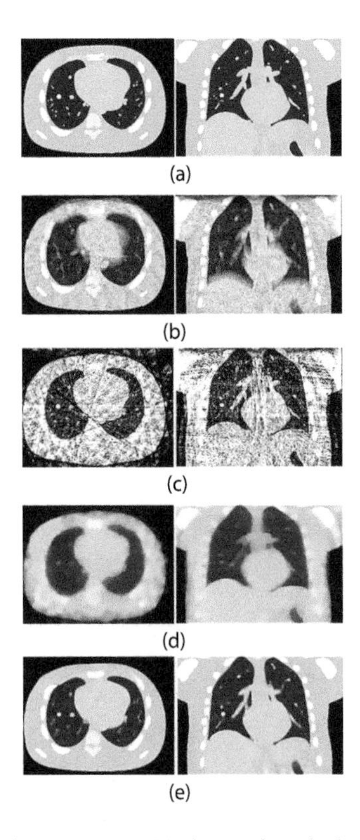

Figure 15.4 Results of 4D-NCAT phantom. Row (a) shows digital phantom at end-expiration phase; row (b) shows 3D-CBCT reconstructed from all projections by FDK; rows (c) through (e) show 4D-CBCT at end-expiration phase reconstructed by FDK, TV minimization and SMEIR algorithm, respectively. The left and the right column show the trans-axial and coronal views, respectively.

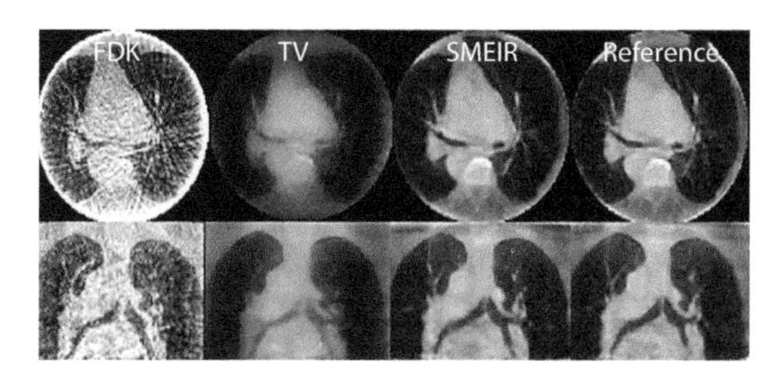

Figure 15.5 Reconstructed phase 0% images of a lung cancer patient using different algorithms (including FDK, TV, and SMEIR) with average projection number per phase of 33. (Top): transverse; (Bottom): coronal.

effectively preserves fine structures. Tumor tracking analysis showed that the maximum error in tumor position detection was less than 2-mm in SMEIR for all four patients when an average of 20–30 projections per phase was used for reconstruction.

15.2.3 Real-time imaging based on electromagnetic transponders

The Calypso® System (Varian Medical Systems, Inc., Palo Alto, CA) is a commercial device which has been developed and used for target localization or tracking for prostate and lung cancer treatments [42,43]. Electromagnetic transponders are implanted inside the tumor before CT simulation. The locations of the transponders are identified in the planning CT images, and imported into the Calypso 4D tracking station together with the treatment isocenter location. For on-board imaging, the Calypso detector antenna array contains source coils and receiver coils. The source coils generate an oscillating radio-frequency (RF) field, inducing resonances in the transponders. When the field is switched off, the transponder emits signals during relaxation, which is detected by the receiver coils to establish the location of these transponders. The centroid of the transponder locations is calculated and used to represent the location of the tumor.

Calypso can provide real-time monitoring of the tumor location before or during the radiotherapy treatment with no ionizing radiation dose to the patient. The signal from Calypso can be used for gated treatment or dynamic target tracking of the target. However, implanting the electromagnetic transponder in a stable location in the lung tumor proved to be challenging for some patients [43].

15.2.4 On-board MRI

Magnetic resonance imaging (MRI) integrated with a radiotherapy unit has been introduced in recent years for target localization [44–45]. Compared to x-ray imaging techniques, MRI has much better soft-tissue contrast and no ionizing radiation dose to patients, which makes it an attractive modality for daily imaging for both inter and intra-fraction verification. The on-board MRI systems have been developed by integrating the MRI scanner with a linear accelerator or a ^{60}Co treatment machine [44–47]. Most of current commercially available MRI-radiotherapy machines use low-field MRI to reduce interference with radiation therapy delivery and decrease geometric distortion.

Currently, 2D MR cine has been used as the primary technique for real-time target verification during the treatment. However, it doesn't provide volumetric information of the patient, and therefore cannot verify target motion along the direction perpendicular to the cine plane. New approaches have been proposed to accelerate the 2D cine acquisition using under sampling, so that multiple 2D cine images can be acquired rapidly with minimal latency in between to provide volumetric verification of the target location [48]. 4D-MRI is also being developed through either prospective or retrospective approach for 4D verification of the target. Due to limitations of hardware and software, prospective 4D-MRI suffers from poor temporal resolution (~1 s) and poor spatial resolution (4–5 mm) [49,50]. Retrospective 4D-MRI has better temporal and in-plane resolution, but suffers from long acquisition time (5–30 min), and poor plane-to-plane resolution

(3–5 mm slice thickness) [51,52]. To address the limitations of 2D cine MRI and 4D-MRI, a volumetric cine MRI (VC-MRI) technique has been developed recently to generate real-time 3D-MRI images based on patient prior knowledge and motion modeling for real-time target localization or tracking in lung and liver treatments [53].

15.3 ADVANCEMENTS IN TREATMENT DELIVERY TECHNIQUES

The clinical practice of IGRT for lung cancer with an L-shaped Linac, an O-shaped Linac and a robotic arm linac is discussed in Chapters 7, 8 and 9, respectively. The topic of MRI-based IGRT for lung cancer is discussed in Chapter 18. In this section, we will focus on the technical details of real-time tracking.

15.3.1 TRACKING BASED ON L-SHAPED LINAC

Real-time tracking on L-shaped linac can be accomplished by dynamically adjusting the position of the multi-leaf collimator (MLC) to control the radiation field. The idea to synchronize MLC position to target motion was introduced more than 15 years ago. In 2001, Keall et al. [54] demonstrated the feasibility of performing 1D motion compensation with manual synchronization. In 2006, a dynamic MLC tracking system with real-time feedback from an external position monitoring system (RPM, Varian) was integrated on a Varian linac [55] and in 2008 the feasibility of performing 3D motion compensation was demonstrated [56]. MLC tracking was implemented in a research environment on a Siemens linac in 2010 [57] and on a Elekta Linac in 2012 [58]. Dynamic MLC tracking has been guided by kV [59] and MV imaging systems [60,61], as well as wired and wireless electromagnetic transponders [62,63]. The first clinical implementation of electromagnetic transponder-guided MLC tracking was reported in 2013 for a prostate cancer patient treated with dual-arc VMAT [64]. In this study, only rigid tumor translations (not rotations) were corrected for. A noncommercial research code was used to drive the MLC and to control the beam-on status. The algorithm extracts the target location from the electromagnetic transponder signal and dynamically calculates optimal motion-compensated leaf aperture [65]. To minimize radiation leakage through the tips of closed MLC, leaf pairs that are not participating in the tracking process are moved under the nearest jaw. In anomalous situations (such as a large shift in patient position, sudden change in respiratory pattern, bowel movement, swallowing or coughing), a beam-hold status is triggered. Initial studies conducted in phantoms concluded that submillimeter geometric accuracy and very high dosimetric conformity could be achieved using this methodology [56,63,66]. Results on the first clinical trial on 15 prostate cancer patients demonstrated that MLC tracking improves the fidelity between the planned and the delivered dose [67].

15.3.2 TRACKING BASED ON O-SHAPED LINAC

VERO is novel platform for image-guided SBRT developed by BrainLAB (BrainLAB AG, Feldkirchen, Germany) and MHI (Mitsubishi Heavy Industries, Tokyo, Japan) [68]. The system consists of a compact 6 MV C-band linac mounted on an O-ring gantry. The radiation beam is collimated by a fast MLC providing a maximum aperture of 15×15 cm^2 and a maximum leaf speed of 5 cm/second [69]. The linac-MLC assembly is mounted on two orthogonal gimbals that allow panning and tilting the beam up to ± 2.5 degrees with a maximum speed of 9 cm/second and 0.1 mm iso centric accuracy. The beam can be steered quickly (up to ± 4.4 cm) to follow the target, independently from the MLC motion. In this way, target tracking is decoupled by the intensity modulation of the dose. The imaging system consists of a MV electronic portal imaging device and two diagnostic x-ray sources with corresponding flat panel detectors mounted at 45 degree angles relative to the MV beam axis. The stereo kV system can operate in single image or fluoroscopic mode with simultaneous or interlaced acquisition and allow the acquisition of cone beam CT. Real-time tumor motion tracking is achieved by combining the information from the kV imaging system operating in fluoroscopic mode with the signal from infrared markers (ExacTrac®, BrainLAB AG, Feldkirchen, Germany) [70,71]. A patient-specific correlation model is created between the breathing signal (position of IR marker acquired at 50 Hz) and the tumor position. The tumor position is automatically extracted from the kV imaging system using a fiducial detection algorithm. Fiducial-less tracking based on tumor density alone is also possible. The polynomial forward prediction model predicts the target position ahead of time, so the beam can be steered to the anticipated target position within the system latency (~40 ms). The geometric accuracy of tumor motion tracking measured in phantom experiments was <1 mm (tracking error 90th percentile E90% <0.82 mm up to frequencies of 30 breaths per minute) [72]. Similar performances were observed in the pan and tilt directions. Depuydt et al. described the first clinical application of real-time tumor tracking using VERO on a group of 10 patients with lesions in the lung or liver. The authors estimated CTV-PTV margins needed to account for residual uncertainties in treatments with real-time tracking, and quantified the PTV volume reduction compared to the ITV-based approach. Tracking resulted in a 35% PTV volume reduction corresponding to a <1% reduction of lung and liver NTCP [73].

15.3.3 Tracking based on robotic arm linac

The CyberKnife® system (Accuray Inc., Sunnyvale CA) was the first medical device capable of dynamic target tracking, with the clinical implementation of the Synchrony® Respiratory Motion tracking system in 2004 [74,75]. The system consists of a compact X-band linac attached to a robotic arm that enables positioning the radiation source anywhere around the anterior and lateral aspect of the patient positioning system. Synchrony is based on a correlation model between the position of the target (extracted from two orthogonal x-ray camera images acquired at 45 degree angles), and the position of three external markers (LED), placed on the patient chest or abdomen prior to each treatment session. The LED positions are read continuously (~30 Hz) by an optical camera and provide a surrogate representation of the patient breathing pattern. At the beginning of each treatment session, the user builds the synchrony correlation model by acquiring a set of 8–15 x-ray images. In the correlation model, 2 second-order polynomial functions are combined to include hysteresis in the tumor trajectories between inhale and exhale motion [76]. An optimal correlation model is achieved when the model points are evenly distributed, cover >85% of the breathing cycle, include the four main respiratory phases (maximum inhale, maximum exhale, inhale center and exhale center) and have a low correlation error. During treatment, the tumor position is calculated from the position of the external surrogates ~115 ms ahead of time, and the robot is retargeted to the anticipated target location. Radiation delivery is fully synchronized with target motion. X-ray images are acquired periodically and the actual target position is used to update the correlation model to reflect changes in the respiratory pattern. Figure 15.6 shows an example of patient breathing model. A new imaging modality called "image

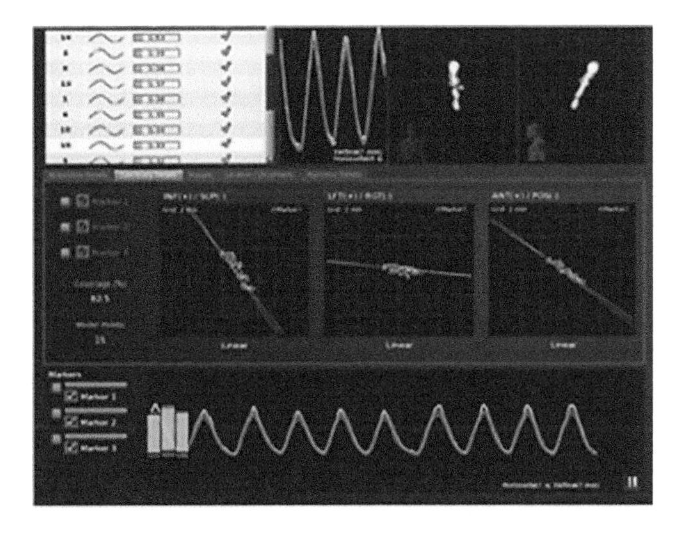

Figure 15.6 Example of patient breathing model showing a graphical representation of the correlation model and breathing pattern.

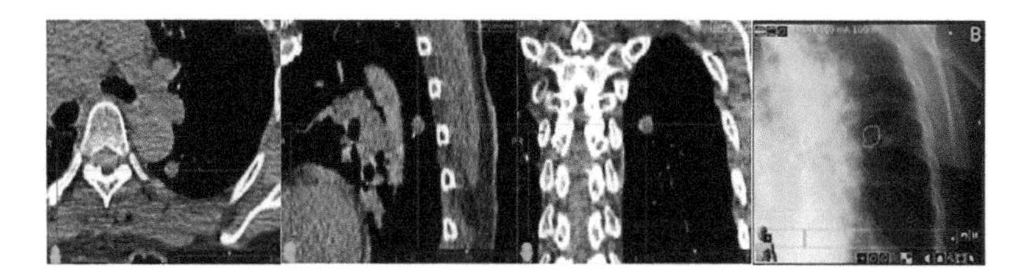

Figure 15.7 Example of a lesion treated using 1-view tracking, axial sagittal and coronal view, and 2D projection image.

burst" enables the user to acquire a continuous sequence of x-ray images (approximately one image pair every second) and to adapt more rapidly to intra-fractional variations in respiratory pattern. One drawback when using image burst, is the increase in imaging dose; the appropriate imaging interval should be evaluated on a case-by-case basis.

Image recognition software calculates the target position based on the location of implanted gold markers (fiducial tracking) or based on the tumor density itself (fiducial-less tracking). Fiducial-less tracking is typically feasible for relatively large lesions (>1 cm in diameter) surrounded by lung parenchyma. Dynamic tracking based on only one camera view (1-view tracking) can be used if the view of the lesion is obstructed by the spine or other central organs in one of the 45-degree projection images. Figure 15.7 shows an example of a lesion treated using 1-view tracking. In 1-view tracking, the component of target motion in the imaging plane is tracked, while the component of target motion perpendicular to the imaging plane (out-of-plane motion) is compensated by a partial ITV expansion. Because of the geometry of the imaging system, the superior-inferior axis is common to both images, and target motion in the superior-inferior direction (often the predominant motion component) can always be tracked.

Targeting accuracy is defined as the ability of the system to deliver a spherical dose distribution to a moving phantom. The manufacturer specification of targeting accuracy for synchrony tracking is <0.95 mm. The first evaluation of the clinical accuracy of Synchrony was carried out by Hoogeman et al. [77]. These authors calculated the difference between the predicted and actual target position and found that the mean correlation error was <0.3 mm and that intra fraction error was <2.5 mm for motion amplitudes up to 2 cm. In a recent publication, Floriano et al. evaluated the global tracking uncertainty and estimated target margins for patients treated with Synchrony [78]. Their results were consistent with previous published studies [79–82] and supported a 5-mm isotropic CTV-to-PTV margin. Jung et al. compared the accuracy of fiducial-less lung tracking with that of fiducial-based tracking in patient-specific lung phantoms. For both tracking modalities, submillimeter tracking errors in all anatomical directions were achieved [83].

15.3.4 Gated-treatment-based on-board MRI

Recent technological breakthroughs have led to the development of MRI-guided radiation therapy devices [84–87], using low-latency cine MR images to account for breathing motion [88–90]. The main advantage of on-board MRI is the superior soft-tissue contrast and the ability to visualize the target without the need for implanted markers. As the target is visualized directly and continuously during treatment, the gating/tracking feedback signal is based on the target motion itself. Direct tracking of the target motion is expected to result in improved treatment accuracy compared to extracting target motion from the positions of external surrogate markers. Moreover, on-board MRI is the only imaging modality that enables visualizing the organs at risk and adapting the treatment prioritizing dose tolerance to the critical structures rather than target coverage.

The use of 2D cine MRI to assess tumor motions was reported in [91]. Paganelli et al. quantified the potential gain of MRI guidance by comparing the motion tracking accuracy of cine MRI with that of surrogate-based tumor tracking [92]. An automatic feature-detection algorithm applied to the cine MRI sequences enabled to directly track the liver with superior accuracy than relying on surrogates. For surrogate-based tracking, tracking errors in the range of 1.0 mm to 3.6 mm were observed depending on the motion amplitude.

The gain of MRI guidance (defined as the fraction of samples whose tracking error was larger than a defined threshold) was less than 10% when accepting a 3-mm threshold, but increased to 30% when requiring a more stringent (1.5 mm) threshold [92].

While prototype systems integrating a 1.5 T MRI scanner with a linear accelerator are currently being developed, the only clinically available MRI-guided radiation therapy system today is MRIdian® (ViewRay, Oakwood Village, Ohio) [84]. The ViewRay® system features a 0.35 T whole-body MRI scanner integrated on a ring gantry with three ^{60}Co heads. Each ^{60}Co head is equipped with independent doubly focused MLC. During treatment, MR images are acquired every 300 ms and compared to the treatment planning images. Gating structures can be set on the target or organs at risk. If deviations in the position of the gating structure are above the user-defined threshold, the beam is paused. Treatment is resumed automatically when the gating structure moves back into the treatment boundary.

Crijns et al. demonstrated the feasibility of using an online MRI signal to gate the output of a linear accelerator [93]. An external control interface allowed establishing real-time communication with the MRI scanner (~10 ms lag time) and the beam was turned off by inhibiting the magnetron from producing RF pulses (pulse rate frequency (PRF) muting) [94]. The same feedback framework can also be used to control gantry rotation and MLC aperture thus enabling real-time tumor motion tracking [58].

15.4 SUMMARY AND FUTURE DIRECTIONS

In image verification, the ideal imaging technique would provide real-time volumetric images of the patient with high temporal and spatial resolution for accurate 3D cine verification of the target. Achieving this goal is challenging, due to the limitation of the acquisition speed of different imaging techniques. In x-ray-based imaging techniques, a method was proposed previously to generate cine CBCT images using a single cone-beam projection and patient modeling [13]. However, the accuracy of the reconstructed cine CBCT is limited by the accuracy of the patient model, which is affected by patient breathing pattern changes from simulation to treatment. The LIVE system addressed this limitation by incorporating free form deformation to correct for any errors in patient modeling [14]. By exploring the continuity of patient respiratory motion, LIVE can potentially further reduce the scan angle needed to achieve quasi-cine CBCT. In MRI, a similar method has been developed to use patient modeling to reconstruct volumetric cine MRI (VC-MRI) images based on a single 2D cine MR image [53]. The accuracy and temporal resolution of VC-MRI can be potentially further improved using free-form deformation and sparse sampling in MRI acquisition. Various 4D-MRI techniques are also being actively investigated to generate high spatial and temporal resolution images with minimal-motion artifacts [95,96].

In delivery tracking, current technologies enable tracking translational and rotational target motion during a breathing cycle. However, lung tumors also undergo deformation. Kyriakou and McKenzie evaluated changes in tumor shapes during respiration using statistical shape modeling and observed a correlation between velocity and strain in deforming tumors [97]. Liu et al. calculated differences in tumor motion using rigid and deformable image registration and observed a difference of up to 2.7 mm in the superior-inferior direction for a patient with a large tumor extending from the upper to the mid lung [98]. For advanced stage diseases with nodal involvement, the relative motion between the primary tumor and the related lymph nodes needs to be considered. Donelly et al. [99] and Panarotto et al. [100] independently observed deformations larger than 10 cm in the composite tumor system. Correcting dynamically for tumor deformation is challenging. Respiratory gating and tracking based on robotic arm linac or O-shaped linac enables holding the beam or moving the beam in a rigid manner, but do not allow compensating for intra-fraction tumor deformation. Dynamic MLC tracking has potentially the ability to compensate for tumor deformation. However, in clinical studies reported so far only rigid tumor displacements were accounted for. Ge et al. explored the feasibility of dynamic MLC tracking to account for tumor deformation, by warping the planned beam aperture to conform to the new tumor shape based on the input from a deformable image registration software [101]. The feasibility and clinical impact of such techniques remain to be further investigated.

REFERENCES

1. Zelefsky, M.J. et al., Improved clinical outcomes with high-dose image guided radiotherapy compared with non-IGRT for the treatment of clinically localized prostate cancer. *Int J Radiat Oncol Biol Phys*, 2012. **84**(1): 125–9.
2. Soike, M. et al., Image guided radiation therapy results in improved local control in lung cancer patients treated with fractionated radiation therapy for stage IIB-IIIB disease. *Int J Radiat Oncol Biol Phys*, 2013. **87**(2): S547–8.
3. Godfrey, D.J. et al., Digital tomosynthesis with an on-board kilovoltage imaging device. *Int J Radiat Oncol Biol Phys*, 2006. **65**(1): 8–15.
4. Dobbins, J.T., 3rd and D.J. Godfrey, Digital x-ray tomosynthesis: Current state of the art and clinical potential. *Phys Med Biol*, 2003. **48**(19): R65–106.
5. Ren, L. et al., Automatic registration between reference and on-board digital tomosynthesis images for positioning verification. *Med Phys*, 2008. **35**(2): 664–72.
6. Feldkamp, L.A., L.C. Davis, and J.W. Kress, Practical cone-beam algorithm. *J Opt Soc Am A Opt Image Sci Vis*, 1984. **1**(6): 612–9.
7. Zhang, Y. et al., Respiration-phase-matched digital tomosynthesis imaging for moving target verification: A feasibility study. *Med Phys*, 2013. **40**(7): 071723.
8. Ren, L. et al., A novel digital tomosynthesis (DTS) reconstruction method using a deformation field map. *Med Phys*, 2008. **35**(7): 3110–5.
9. Zhang, Y. et al., A technique for estimating 4D-CBCT using prior knowledge and limited-angle projections. *Med Phys*, 2013. **40**(12): 121701.
10. Zhang, Y. et al., Preliminary clinical evaluation of a 4D-CBCT estimation technique using prior information and limited-angle projections. *Radiother Oncol*, 2015. **115**(1): 22–9.
11. Zhang, Y., F.F. Yin, and L. Ren, Dosimetric verification of lung cancer treatment using the CBCTs estimated from limited-angle on-board projections. *Med Phys*, 2015. **42**(8): 4783–95.
12. Ren, L. et al., Development and clinical evaluation of a three-dimensional cone-beam computed tomography estimation method using a deformation field map. *Int J Radiat Oncol Biol Phys*, 2012. **82**(5): 1584–93.
13. Li, R. et al., Real-time volumetric image reconstruction and 3D tumor localization based on a single x-ray projection image for lung cancer radiotherapy. *Med Phys*, 2010. **37**(6): 2822–6.
14. Ren, L., Y. Zhang, and F.F. Yin, A limited-angle intrafraction verification (LIVE) system for radiation therapy. *Med Phys*, 2014. **41**(2): 020701.
15. Sonke, J.J. et al., Respiratory correlated cone beam CT. *Med Phys*, 2005. **32**(4): 1176–86.
16. Li, T. et al., Four-dimensional cone-beam computed tomography using an on-board imager. *Med Phys*, 2006. **33**(10): 3825–33.
17. Kriminski, S. et al., Respiratory correlated cone-beam computed tomography on an isocentric C-arm. *Phys Med Biol*, 2005. **50**(22): 5263–80.
18. Purdie, T.G. et al., Respiration correlated cone-beam computed tomography and 4DCT for evaluating target motion in Stereotactic Lung Radiation Therapy. *Acta Oncol*, 2006. **45**(7): 915–22.
19. Lu, J. et al., Four-dimensional cone beam CT with adaptive gantry rotation and adaptive data sampling. *Med Phys*, 2007. **34**(9): 3520–9.
20. Sonke, J.J., J. Lebesque, and M. van Herk, Variability of four-dimensional computed tomography patient models. *Int J Radiat Oncol Biol Phys*, 2008. **70**(2): 590–8.
21. Bergner, F. et al., An investigation of 4D cone-beam CT algorithms for slowly rotating scanners. *Med Phys*, 2010. **37**(9): 5044–53.
22. Leng, S. et al., High temporal resolution and streak-free four-dimensional cone-beam computed tomography. *Phys Med Biol*, 2008. **53**(20): 5653–73.
23. Li, G. et al., Advances in 4D medical imaging and 4D radiation therapy. *Technol Cancer Res Treat*, 2008. **7**(1): 67–81.
24. Bergner, F. et al., Autoadaptive phase-correlated (AAPC) reconstruction for 4D CBCT. *Med Phys*, 2009. **36**(12): 5695–706.

25. Qi, Z. and G.H. Chen, Extraction of tumor motion trajectories using PICCS-4DCBCT: A validation study. *Med Phys*, 2011. **38**(10): 5530–8.
26. Wang, J. and X. Gu, Simultaneous motion estimation and image reconstruction (SMEIR) for 4D cone-beam CT. *Med Phys*, 2013. **40**(10): 101912–23.
27. Solberg, T. et al., Enhancement of 4D cone-beam computed tomography through constraint optimization. *Proceedings of International Conference on the Use of Computers in Radiation Therapy*, 2010.
28. Song, J. et al., Sparseness prior based iterative image reconstruction for retrospectively gated cardiac micro-CT. *Med Phys*, 2007. **34**(11): 4476–83.
29. Chen, G.-H., J. Tang, and S. Leng, Prior image constrained compressed sensing (PICCS): A method to accurately reconstruct dynamic CT images from highly undersampled projection data sets. *Med Phys*, 2008. **35**(2): 660–3.
30. Mc Kinnon, G.C. and R.H. Bates, Towards imaging the beating heart usefully with a conventional CT scanner. *IEEE Trans Biomed Eng*, 1981. **28**(2): 123–7.
31. Rit, S. et al., On-the-fly motion-compensated cone-beam CT using an a priori model of the respiratory motion. *Med Phys*, 2009. **36**(6): 2283–96.
32. Rit, S., D. Sarrut, and L. Desbat, Comparison of analytic and algebraic methods for motion-compensated cone-beam CT reconstruction of the thorax. *IEEE Trans Med Imaging*, 2009. **28**(10): 1513–25.
33. Li, T., A. Koong, and L. Xing, Enhanced 4D cone-beam CT with inter-phase motion model. *Med Phys*, 2007. **34**(9): 3688–95.
34. Zhang, Q. et al., Correction of motion artifacts in cone-beam CT using a patient-specific respiratory motion model. *Med Phys*, 2010. **37**(6): 2901–9.
35. Yamamoto, T. et al., Reproducibility of four-dimensional computed tomography-based lung ventilation imaging. *Acad Radiol*, 2012. **19**(12): 1554–65.
36. Chang, J. et al., Observation of interfractional variations in lung tumor position using respiratory gated and ungated megavoltage cone-beam computed tomography. *Int J Radiat Oncol Biol Phys*, 2007. **67**(5): 1548–58.
37. Wang, J. and X. Gu, High-quality four-dimensional cone-beam CT by deforming prior images. *Phys Med Biol*, 2013. **58**(2): 231–46.
38. Staub, D. et al., 4D Cone-beam CT reconstruction using a motion model based on principal component analysis. *Med Phys*, 2011. 38(12): 6697–709.
39. Yan, H. et al., A hybrid reconstruction algorithm for fast and accurate 4D cone-beam CT imaging. *Med Phys*, 2014. **41**(7): 071903.
40. Lu, W.G. et al., Fast free-form deformable registration via calculus of variations. *Physics in Medicine and Biology*, 2004. **49**(14): 3067–87.
41. Ren, L. et al., A novel digital tomosynthesis (DTS) reconstruction method using a deformation field map. *Med Phys*, 2008. **35**(7): 3110–5.
42. Mantz, C., A phase II trial of stereotactic ablative body radiotherapy for low-risk prostate cancer using a non-robotic linear accelerator and real-time target tracking: Report of toxicity, quality of life, and disease control outcomes with 5-year minimum follow-up. *Front Oncol*, 2014. **4**: 279.
43. Shah, A.P. et al., Real-time tumor tracking in the lung using an electromagnetic tracking system. *Int J Radiat Oncol Biol Phys*, 2013. **86**(3): 477–83.
44. Dempsey, J. et al., A real-time MRI guided external beam radiotherapy delivery system. *Med Phys*, 2006. **33**(6): 2254.
45. Lagendijk, J.J. et al., MRI/linac integration. *Radiother Oncol*, 2008. **86**(1): 25–9.
46. Fallone, B.G. et al., First MR images obtained during megavoltage photon irradiation from a prototype integrated linac-MR system. *Med Phys*, 2009. **36**(6): 2084–8.
47. Raaymakers, B.W. et al., Integrating a 1.5 T MRI scanner with a 6 MV accelerator: Proof of concept. *Phys Med Biol*, 2009. **54**(12): N229–37.
48. Sarma, M. et al., Accelerating dynamic magnetic resonance imaging (MRI) for lung tumor tracking based on low-rank decomposition in the spatial-temporal domain: A feasibility study based on simulation and preliminary prospective undersampled MRI. *Int J Radiat Oncol Biol Phys*, 2014. **88**(3): 723–31.

49. Hu, Y. et al., Respiratory amplitude guided 4-dimensional magnetic resonance imaging. *Int J Radiat Oncol Biol Phys*, 2013. **86**(1): 198–204.
50. Cai, J. et al., Four-dimensional magnetic resonance imaging (4D-MRI) using image-based respiratory surrogate: A feasibility study. *Med Phys*, 2011. **38**(12): 6384–94.
51. Tryggestad, E. et al., Respiration-based sorting of dynamic MRI to derive representative 4D-MRI for radiotherapy planning. *Med Phys*, 2013. **40**(5): 051909.
52. von Siebenthal, M. et al., 4D MR imaging of respiratory organ motion and its variability. *Phys Med Biol*, 2007. **52**(6): 1547–64.
53. Harris, W. et al., A technique for generating volumetric cine-magnetic resonance imaging. *Int J Radiat Oncol Biol Phys*, 2016. **95**(2): 844–53.
54. Keall, P.J. et al., Motion adaptive x-ray therapy: A feasibility study. *Phys Med Biol*, 2001. **46**(1): 1–10.
55. Keall, P.J. et al., The management of respiratory motion in radiation oncology report of AAPM Task Group 76. *Med Phys*, 2006. **33**(10): 3874–900.
56. Sawant, A. et al., Management of three-dimensional intrafraction motion through real-time DMLC tracking. *Med Phys*, 2008. **35**(5): 2050–61.
57. Tacke, M.B. et al., Real-time tumor tracking: Automatic compensation of target motion using the Siemens 160 MLC. *Med Phys*, 2010. **37**(2): 753–61.
58. Crijns, S.P., B.W. Raaymakers, and J.J. Lagendijk, Proof of concept of MRI-guided tracked radiation delivery: Tracking one-dimensional motion. *Phys Med Biol*, 2012. **57**(23): 7863–72.
59. Poulsen, P.R. et al., Dynamic multileaf collimator tracking of respiratory target motion based on a single kilovoltage imager during arc radiotherapy. *Int J Radiat Oncol Biol Phys*, 2010. **77**(2): 600–7.
60. Cho, B. et al., First demonstration of combined kV/MV image-guided real-time dynamic multileaf-collimator target tracking. *Int J Radiat Oncol Biol Phys*, 2009. **74**(3): 859–67.
61. Cho, B. et al., Real-time target position estimation using stereoscopic kilovoltage/megavoltage imaging and external respiratory monitoring for dynamic multileaf collimator tracking. *Int J Radiat Oncol Biol Phys*, 2011. **79**(1): 269–78.
62. Ravkilde, T. et al., Geometric accuracy of dynamic MLC tracking with an implantable wired electromagnetic transponder. *Acta Oncol*, 2011. **50**(6): 944–51.
63. Sawant, A. et al., Toward submillimeter accuracy in the management of intrafraction motion: The integration of real-time internal position monitoring and multileaf collimator target tracking. *Int J Radiat Oncol Biol Phys*, 2009. **74**(2): 575–82.
64. Keall, P.J. et al., The first clinical implementation of electromagnetic transponder-guided MLC tracking. *Med Phys*, 2014. **41**(2): 020702.
65. Keall, P. and D. Ruan, Dynamic multileaf collimator control for motion adaptive radiotherapy: An optimization approach. *IEEE Power Engineering and Automation Conference (PEAM)*, Vol. **3**, 2011, Wuhan, China, pp. 100–3.
66. Krauss, A. et al., Electromagnetic real-time tumor position monitoring and dynamic multileaf collimator tracking using a Siemens 160 MLC: Geometric and dosimetric accuracy of an integrated system. *Int J Radiat Oncol Biol Phys*, 2011. **79**(2): 579–87.
67. Colvill, E. et al., Multileaf collimator tracking improves dose delivery for prostate cancer radiation therapy: Results of the first clinical trial. *Int J Radiat Oncol Biol Phys*, 2015. **92**(5): 1141–7.
68. Kamino, Y. et al., Development of a four-dimensional image-guided radiotherapy system with a gimbaled X-ray head. *Int J Radiat Oncol Biol Phys*, 2006. **66**(1): 271–8.
69. Nakamura, M. et al., Dosimetric characterization of a multileaf collimator for a new four-dimensional image-guided radiotherapy system with a gimbaled x-ray head, MHI-TM2000. *Med Phys*, 2010. **37**(9): 4684–91.
70. Verellen, D. et al., Quality assurance of a system for improved target localization and patient set-up that combines real-time infrared tracking and stereoscopic X-ray imaging. *Radiother Oncol*, 2003. **67**(1): 129–41.
71. Chang, Z. et al., 6D image guidance for spinal non-invasive stereotactic body radiation therapy: Comparison between ExacTrac X-ray 6D with kilo-voltage cone-beam CT. *Radiother Oncol*, 2010. **95**(1): 116–21.
72. Depuydt, T. et al., Geometric accuracy of a novel gimbals based radiation therapy tumor tracking system. *Radiother Oncol*, 2011. **98**(3): 365–72.

73. Depuydt, T. et al., Treating patients with real-time tumor tracking using the Vero gimbaled linac system: Implementation and first review. *Radiother Oncol*, 2014. **112**(3): 343–51.
74. Kilby, W. et al., The CyberKnife robotic radiosurgery system in 2010. *Technol Cancer Res Treat*, 2010. **9**(5): 433–52.
75. Muacevic, A. et al., Technical description, phantom accuracy, and clinical feasibility for single-session lung radiosurgery using robotic image-guided real-time respiratory tumor tracking. *Technol Cancer Res Treat*, 2007. **6**(4): 321–8.
76. Ernst, F. et al., Correlation between external and internal respiratory motion: A validation study. *Int J Comput Assist Radiol Surg*, 2012. **7**(3): 483–92.
77. Hoogeman, M. et al., Clinical accuracy of the respiratory tumor tracking system of the CyberKnife: Assessment by analysis of log files. *Int J Radiat Oncol Biol Phys*, 2009. **74**(1): 297–303.
78. Floriano, A. et al., Retrospective evaluation of CTV to PTV margins using CyberKnife in patients with thoracic tumors. *J Appl Clin Med Phys*, 2014. **15**(6): 4825.
79. Sawkey, D., M. Svatos, and C. Zankowski, Evaluation of motion management strategies based on required margins. *Phys Med Biol*, 2012. **57**(20): 6347–69.
80. Pepin, E.W. et al., Correlation and prediction uncertainties in the CyberKnife Synchrony respiratory tracking system. *Med Phys*, 2011. **38**(7): 4036–44.
81. George, R. et al., On the accuracy of a moving average algorithm for target tracking during radiation therapy treatment delivery. *Med Phys*, 2008. **35**(6): 2356–65.
82. Lu, X.Q. et al., Organ deformation and dose coverage in robotic respiratory-tracking radiotherapy. *Int J Radiat Oncol Biol Phys*, 2008. **71**(1): 281–9.
83. Jung, J. et al., Verification of accuracy of CyberKnife tumor-tracking radiation therapy using patient-specific lung phantoms. *Int J Radiat Oncol Biol Phys*, 2015. **92**(4): 745–53.
84. Mutic, S. and J.F. Dempsey, The ViewRay system: Magnetic resonance-guided and controlled radiotherapy. *Semin Radiat Oncol*, 2014. **24**(3): 196–9.
85. Fallone, B.G., The rotating biplanar linac-magnetic resonance imaging system. *Semin Radiat Oncol*, 2014. **24**(3): 200–2.
86. Keall, P.J. et al., The Australian magnetic resonance imaging-linac program. *Semin Radiat Oncol*, 2014. **24**(3): 203–6.
87. Lagendijk, J.J., B.W. Raaymakers, and M. van Vulpen, The magnetic resonance imaging-linac system. *Semin Radiat Oncol*, 2014. **24**(3): 207–9.
88. Tryggestad, E. et al., 4D tumor centroid tracking using orthogonal 2D dynamic MRI: Implications for radiotherapy planning. *Med Phys*, 2013. **40**(9): 091712.
89. Bjerre, T. et al., Three-dimensional MRI-linac intra-fraction guidance using multiple orthogonal cine-MRI planes. *Phys Med Biol*, 2013. **58**(14): 494350.
90. Kupelian, P. and J.J. Sonke, Magnetic resonance-guided adaptive radiotherapy: A solution to the future. *Semin Radiat Oncol*, 2014. **24**(3): 227–32.
91. Sawant, A. et al., Investigating the feasibility of rapid MRI for image-guided motion management in lung cancer radiotherapy. *Biomed Res Int*, 2014. **2014:** 485067.
92. Paganelli, C. et al., Magnetic resonance imaging-guided versus surrogate-based motion tracking in liver radiation therapy: A prospective comparative study. *Int J Radiat Oncol Biol Phys*, 2015. **91**(4): 840–8.
93. Crijns, S.P. et al., Towards MRI-guided linear accelerator control: Gating on an MRI accelerator. *Phys Med Biol*, 2011. **56**(15): 4815–25.
94. Evans, P.M. et al., Gating characteristics of an Elekta radiotherapy treatment unit measured with three types of detector. *Phys Med Biol*, 2010. **55**(8): N201–10.
95. Liu, Y. et al., Four dimensional magnetic resonance imaging with retrospective k-space reordering: A feasibility study. *Med Phys*, 2015. **42**(2): 534–41.
96. Liu, Y. et al., T2-weighted four dimensional magnetic resonance imaging with result-driven phase sorting. *Med Phys*, 2015. **42**(8): 4460–71.
97. Kyriakou, E. and D.R. McKenzie, Changes in lung tumor shape during respiration. *Phys Med Biol*, 2012. **57**(4): 919–35.

98. Liu, H.H. et al., Assessing respiration-induced tumor motion and internal target volume using four-dimensional computed tomography for radiotherapy of lung cancer. *Int J Radiat Oncol Biol Phys*, 2007. **68**(2): 531–40.
99. Donnelly, E.D. et al., Assessment of intrafraction mediastinal and hilar lymph node movement and comparison to lung tumor motion using four-dimensional CT. *Int J Radiat Oncol Biol Phys*, 2007. **69**(2): 580–8.
100. Pantarotto, J.R. et al., Motion analysis of 100 mediastinal lymph nodes: Potential pitfalls in treatment planning and adaptive strategies. *Int J Radiat Oncol Biol Phys*, 2009. **74**(4): 1092–9.
101. Ge, Y. et al., Toward the development of intrafraction tumor deformation tracking using a dynamic multi-leaf collimator. *Med Phys*, 2014. **41**(6): 061703.

16

Treatment response assessment and response guided adaptive treatment

TIM LAUTENSCHLAEGER, MARTHA MATUSZAK, AND FENG-MING (SPRING) KONG

16.1 INTRODUCTION

Lung cancers are heterogeneous in biological features, clinical presentation and their response to treatments. Some lung cancers respond quickly to radiation therapy (RT), achieving a complete response before the completion of a planned course of RT, while other lung cancers appear to show very limited response to RT.

Many efforts have been executed and have shown promise to be useful in predicting treatment response of individual patients. However, no approach has been widely adapted in clinical routine use, and thus patients and health-care providers are still facing a reality of very significant RT response heterogeneity. Similarly, normal tissue response to radiation therapy varies widely, making radiation toxicity prediction difficult.

Both molecular and imaging biomarkers have been developed over the last decades, improving abilities to measure and predict treatment tumor response. Molecular markers including DNA, RNA, or protein cytokines measured in blood have shown promise as tumor response prediction and measurement tools. Similarly, certain tissue markers have shown promise for upfront prediction of outcomes but are not frequently used to measure response early during treatment, mainly due to the need for repeated biopsies. Molecular and imaging markers also can be used to measure and predict normal tissue response and radiation toxicity.

Personalized adaptive RT (PART) aims to refine RT to maximize the probability of tumor control and minimize the risk of toxicity. PART uses assessment of early tumor response and adjusts dose to tumor and organs-at-risk (OARs) with the goal to optimize outcome. Two potential strategies may be used for PART. The standard dose can be increased or decreased with the aim to have toxicity rates below a predefined threshold. Dose escalation is applied to patients with tumors more resistant to radiation. Patients with small tumor volumes, peripherally located tumors, and tumors far from OARs have a much lower estimated toxicity rate, allowing for increased radiation dose. Dose de-escalation may be applied to tumors that are more sensitive to radiation, or to patients with tumors in an unfavorable locations leading to higher toxicity at standard or increased doses.

16.2 TUMOR RESPONSE

Tumor response can be measured using a variety of methods at many different time points. This chapter reviews and comments on the response assessment after the completion of therapy, as well as during treatment. Response assessment after completion of therapy commonly is used to determine if treatment potentially worked or failed. During-treatment assessment can guide adaptive changes to the ongoing treatment.

16.2.1 Post-treatment tumor response

16.2.1.1 RESPONSE ASSESSMENT METHODS

Response Evaluation Criteria In Solid Tumors (RECIST) were developed in 2000 (RECIST 1.0) [1] and updated in 2009 (RECIST 1.1) to facilitate imaging response assessment [2]. RECIST 1.1 has been widely adapted and represents the current standard for assessment of tumor response using CT or anatomic magnetic resonance imaging (MRI) data. Target lesions (up to two per organ and five total [2]) are identified and the sum of the longest diameter (LD) of each target lesion is recorded. A complete response (CR) is defined as the disappearance of all target lesions, a partial response (PR) as at least a 30% decrease in the sum of the LD of target lesions, progressive disease (PD) as at least a 20% increase in the sum of the LD of target lesions or the appearance of new lesions, and stable disease (SD) as all other scenarios. There are several important changes between RECIST 1.0 and RECIST 1.1 (Table 16.1). Previously, RECIST 1.0 required documenting up to 10 target lesions (5 per organ)—now only 5 lesions (2 per organ) are required. RECIST 1.1 now includes size criteria for lymph nodes. Lymph nodes less than 10 mm short-axis diameter are being considered non-pathological, between 10 and 15 mm they are being considered a non-target lesion, and equal to or greater than 15 mm short axis is considered a target lesion. There now also is a minimum absolute increase of 5 mm in lesions in addition to the 20% increase requirement to call progressive disease (PD). Additionally, PET is now included in RECIST 1.1.

The longest diameter (LD) on predefined planes (axial, coronal, sagittal) is likely dependent on patient positioning as minor changes in patient position can lead to changes of what will be visualized on a CT

Table 16.1 Select changes of RECIST criteria for response evaluation of solid tumors

Criteria	RECIST 1.0	RECIST 1.1
Minimum size	>10mm	>15 mm for target 10–15 mm for nontarget
Number of index lesions	10 (5 per organ)	5 (2 per organ)
Complete response for lymph nodes	Not defined	<10 mm short axis
Progressive disease	20% increase	20% and 5-mm increase or new lesion
Use of PET-CT	Not defined	Used to identify new lesions

plane. As tumors can grow in very irregular shapes, these changes in the image plane can result in significant alterations of the quantification of the LD. Volumetric quantitative assessment of tumor volume on CT is potentially more reproducible than uni or bidirectional tumor measurements [3].

The presence of atelectasis or scar tissue can sometimes represent a challenge when assessing treatment response on CT. In these challenging cases, metabolic imaging using FDG-PET often is very useful to differentiate between recurrence and post-treatment changes [4].

PET has been widely used in treatment response assessment. In addition to the use of PET in RECIST 1.1, FDG-PET has been developed with the goal to standardize response assessment using (18) F-FDG-PET [5]. A fixed small region of interest about 1 cm (3) in volume (1.2-cm diameter) in the most active region of a tumor is selected and SUV lean measurements are used as a continuous variable. A treatment response is defined as a 30% decline in SUV. The European Organization for Research and Treatment of Cancer (EORTC) has developed guidelines for response assessment using PET. EORTC criteria are based on adding max SUV from up to seven target lesions from as many organs as possible. Partial metabolic response (PMR) is defined as a reduction of the sum of max SUV of at least 25% and progressive metabolic disease (PMD) as an increase of the sum of max SUV of at least 25%. A comparison of response assessments using EORTC and PERCIST criteria suggests that that both give similar responses and the association of metabolic response with overall survival is also similar between both criteria [6]. Qualitative assessment methods such as the Peter MacCallum (PM) method of qualitative visual assessment have also been evaluated in comparison to semi quantitative assessment methods. In one study PM identified significantly more CMR than the semi quantitative assessment method from the University of Michigan (38.6% vs 13.6%) [7].

In summary, many methods exist to measure response. They all have different strengths and their ideal use remains to be determined through future studies.

16.2.1.2 POST-RT RESPONSE ASSESSMENT CAN PREDICT LONG-TERM OUTCOMES

Radiation therapy plays an important role for both non-small-cell lung cancer (NSCLC) and small-cell lung cancer (SCLC) and treatment response is often associated with local tumor control and survival.

Radiation therapy responses of NSCLC determined by CT typically require several months. A recent study of 22 NSCLC patients assessing uni- and bi-dimensional tumor extent, as well as tumor volume, showed the average time to the tumor nadir was 11 months from RT completion [8]. Pre-treatment volume of NSCLC is known to be an important predictor of treatment response [9]. NSCLC tumor volumes greater than 100 cc are associated with local control rates of only a few percent [9]. Similarly, NSCLC volumes of 124 cc or greater at 24 months' post-treatment predicts for very poor local control [8]. Good local control is associated with improved cause-specific survival (CSS). In a retrospective study of elderly patients treated with definitive radiation to 66 Gy in 2.2 Gy fractions a 3-year CSS of 45% was observed for patients without local failure versus a 3-year CSS of only 23% for patients, who failed locally [10].

Treatment response for NSCLC after RT assessed by FDG-PET has been shown to be an important prognostic factor [11]. Importantly, the complete response rate assessed by PET is three times higher than that assessed by CT [11]. Assessment of metabolic tumor activity in locally advanced NSCLC after induction chemoRT using a SUV cutoff of 4 was of prognostic significance with a median overall survival of 56 months for patients with tumors with a SUV <4 and only 19 months for patients with SUV >4 [12]. Similarly, post-treatment PET (median of 70 days after definitive RT to 60 Gy in 30 fractions with or without concurrent chemotherapy) predicted for overall survival [13]. Median overall survival after complete metabolic response (CMR) was 31 months in comparison to only 11 months with patients with a non-CMR [13]. Moreover, local failure and distant metastatic failure rates after stable metabolic disease or progressive metabolic disease were significantly worse in comparison to patients with CMR (HR > 2 for both local and distant failure) [13].

There are challenges when adapting PET as a tool for clinical routine use to measure treatment response. Alteration of cutoffs in SUV significantly alters results and different investigators commonly present their results using different cutoffs. In a study evaluating response to neoadjuvant chemotherapy alone for stage III NSCLC a greater than 60% decrease in SUV was associated with an impressive 60% 5-year overall survival while patients who had a lower than 25% decrease in their SUV change had a 5-years-survival lower than 5% [14]. In a cohort of stage III NSCLC treated with neoadjuvant chemoRT, reduction of SUV by at least 80% was associated with favorable outcome [15]. Moreover, sensitivity, specificity and overall accuracy of FDG-PET for the detection of residual tumor after neoadjuvant chemoRT were 94.5%, 80%, and 91% [15]. The presence or absence of an EGFR mutation might also be an important molecular determinant of FDG avidity [16]. Tumors with EGFR mutations might more frequently be less FDG avid than EGFR wild-type tumors [16]. Similarly, different molecular alterations (i.e. VEGF, HIF-1a, or GLUT1) might influence FDG avidity in NSCLC [17]. In patients with advanced NSCLC treated with erlotinib and bevacizumab 18F-FDG-PET as well as H2 (15) O perfusion PET accurately predicted outcomes. In fact, PFS prediction using 18F-FDG-PET classified as reduction or no reduction (9.7 versus 2.8 mo, P=0.01) or perfusion imaging (12.5 versus 2.9 mo, P=0.009) might be more discriminative than CT imaging using RESIST (4.6 for PR versus 2.9 mo for less than PR, P=0.017) [18]. In summary, post-treatment PET for locally advanced and advanced NSCLC is highly correlated with pathologic response, and predicts long term survival and patterns of failure. Post-treatment PET, however, does not provide an opportunity to change the treatment plan.

Treatment response after stereotactic body radiation therapy (SBRT) or stereotactic ablative body radiation (SABR) can be assessed using a variety of imaging modalities.

Metabolic imaging is useful in assessing response to therapy after SBRT. FDG-PET after SBRT can show persistent uptake for up to 2 years after therapy [19], possibly related to persistent inflammation [20]. FDG-PET obtained 1–2 years after SBRT has been reported to predict for local recurrence [21]. Using a cutoff of maximum SUV > 5 there was 100% sensitivity, 91% specificity, a 50% positive predictive value, and a 100% negative predictive value for predicting local recurrence [21]. Similarly, FDG-PET screening scheduled at one year after SBRT and if recurrence was suspected, using SUV cutoffs of 3.2 and 4.2, resulted in 100% sensitivity and specificity of 96%–98% for the prediction of recurrence [22]. Pre-treatment PET metrics have been shown to be associated with outcome in NSCLC after SBRT [23–25].

SCLC is more sensitive to chemotherapy and radiation and often results in excellent imaging responses. A complete response rate of 56% and partial responses in 31% of patients have been reported after standard of care radiation therapy of 45 Gy in 1.5 Gy fractions delivered twice per day (BID) given with concurrent cisplatin and etoposide, resulting in a 5-year overall survival of 26% [26]. Only 10% of patients had stable disease or progressive disease [26]. The primary tumor response of limited disease SCLC to chemo radiotherapy (CRT) also correlates with the duration of brain-metastasis-free survival [27]. For SCLC patients with initial complete response to CRT the median brain-metastasis-free survival averaged 21 months after PCI versus 16 months in patients without PCI [27].

16.2.2 During-treatment tumor response

16.2.2.1 Assessment methods

Available assessment methods include on-board imaging such as cone beam CT (CBCT) or CT on rails as well as CTs in radiation oncology departments dedicated for simulation in addition to those used for post-treatment response assessment (Table 16.2). CBCT is commonly and frequently obtained for difficult cases with target volumes close to critical structures to ensure a high accuracy in patient positioning and limit clinical target volume (CTV) to planning target volume (PTV) expansions. Thus, CBCT is performed already

Table 16.2 Response assessment methods during treatment

Assessment methods	Imaging quality	RT Routine	Effort
Cone beam CT	Poor	Yes	Low
CT on rails	Good	Yes	Medium
Simulation CT	Good	No	High
PET-CT	Good	No	Very high

Note: The table summarizes advantages and disadvantages of during-radiation imaging response assessment methods. Radiation therapy (RT) routine reflects which methods are already obtained frequently as part of standard clinical radiation oncology practice. Effort assessment estimates the additional expenses occurred secondary to additional staff time and equipment cost.

for clinical routine use and is available for adaptive radiation therapy. CBCT image quality, however, does not compare favorably with image quality of CT on rails, CT simulators or diagnostic CT and MRI scans. The lower image quality potentially could have a negative impact on the accuracy of RT response assessment and target and OAR delineation. CT on rails has the advantage of providing diagnostic quality images used for patient positioning. These images are already acquired for clinical routine uses and are available for PRT. One caveat of CT on rails is the need of repositioning for imaging, which limits the wide application of this technology. Additional effort, cost, and availability of CT on rails are factors that can limit its use. Obtaining a new simulation CT for PART is the currently mostly practiced approach. Disadvantages of the approach include the need for additional imaging, associated time commitment from patients and the health-care team, as well as associated costs. PET-based PRT requires a new simulation PET/CT or a diagnostic PET/CT.

An additional difficulty in during-treatment response assessment lies in identifying the most meaningful time points. In one cohort, there was significant intra- and inter-individual heterogeneity in the evolution of tumor maxSUV at early time points at 7 days and 14 days after RT start [28]. Most commonly, PET/CT tumor response assessment during treatment with the goal to adapt RT is conducted around week 4 of a 6-week treatment course. Other time points might be ideal when assessing organs at risk with the goal to predict and ultimately limit toxicity.

16.2.2.2 DURING-TREATMENT RESPONSE AND ITS ASSOCIATION WITH CLINICAL OUTCOME

Assessment of response to therapy after completion of therapy is important as a basis for decision making from that point forward. Post-RT response assessment, however, does not provide the opportunity to alter a course of radiation therapy that is already completed. RT response assessment during RT would provide the opportunity to adjust the RT plan per the assessment well before completion of RT.

Comparing CT and FDG-PET during treatment after two-thirds of treatment were completed, a reduction of metabolic tumor volume of 70% was observed while gross tumor volume (GTV) assessed by CT was reduced only by 41% ($p < 0.001$) [29]. Metabolic tumor volume reduction was more pronounced after two-thirds of a 3D conformal RT course (73% reduction) in comparison to a SBRT course (15% reduction).

FDG-PET/CT obtained after approximately 45 Gy predicts for post-treatment responses in NSCLC [30]. The mean peak tumor FDG activity was 5.2 (95% CI, 4.0–6.4), 2.5 (95% CI, 2.0–3.0), and 1.7 (95% CI, 1.3–2.0) on pre-, during-, and post-RT scans, respectively, and the peak tumor activity during RT correlated strongly with the peak FDG activity 3 months after completion of RT [30]. Interestingly, normalized (to aortic arch) max SUV was lowest in this small study of 15 patients, who were without evidence of disease, and highest in patients who succumbed to their disease [30]. Re-planning based on during–RT PET/CT allowed for a dose escalation of 30–102 Gy (mean, 58 Gy) or a reduction in normal tissue complication probability (NTCP) of 0.4%–3% (mean, 2%) in five of six patients with smaller yet residual tumor volumes [31]. Lack of during–RT PET response also has been reported to be associated with inferior progression-free survival (PFS) for patients receiving hypofractionated RT to 60–66 Gy in 3 Gy fractions [32]. Importantly, there may be a correlation between radiation dose delivered and max SUV at that time with higher max SUV declines with higher radiation doses [33].

Radiation therapy for SCLC often results in excellent imaging responses on CT that can typically be observed before the end of RT. In limited stage SCLC, a median CT-based volume reduction of approximately 70% can be expected before the completion of concurrent chemoRT [34]. Limited stage SCLC patients with greater tumor volume reduction (i.e. >45%) have better loco regional control and longer overall survival than those with less volume reduction [34].

In summary, there is convincing evidence that during-RT tumor assessment predicts long-term outcomes after RT.

16.2.3 TUMOR RESPONSE GUIDED ADAPTIVE TREATMENT

Adaptive radiation therapy started to adapt to setup errors and intrafraction motion [35–37]. After treatment response assessment with PET was developed [30] a first trial assessing the feasibility of PET-guided adaptive treatment was conducted [38]. The study was designed as a prospective single institution (University of

Michigan) phase II clinical trial. Adaptive planning used FDG-PET to measure tumor response after approximately 50 Gy of treatment, and the RT plan was adapted to target the residual metabolic target volume (MTV) for the final 9 fractions. Using an iso-toxicity approach for a 17% risk of grade 3 RILT estimated from a mean lung dose NTCP model, the dose per fraction to the MTV based PTV varied from 2.2 Gy to 3.8 Gy for the adaptive course of treatment. Mature results revealed quite favorable outcomes using this approach [38]. The 2-year rates of in-field loco-regional tumor control (LRTC) was 82% [38].

RTOG 1106 is a phase II clinical trial for patients with locally advanced NSCLC to determine whether residual tumors can be dose-escalated to improve the local-regional progression-free rate at 2 years. FDG-PET/CT is used to measure the tumor response after 18–19 treatments and the final 9 treatments are adjusted to cover residual and/or metabolic tumor volume. The adapted RT plan will be dose-escalated up to 80.4 Gy to the MTV limiting dose per an individualized MLD to 20 Gy and by esophageal and heart tolerance doses. Another strategy of PRT would be to use during-treatment images as a biomarker to predict a patient's radio sensitivity. Patients with greater tumor response may be more radiosensitive, thus requiring a lower dose to control the tumor and allowing to further reduce the risk of toxicity.

Adaptive RT has great potential to improve outcomes after RT. Randomized studies are under way to definitively determine its benefit.

16.3 RESPONSES OF ORGANS-AT-RISK (OARS)

16.3.1 Post-treatment response

Often, various imaging modalities are used to identify the effects of radiation to normal tissue, including MRI, CT, PET, and single photon emission computed tomography (SPECT). Late toxicities are often seen after the fact due to these modalities being used post-radiation rather than during. This is not only for normal lung tissue at risk for toxicity, but also the heart and esophagus. Each imaging modality can detect different responses from different areas. CT is often used to show the direct relationship between how radiopaque the lung tissue is and the lung RT dose resulting in toxicities like cough and shortness of breath as well as radiation pneumonitis [39,40]. Like CT, MRI has been shown to detect radiation pneumonitis by measuring the lung density [41] and unbalanced enhancement of the lung [42]. Esophageal toxicities have been detected via PET scans as FDG uptake was detected in the esophagus following radiation treatment [43–49]. The effects of radiation on the lung as well as the heart have been measured quantifying perfusion and ventilation with SPECT [40,50,51]. A study on 36 esophageal cancer patients identified a very successful linear regression model connecting lung radiation dose and SUV changes [44].

Lung V/Q SPECT is another modality to guide PART with potential benefit in many patients. Lung cancer patients often have ventilation and perfusion defects; V/Q scan are sometimes used to determine if a patient is a surgical candidate. V/Q SPECT data indicates that ventilation and perfusion defects are greater in central then in peripheral tumors [52]. Moreover, apparently normal areas of lung on CT might not function normally as measured by V/Q SPECT [53]. Importantly, regional ventilation and perfusion often improves during RT for centrally located NSCLC [53]. Cardiac SPECT has a long history of visualizing alterations in cardiac perfusion after RT [54–56]. The implications of SPECT abnormalities for individual patients remain to be determined.

Detecting these toxicities early on is ideal; however, most of these imaging modalities are used as post-radiation follow-up imaging, eliminating the opportunity to adjust RT plans before RT completion to limit toxicities to the organs at risk.

16.3.2 During-treatment responses

During a course of radiation therapy, organs at risk are also subject to change, and acquiring imaging during treatment allows for the opportunity to alter the RT plan if needed to aid in limiting toxicities. FDG uptake of normal lung can be observed during RT [30]. In one series, approximately 1–2 weeks into a radiation course, the lung tissue surrounding the GTV was reported to show an uptake of FDG and this was accompanied by shortness of breath in those patients [57]. Several other studies that have reported during-treatment PET assessment do not report data on normal lung SUV, indicating that the meaning of normal lung response remains to be clarified.

Radiation ideally shrinks the tumor away from OARs and adaptive planning could improve RT side effects. CT imaging can detect tumor size alterations during RT. Some data suggest that acquiring a before treatment ventilation and perfusion SPECT can help to denote which lung weaknesses are native to the tumor and a during-treatment SPECT can aid in knowing which dysfunctions may be recuperated following tumor response [58]. FDG-PET can also successfully predict the onset of esophagitis with a median time to onset of 11.6 days after PET and an area under the curve of 0.84 [59].

There also is potential for SPECT guided PART. Identifying functional parts of the lung and sparing them at the expense of non-functioning lung can result in a significant decrease in functional mean lung dose.

Imaging modalities allow for modification of a radiation plan during treatment to focus more on cancer-related dysfunction and treat less otherwise healthy tissue.

16.3.3 OAR imaging guided adaptive treatment

In good practice, radiation therapy normal-tissue dose limits are set to minimize the proportion of patients experiencing bothersome or dangerous toxicities. Thus, radiation dose is determined based on the most sensitive part of the population. Potentially, there are patient determinants for toxicity risk that can be measured, which could allow identification of the most toxicity sensitive and resistant patients. There are no available biomarkers (imaging or molecular) for clinical routine use identifying these patients before RT. OAR evaluation during RT, however, could provide this information.

There are several examples of OAR imaging during RT. Patients with an initially collapsed lung are likely to benefit from reimaging during RT using CT to evaluate if the lung has expanded. If the lung has re-expanded, adaptive planning can limit RT to the expanded lung to limit radiation to the uninvolved lung as much as possible. PET during RT can be used to identify a particularly sensitive OAR. An area of lung identified as particularly sensitive to RT could thus be adaptively spared. Similarly, if PET identifies a particularly sensitive esophagus, we may use IMRT to spare it during the rest of the RT course.

While there clearly is great potential for during-RT assessment to reduce toxicity, and improve cancer control, its benefit remains to be proven in appropriately designed prospective studies.

16.4 TREATMENT RESPONSE OF THE PATIENT

16.4.1 Responses of subjective symptoms

Quality of life (QOL) after radiation therapy for NSCLC has been assessed in several studies. Patients with stage III NSCLC enrolled in RTOG 0617 had a clinically meaningful decline in quality of life as assessed by FACT-LCS [60]. More patients in the 74-Gy arm than in the 60-Gy arm had clinically meaningful decline in FACT-LCS at 3 months (45% vs 30%; P = .02). At 12 months, fewer patients who received IMRT (vs 3D-CRT) had clinically meaningful decline in FACT-LCS (21% vs 46%; $P = .003$), suggesting a possible benefit of IMRT for preservation of patient-reported QOL.

Patients with stage I NSCLC undergoing SBRT have stable QOL as assessed by the European Organization for Research and Treatment of Cancer Quality of Life Questionnaire (EORTC QLQ)-C30 and the lung cancer-specific questionnaire QLQ-LC13 [61]. After treatment with SBRT, there was a slow decline of the global health status over 5 years ($p < 0.0001$). The physical functioning and the role functioning improved slowly over the years ($p < 0.0001$). The emotional functioning (EF) improved significantly at 1 year compared to baseline.

QOL during-treatment assessments could be used similarly to OAR and tumor during-treatment assessment for adaptive treatment. Patients with significant QOL impairment prior to RT start could continue treatment as long their QOL improves significantly and then stop RT to limit toxicities. Patients undergoing definitive treatment could receive dose-escalated RT as long their QOL remains stable.

16.4.2 Responses of biomarkers in the blood

The blood pool is a unique resource that potentially reflects important tumor and OAR characteristics and can be tested repeatedly with minimal effort and risk. As such, it is uniquely suitable for during-treatment testing for tumor response and toxicity risk assessment. Plasma-transforming growth factor-beta1 (TGFβ1) levels at end or during radiotherapy were shown to predict late toxicity of patients with lung carcinoma [62,63]. Other cytokines have also been shown to be of prognostic value [64,65]. Baseline interleukin-8 (IL-8) and radiation induced elevation of TGFβ 1 also have been shown to predict for radiation pneumonitis [66–70]. A combined model of IL-8, TGFβ 1, and mean lung dose (MLD) could predict lung toxicity with an area under the curve of 0.80 [70]. Single nucleotide polymorphisms (SNP) of the TGFβ 1 gene were reported to be associated with risk of radiation pneumonitis in NSCLC patients treated with RT [71]. SNPs in genes for TGFβ, VEGF, TNFα, XRCC1 and APEX1 together with MLD were combined into a normal-tissue complication probability (NTCP) model to predict radiation pneumonitis risk [72]. This NTCP model was evaluated for radiation dose changes using an iso-toxicity approach, and it was found that 59% of patients would have had a change in prescription of 5 Gy or more (either dose escalation or de-escalation), and 19% of patients would have had changes in prescription of 20 Gy or more. SNPs in DNA repair pathways were found to be independently associated with overall survival in NSCLC treated with RT with or without chemotherapy [73].

Micro-RNAs (miRNAs) are noncoding RNAs about 18–25 nucleotides in length and are important post-transcriptional regulators of gene expression. MiRNAs can be reliably measured in serum/plasma [74–80]. A serum miRNA signature consisting of five miRNA markers (miR-15b, miR-34a, miR-221, miR-224, and miR-130b) was found to be associated with OS in NSCLC [81]. Interestingly, patients classified by this miRNA marker as low risk appeared to derive a benefit from dose escalation to >70 Gy, while high-risk patients appeared to derive a benefit if dose was escalated beyond 83 Gy. Serum miR-191 was identified to predict radiation pneumonitis [82].

In summary, several blood biomarkers have shown great promise to predict treatment outcome. More studies are needed to definitively establish and validate the value of these markers.

16.4.3 Blood marker guided adaptive treatment, potential clinical trials

To develop a clinical decision tool for PART, both toxicity and tumor control probability need to be accounted for. Typical metrics used in evaluating new markers (e.g. area under the curve (AUC) for a classification problem) do not directly address the ability of a marker to improve LRTC at a fixed rate of toxicity. In fact, any marker only predicting either tumor control probability or toxicity risk will not be sufficient for a clinical decision tool providing information regarding optimal RT dose. For example, if a RT dose is linearly related to toxicity and LRTC, then one cannot improve tumor control probability without also increasing toxicity. A useful clinical decision tool will be a function of tumor control probability and toxicity risk determined by several biomarkers to select an optimal dose defined as the dose that maximizes tumor control probability and minimizes the sum of weighted toxicity probabilities [83].

A simplistic function F combining tumor control probability P_{LC} and probabilities for toxicity P_{tox} can be expressed as follows:

$$F(x) = aP_{LC}(x) - \left(b_1 P_{toxA}(x) + b_2 P_{toxB}(x) + \ldots\right),$$

where x is the RT dose and a and b_i are weighting factors representing the importance for individual patients and health-care providers.

Considerations for clinical parameters such as performance status or QOL possibly representing an individual patient's maximum tolerated toxicity might prove to be critical in ensuring success of such a clinical decision tool (i.e. $z<y$ for $b_1P_{toxA}(x) + b_2P_{toxB}(x)+\ldots < y$ for KPS 100 patients, and $b_1P_{toxA}(x) + b_2P_{toxB}(x)+\ldots < z$ for KPS 60 patients). Efficacy of biomarker guided adaptive therapy should also be tested prospectively in the clinic.

16.5 FUTURE DIRECTIONS

Lung cancer and normal-tissue responses vary from patient to patient after and during a course of treatment. While post-treatment response is predictive of long-term outcome of tumor control and toxicity, during-treatment response provides an opportunity for adaptive treatment. Anatomical imaging like CT, functional imaging such as FDG-PET for tumor, V/Q SPECT for lung and certain molecular alterations identified in blood can be acquired during treatment, and have shown great promise to guide risks limiting adaptive treatment.

Metabolic tumor response assessment using FDG-PET is a powerful tool measuring and predicting treatment response. In NSCLC, lower pretreatment metabolic activity and complete metabolic response during or after treatment is associated with better local control and longer overall survival. Adaptive re-planning reducing the GTV to the metabolic tumor volume after about two-thirds of treatment often allows for iso toxic dose escalation to the tumor. Such an adaptive RT is currently being prospectively evaluated in a randomized phase II study RTOG1106.

Normal tissue functional images, such as FDG-PET and lung V/Q SPECT-CT have also shown promise in guiding adaptive treatment. Complexity of its application should be anticipated. Randomized studies are needed to further test its clinical benefit.

Molecular blood biomarkers show great promise as tools predicting survival and pneumonitis. In fact, biomarker-adapted RT aiming for iso-toxic RT prescription might lead to important prescription alterations in more than half of stage III NSCLC patients. Similarly, molecular (i.e. ERCC1 SNPs, microRNA) blood signatures might identify patients who benefit from RT dose escalation.

Patient perceived responses to RT (quality of life QOL) are in general favorable. Often patients perceive dramatic improvements in their ability to breathe and their overall QOL. Should QOL improve, the patient may be able to tolerate more intensive treatment.

In summary, response-based adaptive RT shows a great promise to improve cancer control and reduce toxicity of RT. As a first randomized study, RTOG1106 has reached accrual goal of 138 patients in early 2017, and might provide milestone data establishing clinical efficacy of adaptive RT. More prospective and randomized trials are needed to evaluate biomarkers and their potential benefit for adaptive RT. It remains a challenge to combine toxicity prediction and tumor control probability prediction into an adaptive tool that truly optimizes RT for the benefit of the many lung cancer patients in the US and worldwide.

REFERENCES

1. Therasse, P. et al., New guidelines to evaluate the response to treatment in solid tumors. European Organization for Research and Treatment of Cancer, National Cancer Institute of the United States, National Cancer Institute of Canada. *J Natl Cancer Inst*, 2000. **92**(3): 205–16.
2. Eisenhauer, E.A. et al., New response evaluation criteria in solid tumours: Revised RECIST guideline (version 1.1). *Eur J Cancer*, 2009. **45**(2): 228–47.
3. Nishino, M. et al., CT tumor volume measurement in advanced non-small-cell lung cancer: Performance characteristics of an emerging clinical tool. *Acad Radiol*, 2011. **18**(1): 54–62.
4. Juweid, M.E. and B.D. Cheson, Positron-emission tomography and assessment of cancer therapy. *N Engl J Med*, 2006. **354**(5): 496–507.
5. Wahl, R.L. et al., From RECIST to PERCIST: Evolving considerations for PET response criteria in solid tumors. *J Nucl Med*, 2009. **50**(Suppl. 1): 122S–50.
6. Skougaard, K. et al., Comparison of EORTC criteria and PERCIST for PET/CT response evaluation of patients with metastatic colorectal cancer treated with irinotecan and cetuximab. *J Nucl Med*, 2013. **54**(7): 1026–31.
7. Wang, J. et al., Metabolic response assessment with F-FDG PET/CT: Inter-method comparison and prognostic significance for patients with non-small cell lung cancer. *J Radiat Oncol*, 2015. **4**(3): 249–56.

8. Werner-Wasik, M. et al., Assessment of lung cancer response after nonoperative therapy: Tumor diameter, bidimensional product, and volume. A serial CT scan-based study. *Int J Radiat Oncol Biol Phys*, 2001. **51**(1): 56–61.
9. Willner, J. et al., Dose, volume, and tumor control prediction in primary radiotherapy of non-small-cell lung cancer. *Int J Radiat Oncol Biol Phys*, 2002. **52**(2): 382–9.
10. Joo, J.H. et al., Definitive radiotherapy alone over 60 Gy for patients unfit for combined treatment to stage II-III non-small cell lung cancer: Retrospective analysis. *Radiat Oncol*, 2015. **10**(1): 250.
11. Mac Manus, M.P. et al., Positron emission tomography is superior to computed tomography scanning for response-assessment after radical radiotherapy or chemoradiotherapy in patients with non-small-cell lung cancer. *J Clin Oncol*, 2003. **21**(7): 1285–92.
12. Hellwig, D. et al., Value of F-18-fluorodeoxyglucose positron emission tomography after induction therapy of locally advanced bronchogenic carcinoma. *J Thorac Cardiovasc Surg*, 2004. **128**(6): 892–9.
13. Mac Manus, M.P. et al., Metabolic (FDG-PET) response after radical radiotherapy/chemoradiotherapy for non-small cell lung cancer correlates with patterns of failure. *Lung Cancer*, 2005. **49**(1): 95–108.
14. Eschmann, S.M. et al., Repeat 18F-FDG PET for monitoring neoadjuvant chemotherapy in patients with stage III non-small cell lung cancer. *Lung Cancer*, 2007. **55**(2): 165–71.
15. Eschmann, S.M. et al., 18F-FDG PET for assessment of therapy response and preoperative re-evaluation after neoadjuvant radio-chemotherapy in stage III non-small cell lung cancer. *Eur J Nucl Med Mol Imaging*, 2007. **34**(4): 463–71.
16. Kaira, K. et al., Prognostic impact of 18F-FDG uptake on PET in non-small cell lung cancer patients with postoperative recurrence following platinum-based chemotherapy. *Respir Investig*, 2014. **52**(2): 121–8.
17. Kaira, K. et al., Biological significance of 18F-FDG uptake on PET in patients with non-small-cell lung cancer. *Lung Cancer*, 2014. **83**(2): 197–204.
18. de Langen, A.J. et al., Monitoring response to antiangiogenic therapy in non-small cell lung cancer using imaging markers derived from PET and dynamic contrast-enhanced MRI. *J Nucl Med*, 2011. **52**(1): 48–55.
19. Hoopes, D.J. et al., FDG-PET and stereotactic body radiotherapy (SBRT) for stage I non-small-cell lung cancer. *Lung Cancer*, 2007. **56**(2): 229–34.
20. Cuaron, J., M. Dunphy, and A. Rimner, Role of FDG-PET scans in staging, response assessment, and follow-up care for non-small cell lung cancer. *Front Oncol*, 2012. **2**: 208.
21. Zhang, X. et al., Positron emission tomography for assessing local failure after stereotactic body radiotherapy for non-small-cell lung cancer. *Int J Radiat Oncol Biol Phys*, 2012. **83**(5): 1558–65.
22. Takeda, A. et al., Evaluation for local failure by 18F-FDG PET/CT in comparison with CT findings after stereotactic body radiotherapy (SBRT) for localized non-small-cell lung cancer. *Lung Cancer*, 2013. **79**(3): 248–53.
23. Abelson, J.A. et al., Metabolic imaging metrics correlate with survival in early stage lung cancer treated with stereotactic ablative radiotherapy. *Lung Cancer*, 2012. **78**(3): 219–24.
24. Lee, P. et al., Metabolic tumor volume is an independent prognostic factor in patients treated definitively for non-small-cell lung cancer. *Clin Lung Cancer*, 2012. **13**(1): 52–8.
25. Liao, S. et al., Prognostic value of metabolic tumor burden on 18F-FDG PET in nonsurgical patients with non-small cell lung cancer. *Eur J Nucl Med Mol Imaging*, 2012. **39**(1): 27–38.
26. Turrisi, A.T., 3rd, et al., Twice-daily compared with once-daily thoracic radiotherapy in limited small-cell lung cancer treated concurrently with cisplatin and etoposide. *N Engl J Med*, 1999. **340**(4): 265–71.
27. Manapov, F. et al., Primary tumor response to chemoradiotherapy in limited-disease small-cell lung cancer correlates with duration of brain-metastasis free survival. *J Neurooncol*, 2012. **109**(2): 309–14.
28. van Baardwijk, A. et al., Time trends in the maximal uptake of FDG on PET scan during thoracic radiotherapy. A prospective study in locally advanced non-small cell lung cancer (NSCLC) patients. *Radiother Oncol*, 2007. **82**(2): 145–52.
29. Mahasittiwat, P. et al., Metabolic tumor volume on PET reduced more than gross tumor volume on CT during radiotherapy in patients with non-small cell lung cancer treated with 3DCRT or SBRT. *J Radiat Oncol*, 2013. **2**(2): 191–202.
30. Kong, F.M. et al., A pilot study of [18F]fluorodeoxyglucose positron emission tomography scans during and after radiation-based therapy in patients with non small-cell lung cancer. *J Clin Oncol*, 2007. **25**(21): 3116–23.

31. Feng, M. et al., Using fluorodeoxyglucose positron emission tomography to assess tumor volume during radiotherapy for non-small-cell lung cancer and its potential impact on adaptive dose escalation and normal tissue sparing. *Int J Radiat Oncol Biol Phys*, 2009. **73**(4): 1228–34.
32. Harris, J.P. et al., Outcomes of modestly hypofractionated radiation for lung tumors: Pre- and midtreatment positron emission tomography-computed tomography metrics as prognostic factors. *Clin Lung Cancer*, 2015. **16**(6): 475–85.
33. Massaccesi, M. et al., 18 F-FDG PET-CT during chemo-radiotherapy in patients with non-small cell lung cancer: The early metabolic response correlates with the delivered radiation dose. *Radiat Oncol*, 2012. 7: 106.
34. Lee, J. et al., Early treatment volume reduction rate as a prognostic factor in patients treated with chemoradiotherapy for limited stage small cell lung cancer. *Radiat Oncol J*, 2015. **33**(2): 117–25.
35. Yan, D. et al., Computed tomography guided management of interfractional patient variation. *Semin Radiat Oncol*, 2005. **15**(3): 168–79.
36. Li, X.A. et al., Interfractional variations in patient setup and anatomic change assessed by daily computed tomography. *Int J Radiat Oncol Biol Phys*, 2007. **68**(2): 581–91.
37. Hugo, G.D., D. Yan, and J. Liang, Population and patient-specific target margins for 4D adaptive radiotherapy to account for intra- and inter-fraction variation in lung tumour position. *Phys Med Biol*, 2007. **52**(1): 257–74.
38. Kong F. M. et al., Effect of midtreatment PET/CT-adapted radiation therapy with concurrent chemotherapy in patients with locally advanced non-small-cell lung cancer: A phase 2 clinical trial. *JAMA oncology*, 2017; PubMed [journal] PMID: 28570742.
39. Mah, K. et al., Acute radiation-induced pulmonary damage: A clinical study on the response to fractionated radiation therapy. *Int J Radiat Oncol Biol Phys*, 1987. **13**(2): 179–88.
40. Boersma, L.J. et al., Recovery of overall and local lung function loss 18 months after irradiation for malignant lymphoma. *J Clin Oncol*, 1996. **14**(5): 1431–41.
41. Yankelevitz, D.F. et al., Lung cancer: Evaluation with MR imaging during and after irradiation. *J Thorac Imaging*, 1994. **9**(1): 41–6.
42. Ogasawara, N. et al., Perfusion characteristics of radiation-injured lung on Gd-DTPA-enhanced dynamic magnetic resonance imaging. *Invest Radiol*, 2002. **37**(8): 448–57.
43. Hicks, R.J. et al., Early FDG-PET imaging after radical radiotherapy for non-small-cell lung cancer: Inflammatory changes in normal tissues correlate with tumor response and do not confound therapeutic response evaluation. *Int J Radiat Oncol Biol Phys*, 2004. **60**(2): 412–8.
44. Guerrero, T. et al., Radiation pneumonitis: Local dose versus [18F]-fluorodeoxyglucose uptake response in irradiated lung. *Int J Radiat Oncol Biol Phys*, 2007. **68**(4): 1030–5.
45. Hart, J.P. et al., Radiation pneumonitis: Correlation of toxicity with pulmonary metabolic radiation response. *Int J Radiat Oncol Biol Phys*, 2008. **71**(4): 967–71.
46. Abdulla, S. et al., Quantitative assessment of global lung inflammation following radiation therapy using FDG PET/CT: A pilot study. *Eur J Nucl Med Mol Imaging*, 2014. **41**(2): 350–6.
47. McCurdy, M. et al., The role of lung lobes in radiation pneumonitis and radiation-induced inflammation in the lung: A retrospective study. *J Radiat Oncol*, 2013. **2**(2): 203–8.
48. McCurdy, M.R. et al., [18F]-FDG uptake dose-response correlates with radiation pneumonitis in lung cancer patients. *Radiother Oncol*, 2012. **104**(1): 52–7.
49. Mac Manus, M.P. et al., Association between pulmonary uptake of fluorodeoxyglucose detected by positron emission tomography scanning after radiation therapy for non-small-cell lung cancer and radiation pneumonitis. *Int J Radiat Oncol Biol Phys*, 2011. **80**(5): 1365–71.
50. Seppenwoolde, Y. et al., Regional differences in lung radiosensitivity after radiotherapy for non-small-cell lung cancer. *Int J Radiat Oncol Biol Phys*, 2004. **60**(3): 748–58.
51. Marks, L.B. et al., Radiation-induced pulmonary injury: Symptomatic versus subclinical endpoints. *Int J Radiat Biol*, 2000. **76**(4): 469–75.
52. Yuan, S.T. et al., Semiquantification and classification of local pulmonary function by V/Q single photon emission computed tomography in patients with non-small cell lung cancer: Potential indication for radiotherapy planning. *J Thorac Oncol*, 2011. **6**(1): 71–8.

53. Meng, X. et al., Changes in functional lung regions during the course of radiation therapy and their potential impact on lung dosimetry for non-small cell lung cancer. *Int J Radiat Oncol Biol Phys*, 2014. **89**(1): 145–51.
54. Maunoury, C. et al., Myocardial perfusion damage after mediastinal irradiation for Hodgkin's disease: A thallium-201 single photon emission tomography study. *Eur J Nucl Med*, 1992. **19**(10): 871–3.
55. Prosnitz, R.G. et al., Prospective assessment of radiotherapy-associated cardiac toxicity in breast cancer patients: Analysis of data 3 to 6 years after treatment. *Cancer*, 2007. **110**(8): 1840–50.
56. Zellars, R. et al., SPECT analysis of cardiac perfusion changes after whole-breast/chest wall radiation therapy with or without active breathing coordinator: Results of a randomized phase 3 trial. *Int J Radiat Oncol Biol Phys*, 2014. **88**(4): 778–85.
57. De Ruysscher, D. et al., Increased (18)F-deoxyglucose uptake in the lung during the first weeks of radiotherapy is correlated with subsequent Radiation-Induced Lung Toxicity (RILT): A prospective pilot study. *Radiother Oncol*, 2009. **91**(3): 415–20.
58. Yuan, S.T. et al., Changes in global function and regional ventilation and perfusion on SPECT during the course of radiotherapy in patients with non-small-cell lung cancer. *Int J Radiat Oncol Biol Phys*, 2012. **82**(4): e631–8.
59. Yuan, S. T. et al., Timing and intensity of changes in FDG uptake with symptomatic esophagitis during radiotherapy or chemo-radiotherapy. *Radiat Oncol*, 2014. 9(1):37. doi: 10.1186/1748-717X-9-37. PubMed PMID: 24467939; PubMed Central PMCID: PMC3996188.
60. Movsas, B. et al., Quality of life analysis of a radiation dose-escalation study of patients with non-small-cell lung cancer: A secondary analysis of the radiation therapy Oncology Group 0617 randomized clinical trial. *JAMA Oncol*, 2016 Mar. 2(3):359–67.
61. Ubels, R.J. et al., Quality of life during 5 years after stereotactic radiotherapy in stage I non-small cell lung cancer. *Radiat Oncol*, 2015. **10**: 98.
62. Kong, F. et al., Plasma transforming growth factor-beta1 level before radiotherapy correlates with long term outcome of patients with lung carcinoma. *Cancer*, 1999. **86**(9): 1712–9.
63. Zhao, L. et al., Changes of circulating transforming growth factor-beta1 level during radiation therapy are correlated with the prognosis of locally advanced non-small cell lung cancer. *J Thorac Oncol*, 2010. **5**(4): 521–5.
64. Ujiie, H. et al., Serum hepatocyte growth factor and interleukin-6 are effective prognostic markers for non-small cell lung cancer. *Anticancer Res*, 2012. **32**(8): 3251–8.
65. Chang, C.H. et al., Circulating interleukin-6 level is a prognostic marker for survival in advanced non-small cell lung cancer patients treated with chemotherapy. *Int J Cancer*, 2013. **132**(9): 1977–85.
66. Rube, C.E. et al., Increased expression of pro-inflammatory cytokines as a cause of lung toxicity after combined treatment with gemcitabine and thoracic irradiation. *Radiother Oncol*, 2004. 72(2): 231–41.
67. Anscher, M.S. et al., Plasma transforming growth factor beta1 as a predictor of radiation pneumonitis. *Int J Radiat Oncol Biol Phys*, 1998. **41**(5): 1029–35.
68. Arpin, D. et al., Early variations of circulating interleukin-6 and interleukin-10 levels during thoracic radiotherapy are predictive for radiation pneumonitis. *J Clin Oncol*, 2005. **23**(34): 8748–56.
69. Chen, Y. et al., Interleukin (IL)-1A and IL-6: Applications to the predictive diagnostic testing of radiation pneumonitis. *Int J Radiat Oncol Biol Phys*, 2005. **62**(1): 260–6.
70. Stenmark, M.H. et al., Combining physical and biologic parameters to predict radiation-induced lung toxicity in patients with non-small-cell lung cancer treated with definitive radiation therapy. *Int J Radiat Oncol Biol Phys*, 2012. **84**(2): e217–22.
71. Yuan, X. et al., Single nucleotide polymorphism at rs1982073:T869C of the TGFbeta 1 gene is associated with the risk of radiation pneumonitis in patients with non-small-cell lung cancer treated with definitive radiotherapy. *J Clin Oncol*, 2009. **27**(20): 3370–8.
72. Tucker, S.L. et al., Incorporating single-nucleotide polymorphisms into the Lyman model to improve prediction of radiation pneumonitis. *Int J Radiat Oncol Biol Phys*, 2013. **85**(1): 251–7.
73. Wang, W. et al., Single nucleotide polymorphisms in DNA repair genes may be associated with survival in patients with non-small cell lung cancer treated with definitive radiation therapy. *Int J Radiat Oncol Biol Phys*, 2012. **84**(3): S69.

74. Landi, M.T. et al., MicroRNA expression differentiates histology and predicts survival of lung cancer. *Clin Cancer Res*, 2010. **16**(2): 430–41.
75. Yu, S.L. et al., MicroRNA signature predicts survival and relapse in lung cancer. *Cancer Cell*, 2008. **13**(1): 48–57.
76. Vosa, U. et al., Identification of miR-374a as a prognostic marker for survival in patients with early-stage nonsmall cell lung cancer. *Genes Chromosomes Cancer*, 2011. **50**(10): 812–22.
77. Hermeking, H., The miR-34 family in cancer and apoptosis. *Cell Death Differ*, 2010. **17**(2): 193–9.
78. Sen, C.K. et al., Micromanaging vascular biology: Tiny microRNAs play big band. *J Vasc Res*, 2009. **46**(6): 527–40.
79. Yang, C. et al., Epigenetic silencing of miR-130b in ovarian cancer promotes the development of multidrug resistance by targeting colony-stimulating factor 1. *Gynecol Oncol*, 2012. **124**(2): 325–34.
80. Franchina, T. et al., Circulating miR-22, miR-24 and miR-34a as novel predictive biomarkers to pemetrexed-based chemotherapy in advanced non-small cell lung cancer. *J Cell Physiol*, 2014. **229**(1): 97–9.
81. Bi, N. et al., Serum miRNA signature to identify a patient's resistance to high-dose radiation therapy for unresectable non-small cell lung cancer., in 2013 ASCO Annual Meeting. 2013, *J Clin Oncol*. suppl; abstr 7580.
82. Bi, N. et al., Serum microRNA as a predictive marker for radiation pneumonitis in patients with inoperable/unresectable non-small cell lung cancer (NSCLC). *Int J Radiat Oncol Biol Phys*, 2013. **87**(2): S93.
83. Schipper, M.J. et al., Personalized dose selection in radiation therapy using statistical models for toxicity and efficacy with dose and biomarkers as covariates. *Stat Med*, 2014. **33**(30): 5330–9.

17

Adaptive radiation therapy for lung cancer

MARTHA MATUSZAK, KRISTY K. BROCK,
AND FENG-MING (SPRING) KONG

17.1 INTRODUCTION

There is great potential for change during a course of radiation therapy for lung cancer patients. As discussed in Chapter 12, there are many different sources of uncertainty in image-guided lung radiation therapy, making it possible that the desired treatment plan may not be fully realized from the initial planning. As discussed in Chapter 16, lung tumors and normal tissues respond to treatment, which could render the original plan unable to meet the original goals of radiation therapy or prompt the treatment team to alter the original plan goals to better customize therapy to the individual patient. Table 17.1 summarizes some of the sources of data that can be used to trigger or drive a plan adaption for lung cancer.

Depending on the time scale and potential impact of changes noted during lung radiation therapy, different types of interventions are possible. The earliest form of adaptive therapy, which we now consider simple image-guided radiation therapy (IGRT), would be translating or rotating the patient based on daily imaging. More recently, adaptive therapy is an intervention that changes or adapts the patient's current treatment plan. Adaptations to treatment plans largely fall into categories of online and offline. Online adaptations, which are discussed in Section 17.2.1, are applied at the time of treatment, in a time-frame on the order of minutes. As shown in Figure 17.1, online adaptations are considered a tight inner loop closely tied to the original or

Table 17.1 Sources of data that may motivate adaptive radiation therapy

Category	Description	Scope	Example
Relative geometric	Change in patient geometry that alters the relative relationship between structures	Local	Esophagus position shifted toward target
Absolute geometric	Change in patient geometry that alters the viability of the dose calculation	Local or Global	Change in atelectasis or pleural effusion
Relative global biomarker	Change in biomarker value versus baseline that indicates a difference in patient's radio-sensitivity	Global	Week 4 Baseline cytokine value that indicates greater risk for pneumonitis
Local functional	Measurement of local tumor or normal tissue function	Local	Metabolic imaging of tumor or ventilation imaging of lung

initial treatment plan. Typically, online adaptations are designed to preserve the original treatment goals and correct for geometric differences between the treatment planning scan and the patient's geometry at the time of treatment. Offline adaptations are typically performed on the timescale of days, and shown outside of the daily treatment loop in Figure 17.1. These adaptations could also be applied to account for geometric differences, but those that are likely to be persistent over multiple treatments. In addition, many radiation therapy centers do not have the resources to apply online adaptations and therefore rely on offline adaptation (discussed in Section 17.2.2) to correct for daily uncertainty that has accumulated. Offline adaptive therapy can also be initiated to account for treatment response. This response could be global, such as a change in a blood biomarker, or local, such as a change identified in a functional image dataset. Chapter 16 covered a variety of tumor and normal-tissue response imaging and metrics that can serve as the motivation for an offline adaptation for lung cancer. It is more common in offline adaptive therapy that the treatment goals will change based on new information and the baseline treatment planning goals will become obsolete or updated.

Online and offline adaptation require many of the same tools, but also many unique ones. Both strategies and the tools and resources required to perform them will be covered throughout this chapter. In Section 17.2, online and offline adaptive strategies and requirements will be described. Section 17.3 will cover the tools needed to perform adaptive therapy effectively, including image registration, treatment planning, and dose accumulation. Finally, Section 17.4 will focus on the topic of quality assurance for adaptive treatments.

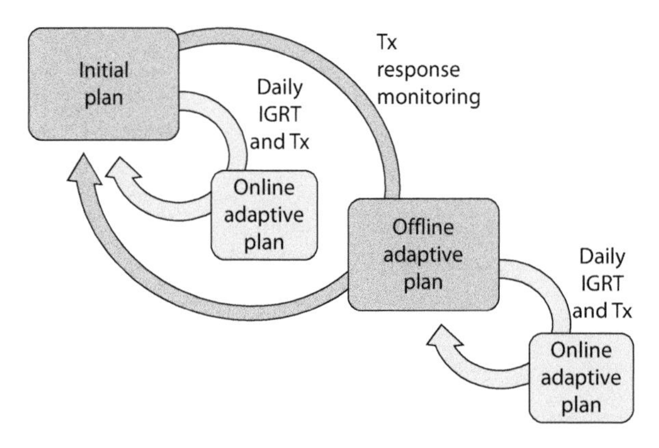

Figure 17.1 The timescale loops of adaptive therapy showing an online adaptive plan tightly coupled to the initial treatment planning and daily IGRT cycle as well as the offline adaptive loop, happening on an extended loop outside of the daily treatment process.

17.2 STRATEGIES FOR ADAPTIVE THERAPY

17.2.1 ONLINE ADAPTIVE THERAPY

Online adaptive therapy is the utilization of a real-time intervention to the treatment plan and/or delivery to account for changes (i.e. geometric or functional) that are not able to be resolved by image-guided setup with translation or acceptable rotations of the patient. Online adaptation has been well studied in some body sites, such as prostate, due to the ability to dynamically alter the treatment apertures to maximize target coverage while sparing the rectal interface. Similar tracking methods are being studied in lung patients, although beam's-eye view tracking can be challenging without resolvable contrast differences or landmarks for accurate localization. Bryant et al. have shown promising results with a two-dimensional/three-dimensional (2D/3D) tracking method on lung lesions [1]. Such a method could be used for real-time adaptive therapy for lung stereotactic body radiation therapy (SBRT) patients to track real-time breathing motion as well as adapt 3D conformal radiation therapy (3D-CRT) beam apertures to the current target. Such methods with and without the use of markers are currently in use commercially as part of lung SBRT treatment with a robotic linear accelerator [2,3]. Marker-less tracking remains challenging in some patient geometries regardless of imaging improvements such as dual energy imaging [4]. For patients with identifiable tumors based on marker or soft tissue imaging during delivery, online adaptations and tracking can be used to account for changes in respiration excursion at the time of treatment that cannot be mitigated by IGRT treatment couch or patient shifts prior to treatment delivery. Hugo et al. studied changes in diaphragm position in 10 patients and determined that while most changes in daily breathing motion do not require adaptation, some patients may experience larger changes that require intervention beyond IGRT [5]. In some cases, simple aperture-based adaptations may be possible, but more work is needed for target areas with poor contrast or plans that utilize intensity modulation such as intensity-modulated radiation therapy (IMRT) and volumetric modulated arc therapy (VMAT). Similar work by Ruben et al. showed that approximately 19% of SBRT patients studied may experience clinically relevant changes in breathing motion and could benefit from tracking or re-planning [6]. Figure 17.2, from Colvill et al. showed examples of real-time tumor tracking for lung SBRT patients over different platforms [7]. Typical and atypical patterns of respiratory motion and excursion are possible. In the Colvill study, 10 participating institutions with varying equipment could adapt based on tracking methods. Each institution is summarized in Table 17.2.

Tracking-based methods aim to track the tumor during respiratory motion by moving the patient or the treatment beam. Such methods do not typically require a recalculation or a optimization of the treatment plan, and have been proven, across different platforms, to be accurate within conventionally acceptable patient-specific quality assurance passing rates. Use of tracking-based adaptations in early-stage lung cancer in the context of few fraction SBRT treatments can reduce the amount of normal lung (and potentially other organs-at-risk [OAR]) in the treatment beam thus minimizing the irradiated area without unduly increasing the chances for a geometric miss. Such systems must have accurate imaging and tracking algorithms.

While tracking-based adaptations can be highly successful in early-stage lung cancer radiotherapy, tracking more advanced stage disease is potentially more challenging due to the increased chance for larger anatomic changes and tumor response over the increased time course of treatment. Conditions such as atelectasis and pleural effusion also may not only drastically alter the local anatomy, but can also affect the viability of the dose calculated on the treatment planning CT. Therefore, online adaptive therapy for many lung cancer patients requires the ability to perform fast-dose calculations and re-planning. Figure 17.3 demonstrates a more advanced online adaptive planning strategy, in which the daily patient characteristics are monitored which may or may not trigger an adaptation. With the increasing use of advanced intensity modulated techniques for lung cancer treatment, fast optimization or inverse planning is generally required during the adaptive planning step. The technology for real-time dose calculation and optimization is available, although commercial implementations are limited. Graphics Processing Units (GPU) and cloud-computing strategies have both shown promise in this area, with dose calculations and plan optimization times on the orders of seconds to less than 3 minutes [8,9]. Online re-planning with inverse optimization requires updated input

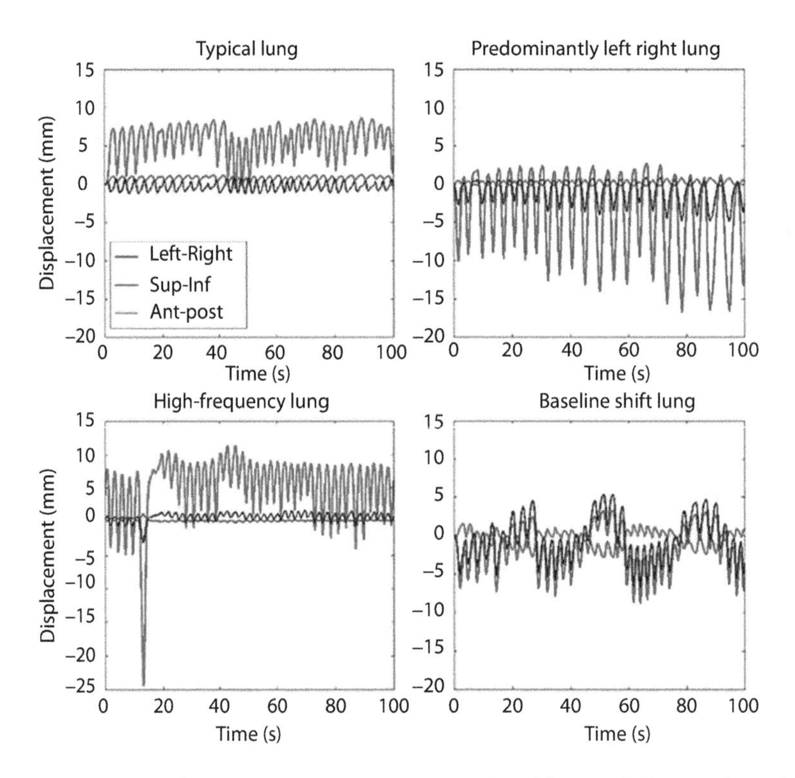

Figure 17.2 Patient-measured lung SBRT tumor traces. (Reproduced from Colvill, E. et al., *Radiother Oncol*, 119, 159–165, 2016, under open-access permissions.)

from the online information, typically in the form of updated segmentation or contours. Physician contouring for real-time adaptation is likely to be too time-consuming to be used for online re-planning. Therefore, some level of automation with respect to segmentation is necessary for efficient re-planning. Transfer of contours via deformable image registration (DIR) (to be discussed further in Section 17.3.2) with a validated algorithm is a common approach. Fast image registration and segmentation methods are becoming available through modern computing and have been quoted on the order of seconds [10]. While review of automatically segmented or transferred volumes is essential to the online adaptive quality assurance process, automated methods continue to improve and clinical use and acceptance of accurate, fast methods for automated segmentation are likely to become more widespread soon [11].

17.2.2 Offline adaptive therapy

As described in Figure 17.1, offline adaptive therapy is performed on a longer timescale than online adaptive therapy. Both correction-based and response-based adaptations can be done via offline adaptive radiation therapy. Generally, if the goal of adaptation is to preserve the baseline planning goals, then the adaption is performed due to geometric changes and considered a correction-based adaptation. This means that the baseline goal has not changed, although the geometry has altered so that the baseline goals may no longer be able to be achieved. Correction-based adaptations can also be made via online adaptive therapy, but large geometric changes that require additional evaluation that cannot be achieved in a short time frame may warrant an offline approach. Figure 17.4 illustrates a generic offline adaptive planning approach in which updated information is considered to determine whether a re-planning is required. Then, the adaptive planning is executed while the original plan continues until the quality assurance on the adaptive plan is complete.

The extreme version of a correction-based offline adaptation would be re-planning prior to each treatment fraction to account for dose errors that have accumulated to-date. This would require methods to (1) track the breathing motion and patient geometry at the time of treatment and (2) calculate and accumulate dose-to-date

Table 17.2 Institution-Specific Materials and Methods for Adaptive Tracking

Adaption type	Institution	System version	Planning system	Treatment type	Motion guidance	Motion platform	Dosimetry phantom	Degrees of Freedom (Lung/ Prostate)
Robotic tracking	University Clinic Schleswig-Holstein	CyberKnife®	Multiplan	Robotic	kV and optical imaging	Custom	Octavius	3D/3D
	Stanford University	CyberKnife	Multiplan	Robotic	kV and optical imaging	CIRS dynamic phantom	Stereotactic dose verification phantom	1D/1D
Gimbaled tracking	Kyoto University Hospital	Vero	iPLAN	IMRT	kV and optical imaging	Quasar (prostate) Custom (lung)	IMRT	4D/1D
	University Hospital, Brussels	Vero	iPLAN	Conformal	kV and optical imaging	BrainLab gating phantom	Quasar respiratory phantom	1D
MLC tracking	Nortern Sydney Cancer Centre	Varian Trilogy Millennium MLC	Eclipse	VMAT	Calypso®	HexaMotion	Delta4	3D/3D
	Aarhus University Hospital	Varian Truebeam Millennium MLC	Eclipse	VMAT	Calypso	HexaMotion	Delta4	3D/3D
	Rigshospitalet, Copenhagen	Varian Novalis Tx HD MLC	Eclipse	VMAT	Optical ExacTrac®	HexaMotion	Delta4	3D/3D
	Institute of Cancer Research, London	Elekta Synergy Agility MLC	Pinnacle	IMRT	Motion platform	Custom	Delta4	3D/3D
Couch tracking	University Hospital, Zurich	Varian Trilogy Protura couch	Eclipse	VMAT	Optical	HexaMotion	Delta4	4D/2D
	University Hospital of Würzburg	Elekta Synergy HexaPod couch	Pinnacle	VMAT	Optical	HexaPod	ArcCHECK	3D/3D

Source: Reproduced with open-access permissions from Colvill, E. et al., *Radiother Oncol*, 119, 159–165, 2016.
IMRT = Intensity modulated radiation therapy.
VMAT = Volumetric modulated are therapy.
kV = kilovoltage.
D = Degrees of freedom.
4D = Three degrees of freedom of dosimeter with 1D external surrogate motion.

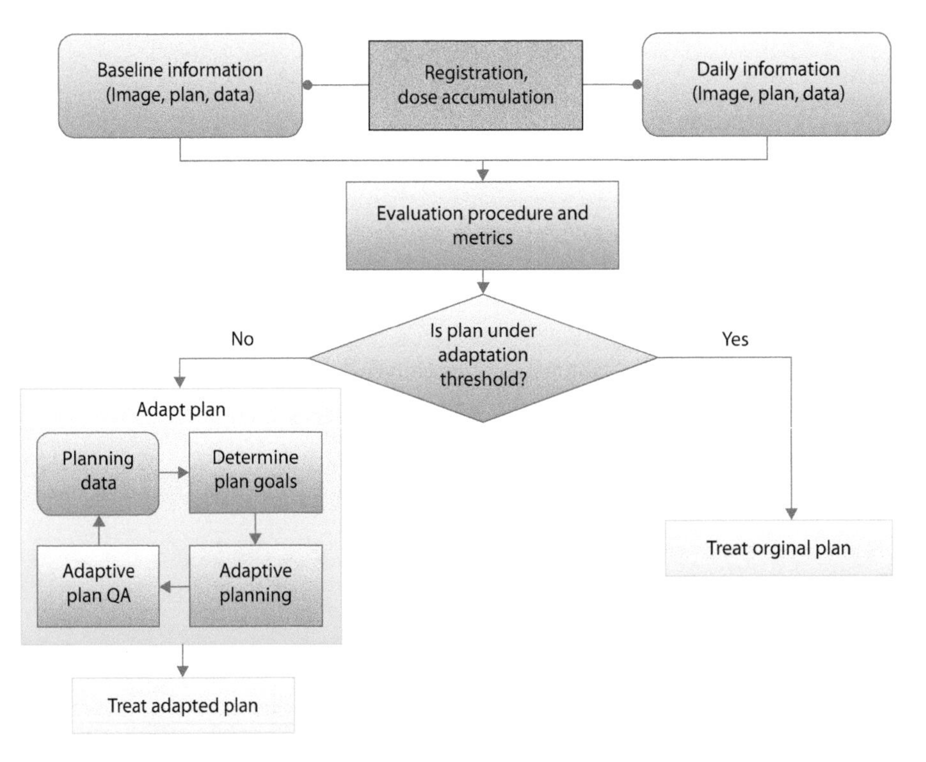

Figure 17.3 Workflow for daily plan evaluation and potential adaptation.

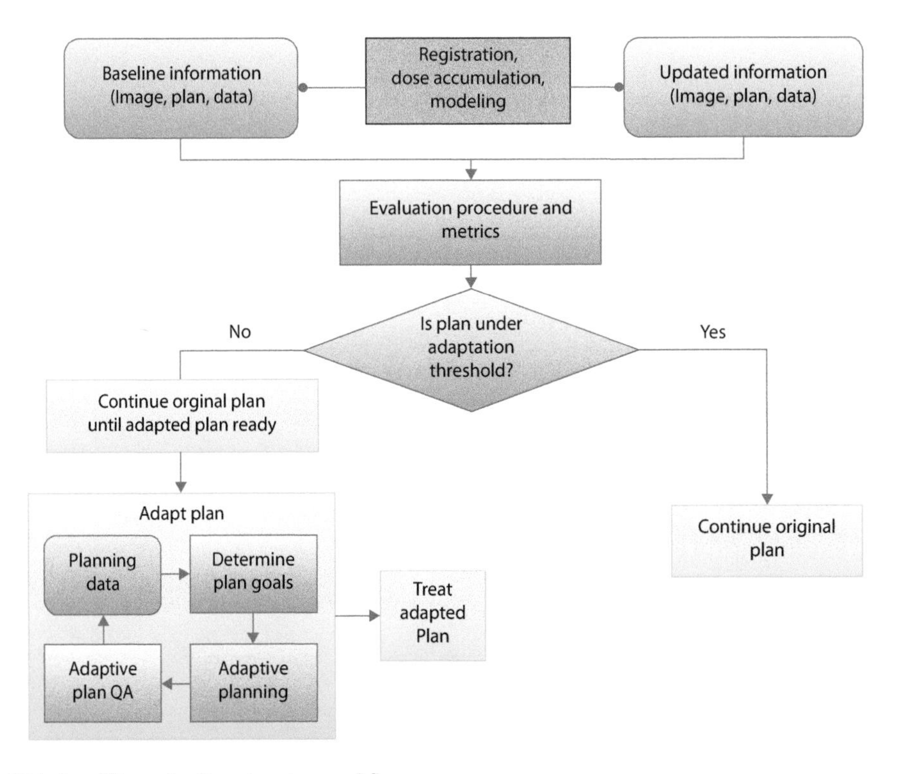

Figure 17.4 An offline adaptive planning workflow.

using image registration techniques and (3) re-plan considering the current dose and cumulative limits. While a seemingly idealized adaptive treatment scenario, Mišić and Chan caution planners about employing such a strategy to account for respiration-based changes [12]. As one would expect, daily dose-reactive planning, can accumulate tumor under and overdoses throughout treatment, potentially leading to a more heterogeneous, and potentially less biologically effective composite treatment. Thus, proper biologically corrected objectives that penalize unwanted features of the composite dose distribution must be applied to circumvent deleterious side effects of adaptive planning. In addition, the benefits of daily re-planning, even when including response-based adaptation may be small in magnitude relative to the benefits of a single adaptation or weekly adaptations [13]. However, Kim and Philips demonstrated the potential improvements in tumor control probability when performing daily re-planning in the lung, using a predictive model to describe tumor shrinkage [14]. Re-planning daily showed an improvement in tumor equivalent uniform doses, although the feasibility of online planning was not addressed. Typically, stochastic optimization algorithms, such as the one employed by Kim and Philips, are better suited for offline timescales.

Correction-based adaptations are common, if not required, in proton therapy. In proton treatment for lung cancer, at least weekly evaluation of the patient's geometry is highly recommended to evaluate the impact of geometric changes on the proton dose distribution. While robust planning methods can improve the viability of the original plan, rescanning and adaptation of treatment are necessary in many lung cancer patients treated with protons [15]. Figure 17.5 shows a typical adaptive process undertaken in a proton therapy setting, with many similarities to current mainstream adaptive photon therapy. Here, a lung plan is shown on the original CT geometry. After an adaptive simulation CT, dose from the original plan can be

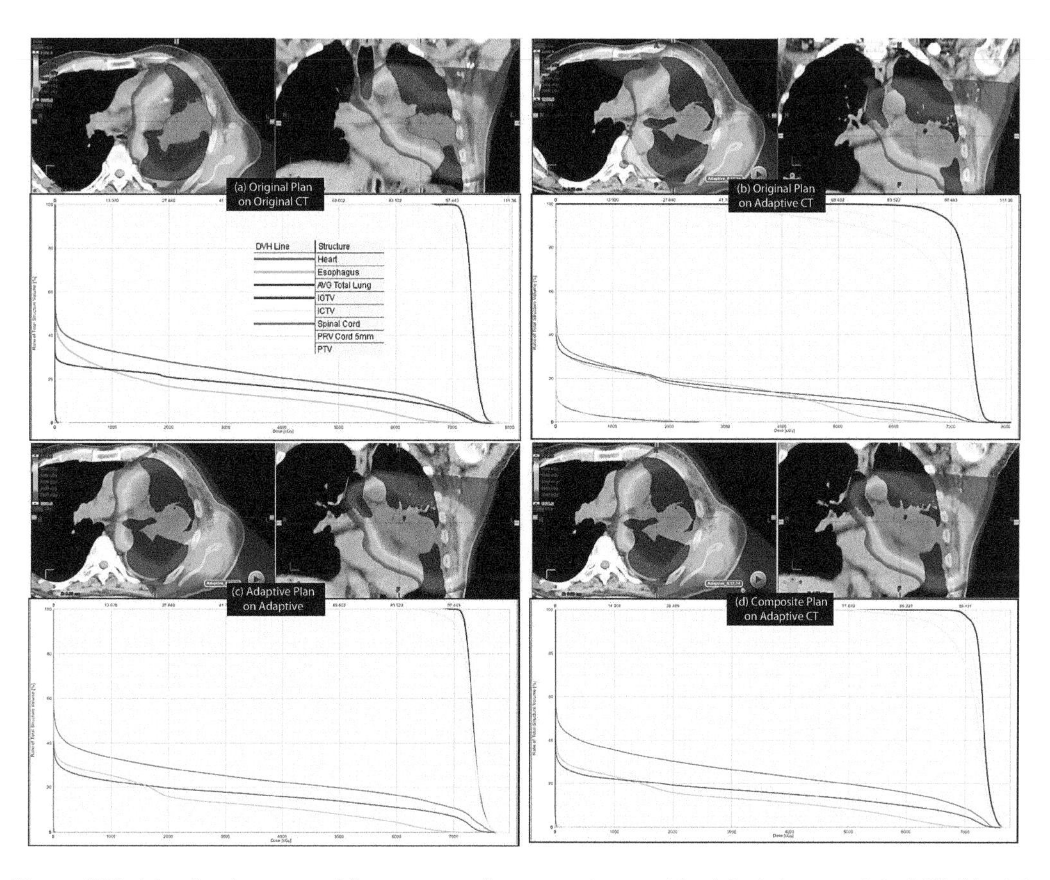

Figure 17.5 Adaptive therapy workflow common for proton therapy. (a) original plan on original CT, (b) original plan calculated on the adaptive CT, (c) an adaptive plan displayed on the adaptive CT and (d) composite dose accumulated and displayed on adaptive CT. (Courtesy of Cody Wages and Radhe Mohan, MD Anderson Cancer Center.)

calculated on the adaptive CT for dose evaluation (b) and potential re-planning (c). Finally, multiple methods can be used to compute the composite dose (d).

A response-based adaptation is defined as the process of generating an adapted treatment plan to account for observed response of the target(s) and/or normal tissue(s). Although there is potential for an online response-based adaptive workflow, there is little work describing such a procedure and none are currently implemented in clinical practice.

The full workflow for an ideal generalized offline adaptation is shown in Figure 17.4. Starting with an existing treatment plan calculated on the simulation image, new information about the patient becomes available that makes the initial treatment plan no longer acceptable. That information usually falls into one of the categories listed in Table 17.1.

There are several reasons for choosing an offline adaptation over an online procedure. First, the type of data triggering the adaptation may be gathered over time, or not available until a given time in treatment. Second, there are challenges with online adaptation that are alleviated by eliminating the need to re-plan while the patient is on the table for treatment.

Weiss et al. studied the potential for dose escalation via offline adaptive therapy by retrospectively re-planning 10 cases at two time points during conventionally fractionated treatment [16]. DIR (see Section 17.3.2.2) was used to propagate the initial clinical target volume (CTV) from the pre-treatment planning CT to the week 2 and week 4 scans. The mid-ventilation phase from four-dimensional CT (4D-CT) was used in all cases. A simultaneous integrated boost was tested in the last 8 fractions. This study showed considerable reduction of the primary tumor and lymph node volumes (39% and 51%), which were like reductions noted by Kataria et al. in a prospective 15-patient study and Berkovic in a 41-patient report [17,18]. Weiss et al. found relatively smaller changes in the warped CTVs from baseline to week 4 (179 cc versus 184 cc). Attributable to this small difference in CTV, the difference in target dose for the non-adapted and adapted PTVs was only 1 Gy. When dose escalating up to iso-toxic levels, there was a strong potential to increase the dose to the week 4 primary tumor volumes. However, this was possible only when treating up to the normal tissue tolerance levels. Other authors have proposed the use of alternate imaging modalities, such as fludeoxyglucose Positron Emission Tomography (FDG-PET) or fluorothymidine PET (FLT-PET), to define a boost region for adaptive lung radiotherapy. These potentially smaller adaptive targets may allow for boosting without having to increase dose to normal tissues compared to the conventional 60 Gy in 30 fractions that is considered the current standard of care in locally advanced non-small-cell lung cancer (NSCLC) [19]. One such example of applying an FDG-PET response-based offline adaptation is Radiation Therapy Oncology Group (RTOG) Trial 1106, in which a 30-fraction treatment course for definitive NSCLC patients is adapted after the first 21 fractions based on an adaptive PET scan. In this trial, the adaptive PET imaging is acquired approximately 3 days prior to the start of the adaptive plan. An adaptive PET boost target is defined and transferred back to the original treatment planning CT using rigid image registration prior to adaptive planning.

Berkovic stratified patients using sequential versus concurrent chemotherapy and determined that the most favorable time point for adaptation in a 35 fraction course was at 15–20 fractions based on the maximum possible gain calculated in normal lung metrics after re-planning at various time points. Re-planning in this study did not consider density changes, and used only rigid alignment.

In the study by Kataria et al. adaptive planning was performed after 44–46 Gy with re-planning done on the new scan only with manual re-contouring, and no attempt to cover the original CTV volume. In their study, reductions in normal tissue dose metrics were considerable, with improvements ranging from 19% to 81% in various metrics for lung, heart, esophagus, and spinal cord. However, it is important to note that the study did not utilize 4DCT simulation and relied on internal target volume (ITV) expansions to account for motion. When not attempting dose escalation or considering an initial clinical tumor volume, re-planning based on a reduction in tumor volume alone, such as performed retrospectively on 40 lung SBRT patients by Qin et al., may result in an appreciable decrease in normal tissue doses and thus potentially decrease the risk of toxicity [20]. In their study of 3–5 fraction lung SBRT patients, the average ITV decrease was approximately 20% although there was a large range and 15% of patients saw growth in the ITV. Similar reductions were noted in 25 tumors by Bhatt et al. with all tumors responding [21]. Retrospective re-planning showed a reduction in fractional dose to chest wall and lung of 10%–30%. This highlights the importance of monitoring, as both increased and decreased ITV may signal a need for adaptation. In the Qin study, adaptive planning was performed using the same coverage and conformity goals as the initial treatment using cone beam CT (CBCT). The latter can be challenging in situations where the smaller CBCT field of view (FOV) and difference in CT number histogram make it difficult to perform accurate dose calculation. Mitigations of these issues are discussed in Section 17.3.1. In work by Persoon et al., the electronic portal imaging device (EPID) was used to monitor patients with atelectasis and trigger further evaluation and re-planning if needed [22]. Out of five patients monitored with atelectasis, four needed adaptations due to changes in CTV coverage attributed to deformations and shifts caused by a change in the atelectasis. In this work, the EPID dose evaluation and CBCT anatomic images were used as triggers for re-planning. Adaptive planning was performed on newly acquired FDG-PET/CT simulation scans after manual contouring. In a larger study of 163 lung patients with CBCTs, 23% of patients were scored as having lung changes attributed to atelectasis, pleural effusion, or pneumonia/pneumonitis on a retrospective evaluation [23]. Slightly over half (12% total) benefitted from an adaptive plan and most of those were due to atelectasis. Significant density changes altering the dose calculations were noted in 9% of patients (Figure 17.6). This study highlights the importance of monitoring that can quickly and appropriately trigger an adaptive planning process in cases that would benefit.

Kwint et al. have implemented such a fast evaluation protocol and presented its performance on 177 conventionally fractionated and slightly hypo-fractionated lung cancer patients [24]. One-hundred-twenty-eight patients were found to have thoracic changes during treatment. Table 17.3 summarizes the changes observed. Of the changes noted, 12% were classified as requiring immediate response while 8% of patients were classified as requiring re-planning after obtaining a new CBCT scan.

Brink et al., for example, commissioned an automated, de-formable, image registration–based technique to predict CBCT measured tumor response, which appeared to be correlated to individual patient and tumor characteristics [25]. Somewhat surprisingly, in their work, large tumor regressions were associated with poor local control and overall survival. Further analyses such as these will become important not only in monitoring patients to signal a need for adaptation, but also in helping to personalize the adaptation for an individual patient.

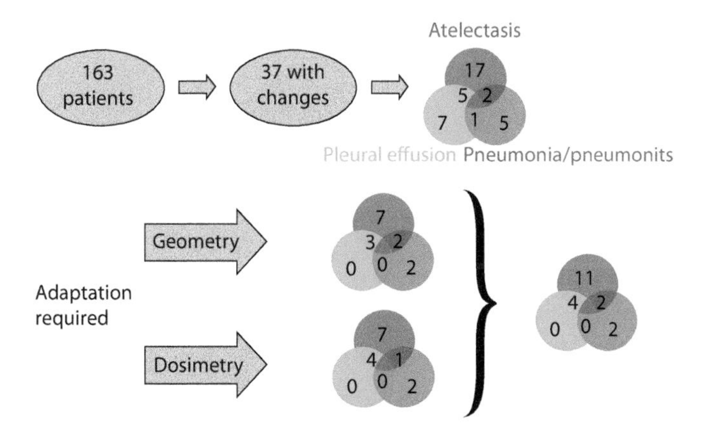

Figure 17.6 Diagram showing 37 out of 163 patients with lung density changes. In the upper part, 37 patients were divided into three types: atelectasis (red circle), pneumonia/pneumonitis (blue circle), and pleural effusion (green circle). Some patients have two different types of changes represented by a number in the overlap zone of the two circles, e.g., 5 patients have both an atelectasis and a pleural effusion. The lower part shows the results of the geometric and dosimetric evaluation of the 37 patients. The geometry- and the dosimetry-arrows lead to two Venn diagrams, dividing the changes with geometric or dosimetric impact into the three types. The final Venn diagram shows the total number of patients in the different categories requiring an adaptive treatment plan due to either dosimetry, geometry or both. (Reproduced with permissions from Møller, D.S. et al., *Radiother Oncol*, 110, 517–22, 2014.)

Table 17.3 Intrathoracic anatomical changes (N = 210) in 128 patients

ITACs	N (%)
Atelectasis developing/ increasing	28 (13)
Atelectasis resolving/decreasing	12 (6)
Tumor baseline shift	56 (27)
Infiltrative changes	6 (3)
Tumor regression	73 (35)
Tumor progression	22 (10)
Pleural effusion	13 (6)
Total	210 (100)

Source: Reproduced with permission from Kwint, M. et al., *Radiother Oncol*, 113, 392–397, 2014.

17.3 TOOLS FOR ADAPTIVE THERAPY

17.3.1 Imaging

Reliable task-oriented imaging is an important component of adaptive therapy. For patients with lung cancer, as well as most other sites treated with radiation therapy, CT imaging serves as a modality to provide electron density information for dose calculations for initial and adaptive planning. 4DCT can be used to evaluate changes in breathing motion or tumor excursion during treatment. Since changes in lung function are common, and many times are the reason for an adaptation in lung cancer therapy, repeat evaluation of respiratory motion is essential. Figure 17.7 demonstrates the change in excursion noted on 4DCT after approximately two-thirds of a course of concurrent chemo radiotherapy for a NSCLC patient being treated over 30 fractions.

Tumor response is commonly imaged not only via CT, but also with FDG-PET imaging, as discussed in more detail in Chapter 16. Thus, PET/CT is an important modality in adaptive lung radiotherapy based on tumor response. The Radiation Therapy Oncology Group (RTOG, now part of NRG Oncology) trial 1106 is currently studying PET adaptive radiation therapy versus standard radiation therapy in locally advanced NSCLC patients. It is important to note that delineation of tumor volumes based on PET is subject to volume averaging effects in smaller and more mobile tumors. Thus, 4DCT PET can be considered to mitigate motion effects. Other imaging modalities that can be used to measure tumor response are covered in Chapter 16.

Finally, imaging for normal tissue function can also be an important aspect of adaptive therapy, especially when the adaptation is based on functional avoidance or response. For example, CT, PET, and single-photon emission computed tomography (SPECT) can each be used for ventilation and perfusion imaging of the lung. Such information can be used in functional avoidance planning and adaptation. Care should be taken in image registration and segmentation with respect to the breathing state at acquisition and for treatment planning and delivery. More detail on functional imaging modalities in lung is given in Chapter 16.

17.3.2 Image registration for adaptation therapy

Image registration is an essential step in adaptive therapy. Image guidance is discussed throughout this book and image registration is a key component. For adaptive therapy, selection of an appropriate image registration strategy, commissioning of the chosen strategy, and proper clinical use, is extremely important. For tracking applications or daily alignment of adaptive patients, rigid image registration is generally acceptable. However, lung patients often experience tumor shrinkage and potentially drastic changes in normal tissue anatomy that render rigid registration inadequate [14,26–29]. In these situations, which can be the trigger

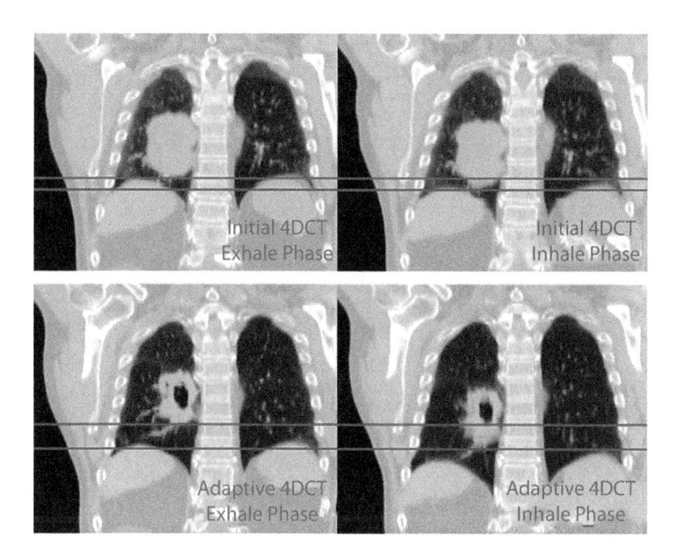

Figure 17.7 Notable change in tumor excursion during treatment for an adaptive lung patient imaged with 4DCT.

for an adaptation, DIR is needed. DIR can be applied to map either contours or doses from one dataset to another. Image registration can also aid in fusing information from multi-modality images together to better use the information for adaptive planning. To use image registration for either purpose, one must choose (1) a similarity metric to judge the "goodness" of the registration process, (2) a transformation method to describe the voxel to voxel transformation between two image sets, and (3) an optimization algorithm to find the best parameters for the transformation that result in the maximum similarity metric between the two datasets [30,31]. The question of how "good" is "good enough" is often raised in the discussion of DIR. This is a question that is complex to answer, with many factors dictating the impact of the uncertainty [32]. Ideally, the DIR algorithm is accurate in all areas to within an imaging voxel. This would ensure that all contours and dose assessments were not influenced by error. However, as with all processes, we must balance uncertainty with impact. The impact of DIR uncertainty depends on the application and the relationship of the uncertainty to the quantity that is being impacted by the DIR uncertainty. For example, DIR uncertainty for dose assessment of more than 1 voxel in a high-dose gradient for evaluation of the dose in a serial structure, such as the spinal cord, may have significant clinical consequences [32–35]. However, DIR uncertainty for contour propagation for daily dose assessment in a parallel structure, such as the lung, may have less of an impact. This is still an area of investigation and we must be mindful of the uncertainties in DIR and their propagation into the applications that use DIR results. DIR has three main applications in adaptive lung radiotherapy: (1) contour propagation, (2) multi-modality image registration, and (3) dose mapping and accumulation. The accuracy requirements are different for each application.

17.3.2.1 CONTOUR PROPAGATION

Adaptive treatment planning increases the contour burden as the number of adaptations increases. To manage the time required for contouring on the new treatment planning image, DIR can be used to propagate the contours from the initial planning scan onto the secondary treatment planning scan. Intensity-based image registration algorithms (e.g. normalized correlation coefficient or mean squared difference) are often employed for this purpose [36–38]. The rich contrast inherent to the lung CT image increases the probability that the registration at the boundary of the structures (e.g. the tumor within the lung, the boundary of the lung, and the spinal canal) will have a high level of accuracy. The accuracy requirements for DIR used for contour propagation is less stringent than that needed for multi-modality image registration and dose mapping and accumulation, as the accuracy is only relevant at the boundary of the structure. In addition, unlike the other two applications, certain areas that lack accuracy can be manually adjusted.

Commissioning of DIR for contour propagation should demonstrate the following three criteria: (1) the integrity of the propagated structure is maintained, (2) the accuracy of the propagated contour is within the inter-observer contour variation, and (3) the propagation process leads to a more efficient clinical workflow.

To determine the integrity of the propagated structure, registrations with different degrees of deformation should be performed between images of the same and different slice thicknesses. The propagated structures should be evaluated to ensure that the structure is properly recognized by the treatment planning system (e.g. volume, center of mass, etc. are correct), and that the application of the DIR to the structure does not result in a disruption to the boundary of the contour (e.g. holes within the contour, fragments, or artifacts).

Quantifying the accuracy of the propagated contour should be performed relative to the inter-observer contour variation when the accuracy is assessed on a clinical image where the ground truth is not known. That is, given the statistical distribution of variations observed between experts contouring the same structure on the same image, if the distribution does not change when replacing a randomly selected observer with the results of the DIR propagated contour, then the accuracy of the DIR algorithm to propagate the contour is within the accuracy of the inter-observer uncertainty. If this can be demonstrated to be a consistent result for a structure and registration method, then the propagated contours can be used without modification. If this criterion cannot be met, the contours should be carefully reviewed by a trained expert and edited as needed.

The final step in commissioning DIR for contour propagation is to ensure that the process improves clinical efficiency. If the DIR propagated contours require substantial editing and the editing tools are not well developed, the process may not improve efficiency. It is, therefore, important to study the impact of the DIR-based contour propagation on the clinical workflow when establishing the adaptive radiotherapy in lung cancer.

17.3.2.2 MULTI-MODALITY IMAGE REGISTRATION

Adaptive radiotherapy in the lung is often performed based on functional imaging, specifically PET, to identify the active region of the tumor and/or function of the lung. Typically, PET images are obtained in combination with CT images, which can then be used to guide the registration. The PET image itself, which is typically obtained during free breathing, is challenging to use directly for the registration given the lack of anatomical information as well as the incorporation of breathing motion into the image. Registration, either rigid or deformable, of the functional image (via the CT associated with the PET) to the planning CT image at the time of initial treatment planning is relatively straightforward.

Several DIR algorithms have been shown to have an average accuracy on the order of 1–2 voxel, including intensity-based methods that rely on spline-based transformation or free-form deformation and biomechanically-based models [26,27,39,40]. However, many algorithms also report maximum errors on the order of several voxels [41–43]. Commissioning of DIR between CT and PET-CT has two primary requirements: (1) accuracy in the DIR determined using target registration error (TRE) as well as contour propagation assessment, described above; and (2) accuracy in the application of the DIR to the functional image (e.g. the PET).

Standard DIR commissioning techniques can be employed to evaluate the registration of the CT to CT component of the registration. TRE can be easily performed in the lung, given the wealth of anatomical landmarks that can be identified using the bronchial bifurcations. Most commercial deformable registration algorithms allow the users to select points and efficiently evaluate the registration results within the software. It is important to assess the accuracy of the DIR for multi-modality image registration in the context of the use of the final images. If the functional image is being utilized to define the boundary of the tumor volume, then the accuracy around the boundary of the tumor is the area of importance and should be carefully evaluated. However, if the functional image is to be used to evaluate the local function of the lung, for functional avoidance of dose, then the overall accuracy of the DIR is important and should be carefully assessed, paying special attention to areas of maximum uncertainty.

The application of the DIR results to the functional component of the image (e.g. PET or SPECT) can be more challenging as the user must ensure that the new voxel values of the functional image maintain consistency in the overall level of function, e.g. the overall functional uptake represented in the image must maintain consistency. Definition of functional lungs could be challenging, and should be performed by experienced professionals.

17.3.2.3 DOSE MAPPING AND ACCUMULATION

Arguably, one of the most critical components of adaptive radiotherapy of the lung is the mapping of dose from the initial treatment planning image onto the adaptive planning image for dose accumulation. Here, DIR algorithms are challenged due to the often-dramatic changes in the lung structure and tumor volume. In addition, studies have documented the complex nature of tumor response highlighting the need for DIR algorithms to be able to handle an elastic response of the tumor as well as the 'erosion' of the tumor [26,44,45]. In the elastic response of the tumor, the relationship between the tumor boundary and the normal tissue has consistency, that is, as the tumor responds in size the normal tissue tracks with it. In the eroding response of the tumor, the normal tissue stays stationary and the tumor responds, leading to the hypothesis that microscopic disease may still be present even when bulky tumor is no longer visible. The physician must decide on the dose needed to control these targets, which may be microscopic during the adaptive course and macroscopic during the initial planning. In addition to overcoming the challenges in DIR for dose accumulation, one must also consider if updates to toxicity models are necessary when applying conventional dose constraints to during-treatment imaging-based dose calculations and volumes versus pre-treatment volumes. This is especially true for structures in which substantial changes can be expected, such as the normal lung (lungs minus gross tumor volume). The commissioning of DIR for dose mapping is consistent with that for multi-modality image registration. Volumetric assessment of the accuracy is important since the dose will be accumulated at all points in the volume; therefore, TRE is an appropriate and reasonable metric. The goal is for consistent accuracy across the entire region to within a voxel. However, the impact of uncertainties will be greatest in the regions of high-dose gradients. Research has shown that changes in the average uncertainty in the DIR algorithm of even 1.6 mm may have a clinically relevant impact on the decision-making metrics for lung cancer (e.g. minimum dose to the tumor).

The use of DIR to map and accumulate dose in the adaptive setting is also challenging due to the loss of tissue, presenting the question: how do we accumulate dose in tissue that is no longer there? This is a question that does not have a clear answer. As the field explores the answer to this question, caution should be used in the interpretation of dose accumulation in responding tissues, acknowledging the limitations in the determination of the accuracy in this area.

17.3.3 TREATMENT PLANNING

Treatment planning for adaptive therapy requires the same tools as initial treatment planning along with some additional adaptively focused functions. Treatment planning can vary slightly depending on whether you are performing an online adaptation or an offline adaptation. As in many of the other areas, online adaptive tools must be as efficient and independent of required user intervention as possible.

17.3.3.1 TREATMENT PLANNING FOR ONLINE ADAPTIVE THERAPY

Online adaptations may or may not require online treatment planning. In most tracking-based online adaptations, 3D-CRT plans are generated at a static state of the patient's breathing. During delivery, the patient or beam is adjusted to match the current breathing trace and reproduce, as closely as possible, the originally intended treatment plan delivery. For lung patients in whom tracking-based adaptations are not performed, or there is no sufficient to account for observed anatomic changes, a library of plans can be created prior to treatment and a "plan of the day" can be chosen or perhaps more common, adaptive re-planning can be performed. Online adaptations such as these, are referred to as instances of online re-planning or online adaptive planning. In almost all published instances of online adaptive re-planning, treatment planning is performed via inverse planning. Intensity modulated strategies such intensity modulated radiation therapy (IMRT), volumetric modulated arc therapy (VMAT), a tomographic IMRT delivery, or other specialized intensity modulation techniques are common when using inverse planning although simpler 3D-CRT plans can also be inversely optimized. A physical compensation technique would likely not be feasible due to the time required for fabrication of the compensators. Inverse planning is a common requirement for online re-planning because online forward planning is resource intensive and difficult to automate due to the need for user interaction.

Several different treatment planning strategies for online re-planning have been reported. Ahunbay and Li have published an in-house technique called "Gradient Maintenance" which attempts to lessen the time burden of adaptive segmentation by only requiring delineation of the target volume of the day [46]. The algorithm then attempts to maintain the gradients around organ-at-risk regions that were present in the original plan. This method has shown promise in pelvic cases, although its utility in lung cases would be dependent on how drastic the anatomic changes were. In cases of significant tumor and OAR changes, additional segmentation and more extensive re-planning techniques may be needed. For VMAT, a recent report by Crijns et al. highlights the various levels of online adaptation possible from aperture morphing to full re-planning [47].

Zarepisheh et al. have presented a voxel-based planning algorithm that can drive an adaptive plan to the dose volume histograms achieved in the initial plan or previously achieved plan from a library [48]. Such a method could be used to safely adapt a plan with large anatomic changes to meet the objectives in the original plan. If such a plan is not Pareto optimal, then an improved Pareto-optimal plan will be chosen. With the use of GPU architecture, planning times were on the order of 10 seconds for reasonably sized patient geometries and beams. Further potential improvements in the plan due to drastic changes could then be further addressed using an offline re-planning approach where more time and consultation with the physician regarding the updated goals is possible.

17.3.3.2 TREATMENT PLANNING FOR OFFLINE ADAPTIVE THERAPY

Offline adaptive treatment planning strategies are most commonly based on re-planning or re-optimization for the remaining fractions based on updated patient geometry. There are very few reports on more sophisticated techniques that consider what was delivered to the patient previously and even fewer that attempt to consider predicted changes based on the observed trajectory of tumor shrinkage. Zhang et al. recently reported on an adaptive treatment planning strategy that incorporates predicted tumor shrinkage models [49]. Using this technique, they demonstrated a potential for increase dose escalation to the predicted residual tumor volume compared to simple mid-treatment re-planning. Although the prediction model is preliminary, the performance was promising with dice coefficients of predicted and actual residual GTV on the order of inter-observer target delineation of approximately 0.7. Another promising tumor shrinkage model, developed by Tariq et al., further demonstrates the feasibility of predicting patient response and using model-based tumor shrinkage for re-planning [50]. However, using predicted tumor shrinkage as a basis for volume reduction is clinically unstudied, and may not be accepted in clinical trials without further validation.

As more advanced technologies and techniques are applied in treatment planning, such as maximizing biologically effective doses, it will be imperative for the physicists or adaptive plan developers to work with radiation biologists and clinicians to ensure the proper parameters, such as the alpha/beta ratio are validated for different lung cancer types, including NSCLC and small-cell lung cancer (SCLC), but also even into the subclassifications of these diseases based on histology as well as the potential effects of different targeted therapies that may be applied.

17.4 QUALITY ASSURANCE

Quality assurance (QA) for adaptive radiation therapy is multifaceted, in that quality control is required for many distinct steps at varying time scales. Table 17.4 summarizes some of the quality assurance categories recommended for adaptive therapy and where to find additional guidance, such as in AAPM Task Group Reports. Many QA tasks related to imaging and image registration and segmentation share requirements with standard non-adaptive planning. However, to gain the speed necessary for online re-planning and adaptation, quality and capabilities can be sacrificed. Thus, comprehensive QAs, using the adaptive therapy settings are extremely important to ensure safety and proper operation.

The strategies used for patient-specific plans quality assurance vary from clinic to clinic regardless of the use of online versus offline treatment planning. Clinics that employ offline planning may choose to simply employ the same techniques for patient-specific QA that are used for initial plans. These techniques range from measurements of the intended plan compared to calculations on a specialty phantom, delivery to the

Table 17.4 Summary of quality assurance categories for adaptive radiation therapy

Category	Description	Guidance
Online image acquisition	Image quality for the online image	AAPM TG142
Online image localization	Localization of online image	AAPM TG142
Image registration	Accuracy of registration for adaptation situation	AAPM TG132
Image segmentation	Accuracy of segmentation for relevant anatomy	AAPM TG53, TG132
Performance of inverse planning	Speed and quality of treatment planning algorithm	AAPM TG53
Patient specific adaptive plan QA	Verification of patient plan accuracy and deliverability	AAPM TG119, TG120

EPID, or independent (from the treatment planning system) calculation-based QA on the patient geometry. Certainly, online re-planning requires a likely departure from more conventional measurement-based QA techniques due to the patient being on the table and the need for efficiency. Thus, fast, independent calculation-based methods may be considered.

As adaptive planning becomes more common in clinical practice, all-in-one quality assurance tools designed especially for the needs of adaptive planning, may be used more frequently. A tool developed and reported on by Chen et al. is designed to check plan parameters, plan quality, verify data transfer between the planning and record and verify system, provide a secondary independent monitor unit check, and validate the treatment delivery record [51].

REFERENCES

1. Bryant, J.H. et al., Registration of clinical volumes to beams-eye-view images for real-time tracking. *Med Phys*, 2014. **41**(12): 121703.
2. Descovich, M. et al., Comparison between target margins derived from 4DCT scans and real-time tumor motion tracking: Insights from lung tumor patients treated with robotic radiosurgery. *Med Phys*, 2015. **42**(3): 1280–7.
3. Jung, J. et al., Verification of accuracy of CyberKnife tumor-tracking radiation therapy using patient-specific lung phantoms. *Int J Radiat Oncol Biol Phys*, 2015. **92**(4): 745–53.
4. Menten, M.J. et al., Using dual-energy x-ray imaging to enhance automated lung tumor tracking during real-time adaptive radiotherapy. *Med Phys*, 2015. **42**(12): 6987–98.
5. Hugo, G. et al., Changes in the respiratory pattern during radiotherapy for cancer in the lung. *Radiother Oncol*, 2006. **78**(3): 326–31.
6. Ruben, J.D. et al., Variation in lung tumour breathing motion between planning four-dimensional computed tomography and stereotactic ablative radiotherapy delivery and its dosimetric implications: Any role for four-dimensional set-up verification? *Clin Oncol (R Coll Radiol)*, 2016. **28**(1): 21–7.
7. Colvill, E. et al., A dosimetric comparison of real-time adaptive and non-adaptive radiotherapy: A multi-institutional study encompassing robotic, gimbaled, multileaf collimator and couch tracking. *Radiother Oncol*, 2016. **119**(1): 159–65.
8. Na, Y.H. et al., Toward a web-based real-time radiation treatment planning system in a cloud computing environment. *Phys Med Biol*, 2013. **58**(18): 6525–40.
9. Tian, Z. et al., A GPU OpenCL based cross-platform Monte Carlo dose calculation engine (goMC). *Phys Med Biol*, 2015. **60**(19): 7419–35.
10. Yu, G. et al., Accelerated gradient-based free form deformable registration for online adaptive radiotherapy. *Phys Med Biol*, 2015. **60**(7): 2765–83.

11. Sharp, G. et al., Vision 20/20: Perspectives on automated image segmentation for radiotherapy. *Med Phys*, 2014. **41**(5): 050902.
12. Misic, V.V. and T.C. Chan, The perils of adapting to dose errors in radiation therapy. *PLOS ONE*, 2015. 10(5): e0125335.
13. Dial, C. et al., Benefits of adaptive radiation therapy in lung cancer as a function of replanning frequency. *Med Phys*, 2016. **43**(4): 1787.
14. Kim, M. and M.H. Phillips, A feasibility study of dynamic adaptive radiotherapy for nonsmall cell lung cancer. *Med Phys*, 2016. **43**(5): 2153.
15. Li, H. et al., Robust optimization in intensity-modulated proton therapy to account for anatomy changes in lung cancer patients. *Radiother Oncol*, 2015. **114**(3): 367–72.
16. Weiss, E. et al., Dose escalation for locally advanced lung cancer using adaptive radiation therapy with simultaneous integrated volume-adapted boost. *Int J Radiat Oncol Biol Phys*, 2013. **86**(3): 414–9.
17. Berkovic, P. et al., Adaptive radiotherapy for locally advanced non-small cell lung cancer, can we predict when and for whom? *Acta Oncol*, 2015. **54**(9): 1438–44.
18. Kataria, T. et al., Adaptive radiotherapy in lung cancer: Dosimetric benefits and clinical outcome. *Br J Radiol*, 2014. **87**(1038): 20130643.
19. Bradley, J.D. et al., Standard-dose versus high-dose conformal radiotherapy with concurrent and consolidation carboplatin plus paclitaxel with or without cetuximab for patients with stage IIIA or IIIB non-small-cell lung cancer (RTOG 0617): A randomised, two-by-two factorial phase 3 study. *Lancet Oncol*, 2015. **16**(2): 187–99.
20. Qin, Y. et al., Adaptive stereotactic body radiation therapy planning for lung cancer. *Int J Radiat Oncol Biol Phys*, 2013. **87**(1): 209–15.
21. Bhatt, A.D. et al., Tumor volume change with stereotactic body radiotherapy (SBRT) for early-stage lung cancer: Evaluating the potential for adaptive SBRT. *Am J Clin Oncol*, 2015. **38**(1): 41–6.
22. Persoon, L.C. et al., First clinical results of adaptive radiotherapy based on 3D portal dosimetry for lung cancer patients with atelectasis treated with volumetric-modulated arc therapy (VMAT). *Acta Oncol*, 2013. **52**(7): 1484–9.
23. Møller, D.S. et al., Adaptive radiotherapy of lung cancer patients with pleural effusion or atelectasis. *Radiother Oncol*, 2014. **110**(3): 517–22.
24. Kwint, M. et al., Intra thoracic anatomical changes in lung cancer patients during the course of radiotherapy. *Radiother Oncol*, 2014. **113**(3): 392–7.
25. Brink, C. et al., Locoregional control of non-small cell lung cancer in relation to automated early assessment of tumor regression on cone beam computed tomography. *Int J Radiat Oncol Biol Phys*, 2014. **89**(4): 916–23.
26. Cazoulat, G. et al., Biomechanical deformable image registration of longitudinal lung CT images using vessel information. *Phys Med Biol*, 2016. **61**(13): 4826–39.
27. Veiga, C1., First clinical investigation of cone beam computed tomography and deformable registration for adaptive proton therapy for lung cancer. *Int J Radiat Oncol Biol Phys*, 2016. **95**(1): 549–59.
28. Badawi, A.M. et al., Classifying geometric variability by dominant eigenmodes of deformation in regressing tumours during active breath-hold lung cancer radiotherapy. *Phys Med Biol*, 2012. **57**(2): 395–413.
29. Sonke, J.J. and J. Belderbos, Adaptive radiotherapy for lung cancer. *Semin Radiat Oncol*, 2010. **20**(2): 94–106.
30. Brock, K.K., Image registration in intensity-modulated, image-guided and stereotactic body radiation therapy. *Front Radiat Ther Oncol*, 2007. **40**: 94–115.
31. Kessler, M.L., Image registration and data fusion in radiation therapy. *Br J Radiol*, 2006. **79** (Spec No 1): S99–108.
32. Samavati, N., M. Velec, and K.K. Brock, Effect of deformable registration uncertainty on lung SBRT dose accumulation. *Med Phys*, 2016. **43**(1): 233.
33. Guy, C.L. et al., Effect of atelectasis changes on tissue mass and dose during lung radiotherapy. *Med Phys*, 2016. **43**(11): 6109.
34. Szeto, Y.Z. et al., Effects of anatomical changes on pencil beam scanning proton plans in locally advanced NSCLC patients. *Radiother Oncol*, 2016. **120**(2): 286–92.

35. Cunliffe, A.R. et al., Effect of deformable registration on the dose calculated in radiation therapy planning CT scans of lung cancer patients. *Med Phys*, 2015. **42**(1): 391–9.
36. Fatyga, M. et al., A voxel-by-voxel comparison of deformable vector fields obtained by three deformable image registration algorithms applied to 4DCT lung studies. *Front Oncol*, 2015. **5**: 17.
37. Wu, Q. et al., Deformable image registration of CT images for automatic contour propagation in radiation therapy. *Biomed Mater Eng*, 2015. **26** (Suppl. 1): S1037–44.
38. Reboucas Filho, P.P. et al., Novel and powerful 3D adaptive crisp active contour method applied in the segmentation of CT lung images. *Med Image Anal*, 2017. **35**: 503–16.
39. Heinrich, M.P. et al., Deformable image registration by combining uncertainty estimates from supervoxel belief propagation. *Med Image Anal*, 2016. **27**: 57–71.
40. Zhong, H. et al., Evaluation of adaptive treatment planning for patients with non-small cell lung cancer. *Phys Med Biol*, 2017. 62.
41. Brock, K.K. and Deformable Registration Accuracy Consortium, Results of a multi-institution deformable registration accuracy study (MIDRAS). *Int J Radiat Oncol Biol Phys*, 2010. **76**(2): 583–96.
42. Kashani, R. et al., Objective assessment of deformable image registration in radiotherapy: A multi-institution study. *Med Phys*, 2008. **35**(12): 5944–53.
43. Kadoya, N. et al., Multi-institutional validation study of commercially available deformable image registration software for thoracic images. *Int J Radiat Oncol Biol Phys*, 2016. **96**(2): 422–31.
44. Robertson, S.P., E. Weiss, and G.D. Hugo, A block matching-based registration algorithm for localization of locally advanced lung tumors. *Med Phys*, 2014. **41**(4): 041704.
45. Hardcastle, N. et al., Accuracy of deformable image registration for contour propagation in adaptive lung radiotherapy. *Radiat Oncol*, 2013. **8**: 243.
46. Ahunbay, E.E. and X.A. Li, Gradient maintenance: A new algorithm for fast online replanning. *Med Phys*, 2015. **42**(6): 2863–76.
47. Crijns, W. et al., Online adaptation and verification of VMAT. *Med Phys*, 2015. **42**(7): 3877–91.
48. Zarepisheh, M. et al., A multicriteria framework with voxel-dependent parameters for radiotherapy treatment plan optimization. *Med Phys*, 2014. **41**(4): 041705.
49. Zhang, P. et al., Predictive treatment management: Incorporating a predictive tumor response model into robust prospective treatment planning for non-small cell lung cancer. *Int J Radiat Oncol Biol Phys*, 2014. **88**(2): 446–52.
50. Tariq, I. et al., Mathematical modelling of tumour volume dynamics in response to stereotactic ablative radiotherapy for non-small cell lung cancer. *Phys Med Biol*, 2015. **60**(9): 3695–713.
51. Chen, G.P., E. Ahunbay, and X.A. Li, Technical Note: Development and performance of a software tool for quality assurance of online replanning with a conventional Linac or MR-Linac. *Med Phys*, 2016. **43**(4): 1713.

18

MRI-based IGRT for lung cancer

ROJANO KASHANI AND LAUREN HENKE

18.1 INTRODUCTION

Magnetic resonance imaging (MRI) has been finding its way into clinical use for target delineation in radiotherapy due to its superiority in soft-tissue definition compared to other imaging modalities, with demonstrated benefits in some disease sites [1–4]. The use of MRI in lung cancer and lung radiotherapy, however, has been limited by two main factors: the increased magnetic susceptibility artifacts caused by low proton density in the lung, and the presence of respiratory motion. The recent advancements in MRI pulse sequence development have reduced the impact of susceptibility artifact, as well as minimizing motion artifacts through faster image acquisition allowing for breath-hold scans or volumetric interpolated breath-hold scans [1]. Recent studies have evaluated the sensitivity of MRI in identifying lung lesions for diagnostic purposes, and have shown comparable results to positron emission tomography (PET) for larger lesions, but lower sensitivity in identifying lesions smaller than 5 mm [5]. Other studies have investigated the correlation between the functional signal from diffusion-weighted MR with the standard uptake value (SUV) from PET [6]. In addition to the use of MRI for diagnostic purposes, the interest in using MRI as the sole modality for patient simulation in place of computed tomography (CT), which is the current clinical standard for patient simulation, has increased significantly in recent years. The application of an MRI-sim only approach has been limited to a few sites and further evaluation of target delineation in lung based on MRI is warranted prior to utilization of this technique [2]

While the use of MRI for patient simulation and target delineation was a natural extension from diagnostic imaging, the introduction of the MR into the treatment room is an important and exciting development that could introduce a paradigm change in in-room image-guidance. Some of the obvious advantages of MR image-guidance include high soft-tissue contrast, fast volumetric imaging allowing for breath-hold imaging, and the absence of radiation dose from the imaging procedures. Further development in clinical implementation and use of these systems is needed to identify the true benefits over the current standard of practice in-room x-ray imaging. Some potential advantages may be the availability of functional as well as response information on a regular basis through the course of treatment, thus allowing for intervention in the treatment course early on and as needed.

18.2 SYSTEMS FOR MAGNETIC RESONANCE IMAGE GUIDED RADIATION THERAPY (MR-IGRT)

The integration of MRI and external beam radiotherapy has been under investigation and development by several institutions, each with a unique approach to addressing the many design challenges posed by combining the two modalities. Currently, there are five groups that are working on MR-IGRT systems. One system has been in clinical use since 2014 [7] while the installation of another system was completed in October 2015, and this system is expected to be ready for clinical use soon. Even though the clinical deployment is still limited, there is sufficient preliminary data indicating potential superiority of these systems for some indications [8,9]. In this section, we provide a brief description of each system in its current state of development based on published data from each group.

18.2.1 Magnetic resonance imaging-linac system

The MR-linac system from the University Medical Center Utrecht, the Netherlands, was developed in collaboration with Philips Medical Systems (Best, The Netherlands), and Elekta AB (Stockholm, Sweden) [10,11]. This system consists of 1.5 Tesla Philips MRI scanner, modified to allow the incorporation of a 6 mega-voltage (MV) Elekta linear accelerator on a ring in the transverse midplane [11,12]. The accelerator head is equipped with a multileaf collimator (MLC) and can rotate in either direction [10] enabling delivery of intensity-modulated radiotherapy (IMRT). This system does not allow for couch shifts to correct for patient setup; however, it uses a virtual couch-shift technique where the treatment plan is adjusted daily based on the anatomy of the day accounting for any translations, rotations, or deformations [11,12]. The treatment planning system for the MR-linac has a Monte Carlo dose calculation algorithm capable of simulating the magnetic field and accounting for the electron return effect in the dose calculation. This is an important part of any MR-IGRT system, as it can have a significant impact on the dose distribution at interfaces, depending on the strength of the magnetic field, its orientation relative to the beam, and other patient- and field-specific parameters [13–15]. In this design the MR and the RT systems share an isocenter, thus allowing for image acquisition during treatment delivery. Proof-of-concept studies were performed showing the system's capability to track the target in phantom geometry; however, additional details regarding the latency and spatial resolution of these images, as well as practical considerations for applications to human subjects, are needed prior to clinical deployment [16,17].

Other considerations in designing these hybrid systems include the radiofrequency (RF), and magnetic interference and shielding. In this system, the issue of RF inference between the accelerator and the image acquisition system was addressed by modifying the Faraday cage such that the linear accelerator was placed outside the Faraday cage [11,12]. The magnetic interference between the MR and the accelerator was also a concern in designing this system. This issue was addressed by modifying the active magnetic shielding of the MR to create a region in the transverse plane where the accelerator ring is placed, thus allowing for magnetic decoupling of the two systems [11,12,17].

18.2.2 Magnetic resonance cobalt-60 system

The MRIdian® system (ViewRay Inc., Oakwood Village Ohio) is an integrated MR-IGRT system that combines a vertically gapped 0.35 Tesla whole-body MR scanner with three Cobalt-60 heads, allowing for simultaneous imaging and treatment delivery [7]. Each of the three Cobalt-60 heads is equipped with fast pneumatic source mechanism, and doubly divergent MLCs, allowing for IMRT as well as conformal treatment delivery. The three treatment heads are 120° apart, and can be used for treatment simultaneously. The system is capable of fast volumetric imaging prior to treatment for patient setup, with imaging times ranging from 17 seconds to over 3 minutes, depending on the desired field of view and resolution [18]. In addition to the volumetric imaging for setup, the system allows for acquisition of planar images in the sagittal plane during the treatment delivery, which can be used for gating based on internal patient anatomy. Details of the gating capabilities are described in the next section in this chapter. The system also has an integrated treatment planning system with fast dose calculation and plan re-optimization, which is fully accessible from the treatment delivery workspace, allowing for seamless online treatment plan adaptation based on the daily setup MR image [7,9,18].

One consideration with this system is the low-field MR, which results in images with lower signal-to-noise ratio. This issue can be addressed by optimizing the sequences to acquire high-quality images, sufficient for localization of soft-tissue contour delineation during treatment-plan adaptation. The lower magnetic field strength can be considered to have some potential benefits. One is the reduced magnetic field susceptibility artifacts and smaller geometric distortion in the patient as described by Stanescu et al. [19]. Another is the lower impact of the magnetic field on the dose distribution due to the electron return effect at tissue interfaces inside the body and at the skin [7,13,14]. It is important to recognize that both effects mentioned here can be estimated and corrected for, even in systems with higher magnetic field, and therefore should not be a considered a direct limitation of other high-field systems. The use of Cobalt-60 sources instead of a linear accelerator in this system is perceived as a drawback due to the lower dose rate and the implications on plan quality. Wooten el al. showed clinically equivalent plans between Cobalt-60 IMRT and standard linac-based plans for a variety of sites [20]. In the next generation of the MRIdian system, the three Cobalt-60 sources will be replaced with a single 6 MV linac, thus eliminating such concerns.

18.2.3 Magnetic resonance-guided facility at Princess Margaret Hospital

The MR-guided facility at the Princess Margaret Hospital consists of a standard TrueBeam linear accelerator (Varian Medical Systems, Paolo Alto, CA) with a modified treatment couch and a 1.5 Tesla Siemens Espree MRI (Siemens, USA) on rails that can be brought into the treatment room for imaging prior to treatment [21]. Image acquisition involves moving the patient 3.1 meters away from the linac isocenter to the imaging isocenter, followed by advancing the MR on rails over the patient. In this design, a set of radio frequency isolation doors separate the MR scanner from the linac, to avoid artifacts on the MR images caused by the linac. Additional safety measures and tools are in place to reduce the potential for collisions between the moving MR scanner and the patient. Once the image acquisition is complete, the MR images are routed to the image registration system to determine the shifts, which in turn are sent to the control system for adjusting the couch prior to treatment [21]. One of the main drawbacks of such a system is that MR imaging is available only prior to the treatment and cannot be used for monitoring the patient during treatment delivery. However, it may be possible to combine the daily MR information with the standard imaging capabilities on the linac, to provide real-time monitoring of the patient during delivery.

18.2.4 Rotating bi-planar linac–magnetic resonance imaging system

The rotating bi-planar linac MR system at the Cross-Cancer Institute is a 0.6 Tesla gapped MRI, with a 6 MV linac that can be positioned either in-line with the magnet, or perpendicular to the magnet with the beam going through the gap [11,12,22]. In this system, the accelerator is passively shielded from the magnetic field, which in turn requires the magnet to be shimmed in the presence of the accelerator passive shielding. The accelerator and the magnet rotate together to treat from different angles. With the final design still under development, some initial results from the bench-top prototype system were published by Fallone et al. in 2009 [23].

18.2.5 The Australian magnetic resonance imaging-Linac program

The Australian MR-linac system consists of a 1 Tesla open bore MR and a 6 MV linac. The system was specifically designed with the intention to allow for evaluation of both the inline and the perpendicular configurations to determine which setup would be superior [24]. In the inline configuration, either the entire magnet assembly needs to rotate around the patient, or the patient and the couch would need to rotate relative to a fixed magnet and accelerator [24]. The final design is favoring an inline configuration with the possibility of a rotating treatment couch assembly, which is currently under evaluation by the same group.

18.3 MRI-BASED RESPIRATORY-INDUCED MOTION MANAGEMENT

As the precision of radiation delivery and planning improves, the importance of management of patient motion and accuracy of target localization in treatment delivery for lung cancers are increasingly recognized. While simple dose-escalations of therapy appeared promising for the improvement of survival outcomes and disease control in several studies within the past decade, a subsequent randomized controlled trial of dose-escalated treatment failed to demonstrate improvement in outcomes for the dose escalation arm [25–27]. Subsequent analysis has demonstrated that higher cardiac dose in the dose-escalation arm may have undermined any benefit of higher dose to the tumor itself [28]. We increasingly recognize that minimization of dose to surrounding organs-at-risk (OARs), such as the heart, may play just as an impactful role in patient outcomes as the tumor itself. It is possible that use of patient-specific dose levels based on the proximity of surrounding critical structures may be advantageous [29–31]. Maximization of the therapeutic index thus requires minimizing the OAR dose while still offering high-dose tumor coverage on an individualized basis. This necessitates precise and reproducible management of individual patient motion during thoracic radiation for accurate treatment delivery.

In the treatment of lung cancer, respiratory motion is a particularly significant source of intrafraction positional uncertainty. Poor tracking of tumor and OAR motion may narrow the therapeutic index through insufficient tumor coverage and increase in unplanned dose to OARs. Current CT-based modalities for image-guided radiation therapy (IGRT) to address respiratory motion, including 4DCT, CBCT, fiducial markers, and external surrogates of motion are insufficient. These approaches, while not without benefit, rely on limited pre-treatment delivery patient data sampling and limited imaging quality during treatment delivery, and do not fully account for obstacles such as internal target volume (ITV) instability, the effects of respiratory variability on gating structure reproducibility, and tumor/OAR deformation [32–35]. Thus, precision and accuracy of CT-based treatment delivery may be limited in some scenarios. Recent studies have also suggested that dynamic 2D lung MRI in the sagittal and coronal direction was better at characterizing lung tumor motion over longer time periods compared to the 4DCT [36–38]. Applying the same concepts to in-room imaging, has the potential to improve measurement and analysis of lung tumor motion inside the treatment room, and to utilize that knowledge in improving motion management strategies. In contrast to CT-based techniques, MR-based IGRT can account for respiratory motion throughout the course of an entire treatment fraction by permitting direct target visualization and continuous gating or tracking on the tumor itself, thus minimizing uncertainty of the target position.

In the previous section, we described various MR-IGRT technologies under development. In this section, we will focus on the system that is currently commercially available and clinically implemented, the MRIdian system from ViewRay®. We will also discuss briefly the reported specification from the Elekta MR-Linac from UMC Utrecht, based on simulated and phantom studies described so far.

18.3.1 Imaging considerations for tracking and gating

Detection of the tumor position remains the most challenging step in the motion management process regardless of the modality used. Due to the large motion of targets in the lung, even small delays between measuring the motion and correcting for it, regardless of the technique used, can result in large dosimetric errors [39]. Consequently, maintaining the optimal delivery accuracy requires the use of predictive algorithms that can estimate future position of the target, or use of a gating or breath-hold techniques with a sufficient safety margin that would ensure target coverage even in the presence of larger than desired delays in the overall process.

With the use of MR as the imaging modality for detection of the target position, the inherent delay in the image acquisition is larger compared to fluoroscopic imaging. Standard fluoroscopic imaging is acquired at a frame rate of approximately 30 milliseconds (ms) [39], whereas planar cine MR imaging is generally acquired at 4–8 frames per second (fps), which equates to an added inherent latency of 125 ms–250 ms for image acquisition alone. Yun et al. reported on a phantom simulation of dynamic low-field MR acquisition at 275 ms followed by auto-segmentation of the target in 5 ms [40]. Similar feasibility studies performed by the group at UMC Utrecht, with 1.5 Tesla MR, suggest the use of MR pencil-beam navigators, which can be acquired at approximately 15 ms [41]. Another MR-based imaging technique that can be used for gated treatment delivery, or to monitor voluntary breath-hold, is cine imaging. This technique is currently used by the MRIdian system from ViewRay, which allows for imaging in the sagittal plane only. Details of imaging frequency and latency from the MRIdian system are described in the next section.

18.3.2 MR navigators for tracking

The use of MR navigators for motion detection originated in breathing correlated diagnostic MR, where diaphragm position determined by a navigator was used as surrogate for the motion of other internal organs [42,43]. MR pencil-beam navigators have the advantage of being very fast in detecting the motion (15 ms), and can be placed directly on the tumor or organ of interest without the need for an internal or external surrogate. While this is a one-dimensional MR acquisition, the navigators can be placed in any arbitrary orientation such that the maximum motion of the target or the surrogate is realized and can be used for motion management. A study by Stam et al. evaluated the accuracy of such navigators in determining organ motion at various interfaces between water, air, and fat in a moving phantom [41]. In the same study, the use of navigators for tracking kidney motion in volunteers was investigated by acquiring alternating navigators and planar sagittal images of the kidney with an acquisition time of 390 ms using a 1.5 T MR scanner. They determined the mean deviation between the navigator and the 2D images to be 0.6 mm, with a maximum of 1.4 mm, which was attributed to the motion of the kidneys during the time required to acquire the 2D images (390 ms) [41]. Using the techniques evaluated in this study, the MR-linac group from UMC Utrecht aims to implement a tracking technique by adapting the collimation system to the position and shape of the target during breathing [17]. In a proof of concept study performed by Crijns et al. the motion tracking on MR was achieved through edge detection on pencil-beam navigators. This prototype system has an MLC controller that allows for rigid translation of the MLC aperture based on the detected position of the target. They measured the latency between the MLC aperture and the target position to be approximately 150 ms, not inclusive of the image acquisition and communication lag (50 ms), adding up to an inherent latency of larger than 200 ms [17]. The latency can be addressed by use of predictive motion models, or optimizing the control system for the MLC feedback loop, both of which are under further development as the final clinical version of the system is being deployed.

In this prototype system, the motion in the target was tracked by pencil-beam navigators and corrected by rigid translations in the MLC aperture. However, given that the motion in the abdomen and lung is more complex than the simple rigid one-dimensional shift, more advanced MR imaging such as 2D planar cine images, or combination of navigators and volumetric imaging, may be necessary to determine and correct for deformation in the target. Characterization of these systems will be fully realizable only after final release of this system for clinical use.

18.3.3 Cine MR for gating

The MRIdian system utilizes a gating technique based on 2D planar cine MR images for motion management. This system is capable of acquiring both high-resolution volumetric setup MR images as well as "cine" planar images in the sagittal plane at a rate of four frames per second (fps), or alternatively, three parallel sagittal planes at two fps with sequential acquisition of planes over a 0.5 second time interval. In-plane image resolution is 3.5 mm × 3.5 mm, with slice thickness of 0.5, 0.7, or 1.0 cm. This allows for direct tumor visualization during radiotherapy delivery, and subsequent tumor delineation on each frame via deformable registration, which can be used for gating the treatment beam.

In the MR-based gating process, like the standard gating workflow, the patient first undergoes a daily setup onboard volumetric imaging that is obtained immediately prior to treatment fraction delivery. The volumetric daily MR is acquired at breath-hold with the patient in the treatment position at isocenter. With the MRIdian system, the fastest presently available volumetric scan requires 17 seconds, thus allowing for acquisition of a breath-hold scan for the initial setup. This scan is used for direct target-based localization. Examples of breath-hold scans of lung and the abdomen are shown in Figure 18.1.

After the initial alignment, all the planning contours are rigidly or deformably transferred from the reference treatment planning image to the daily setup MR. The operator of the system, will then select the reference plane(s) to be used for gating during the treatment as well as the structure contour to be used as the gating target. While the gating target is typically the gross tumor volume (GTV), it can alternatively be a normal tissue or a combination of multiple structures that have been added to create a single gating target contour. The gating target is then transferred from the reference plane to each frame acquired during treatment delivery via deformable registration, and the deformed contour is used by the system to determine if the gating target is inside the gating boundary. The gating boundary is defined either by selection from within the structures defined on the volumetric daily setup image, such as the PTV, or by creation of a symmetric or asymmetric margin around the gating target. During the treatment, the gating target contour is deformably transferred from the reference plane to each frame acquired. If the gating target contour is outside the gating boundary, the system turns off the beam automatically by moving the source to the shielded position. Figure 18.2 shows an example of gating plane selection, and parameter setup.

Prior to initiation of the treatment delivery, the system performs a "Preview" scan to allow the user to evaluate the quality of the deformed gating target on several sample image frames, to determine the quality of the gating, and adjust the gating parameters accordingly. During the "Preview" phase, several frames are acquired and the gating target contour is transferred to each frame via deformable registration. The user then qualitatively evaluates the match between the actual target on each image frame, and the contour transferred by the system as the target. If the match between the two is accurate, no changes in the gating parameters are necessary. In most cases, however, due to the noise in the cine MR images, the deformed gating target contour does not match the actual target perfectly. To reduce the impact of the noise on gating accuracy and overall duty cycle, the user can adjust the percentage of the gating target area that can be outside the gating boundary before the beam is turned off. Typically, this parameter is set to 1%–5% to account for the tracking

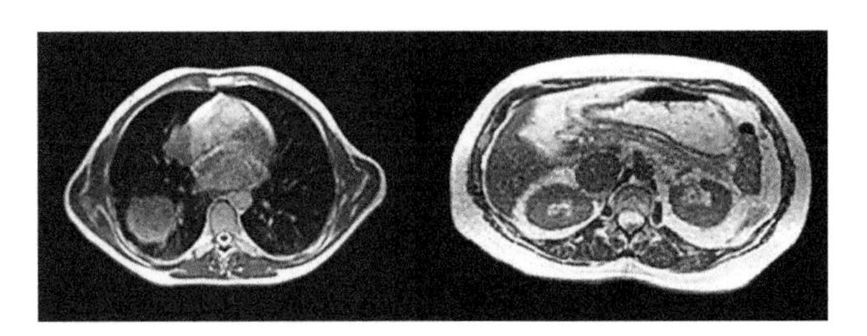

Figure 18.1 Lung tumor and abdominal tumor on a 0.35 T MR-IGRT system.

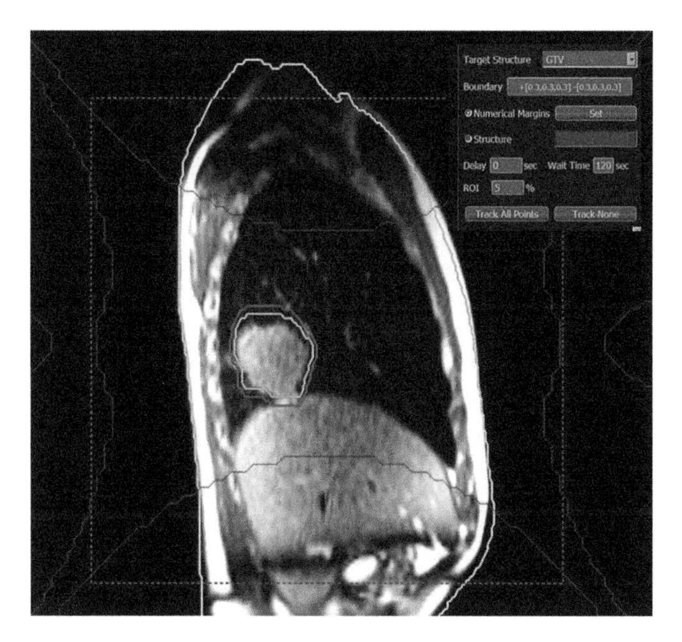

Figure 18.2 Gating setup on the MRIdian® MR-IGRT system. The pink contour is the gating target which will be deformed to each MR cine frame, and the red contour is the gating boundary.

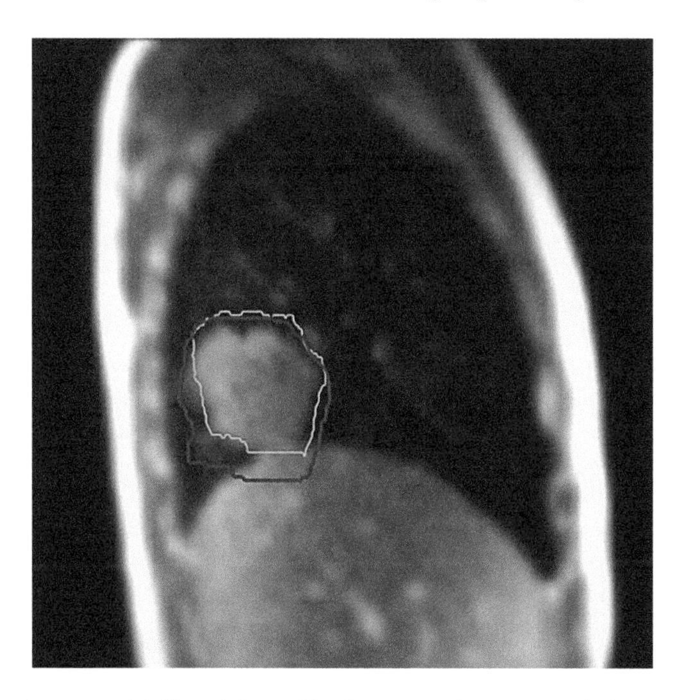

Figure 18.3 The gating target (pink) as deformed by the system does not match the tumor perfectly. In this figure, the superior portion of the gating target is outside of the gating boundary, while the target itself is physically within the gating boundary.

contour occasionally not perfectly matching the actual anatomy being tracked by a few pixels. However, if a lesion is poorly tracked and the user is confident in tumor position, this can be altered. Figure 18.3 shows an example cine MR where the target is physically inside the gating boundary, but the gating target contour as estimated by the system is outside.

The use of low-field 2D cine MR imaging for target tracking and gating is not limited to the MRIdian system. Developers of the rotating bi-planar MR-linac at the Cross-Cancer Institute have also described the use of dynamic planar MR images in determining the position and shape of lung tumors during treatment delivery [40]. In this system, the planar MR imaging is not limited to the sagittal plane, and will be selected such that the maximum dimension of the tumor can be visualized in each beam's-eye view. An auto-contouring algorithm is utilized in this system for target definition on each frame. Initial simulation studies indicate an image acquisition time of 275 ms followed by auto-contouring the lung tumor in 5 ms [40]. Further detail on the correction strategy and the overall latency may be needed prior to clinical deployment of the system.

18.3.4 Temporal resolution and latency

Per the recommendations of Task Group 76 of the American Association of Physicists in Medicine, the overall system latency for lung tumor tracking or gating should be less than 500 ms [44]. This includes the time required for identifying the target location, processing and transfer of the information, and the time required for correcting the beam whether through beam-holds or beam repositioning. Acquisition of planar cine MR images has an inherent latency of approximately 200–300 ms [40,41,44], with most systems capable of planar imaging at 4 fps. The processing time varies with the system in use and the technique, but has been reported to be on the order of a few milliseconds by various groups. The response time also varies among systems and depends on whether gating or tracking is employed. In general, gating the beam, where the beam is turned on/off as the target goes in and out of a predefined boundary, has a lower latency compared to tracking where the beam is adjusted to the position and/or shape of the target. However, the latency in the response of the system can be addressed with different techniques such as use of predictive models for the motion, or use of safety margins.

18.3.5 Clinical workflow considerations

Currently, the only system that is clinically implemented and used for patient treatment is the MRIdian system from ViewRay, which utilizes a gating technique. Real-time MRI guidance with cine MRI gating is presently used in two general clinical scenarios: coached breath-hold and free-breathing techniques. When breath-hold delivery techniques are desired, patients' pre-treatment simulation/planning images should be acquired at maximum inhalation breath-hold (MIBH) or exhale breath-hold breathing states. However, before decision for breath-hold versus free-breathing treatment, each patient's tumor motion, breath-hold reproducibility, and breath-hold tolerance must be evaluated at simulation. Patients should therefore all undergo simulation with a free-breathing, max inspiratory breath-hold, and/or a shallow breathing method for evaluation of the optimal strategy on an individualized basis. If a patient tolerates breath-hold and it is the physician's preference, the breath-hold simulation scans will be selected for use for planning and all subsequent daily set-up images will be acquired at the appropriate matching stage of inhalation or exhalation. For patient comfort, a MIBH simulation and treatment modality is often selected.

During treatment delivery, patients treated using breath-hold techniques are coached with audio or visual feedback to optimize tumor/target time within the boundary structure. For audio feedback, the therapist outside of the treatment room visualizes the position of the target within the gating boundary and encourages the patient to acquire a smaller or larger air volume for their MIBH positioning. With some practice, this can be successfully implemented. Visual feedback may provide a preferable and more direct method for patients to optimize tumor/target time within the boundary. Some centers utilize a projected image of a patient's tumor and boundary structure to the patient; other centers may opt for use of projected animations to guide patient breath hold depth. Although both audio and visual coaching require some element of patient participation in the treatment delivery, a patient may appreciate an active role in therapy.

Apart from potential improvements in image quality when a patient is treated at breath-hold position, there are several additional benefits to this strategy. First, the efficiency of treatment delivery may be improved compared with a free-breathing gating technique. When a patient is treated at breath-hold, the beam-on time (the time where the GTV is within the boundary region) is maximized. Any potential difficulty in target tracking or beam gating by the system is also minimized in this approach. A breath-hold approach also minimizes the number of beam on-off events, which in turn reduces the dosimetric impact of the overall latency in the system.

Disadvantages of the breath-hold approach relate primarily to patient comfort and the requirements for coaching and visual feedback. In the setting of primary lung malignancies, patients may frequently have poor underlying lung capacity, in addition to air-space occupying lesions. Repeated breath-holds, often over the course of an extended treatment delivery time, may be excessively tiring and may not be physically possible for many thoracic patients. Similarly, patients with reduced health and capacity for attention may have difficulty complying with auditory coaching or have trouble visualizing tumor position within projected images for vision-based feedback. In these scenarios, it may be prudent to instead select a free-breathing technique.

For implementation of free-breathing gating techniques, the initial steps for patient simulation, and setup imaging acquisition are parallel to those used for breath-hold techniques. Transfer and selection of the gating structure and boundary, and structure tracking settings are also like those employed for breath-hold. However, some distinctions should be made in several of these steps when free-breathing is to be used.

First, patient simulation differs in some regards. At time of simulation, emphasis should be placed on instructions for shallow free-breathing by the patient. This allows for maximization of the efficiency of subsequent treatment delivery and allows the clinician to accurately assess the degree of target motion related to the respiratory cycle. In a manner that is identical to the breath-hold process, but more pertinent in the setting of free-breathing, each time a cine image is acquired, the gating target contour is compared to a user-defined gating boundary; if the contour is determined to be outside this boundary, the beam is turned off.

One key consideration in the free-breathing approach to respiratory gating is that the user-defined gating boundary is often designed to be smaller than the expansion from the GTV to the planning target volume (PTV), thus introducing a safety margin. For example, if the GTV to PTV expansion is 5 mm, the GTV to gating boundary expansion may be 3 mm. This is due to inherent lag time in cine imaging acquisition and processing as described earlier in this section. By selecting a gating window smaller than the PTV expansion, one conservatively ensures that the target structure (e.g., the GTV) remains within irradiated volume while the beam is on. Given the more continuous nature of respiratory motion while the patient is free-breathing as opposed to breath-holding, such a conservative approach is of greater merit for free-breathing. This minimizes marginal misses and unintentional dose to OARs [45].

Finally, when treated at free-breathing, a patient needs only to lie still within the treatment machine. For patients with limited lung capacity, there is no burden of breath-hold that may result in patient exhaustion and intolerance to therapy. Similarly, free-breathing patients may still be provided with some auditory coaching, such as the suggestion to breathe more shallowly to improve efficiency, but the patient does not need to play an active role in therapy. Patients with poor attention span, limited vision, hearing, or capacity can be treated in this manner without additional difficulty.

18.4 ON-BOARD MR IMAGING FOR TREATMENT ADAPTATION

Application of adaptive radiation therapy (ART) for lung cancer was discussed in the previous chapter. Several studies have evaluated anatomical changes in the tumor and the surrounding normal tissues in lung cancer patients based on daily or weekly in-room cone beam CT (CBCT), as well as repeat CT scans at different time points during the course of treatment [46,47]. There are various anatomical changes that can be observed in lung cancer patients during radiotherapy. These include changes in baseline tumor position, atelectasis, and pleural effusion [48,49], as well as changes in tumor size in response to treatment. Such anatomical changes can impact the treatment by affecting not only the lung density, but also the motion characteristics of the tumor [49]. While there are some studies that evaluated the variations in the magnitude of intra- and interfractional tumor motion, there are few studies that have investigated the dosimetric impact of these changes on the tumor coverage and dose to the surrounding normal tissue. Schmidt et al. investigated how the intrafractional respiratory motion, the interfractional baseline shifts and anatomical changes, affected the delivered dose. They concluded that anatomical changes had a larger impact on the dose distribution in the target, compared to the internal target motion [49]. In some situations, the changes in the target or the lung anatomy during treatment, results in repositioning of the organs at risk into the high-dose regions of the initial plan. In such cases, when the patient is aligned based on their tumor, the target coverage will remain as planned; however, critical organs near the target may fall into the high-dose region, thus receiving much higher than anticipated doses compared to the initial plan. Henke et al. showed that even in patients undergoing stereotactic radiotherapy to lung, where minimal changes in anatomy are expected given the short course of treatment, it is possible to exceed OAR tolerances from day to day [8]. These findings among the many other studies that evaluate changes in the target, and the surrounding normal tissues in lung patients, all point to the potential role of both online and offline adaptive radiotherapy in improving target coverage while reducing or maintaining organ at risk doses in treatment of lung cancer patients [8,46,47].

In the era of integrated MR radiotherapy systems, information on inter- and intrafraction variations in tumor as well as normal tissue anatomy will be readily available at each fraction, without the need for clinical protocols to acquire additional imaging during treatment. This will allow the clinicians to act on the observed changes by not only correcting for the setup differences, but also adjusting the treatment plan as necessary. In this section, we evaluate the role of onboard MR image-guidance in plan evaluation and online plan adaptation, the availability of necessary tools within the MR image-guided systems, as well as workflow considerations and potential applications in lung cancer.

The concept of online adaptive radiotherapy has been under investigation and development for more than two decades without significant progress in clinical implementation due to the complexity of the overall process and the requirements for speed and automation in each step from imaging to contouring, re-planning, and quality assurance [50–57]. A practical online adaptive therapy system should include imaging capabilities, automated contouring tools, fast plan re-optimization and dose calculation, and patient-specific quality assurance (QA). Implementation of online adaptive radiotherapy requires a system with high-quality volumetric images with high spatial integrity, and good soft-tissue contrast for both target and OAR definition. It is also important that the onboard imaging system has a large enough field of view (FOV) such that the external surface of the patient can be captured in the region of interest to accommodate accurate dose calculation. These requirements may not be achievable with the current image quality of most commercial cone beam CT systems. Instead, systems that provide a volumetric in-room fan-beam CT scan or a volumetric onboard MR imaging of the patient in the treatment position could provide the necessary information for online plan adaptation.

In addition to imaging capabilities, an online ART system should provide image-processing tools that enable contour transfer from the initial reference image to the image of the day. This can be achieved through rigid or deformable registration, or by using auto-segmentation techniques. Given the uncertainties associated with both techniques [58–62], the system should also enable online verification and manual contour modification by the user. Once contour transfer and edits have been completed, the system should allow for fast calculation of the original reference plan on the anatomy of the day, followed by fast plan re-optimization as necessary.

The first commercially available MR-IGRT system (MRIdian, ViewRay Inc) was implemented clinically in January 2014 and has been in use for online adaptive radiotherapy at Washington University in St. Louis [7]. This system has an integrated treatment planning system, with a fast Monte Carlo (MC) dose calculation algorithm, which accounts for dose perturbation due to the magnetic field, and an inverse optimization engine capable of generating and calculating IMRT plans in less than 2 minutes. The treatment planning system is directly accessible from the delivery workflow, allowing the user to adjust the plan based on the volumetric daily MR image acquired at the time of patient setup. Once the new plan is generated and treatment delivery is initiated, all corrections for anatomical variations resulting from organ motion are handled through a gated treatment approach as described in the previous section in this chapter [9]. The current version of the system does not allow for further plan adjustments to account for intrafraction organ motion.

The MR-linac currently under development at University Medical Center Utrecht is another system that is expected to allow for online plan adaptation. As described by the developers of the system, it will have capabilities for online plan adaptations to account for both inter- and intrafraction variations in the target and OARs [49]. While the specifications of the system will not be fully clear until it is deployed in the clinic, some initial publications on the various components of the system describe an iterative sequencing loop with adaptation scheme for both inter- and intrafractional variations in the anatomy [49]. In this system, couch corrections are not possible in the lateral and vertical directions, consequently, the daily patient setup variations, including any rotations or deformations in the target will be corrected for by adjusting the beam apertures, followed by tracking techniques to account for motion and deformation caused by breathing as described in the previous section [16,17,49].

18.5 IMAGING CONSIDERATIONS FOR MR-BASED PLAN ADAPTATION

In current clinical practice, treatment plan adaptation is generally performed offline, and involves a re-simulation of the patient with a subset of imaging studies performed at the time of initial planning. With MR-IGRT systems, the availability of high-resolution volumetric MR images of the patient in the treatment position enables the transition from offline adaptation to real-time online plan adjustment prior to treatment. Use of MR plan adaptation requires consideration of several factors, such as the lack of electron density information in the MR image. In standard clinical practice, a CT scan is acquired to provide electron density information for dose calculation. While a CT scan is the easiest and most accurate way of deriving electron density information, the use of MR images for generation of electron density maps has been investigated and clinically implemented for some treatment sites such as brain and prostate [63,64]. For more complex and highly heterogeneous anatomy such as the lungs, the generation of electron density information from MR images alone is more complex and further development may be needed prior to clinical use. Another potential approach is segmentation of anatomy on the MR image, followed by assignment of the electron density to each tissue type. This however requires accurate segmentation of various tissues and organs, and may not be feasible in an online setting with the patient on the table. Other possibilities include the use of rigid or deformable registration to map the initial CT simulation image and the corresponding electron density map, to the MR image of the day. The uncertainties in deformable image registration will affect the accuracy of the electron density maps generated with this technique, and may require manual correction to the resulting electron density distribution. An example of a deformation uncertainty and how it affects the mapping of the electron density is shown in Figure 18.4.

One of the main issues that need to be addressed is the spatial integrity of the MR images, and the intrinsic image distortions that can impact the accuracy of target and organ at risk definition used for plan adaptation. There are two main types of distortions: those that are caused by the inhomogeneity in the main magnetic field and are related to the scanner itself, and those which are patient-specific and are induced by the susceptibility variations at the interface of various tissues inside the patient. Magnetic susceptibility, which describes the ability of an object to become magnetized inside of a magnetic field, varies depending the structural

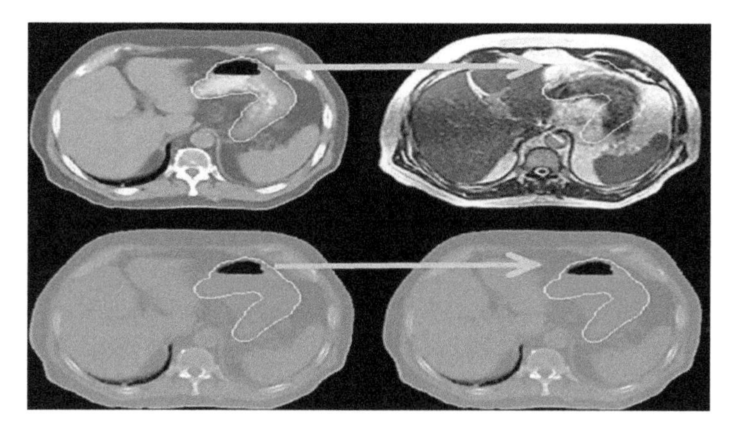

Figure 18.4 Top row indicates the initial CT scan and the stomach as it was deformed to the daily MR. The error in the deformation translates directly to the corresponding electron density maps shown in the bottom row.

composition of various tissues. Susceptibility artifacts are a consequence of perturbations in the local magnetic field at the boundary of various tissues that impacts the spatial correlation of the signal from this region, resulting in distortion in the reconstructed image. Stanescu et al. have shown the magnitude of geometric distortions caused by susceptibility artifacts at various interfaces inside the patient for different magnetic field strengths and orientation [19]. They demonstrated that with the proper corrections, these errors can be reduced to accepted levels for radiation therapy treatment and planning.

Other considerations in imaging for plan adaptation include field of view, and motion artifacts. The field of view needs to be large enough to include the patient's external surface, and extend past the target in the longitudinal direction for accurate dose calculation. This is often a trade-off with the image acquisition time, which needs to be fast enough to reduce motion artifacts caused by breathing. A high-quality image free of artifacts is a requirement.

18.6 SUMMARY

In-room MR image guidance is a promising new advancement in Radiation Oncology, with significant potential to not only improve patient setup and motion management, but also provide the possibility of day to day plan adaptation based on tumor response and changes in normal tissue anatomy. This technology, which has been under development for some time, has only recently found its way to the clinic and therefore the true benefits of such systems in improving outcomes and lowering adverse effects in various treatment sites will be realized in the next few years.

REFERENCES

1. Kumar, S. et al., Magnetic resonance imaging in lung: A review of its potential for radiotherapy. *Br J Radiol*, 2016. **89**(1060): 20150431.
2. Khoo, V.S. and D.L. Joon, New developments in MRI for target volume delineation in radiotherapy. *Br J Radiol*, 2006. **79 Spec No 1**: S2–15.
3. Liney, G.P. et al., Commissioning of a new wide-bore MRI scanner for radiotherapy planning of head and neck cancer. *Br J Radiol*, 2013. **86**(1027): 20130150.
4. Dirix, P., K. Haustermans, and V. Vandecaveye, The value of magnetic resonance imaging for radiotherapy planning. *Semin Radiat Oncol*, 2014. **24**(3): 151–9.
5. Chandarana, H. et al., Pulmonary nodules in patients with primary malignancy: Comparison of hybrid PET/MR and PET/CT imaging. *Radiology*, 2013. **268**(3): 874–81.
6. Schmidt, H. et al., Correlation of simultaneously acquired diffusion-weighted imaging and 2-deoxy-[18F] fluoro-2-D-glucose positron emission tomography of pulmonary lesions in a dedicated whole-body magnetic resonance/positron emission tomography system. *Invest Radiol*, 2013. **48**(5): 247–55.
7. Mutic, S. and J.F. Dempsey, The ViewRay system: Magnetic resonance-guided and controlled radiotherapy. *Semin Radiat Oncol*, 2014. **24**(3): 196–9.
8. Henke, L. et al., Simulated online adaptive magnetic resonance-guided stereotactic body radiation therapy for the treatment of oligometastatic disease of the abdomen and central thorax: Characterization of potential advantages. *Int J Radiat Oncol Biol Phys*, 2016. **96**(5): 1078–86.
9. Acharya, S. et al., Online magnetic resonance image guided adaptive radiation therapy: First clinical applications. *Int J Radiat Oncol Biol Phys*, 2016. **94**(2): 394–403.
10. Lagendijk, J.J. et al., MRI/linac integration. *Radiother Oncol*, 2008. **86**(1): 25–9.
11. Lagendijk, J.J., B.W. Raaymakers, and M. van Vulpen, The magnetic resonance imaging-linac system. *Semin Radiat Oncol*, 2014. **24**(3): 207–9.
12. Lagendijk, J.J. et al., MR guidance in radiotherapy. *Phys Med Biol*, 2014. **59**(21): R349–69.
13. Raaymakers, B.W. et al., Integrating a MRI scanner with a 6 MV radiotherapy accelerator: Dose deposition in a transverse magnetic field. *Phys Med Biol*, 2004. **49**(17): 4109–18.

14. Raaijmakers, A.J., B.W. Raaymakers, and J.J. Lagendijk, Integrating a MRI scanner with a 6 MV radiotherapy accelerator: Dose increase at tissue-air interfaces in a lateral magnetic field due to returning electrons. *Phys Med Biol*, 2005. **50**(7): 1363–76.
15. Raaijmakers, A.J., B.W. Raaymakers, and J.J. Lagendijk, Magnetic-field-induced dose effects in MR-guided radiotherapy systems: Dependence on the magnetic field strength. *Phys Med Biol*, 2008. **53**(4): 909–23.
16. Crijns, S.P. et al., Towards MRI-guided linear accelerator control: Gating on an MRI accelerator. *Phys Med Biol*, 2011. **56**(15): 4815–25.
17. Crijns, S.P., B.W. Raaymakers, and J.J. Lagendijk, Proof of concept of MRI-guided tracked radiation delivery: Tracking one-dimensional motion. *Phys Med Biol*, 2012. **57**(23): 7863–72.
18. Hu, Y. et al., Characterization of the onboard imaging unit for the first clinical magnetic resonance image guided radiation therapy system. *Med Phys*, 2015. **42**(10): 5828–37.
19. Stanescu, T., K. Wachowicz, and D.A. Jaffray, Characterization of tissue magnetic susceptibility-induced distortions for MRIgRT. *Med Phys*, 2012. **39**(12): 7185–93.
20. Wooten, H.O. et al., Quality of intensity modulated radiation therapy treatment plans using a ^{60}Co magnetic resonance image guidance radiation therapy system. *Int J Radiat Oncol Biol Phys*, 2015. **92**(4): 771–8.
21. Jaffray, D.A. et al., A facility for magnetic resonance-guided radiation therapy. *Semin Radiat Oncol*, 2014. 24(3): 193–5.
22. Fallone, B.G., The rotating biplanar linac-magnetic resonance imaging system. *Semin Radiat Oncol*, 2014. **24**(3): 200–2.
23. Fallone, B.G. et al., First MR images obtained during megavoltage photon irradiation from a prototype integrated linac-MR system. *Med Phys*, 2009. **36**(6): 2084–8.
24. Keall, P.J. et al., The Australian magnetic resonance imaging-linac program. *Semin Radiat Oncol*, 2014. **24**(3): 203–6.
25. Socinski, M.A. et al., Randomized phase II trial of induction chemotherapy followed by concurrent chemotherapy and dose-escalated thoracic conformal radiotherapy (74 Gy) in stage III non-small-cell lung cancer: CALGB 30105. *J Clin Oncol*, 2008. **26**(15): 2457–63.
26. Kong, F.M. et al., High-dose radiation improved local tumor control and overall survival in patients with inoperable/unresectable non-small-cell lung cancer: Long-term results of a radiation dose escalation study. *Int J Radiat Oncol Biol Phys*, 2005. **63**(2): 324–33.
27. Bradley, J.D. et al., Standard-dose versus high-dose conformal radiotherapy with concurrent and consolidation carboplatin plus paclitaxel with or without cetuximab for patients with stage IIIA or IIIB non-small-cell lung cancer (RTOG 0617): A randomised, two-by-two factorial phase 3 study. *Lancet Oncol*, 2015. **16**(2): 187–99.
28. Speirs, C.K. et al., Heart dose is an independent dosimetric predictor of overall survival in locally advanced non-small cell lung cancer. *J Thorac Oncol*, 2017. 12(2): 293–301.
29. Cox, J.D., Are the results of RTOG 0617 mysterious? *Int J Radiat Oncol Biol Phys*, 2012. **82**(3): 1042–4.
30. Glide-Hurst, C.K. and I.J. Chetty, Improving radiotherapy planning, delivery accuracy, and normal tissue sparing using cutting edge technologies. *J Thorac Dis*, 2014. **6**(4): 303–18.
31. RTOG 1106/ACRIN 6697, Randomized Phase II Trial of Individualized Adaptive Radiotherapy Using During-Treatment FDG-PET/CT and Modern Technology in Locally Advanced Non-Small Cell Lung Cancer (NSCLC). Available at: http://www.rtog.org/ClinicalTrials/, 2012.
32. Cai, J. et al., Effects of breathing variation on gating window internal target volume in respiratory gated radiation therapy. *Med Phys*, 2010. **37**(8): 3927–34.
33. Yan, H. et al., The investigation on the location effect of external markers in respiratory-gated radiotherapy. *J Appl Clin Med Phys*, 2008. **9**(2): 2758.
34. James, S.S. et al., Quantifying ITV instabilities arising from 4DCT: A simulation study using patient data. *Phys Med Biol*, 2012. **57**(5): L1–7.
35. Lu, X.Q. et al., Organ deformation and dose coverage in robotic respiratory-tracking radiotherapy. *Int J Radiat Oncol Biol Phys*, 2008. **71**(1): 281–9.
36. Cai, J. et al., Evaluation of the reproducibility of lung motion probability distribution function (PDF) using dynamic MRI. *Phys Med Biol*, 2007. **52**(2): 365–73.

37. Cai, J. et al., Reproducibility of interfraction lung motion probability distribution function using dynamic MRI: Statistical analysis. *Int J Radiat Oncol Biol Phys*, 2008. **72**(4): 1228–35.
38. Cai, J., P.W. Read, and K. Sheng, The effect of respiratory motion variability and tumor size on the accuracy of average intensity projection from four-dimensional computed tomography: An investigation based on dynamic MRI. *Med Phys*, 2008. **35**(11): 4974–81.
39. Murphy, M.J., Tracking moving organs in real time. *Semin Radiat Oncol*, 2004. **14**(1): 91–100.
40. Yun, J. et al., Evaluation of a lung tumor autocontouring algorithm for intrafractional tumor tracking using low-field MRI: A phantom study. *Med Phys*, 2012. **39**(3): 1481–94.
41. Stam, M.K. et al., Navigators for motion detection during real-time MRI-guided radiotherapy. *Phys Med Biol*, 2012. **57**(21): 6797–805.
42. Kozerke, S. et al., Volume tracking cardiac 31P spectroscopy. *Magn Reson Med*, 2002. **48**(2): 380–4.
43. Song, R. et al., Evaluation of respiratory liver and kidney movements for MRI navigator gating. *J Magn Reson Imaging*, 2011. **33**(1): 143–8.
44. Keall, P.J. et al., The management of respiratory motion in radiation oncology report of AAPM Task Group 76. *Med Phys*, 2006. **33**(10): 3874–900.
45. Green, O. et al., Implementation of real-time, real-anatomy tracking and radiation beam control on the first MR-IGRT clinical system. *Int J Radiat Oncol Biol Phys*, 2015. 93(3): S115.
46. Tvilum, M. et al., Clinical outcome of image-guided adaptive radiotherapy in the treatment of lung cancer patients. *Acta Oncol*, 2015. **54**(9): 1430–7.
47. Schmidt, M.L. et al., Dosimetric impact of respiratory motion, interfraction baseline shifts, and anatomical changes in radiotherapy of non-small cell lung cancer. *Acta Oncol*, 2013. **52**(7): 1490–6.
48. Knap, M.M. et al., Daily cone-beam computed tomography used to determine tumour shrinkage and localisation in lung cancer patients. *Acta Oncol*, 2010. **49**(7): 1077–84.
49. Kontaxis, C. et al., A new methodology for inter- and intrafraction plan adaptation for the MR-linac. *Phys Med Biol*, 2015. **60**(19): 7485–97.
50. Yan, D., Adaptive radiotherapy: Merging principle into clinical practice. *Semin Radiat Oncol*, 2010. **20**(2): 79–83.
51. Court, L.E. et al., An automatic CT-guided adaptive radiation therapy technique by online modification of multileaf collimator leaf positions for prostate cancer. *Int J Radiat Oncol Biol Phys*, 2005. **62**(1): 154–63.
52. Court, L.E. et al., Automatic online adaptive radiation therapy techniques for targets with significant shape change: A feasibility study. *Phys Med Biol*, 2006. **51**(10): 2493–501.
53. Feng, Y. et al., Direct aperture deformation: An interfraction image guidance strategy. *Med Phys*, 2006. **33**(12): 4490–8.
54. Fu, W. et al., A cone beam CT-guided online plan modification technique to correct interfractional anatomic changes for prostate cancer IMRT treatment. *Phys Med Biol*, 2009. **54**(6): 1691–703.
55. Mohan, R. et al., Use of deformed intensity distributions for on-line modification of image-guided IMRT to account for interfractional anatomic changes. *Int J Radiat Oncol Biol Phys*, 2005. **61**(4): 1258–66.
56. La Macchia, M. et al., Systematic evaluation of three different commercial software solutions for automatic segmentation for adaptive therapy in head-and-neck, prostate and pleural cancer. *Radiat Oncol*, 2012. **7**: 160.
57. Li, G. et al., Clinical assessment of 2D/3D registration accuracy in 4 major anatomic sites using on-board 2D kilovoltage images for 6D patient setup. *Technol Cancer Res Treat*, 2015. **14**(3): 305–14.
58. Brock, K.K. et al., Accuracy of finite element model-based multi-organ deformable image registration. *Med Phys*, 2005. **32**(6): 1647–59.
59. Greenham, S. et al., Evaluation of atlas-based auto-segmentation software in prostate cancer patients. *J Med Radiat Sci*, 2014. **61**(3): 151–8.
60. Kashani, R. et al., Objective assessment of deformable image registration in radiotherapy: A multi-institution study. *Med Phys*, 2008. **35**(12): 5944–53.
61. Thomson, D. et al., Evaluation of an automatic segmentation algorithm for definition of head and neck organs at risk. *Radiat Oncol*, 2014. **9**: 173.
62. Yang, J. et al., A statistical modeling approach for evaluating auto-segmentation methods for image-guided radiotherapy. *Comput Med Imaging Graph*, 2012. **36**(6): 492–500.

63. Kim, J. et al., Implementation of a novel algorithm for generating synthetic CT images from magnetic resonance imaging data sets for prostate cancer radiation therapy. *Int J Radiat Oncol Biol Phys*, 2015. **91**(1): 39–47.
64. Zheng, W. et al., Magnetic resonance-based automatic air segmentation for generation of synthetic computed tomography scans in the head region. *Int J Radiat Oncol Biol Phys*, 2015. **93**(3): 497–506.

Index

E

F

G

H

I

K

L

M

N

S